Univentricular Congenital Heart Defects and the Fontan Circulation

Paul Clift · Konstantinos Dimopoulos
Annalisa Angelini

Editors

Univentricular Congenital Heart Defects and the Fontan Circulation

Practical Manual for Patient Management

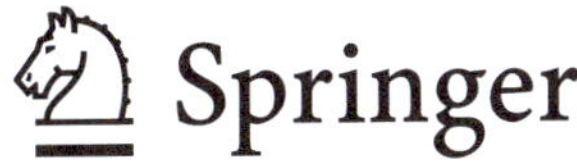

Editors
Paul Clift
Adult Congenital Heart Disease Unit
Queen Elizabeth Hospital Birmingham
Birmingham, UK

Konstantinos Dimopoulos
Royal Brompton Hospital
Imperial College London
London, UK

Annalisa Angelini
Dept of Cardiac Thoracic & Vascular
Sciences and Public Health
University of Padua
Padova, Italy

ISBN 978-3-031-36210-1   ISBN 978-3-031-36208-8   (eBook)
https://doi.org/10.1007/978-3-031-36208-8

This Springer imprint is published by the registered company Springer Nature Switzerland AG
The registered company address is: Gewerbestrasse 11, 6330 Cham, Switzerland

Acknowledgements

The editors would like to express their gratitude to all the authors for their contributions. Much of this book was written during the global COVID-19 pandemic during which many authors worked tirelessly and with great personal sacrifice.

Sadly, our colleague Dr Vish Rasaiah died in the first COVID wave that struck the UK in 2020, shortly after the completion of the first draft of the chapter he co-authored with Dr Mike Harris. Vish was a devoted husband and father, a highly respected neonatologist, a mentor, and friend to many, and like every great teacher, always seeking to increase his own knowledge. He is deeply missed.

We thank all the patients and families with a single ventricle circulation; they are the inspiration for this piece of work.

Finally, we thank our families, whose support to allow us to spend the time to complete this work is greatly appreciated, thank you.

Contents

Part III Surgical Management

Part IV The Fontan Physiology

Part V Follow Up in Childhood of Fontan Patients

Part VI Transition, Education and Lifestyle

Part VII Follow Up in Adult Life

Part VIII A Multi-system Disorder

Part IX The Failing Adult Fontan Patient

The Univentricular Heart: Past, Present and Future

1

Michael L. Rigby

No group of cardiac anomalies has given rise to such argument and controversy as those with 'single ventricle' or 'univentricular heart'. It is true that much past controversy was generated by cardiac morphologists in North America, Europe and the United Kingdom, but they were joined by many influential cardiologists and cardiac surgeons.

In the early years of clinical paediatric cardiology, the presence of a 'double inlet ventricle' was taken as the only criterion of 'single ventricle' (Van Praagh, Ongley and Swan 1964, Lev et al. 1969) [1, 2]. On this basis, it was generally accepted that a single ventricle was a heart in which a left ventricle received two atrioventricular valves or a common valve, in the presence of a rudimentary 'infundibular' chamber. It was also recognised that rarely, hearts were found in which the chamber supporting the atrioventricular valves was a morphologically right ventricle, resembled a biventricular heart with a huge ventricular septal defect or was of indeterminate morphology (Van Praagh et al. 1964). Later it was recognised with increasing frequency that occasionally hearts were encountered with double inlet right ventricle in the presence of a second rudimentary ventricle of left ventricular morphology (Anderson et al. 1979) [3].

Confronted, with evidence that a form of single ventricle of right ventricular morphology could exist with a rudimentary hypoplastic left ventricle, Van Praagh and colleagues proposed a complex definition for a 'true' single ventricle [4] Arguments presented, quite correctly, that the ventricular mass in hearts with absence of the right or left atrioventricular connection 'tricuspid and mitral atresia' was identical to that found in double inlet ventricle and should be classified as 'single ventricle', also fuelled controversy.

The most important contribution to understanding, was the realisation that almost all the hearts with double inlet ventricle or absent atrioventricular connection possess two ventricles, one dominant and the other rudimentary [5]. The small or rudimentary ventricle has a distinct right or left ventricular morphology and, as such, should not be described as an 'outlet chamber' or 'infundibular' chamber or 'pouch'. In reality, from the morphological standpoint, hearts are rarely univentricular, the exception being those rare examples of a solitary ventricle of 'indeterminate' morphology. Thus, 3 distinct types of ventricular morphology can be found, left, right and indeterminate, each of which can not only be recognised by a morphologist with the heart in their hand, but also are readily identified by modern imaging techniques, particularly echocardiography and magnetic resonance. I will address later the issue of the term univentricular heart used for the title of this book.

M. L. Rigby (✉)
The Royal Brompton Hospital, London, UK
e-mail: M.Rigby@rbht.nhs.uk

It was the recognition, that the group of hearts with double inlet ventricle or absent atrioventricular connection, exhibit a univentricular atrioventricular connection rather than being univentricular hearts, which clarified the situation enabling the description of these anomalies in a logical fashion [6]. Of course, the term 'univentricular atrioventricular connection' was never a diagnosis because there are much more precise ways of describing the individual lesions themselves. The concept of the univentricular connection was simply a means of grouping together hearts with comparable morphologies across the atrioventricular junction and separating them from the much larger group of hearts with a biventricular connection.

In essence when Anderson and colleagues introduced their classification of hearts with a univentricular atrioventricular connexion, they emphasised the possibility of any of 4 types of atrial arrangement, solitus, inversus (mirror image) and right or left isomerism, although usual atrial arrangement (situs solitus) is much the most common. They also stipulated the three possible types of atrioventricular connection, absent right, absent left and double inlet, three morphological patterns of the dominant ventricle, left, right and indeterminate and any form of ventriculo-arterial connection, concordant, discordant, double outlet ventricle and single outlet with pulmonary or aortic atresia.

Considering first the most common form of hearts with situs solitus and absence of the right AV connection, also known as tricuspid atresia [7], the only egress of blood from the morphologically right atrium is across a defect in the oval fossa and the left atrium connects directly with a morphologically left ventricle through a left sided AV valve. The rudimentary right ventricle is anterior and right sided. Rarely however, the left atrium connects to a morphologically right ventricle, or even a solitary indeterminate ventricle. With a dominant right ventricle there is usually a posterior and right sided rudimentary left ventricle. Neither of these additional examples could be correctly called 'tricuspid atresia', which is why the use of the term 'absent connection' was preferred.

In contrast, although hearts with normal situs and absent left AV connection frequently have the right atrium connecting to the morphologically right ventricle with the rudimentary left ventricle posterior and left sided ('mitral atresia'), in a significant minority there is a dominant morphologically left ventricle with anterior left sided rudimentary right ventricle [8]. Of course, absent left connection can also rarely co-exist with a solitary indeterminate ventricle. An important message was that absence of an AV connection does not reliably allow us to determine ventricular morphology. When the AV connection is double inlet, both atria connect directly with the same ventricle but the morphology of the atrioventricular valves is rarely that of a normal mitral and tricuspid [9].

Thus, it was believed the atrioventricular connection was univentricular. But therein lay the problem: a dividing line between hearts with biventricular and univentricular AV connection, which seemed so logical from an imaging and morphology point of view, has become outdated in an era in which we talk of the 'univentricular circulation'. Conditions including many variants of the hypoplastic left heart syndrome or hypoplastic right heart, in which there is clearly a biventricular atrioventricular connection, but with hypoplastic left or right ventricle and small mitral or tricuspid valve, are managed surgically to achieve the univentricular circulation. These variants of the 'Fontan' operation or 'total caval pulmonary connection' (TCPC) with the SVC and IVC usually connected directly to the pulmonary arteries, are described as having a functionally single left or right ventricle, no matter what the original atrioventricular connection. Other examples of hearts with biventricular atrioventricular connection, but only suitable for the Fontan operation, include AVSD with hypoplastic left or right ventricle, cases of double outlet right ventricle (DORV) and some hearts with atrial isomerism with complete AVSD and DORV.

If arguments regarding cardiac morphology are unquestionably part of the past, surgical management inevitably straddles the junction between past and present. In 1971 Fontan and Baudet described, for the first time, the successful palliation of patients with tricuspid atresia [10]. Subsequently the technique was used for most forms of functional single ventricle and, over the years, various modifications of the original 'Fontan' operation were described [11, 12]. The most revolutionary of these were the lateral tunnel technique and later the use of an extracardiac conduit [13, 14]. It was the intention of the Fontan operation to separate the systemic and pulmonary venous return and, thus, avoid the disadvantages of long-term hypoxaemia, preserving ventricular function; but it became clear relatively quickly that, while on the one hand the Fontan procedure did convey benefits to many patients, in the early years especially there was a high perioperative mortality [15], which gradually improved but adverse outcomes are still not uncommon, including premature death, systolic and diastolic ventricular failure, acquired cyanosis, thromboembolic disease, arrhythmias, progressive and fatal liver disease and protein losing enteropathy.

There were two extremely important historical landmarks in the management of patients with single ventricle:

- The first was the description the neonatal palliation of hypoplastic left heart syndrome, which became known as the 'Norwood operation' [16]. For the first time successful treatment was described for what was considered to have been a uniformly fatal condition in very early infancy. These patients were then included in the management protocols for single ventricle.
- Secondly, the introduction of the two-stage total caval pulmonary connection (TCPC) during the first 3–4 years of life, some 20 years following the original description of the Fontan operation, had a profound influence in reducing the operative mortality and delaying

the onset of late complications [17], although earlier results indicated a higher mortality in patients who had undergone the Norwood operation. The first stage was the creation of a bidirectional Glenn anastomosis (superior cavo-pulmonary shunt) in late infancy, while the second stage was the inferior cavo-pulmonary anastomosis, usually via an external conduit performed 2–3 years later.

In a long-term study of over 1000 patients undergoing the Fontan operation from 1973 [18] onwards, 40% of patients had died by the last follow-up. Of the patients known to be alive, transplant-free survival was documented in 68%. In this group of patients, the median age at initial operation was 7 years. Not surprisingly, the authors found that the era effect was important. When surgery was performed in the era 1991 to 2000, 10 year survival was 89% although 20 year survival was only 74%. In the era after 2000, 10 years-survival was 95%. Thus, early mortality has continued to fall and medium-term survival has improved. However, this impressive improvement is not accompanied by normal life expectancy because of the chronic effects of high systemic venous pressure and raised lymphatic pressures, inevitably resulting from a Fontan operation. The role of cardiac transplantation will become increasingly important in these patients.

Although the era effect was important, the type of procedures performed greatly impacted on survival: those with an extra cardiac conduit had a significantly lower mortality than those with an atrio-pulmonary connection or lateral tunnel. Patients with atrial isomerism had the lowest overall survival, while ventricular morphology, perhaps surprisingly, had no effect on outcome.

Relatively recent studies from Philadelphia, Australia, New Zealand and Birmingham, USA have reported an excellent survival with no increase in late mortality, but on careful analysis, these results were based on the recent surgical era [19–22]: an extracardiac or lateral tunnel operation was performed, usually in younger patients, with a high proportion receiving a fenestration. The survival data at 20 years was based on a very small number of patients having reached this point, hence the data should be interpreted with caution. Certainly, atrial isomerism was a risk factor for premature death [23, 24].

There is, therefore, little doubt that in the current era, the 20-year survival following Fontan surgery will be >85%. However, the future, i.e. the next 20–30 years, for these patients is extremely difficult to predict. Inevitably, the same complications seen previously will emerge and may well become a problem later in life. It is difficult to imagine any management protocols that will prevent the eventual development of systolic ventricular dysfunction and atrioventricular valve regurgitation, diastolic ventricular dysfunction and rising pulmonary artery pressure, rising venous pressure with the development of hepatic dysfunction and cirrhosis as well as protein losing enteropathy [25–34]. Recurrent and refractory atrial and ventricular arrhythmias in many patients will be inevitable and can present a huge management challenge.

The million-dollar question is what will be the key to improved survival in these patients? It goes without saying that a multidisciplinary team is required for the early detection and treatment of any complications. Mental health problems requiring specialised understanding and treatment will be common. Experts in the management of heart failure, pulmonary hypertension and complex arrhythmias, electrophysiologists, interventional cardiologists, congenital cardiac surgeons, all with an understanding of complex congenital heart disease and physiology, will be essential. Multidisciplinary multidimensional imaging, ultrasound, angiography, CT and resonance imaging will be needed. Experts in the management of Fontan associated liver disease and protein losing enteropathy are also going to be required. It is not going to be cheap. Inevitably some patients will lose their jobs, at times be unable to work, frequently unable to obtain comprehensive health insurance, but no developed country or government should deny these individuals the care they need, yet no doubt some will.

However, these patients must also be given the tools, opportunity and information to manage themselves. Most important is lifestyle changes to avoid obesity, to learn how to exercise regularly, always to walk or cycle rather than drive a car and adhere to careful dietary routines. Knowing that hepatic dysfunction is inevitable, patients should be advised to avoid alcohol consumption or at least consume in extreme moderation. What is the point of receiving excellent care, advice and treatment during childhood and adolescence, only to go on to be life-limited by severe obesity, a sedentary lifestyle, poor diet and an alcoholic liver?

Another major challenge for which there is no uniform consensus is thromboprophylaxis. There is no doubt that the relatively sluggish Fontan circulation predisposes to thrombus formation with pulmonary and systemic embolus risk. We are aware that any arrhythmia at any time immediately increases that risk. These risks increase with time after the Fontan surgery. Every patient requires some form of thromboprophylaxis. The challenge is choosing the correct prophylaxis for an individual patient at particular stages of their life.

Crucial to the future management of these patients is the role of cardiac transplantation, a particularly complex field that involves patients who have had several operations with extensive intrathoracic adhesions and may have anomalies of venous connection, abnormal cardiac position and location, malposition of great arteries and large veins together with pulmonary arterial abnormalities [35–38]. We are becoming aware that, in the Fontan patient, liver failure may precede Fontan failure, hence early cardiac transplantation might sometimes be the best option to avoid deteriorating liver function [39, 40]. It is probably best to presume single ventricle patients will eventually require cardiac transplantation and prepare for that eventuality. With this assumption, the avoidance of blood products during early heart surgery, whenever possible, should be the goal. The patients and families must also be prepared for all late complications. Guidelines for the management of adolescents and adults can be helpful, but individualised protocols specific to the needs of each patient will be essential.

References

1. Van Praagh R, Ongley PA, Swan HJC. Anatomic types of common or single ventricle in man; morphological and geometric aspects of sixty necropsied cases. Am J Cardiol. 1964;13:367–86.
2. Lev M, Liberthson RR, Kirkpatrick JR, Eckner FAO, Arcilla RA. Single (primitive) ventricle. Circulation. 1969;39:577–91.
3. Anderson RH, Becker AE, Freedom RM, Quero-Jimenez M, Macartney FJ, Macartney FJ, Shinebourne EA, Wilkinson JL, Tynan MJ. Problems in the nomenclature of the univentricular heart. Hertz. 1979;4:97–106.
4. Van Praagh R, Plett JA, Van Praagh S, Single ventricle. Pathology, embryology, terminology and classification. Hertz. 1979;4:113–50.
5. Anderson RH, Macartney FJ, Tynan M, Becker AE, Freedom RM, Godman MJ, Hunter S, Quero-Jimenez M, Rigby ML. Univentricular atrioventricular connection: the single ventricle trap unsprung. Pediatr Cardiol. 1983;4:273–80.
6. Anderson RH, Becker AE, Tynan M, Macartney FJ, Rigby ML, Wilkinson JL. The univentricular atrioventricular connexion: getting to the root of a thorny problem. Am J Cardiol. 1984;54:822–8.
7. Anderson RH, Shinebourne EA, Becker EA, Macartney FJ, Wilkinson JL, Tynan MJ. Tricuspid atresia and univentricular heart. Pediatr Cardiol. 1979;1:57–62.
8. Restivo A, Ho SY, Anderson RH, Cameron H, Wilkinson JL. Absent left atrioventricular connection with right atrium connected to morphologically left ventricular chamber and ventriculoarterial discordance. Problem of mitral versus tricuspid atresia. Br H Journal. 1982;48:240–8.
9. Doherty A, Ho SY, Anderson RH, Rigby ML. The morphological nature of the atrioventricular valves in hearts with double inlet ventricle. Pediatr Pathol. 1989;9:521–9.
10. Fontan F, Mounicot FB, Baudet E, et al. "Correction" of tricuspid atresia. 2 cases "corrected" using a new surgical technic. Ann Chir Thorac Cardiovasc. 1971;10:39–47.
11. Kreutzer G, Galindez E, Bono H, et al. An operation for the correction of tricuspid atresia. J Thorac Cardiovasc Surg. 1973;66:613–21.
12. Russo P, Danielson GK, Puga FJ, et al. Modified Fontan procedure for biventricular hearts with complex forms of double-outlet right ventricle. Circulation. 1988;78:III20–5.
13. Mayer JE, Helgason H, Jonas RA, et al. Extending the limits for modified Fontan procedures. J Thorac Cardiovasc Surg. 1986;92:1021–8.
14. Puga FJ. Modified Fontan procedure for hypoplastic left heart syndrome after palliation with the Norwood operation. J Am Coll Cardiol. 1991;17:1150–1.
15. Cetta F, Feldt RH, O'Leary PW, et al. Improved early morbidity and mortality after Fontan operation: the Mayo Clinic experience, 1987 to 1992. J Am Coll Cardiol. 1996;28:480–6.
16. Norwood WI, Jacobs ML, Murphy JD. Fontan procedure for hypoplastic left heart syndrome. Ann Thorac Surg. 1992;54:1025–30.
17. Iyengar AJ, Winlaw DS, Galati JC, et al. The extracardiac conduit Fontan procedure in Australia and New Zealand: hypoplastic left heart syndrome predicts worse early and late outcomes. Eur J Cardiothorac Surg. 2014;46:465–73.
18. Pundi KN, Johnson JN, Dearani JA, Pundi KN, Li Z, Hinck CA, Dahl SH, Cannon BC, O'Leary PW, Driscoll DJ, Cetta F. 40 year follow-up after the fontan operation: long-term outcomes of 1,052 patients. JACC. 2015;66:1700–10.
19. Dabal RJ, Kirklin JK, Kukreja M, et al. The modern Fontan operation shows no increase in mortality out to 20 years: a new paradigm. J Thorac Cardiovasc Surg. 2014;148:2517–24.
20. Driscoll DJ, Offord KP, Feldt RH, et al. Five- to fifteen-year follow-up after Fontan operation. Circulation. 1992;85:469–96.
21. d'Udekem Y, Iyengar AJ, Galati JC, et al. Redefining expectations of long-term survival after the Fontan procedure: twenty-five years of follow-up from the entire population of Australia and New Zealand. Circulation. 2014;130:S32–8.
22. Khairy P, Fernandes SM, Mayer JE, et al. Long-term survival, modes of death, and predictors of mortality in patients with Fontan surgery. Circulation. 2008;117:85–92.
23. Humes RA, Feldt RH, Porter CJ, et al. The modified Fontan operation for asplenia and polysplenia syndromes. J Thorac Cardiovasc Surg. 1988;96:212–8.
24. Bartz PJ, Driscoll DJ, Dearani JA, et al. Early and late results of the modified Fontan operation for heterotaxy syndrome: 30 years of experience in 142 patients. J Am Coll Cardiol. 2006;48:2301–5.
25. Deal BJ, Jacobs ML. Management of the failing Fontan circulation. Heart. 2012;98:1098–104.
26. Mavroudis C, Deal BJ, Backer CL, et al. J. Maxwell chamberlain memorial paper for congenital heart surgery. 111 Fontan conversions with arrhythmia surgery: surgical lessons and outcomes. Ann Thorac Surg. 2007;84:1457–66.

27. Mertens L, Hagler DJ, Sauer U, et al. For the PLE study group: protein-losing enteropathy after the Fontan operation: an international multicenter study. J Thorac Cardiovasc Surg. 1998;115:1063–73.
28. Friedrich-Rust M, Koch C, Rentzsch A, et al. Noninvasive assessment of liver fibrosis in patients with Fontan circulation using transient elastography and biochemical fibrosis markers. J Thorac Cardiovasc Surg. 2008;135:560–7.
29. Ginde S, Hohenwalter MD, Foley WD, et al. Noninvasive assessment of liver fibrosis in adult patients following the Fontan procedure. Congenit Heart Dis. 2012;7:235–42.
30. Yoo BW, Choi JY, Eun LY, et al. Congestive hepatopathy after Fontan operation and related factors assessed by transient elastography. J Thorac Cardiovasc Surg. 2014;148:1498–505.
31. Schwartz MC, Sullivan L, Cohen MS, et al. Hepatic pathology may develop before the Fontan operation in children with functional single ventricle: an autopsy study. J Thorac Cardiovasc Surg. 2012;143:904–9.
32. Samsky MD, Patel CB, DeWald TA, et al. Cardiohepatic interactions in heart failure: an overview and clinical implications. J Am Coll Cardiol. 2013;61:2397–405.
33. Rychik J, Veldtman G, Rand E, et al. The precarious state of the liver after a Fontan operation: summary of a multidisciplinary symposium. Pediatr Cardiol. 2012;33:1001–12.
34. Johnson JA, Cetta F, Graham RP, et al. Identifying predictors of hepatic disease in patients after the Fontan operation: a postmortem analysis. J Thorac Cardiovasc Surg. 2013;146:140–5.
35. Griffiths ER, Kaza AK, Wyler von Ballmoos MC, et al. Evaluating failing Fontans for heart transplantation: predictors of death. Ann Thorac Surg. 2009;88:558–64.
36. Kanter KR, Mahle WT, Vincent RN, et al. Heart transplantation in children with a Fontan procedure. Ann Thorac Surg. 2011;91:823–30.
37. Gambetta K, Backer C, Deal B, et al. Insights into heart transplantation for protein losing enteropathy: a 24 year experience. J Heart Lung Transplant. 2013;32:S193–8.
38. Feldt RH, Driscoll DJ, Offord KP, et al. Protein-losing enteropathy after the Fontan operation. J Thorac Cardiovasc Surg. 1996;112:672–80.
39. Hollander SA, Reinhartz O, Maeda K, et al. Intermediate-term outcomes after combined heart-liver transplantation in children with a univentricular heart. J Heart Lung Transplant. 2013;32:368–70.
40. Daly RC, Topilsky Y, Joyce L, et al. Combined heart and liver transplantation: protection of the cardiac graft from antibody rejection by initial liver implantation. Transplantation. 2013;95:e2–4.

Part I

Anatomy and Epidemiology of the Functionally Univentricular Heart

The Anatomical Substrates of the Univentricular Heart

Marny Fedrigo , Mariavittoria Vescovo ,
Carla Frescura, Gaetano Thiene ,
and Annalisa Angelini

Introduction

Univentricular hearts are a wide spectrum of complex cardiac abnormalities that preclude biventricular surgical repair due to the absence of 2 well-developed ventricles, hence are amenable to a Fontan-type palliation, an operation that reserves the developed ventricle for the systemic circulation [1–4].

Therefore, univentricular hearts include not only hearts with a "solitary ventricle", but also those with one well-developed and one hypoplastic ventricle, which, independently, is unable to support the systemic or pulmonary circulation (functionally univentricular hearts) [5–7].

Solitary Ventricle

A "solitary ventricle" is identified morphologically as a true single ventricle, with only one ventricular cavity within the ventricular mass, of undefined morphology based on the pattern of apical trabeculation. In this setting, there is a double inlet towards, and double outlet from the indeterminate ventricle. A second ventricular cavity is absent and the only septal structure present in such hearts is the muscular outlet septum, interposed between the subarterial outlets (see fig of single ventricle). Such solitary ventricles of indeterminate morphology are usually associated with right isomerism, but can also exist with usual atrial arrangement (Fig. 2.1).

Defects Amenable to Fontan-Type Palliation

A Fontan-type operation is occasionally also performed in patients with a biventricular heart, including:

- Patients in whom septation of the heart may not be possible (e.g. in the presence of a straddling atrioventricular valve, where part of the subvalvar apparatus of the valve crosses the ventricular septal defect and could be disrupted by closure of the defect, (Fig. 2.2)).
- Patients with abnormal ventriculo-arterial connection (and a single outlet)
- Double outlet right ventricle with a non-committed VSD (Fig. 2.3).

M. Fedrigo · C. Frescura · G. Thiene · A. Angelini (✉)
Cardiovascular Pathology, Department of Cardiac,
Thoracic and Vascular Sciences and Public Health,
University of Padua, Padua, Italy
e-mail: marny.fedrigo@aopd.veneto.it;
gaetano.thiene@unipd.it; annalisa.angelini@unipd.it

M. Vescovo
Department of Radiological, Oncological and
Pathological Sciences, Postgraduate medical school,
Institute of Pathology, Sapienza University,
Rome, Italy

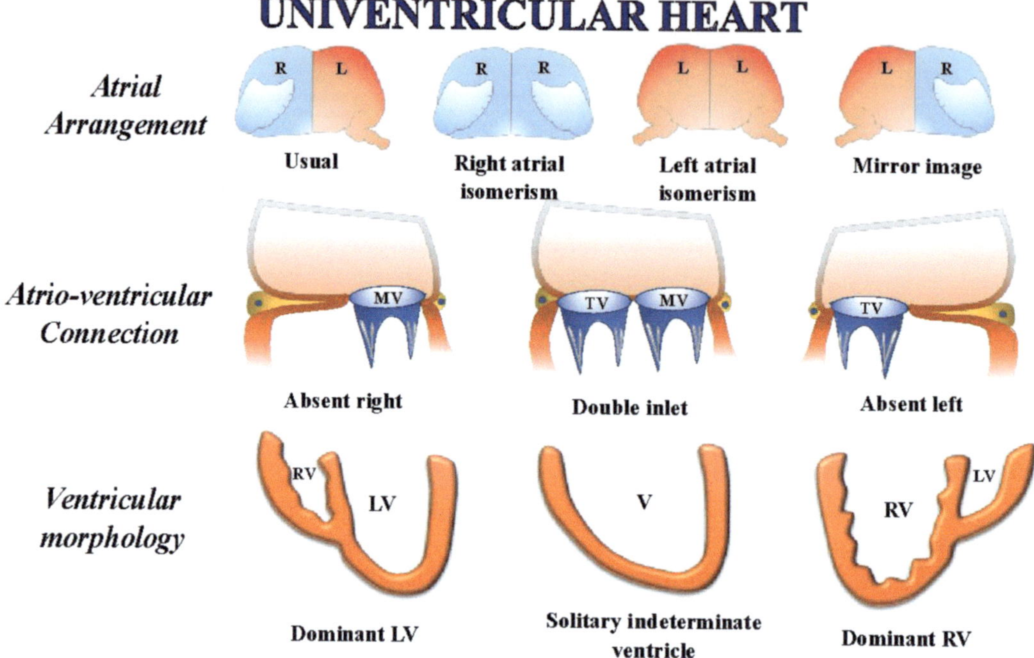

Fig. 2.1 Diagram depicting the types of univentricular hearts in univentricular atrio-ventricular connection, when both atria drain mostly into a single ventricular chamber. On the top the atrial arrangements with the usual, mirror image and right and left atrial isomerism, in the middle the univentricular atrio-ventricular connection with absent right, absent left and double inlet and on the bottom the ventricular morphology with dominant left if the dominant ventricle will be of left morphology, and a small right ventricle, and a dominant right ventricle with a small left ventricular cavity. In the setting of a solitary or indeterminate ventricle we are in the setting of a true uni-ventricular heart or single ventricle. (Courtesy of Prof K. Dimopoulos)

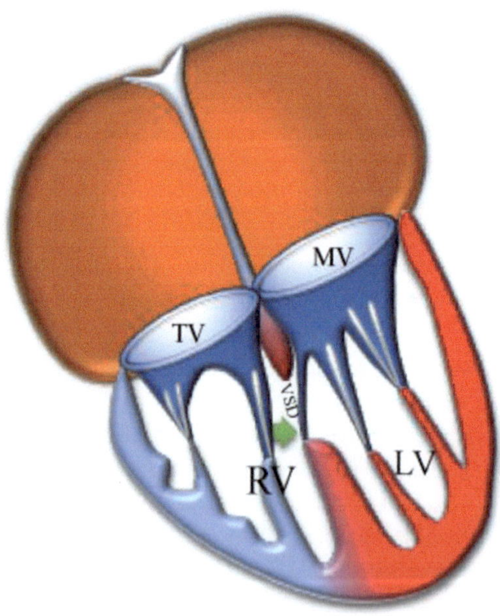

Fig. 2.2 Straddling mitral valve: part of the subvalvar apparatus of the mitral valve crosses the VSD (arrow), precluding patch closure of the defect and a biventricular repair. (Courtesy of Prof K. Dimopoulos)

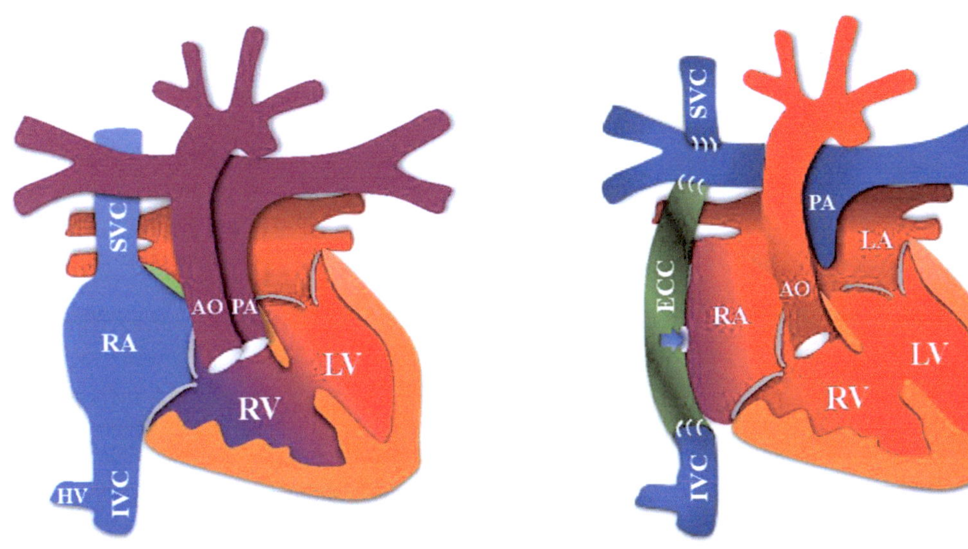

Fig. 2.3 DORV with transposed great arteries and non-committed VSD. (Courtesy of Prof K. Dimopoulos)

Terminology

Definition of a Ventricle

To understand the terminology of univentricular heart, we have to first clarify the morphological definition of what is a ventricle [8, 9]. A normal ventricle is characterised by 3 components, the:

- Inlet,
- Outlet
- Apical trabecular component.

In malformed hearts, what defines a ventricle is the presence of an apical component, which is the most constant structure in the ventricular cavity, and is characterised by a coarse trabecular pattern in the right and a fine trabecular pattern in the left. Even in the absence of the inlet or outlet component, we are still in the presence of a ventricle when the apical component is present.

In some instances, e.g. in pulmonary atresia with intact septum, the three ventricular components of the right ventricle are present, but the ventricle is small due to hypertrophy of the parietal wall and cannot independently support the pulmonary circulation (i.e. biventricular repair of the defect).

Conversely, in the setting of a double outlet right ventricle, even though the outlet of the left ventricle is lacking, the left ventricle may be of good enough size to independently support the systemic or pulmonary circulation.

When the inlet component is lacking, the ventricle is usually hypoplastic and of insufficient size to support the pulmonary or systemic circulation alone.

Hypoplastic Ventricle

The size of the ventricular cavity is important in the decision making process regarding the surgical approach, i.e. biventricular repair versus Fontan-type palliation versus one and half ventricle repair [10].

The one and half ventricle repair is considered when there is mild-moderate hypoplasia of the RV and its valves, allowing the use of the RV as a subpulmonary ventricle that receives blood flow from the inferior vena cava; a superior cavopulmonary shunt, allow flow from the superior vena cava to bypass the heart, directly reaching the lungs, hence providing preload reduction to the hypoplastic RV (Fig. 2.4).

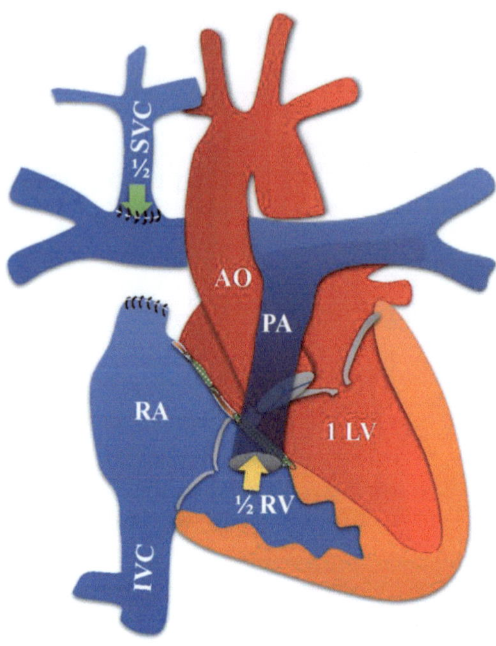

Fig. 2.4 1 and a ½ ventricular repair ("1 LV and ½ RV") which, in effect, is biventricular repair with a superior cavopulmonary shunt. Hence only IVC flow reaches the hypoplastic RV and is "pumped" into the main pulmonary artery, whereas the SVC flow is routed directly to the pulmonary arteries. (Courtesy of Prof K. Dimopoulos)

From a morphological point of view, there are still no established quantitative criteria for differentiating a normal ventricular cavity from a hypoplastic one.

Classification and Nomenclature of Congenital Heart Disease

The simplest approach to the classification and description of congenital heart disease is sequential segmental analysis [11–14], which considers the following mandatory steps in defining the:

1. Atrial situs
2. Atrio-ventricular connection
3. Ventriculo-arterial connection,
4. Ventricular morphology
5. Ventricular topology (d- or l- loop),
6. Associated anomalies
7. Cardiac position.

Using sequential segmental analysis, the univentricular hearts are characterised as follows (Fig. 2.1):

1. Univentricular atrio-ventricular connections: the atrial chambers are connected to only one ventricular cavity in the setting of:
   (a) One normal and one hypoplastic ventricle with:
      - 1 atrio-ventricular valve: Tricuspid atresia or mitral atresia
      - Two atrio-ventricular valves: Double inlet left or right ventricle
      - A common atrio-ventricular valve: Unbalanced AVSD
   (b) A solitary ventricle of indeterminate morphology
2. Biventricular atrioventricular connection: the atrial chambers connect with both ventricular cavity in the setting of:
   (a) 1 normal and one hypoplastic ventricle
      - Single ventriculo-arterial connection: Pulmonary atresia with intact ventricular septum
      - Concordant ventriculo-arterial connection: Severe Ebstein anomaly
   (b) 2 well-developed ventricles
      - Single outlet: Truncus arteriosus
      - Double outlet ventriculo-arterial connection: DORV with non-committed VSD (i.e. one that does not allow the creation of an unobstructed pathway from the left ventricle to one of the great vessels through the VSD, hence not amenable to biventricular repair)

Tricuspid Atresia

Tricuspid atresia is a rare congenital heart defect, present at birth in less than 3% of babies affected by CHD.

It is characterised by an absent connection between the right atrium and the right ventricle. If left untreated, half of the patients die within 10 years of age.

Tricuspid atresia can be distinguished into two phenotypes based on the type of atrioventricular connection: A) univentricular or B) biventricular:

1. Tricuspid atresia with univentricular atrioventricular connection is the classical form, with discontinuity between the atrium and the ventricle in the setting of a muscular floor of the right atrium. The atrioventricular junction is made by a fibro-fatty tissue rim in the atrioventricular groove [15] (Figs. 2.5 and 2.6).
2. Tricuspid atresia with biventricular atrioventricular connection is the rarest form, without fibro-fatty discontinuity between the atrial and ventricular cavity, but rather imperforate valve tissue at the floor of the right atrium.

In both types of tricuspid atresia, the systemic venous blood reaches the right atrium via the superior and inferior vena cava, but can only exit towards the left atrium, through an atrial septal defect, usually an oval fossa (secundum) defect, or patent foramen ovale.

In the left atrium there is a complete (obligatory) mixing of the systemic (deoxygenated) and pulmonary venous (oxygenated) blood and the oxygenated blood from the pulmonary veins.

Therefore, the blood reaching the systemic ventricle and great arteries is partially deoxygenated, causing cyanosis.

The left atrium is connected to the left ventricle via the mitral valve. The left ventricle is well formed in all its tri-partition.

The right ventricle is rudimentary, lacking an inlet, but mostly retaining its apical coarsely-trabeculated component and the outlet, which is connected to a great vessel (see below). Its position is always antero-superior to the left ventricle. The right ventricular size varies, and can be:

- Not extremely small when there is a ventricular septal defect which allows blood flow into the right ventricle, or
- Very small with very thick walls in the setting of an intact ventricular septum.

Ventriculo-arterial connection (Fig. 2.7):

1. In two-third of all cases of tricuspid atresia, there is concordant ventriculo-arterial connection and the right rudimentary ventricle gives rise to the pulmonary trunk and is associated with pulmonary or subpulmonary stenosis (Fig. 2.7) [16, 17].

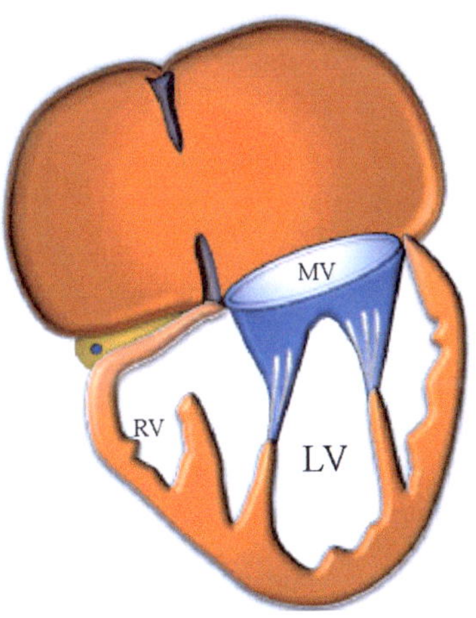

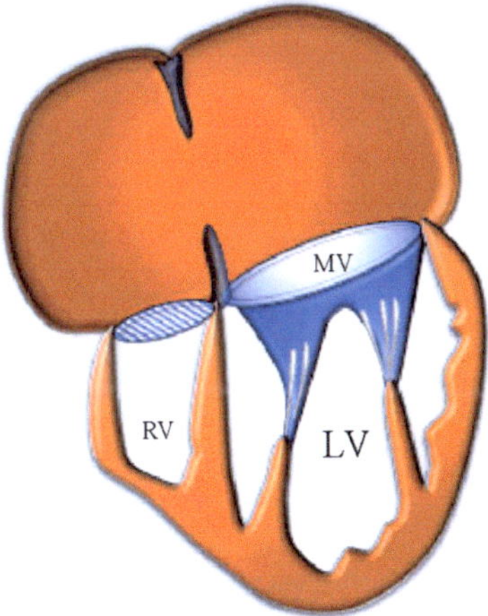

Fig. 2.5 Diagram of tricuspid atresia. On the left there is absent right atrioventricular connection with the muscular floor of the right atrium and the atrioventricular junction represented by a sulcus with fibroadipose tissue; the right cavity is small due to a restricted interventricular septal defect. In the setting of intact septum, the right cavity would be virtual. On the right sided atrioventricular connection will be biventricular (concordant) with an imperforate right tricuspid valve. (Courtesy of Prof K. Dimopoulos)

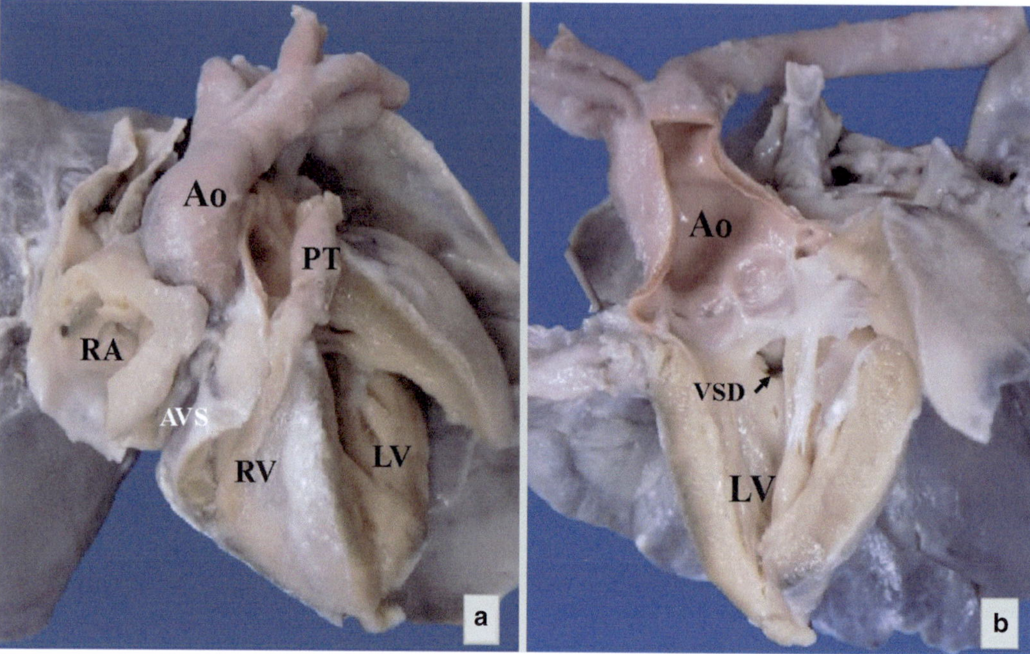

Fig. 2.6 Tricuspid atresia. (**a**) Anterior view of the heart with large right atrium, the atrioventricular sulcus (AVS) and a clear discontinuity between the right atrium (RA) and the right ventricle (RV), which is composed of the apical and outlet part. The left ventricle is reaching the apex of the heart. (**b**) Left oblique view with the well-formed chamber, the interventricular septal defect (arrow) and the aorta with a concordant ventriculo-arterial connection

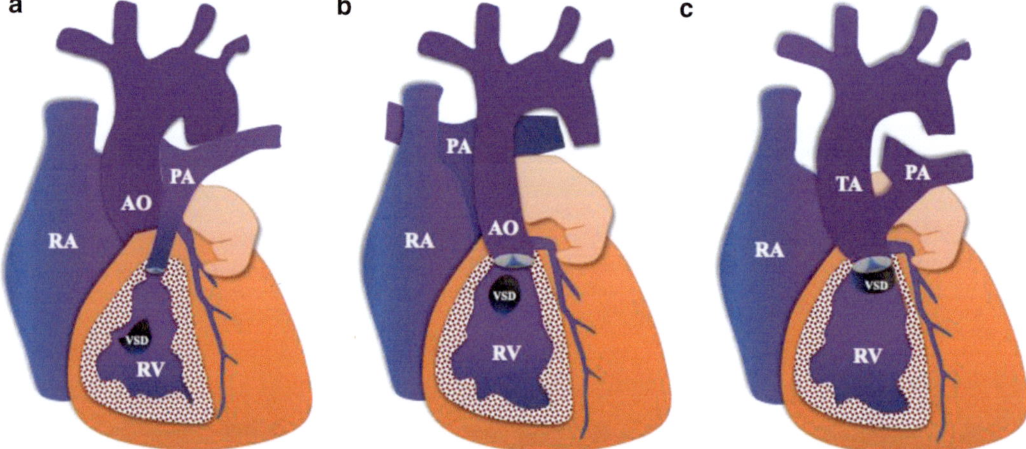

Fig. 2.7 Tricuspid atresia: ventriculoarterial connections. (**a**) Pulmonary or subpulmonary valve stenosis. (**b**) Transposed great arteries, (**c**) Truncus arteriosus.

2. In a third of cases, the ventriculo-arterial connection is:
   (a) discordant (transposition of the great arteries): the pulmonary trunk takes origin from the well-formed left ventricle and is associated again with pulmonary stenosis, while the aorta originates from the rudimentary anterior ventricle result-

ing in obstruction of the aortic flow due to a restrictive ventricular septal defect or a muscular infundibulum;

(b) single outlet vessel, i.e. a common trunk, aorta or pulmonary artery.

Common associated anomalies include dextrocardia, atrial appendage juxtaposition, and a subaortic infundibulum in one out of four cases. Less frequently, there is aortic coarctation.

HLHS

The term HLHS identifies a wide spectrum of congenital cardiac anomalies, characterised by hypoplasia of the left heart with normally aligned great arteries, in the absence of a common atrioventricular valve [18–24]. HLHS includes:

1. Mitral atresia associated with aortic atresia or stenosis
2. Mitral stenosis and aortic atresia
3. Mitral and aortic stenosis
4. Hypoplastic left heart complex (milder end of the spectrum) with a small left ventricle, unable to support the systemic circulation, and a small/hypoplastic ascending aorta.

The following congenital defects are **not** considered HLHS:

- DORV with a hypoplastic LV,
- ccTGA with a large VSD and small LV,
- Unbalanced AVSD with a small LV,
- Long segment-subaortic AS with valvar AS, VSD and aortic arch hypoplasia [25].

The common features of all the congenital abnormalities listed as HLHS are:

- A functional right ventricular chamber
- Hypoplasia of the ascending aortic /aortic arch of varying severity.

The mitral valve and aortic valve are usually maldeveloped and dysplastic, resulting in true valvular stenosis. Only seldomly, the aortic and mitral valve are simply hypoplastic, when the valves are small but not intrinsically stenotic.

During fetal life, the systemic blood flow is provided entirely by the RV via the ductus arteriosus. Thus, a patent ductus arteriosus and adequate mixing of oxygenated and deoxygenated (systemic and pulmonary venous) blood at atrial level are essential for postnatal survival. A restrictive or closed foramen ovale will result in pulmonary edema and severe hypoxia [26, 27].

Left ventricle morphology can vary (Figs. 2.8, 2.9, 2.10 and 2.11), from virtual (slit-like) to dilated and is classified into four subtypes (Fig. 2.12) [28]:

1. Virtual or slit-like left ventricle: a flattened LV without a true cavity, but plastered by endothelium. This type is associated with mitral atresia and aortic atresia. The floor of the left atrium is muscular and no valve tissue is detectable. Its position is in the left-posterior part of the ventricular mass, and can be identified through the left anterior and posterior descending coronary artery encircling the virtual LV on the epicardial surface. The left atrioventricular junction is made of fibrofatty tissue within the atrioventricular groove (Figs 2.8 and 2.9) [29].
2. Miniature LV: the LV is of near-normal size but with severe parietal wall thickness restricting the size of its cavity. The mitral and aortic valves are small, but not stenotic, and can be considered anatomically normal. Dysplastic stenotic valve can sometimes coexist. The cavity does not reach the cardiac apex, which is represented entirely by the right ventricle (Fig. 2.10).
3. Small LV cavity with endocardial fibroelastosis (EFE) and thickened parietal wall. In this setting, there is also mitral stenosis and aortic valve stenosis or atresia. Endocardial fibroelastosis is usually recognizable as a firm whitish layer on the LV endocardium, resulting in a non-compliant cavity. It can be focal, involving the papillary muscles or septum, or diffuse covering the entire ventricular cavity, with severe thickening due to fibroelastic deposition. There is no association between the severity of the endocardial fibroelastosis and the size of the aortic valve (Fig. 2.11).

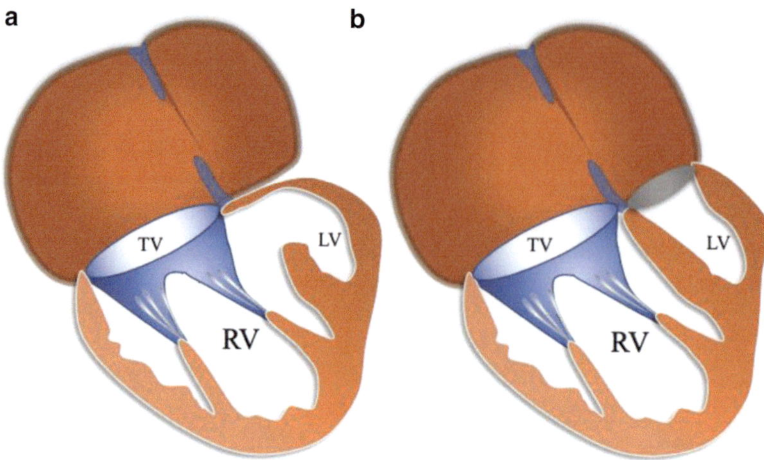

Fig. 2.8 Diagram of mitral atresia. In (**a**), there is absent left atrioventricular connection with muscular floor of the left atrium and the atrioventricular junction represented by a sulcus with fibro-adipose tissue; the left cavity is small due to a restricted interventricular septal defect. In the setting of intact septum (**b**), the left cavity would be quite small or virtual; the atrioventricular connection will be biventricular (concordant) with an imperforate left mitral valve

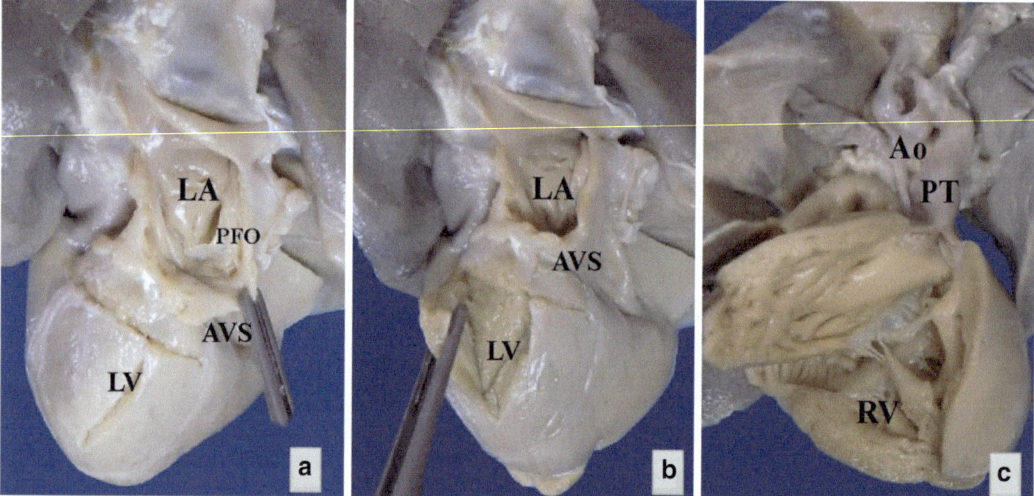

Fig. 2.9 Mitral atresia with slit-like ventricle: (**a**) left posterior view of the heart; there is discontinuity between the left ventricle (cut longitudinally) and the left atrium (with a patent foramen ovale (PFO) and its muscular floor). (**b**) The left ventricle has been opened. Note the lucent endocardium without fibro-elastosis. (**c**) The right ventricle has been opened along the acute margin and the outflow, showing the pulmonary valve. The aorta (Ao) is tiny and atretic. *PT* pulmonary trunk

4. Dilated LV due to mitral regurgitation, with leaflet redundancy, thin LV parietal (free) wall and a giant left atrium, which can produce right atrial compression. In the setting of HLHS, left ventricular dilatation is a paradox anatomically speaking; however, the thin-walled left ventricle is unable to support the systemic circulation (similar to other forms of HLHS) (Fig. 2.12).

The left atrial cavity can be of different sizes, in relation to the morphology of the atrial septum:

- A large left atrium, with a thick septum secundum and a still identifiable thin septum primum, adherent to each other; massively dilated pulmonary veins.
- A small muscular left atrium, with a thick atrial septum but no identifiable secundum and primum components; the pulmonary veins appear small.

- A giant left atrium in the setting of severe mitral regurgitation, with a thin atrial septum, and rightward septal displacement; the pulmonary veins are usually large.

The aortic valve can be atretic or stenotic and, in both cases, there is restricted cusp excursion and post-stenotic dilatation of the ascending aorta. There is a wide spectrum of aortic valve morphological features, from tricuspid dysplastic leaflets to unicuspid and severe stenotic or hypoplastic valve:

- Most often the cusps are dysplastic and rigid, with nodular degeneration and thickening, disruption of the integrity of the fibrosa and mucoid degeneration with secondary fibrosis.
- With unicuspid valves, there is one commissure, an eccentric stenotic commissural orifice, one well-formed interleaflet triangle, a small annulus and dysplastic nodular myxoid excrescences. One or two raphes can be identified as remnants of the commissures.
- A bicuspid aortic valve is not by definition stenotic, but can be stenotic in the setting of leaflet dysplasia. There are two phenotypes:

  - a bicuspid valve with two normal well-formed leaflets and interleaflet triangles,
  - a bicuspid valve with a raphe in one of the leaflets, with an aborted interleaflet triangle.

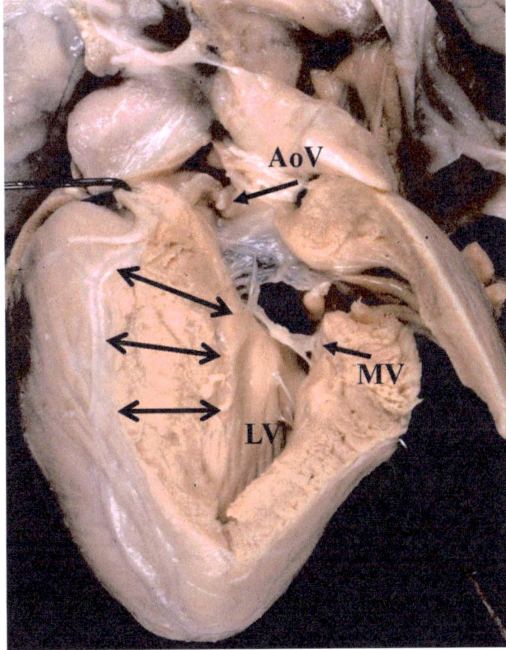

Fig. 2.10 HLHS with a small left ventricle (LV) not forming the apex of the heart, thick parietal wall and severe hypertrophic interventricular septum, small mitral valve and stenotic and dysplastic aortic valve cusps

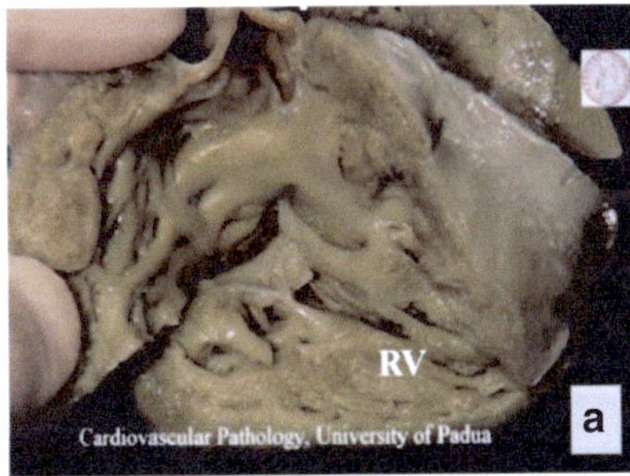

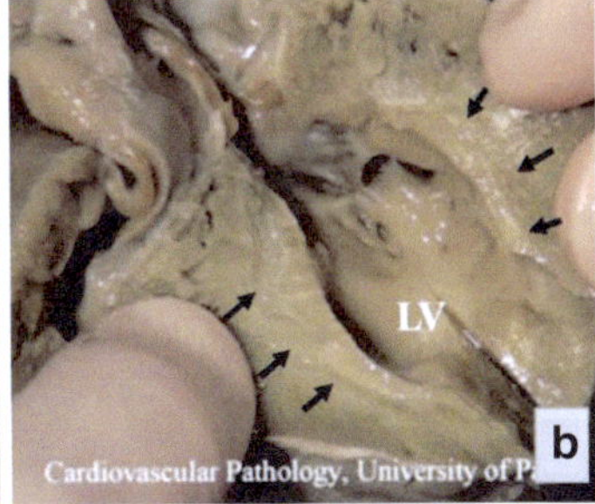

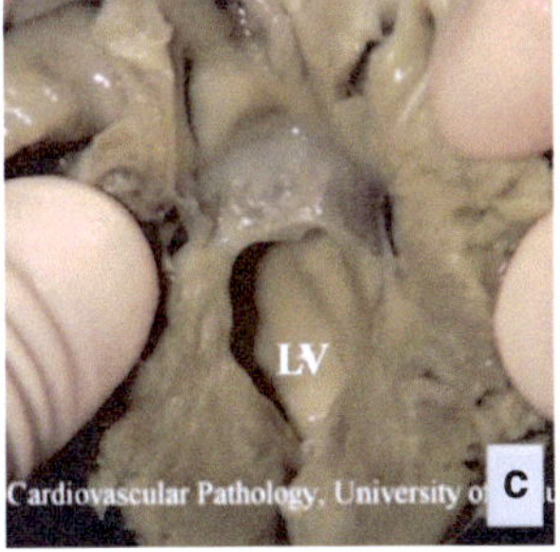

Fig. 2.11 HLHS with a small left ventricle and endocardial fibro-elastosis in the setting of mitral and aortic stenosis. (**a**) Right ventricle of normal size. (**b**) Left ventricular cavity with severe thickening of the endocardium (arrow). Note also the hypertrophy of the parietal wall of the left ventricle. (**c**) The small left ventricle with a stenotic and dysplastic mitral valve with short and fused tendinous cord

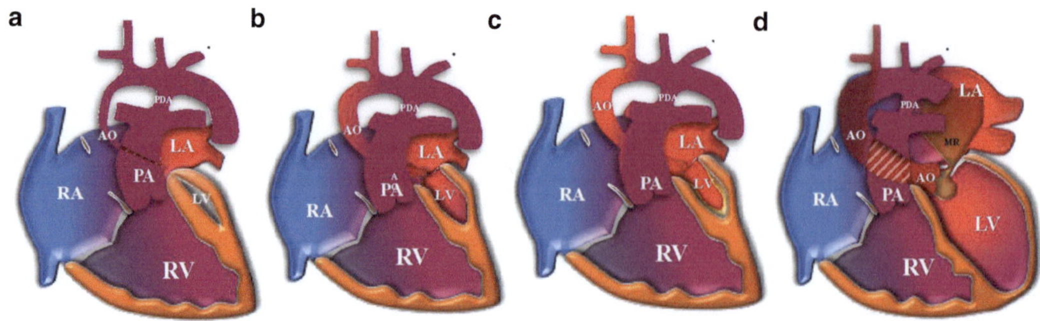

Fig. 2.12 LV morphology variants in HLHS. (**a**): Slit-like LV. (**b**) Severely hypoplastic LV to aorta. (**c**) Small LV with endocardial fibroelastosis, open to the aorta. (**d**) Dilated, thin-walled LV, intact septum and thickened mitral valve with regurgitation

The mitral valve features depend on which of the four types of left ventricles is present:

1. In the slit-like type (in mitral atresia, or mitral and aortic atresia) the valve is usually lacking;
2. In the miniature type, the mitral valve is well formed but globally hypoplastic, with a well differentiated subvalvular apparatus;
3. In the small ventricle associated with EFE the valve can have thick dysplastic leaflets, short chordae, and small papillary muscles again plastered by EFE;
4. In the last type (with left ventricular dilatation) the mitral valve has dysplastic and redundant leaflets, with severe insufficiency.

Associated anomalies:

- In mitral atresia: PDA, aortic arch coarctation, ASD, PFO, VSD, bicuspid aortic valve, bicuspid pulmonary valve, bilateral infundibulum, retroesophageal subclavian artery.
- In aortic atresia with intact septum: Hypoplastic mitral valve, dysplasia of the mitral valve, ASD or PFO, fibroelastosis of the left ventricle and aortic coarctation.

Double Inlet Ventricles

A double inlet ventricle is a condition in which more than 50% of both atria are connected to a dominant ventricle, which can be morphologically left or right. Therefore, the atrioventricular connection is univentricular.

The atrioventricular connection can be through:

- Two separate and patent valves (Figs. 2.13 and 2.14),
- One patent valve and one imperforate valve (left or right),
- A common valve, which may be straddling or overriding (Figs. 2.15 and 2.16) ,
- Two straddling valves, or
- One entirely committed valve and one straddling valve (regardless of morphology), which is connected to the ventricular cavity by more than half its annulus diameter [30].

The atrial arrangement can be in the setting of situs solitus, situs inversus or left/right atrial isomerism.

The dominant ventricle is most commonly of left (~85%, Figs. 2.13 and 2.14) rather than right morphology (~10%, Figs. 2.15 and 2.16), with the corresponding atrioventricular valve (tricuspid valve for the RV and mitral valve for the LV). There is usually a rudimentary or incomplete chamber located anteriorly (morphologically right) or posteriorly (if morphologically left). Very rarely, the ventricular morphology is undetermined (~5%) and a second chamber cannot be clearly identified within the ventricular mass (Fig. 2.17).

The most frequent ventriculoarterial connection is either double-outlet or single outlet from

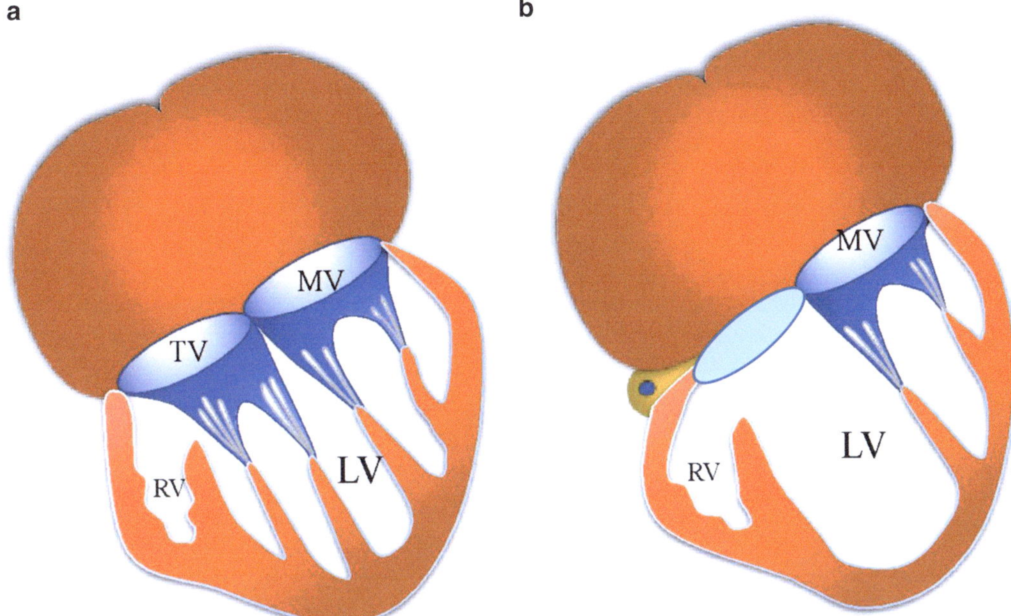

Fig. 2.13 Diagram of the double inlet left ventricle with both atria connected to a well-formed ventricular chamber of left morphology with both atrioventricular valves draining in this chamber while the right ventricle is hypo-plastic . In (**a**) the two atrioventricular valves are open, while in (**b**) one of the two atrioventricular valves is imperforate

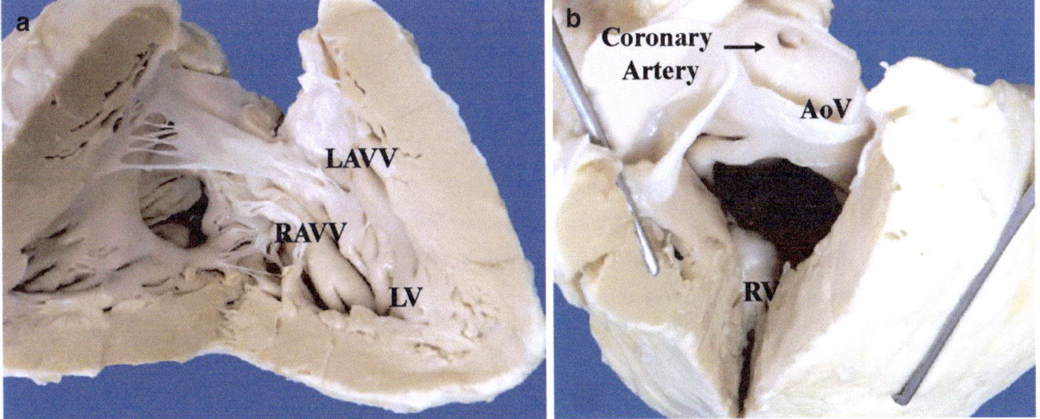

Fig. 2.14 Double inlet left ventricle with TGA. (**a**) View of the left ventricle with both atrioventricular valve draining into this well-formed chamber, an interventricular septal defect and in (**b**) the aorta taking origin from the small hypoplastic right chamber. *LAVV* left atrioventricular valve, *RAVV* right atrioventricular valve, *LV* left ventricle, *AoV* aortic valve. RV: right ventricle

the dominant right ventricle. A rudimentary left ventricular chamber is only composed of its trabecular or apical part. At times, the rudimentary left ventricular chamber can only be identified at histology. The ventricular septum is also hypo-plastic but, different to the double inlet left ventricle, there is a posterior component which is directed towards the crux-cordis. The ventricular septal defect is of membranous type, but can also be muscular.

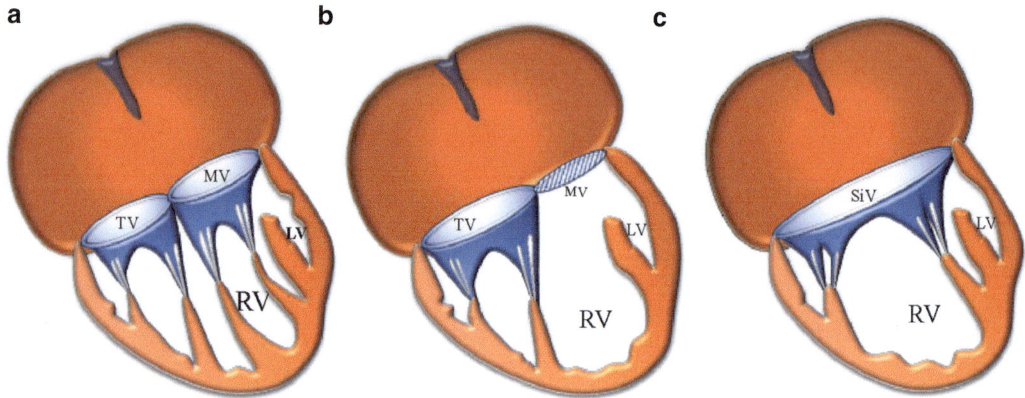

Fig. 2.15 Diagram of the double inlet right ventricle with both atria connected to a well-formed ventricular chamber of right morphology with in (**a**) both atrioventricular valve drain in this chamber while the left ventricle is hypoplastic; in (**b**) One of the two atrioventricular valve is imperforate.; in (**c**) the mode of connection is represented by a common atrioventricular valve

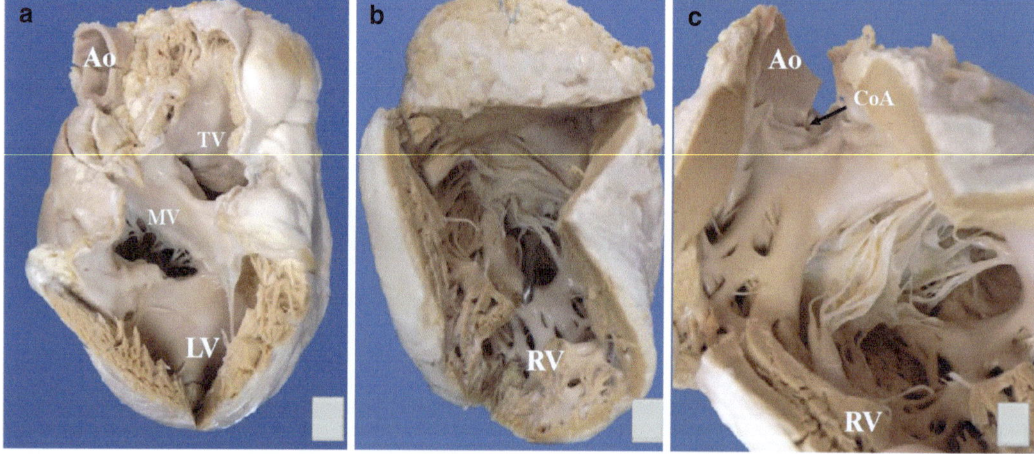

Fig. 2.16 Double inlet right ventricle and TGA. (**a**) The lateral view from the above shows the two well-formed valve, tricuspid and mitral valves draining into a large ventricle, while the left ventricle is hypoplastic. In (**b**) the right ventricle with coarse trabeculations, and the probe from the mitral valve pointing to the RV; in (**c**) outflow tract view from the right chamber with the great vessel represented by the aorta with the origin of the coronary arteries. *CoA* coronary artery

Morphological rules can be of help in the identification of ventricular morphology for the dominant ventricle, such as:

- Apical trabeculation, fine for the left and course for the right ventricle.
- The relative ventricular position within the heart: left posterior and right anterior.
- Atrioventricular valve morphology: Valve morphology can be of help in identifying ventricular morphology and the type of loop, since each valve "belongs" to its ventricle. However, it can at times be difficult to distinguish between the mitral and tricuspid valves; typically, the presence of mural papillary muscles or a cleft in the anterior leaflet identify the mitral valve [31].

Double inlet right ventricle is often associated with right atrial isomerism. The ventricular

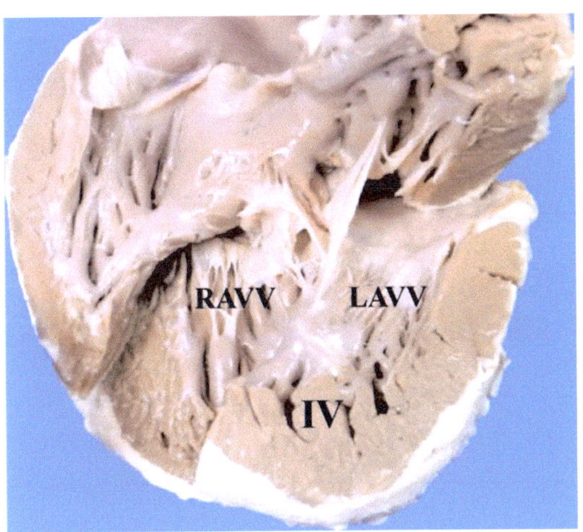

Fig. 2.17 Double inlet indeterminate ventricle with absence of the septal structure, the two valves draining into this chamber. A second small or even virtual cavity was not identified. Note the coarse trabeculations of the indeterminate ventricle (IV). Right atrioventricular valve. Left atrioventricular valve

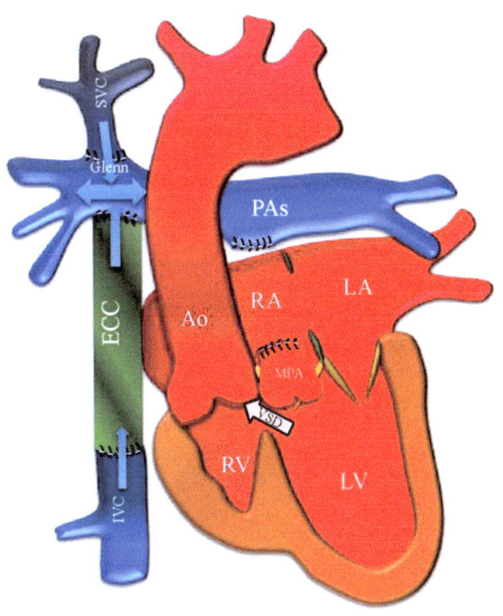

Fig. 2.18 Diagram of double inlet LV with a rudimentary RV and transposed great arteries after total cavopulmonary connection (TCPC) with an extracardiac conduit (ECC) and a bidirectional Glenn anastomosis: the aorta (AO) arises from the right ventricle (RV) and flow of the dominant left ventricle (LV) crosses a restrictive ventricular septal defect (VSD, arrow), which causes "subaortic stenosis". *Glenn* bidirectional Glenn anastomosis, *IVC* inferior vena cava, *LA* left atrium, *MPA* main pulmonary artery, *PAs* pulmonary arteries, *RA* right atrium, *SVC* superior vena cava. (Courtesy of Prof K. Dimopoulos)

chambers communicate through a ventricular septal defect, the so-called "bulboventricular foramen", which is muscular and usually restrictive (i.e. causing obstruction to flow), localized at infundibular level [32, 33].

The ventriculoarterial connection in double inlet ventricles is most commonly discordant (i.e. transposed great arteries). In this setting, the ventricular septal defect can be restrictive, producing subaortic stenosis (Figs. 2.18 and 2.19) [34].

Pulmonary stenosis is also common and may protect the lung vasculature from the development of pulmonary vascular disease. The pulmonary stenosis can be at the level of the valve or subvalvular, at times at the extreme end of the spectrum of stenosis, i.e. pulmonary atresia.

Less commonly, the ventriculoarterial connection can be concordant, defining what is called the "Holmes heart" [35]. Even less commonly, there can be a double outlet from the dominant ventricle.

The "Holmes heart" is characterised by a single morphologically dominant left ventricle, a rudimentary morphologically right ventricle with infundibular outlet chamber, and normally related great arteries, with the pulmonary artery arising from the infundibular outlet chamber and the aorta from the single LV.

A complete morphological evaluation is pivotal for understanding the clinical presentation and surgical management of these patients. The most common morphological pattern is in the setting of situs solitus, double inlet left ventricle positioned posteriorly, and transposition of the great arteries with the aorta arising from the anterior rudimentary chamber, which precludes biventricular surgical repair. There is a single or multiple ventricular septal defects.

Associated anomalies are common and mainly involve the valves. This can be atrioventricular valve stenosis or incompetence due to hypoplasia, straddling, dysplasia or clefting. Pulmonary stenosis can be due either to leaflet dysplasia or a hypoplastic annulus. Subpulmonary stenosis can be due to muscle hypertrophy, infundibular hypoplasia, ventricular septal displacement or a restrictive ventricular septal defect. The latter can

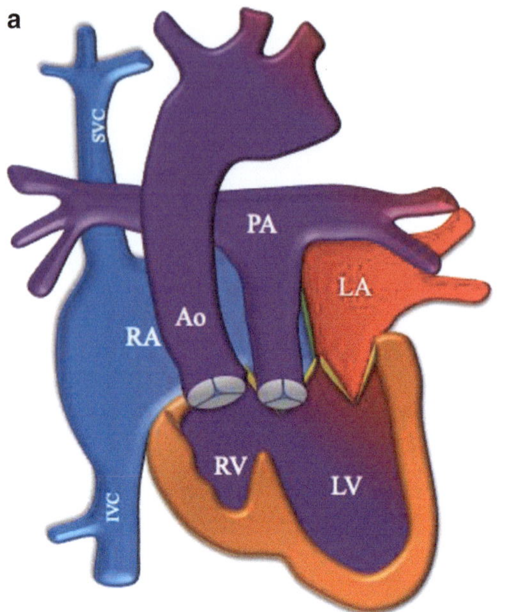

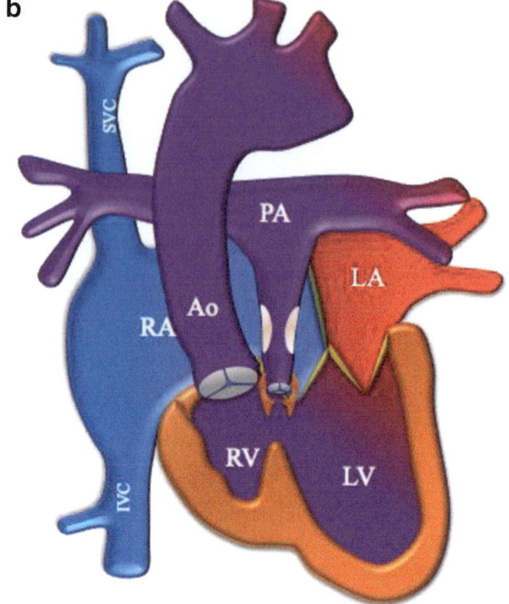

Fig. 2.19 Diagram of DILV with transposed great arteries and (**a**) no pulmonary stenosis or (**b**) severe subvalvar, valvar or supravalvar stenosis. In the absence of pulmonary stenosis, the pulmonary circulation is exposed to increase flow and pressure, resulting in pulmonary vascular disease. Significant pulmonary stenosis "protects" the pulmonary circulation, but may be detrimental if there is insufficient pulmonary blood flow. Courtesy of Prof K. Dimopoulos

produce subpulmonary or subaortic stenosis, depending on the type of ventriculo-arterial connection (concordant vs discordant). An interrupted aortic arch or aortic coarctation may also be present.

Functional Univentricular heart Variants

"Functional univentricular heart" is the term introduced to include cardiac abnormalities with biventricular atrio-ventricular connection, in which there are two ventricular cavities possessing all three components (inlet, apical and outlet), but one of the ventricles is unable to sustain the systemic or pulmonary circulation, hence biventricular repair is not possible.

A ventricle may not be able to support the circulation even in the presence of all three components:

- In pulmonary atresia with intact ventricular septum, the right ventricle possesses all components, but the ventricular cavity may be quite small, or even virtual, due to the extreme hypertrophy of the lateral free wall [36].
- In severe Ebstein anomaly of the tricuspid valve, there is atrialization of a large portion of the right ventricle, which has a papyraceous parietal wall; there is biventricular atrioventricular connection (each atrium connected to its respective ventricle) but the right atrium is severely enlarged, incorporating part of the right ventricular cavity [37–39]. The remaining (functional) right ventricle below the apically

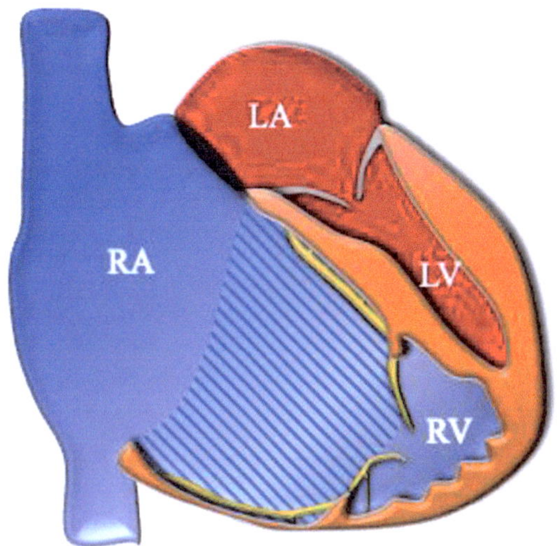

Fig. 2.20 Diagram of severe Ebstein anomaly, with a large portion (striped area) of "atrialised" right ventricle (RV) and a severely apically displaced tricuspid valve (in yellow). The "functional RV is limited to the apex and outflow portions and may be too small to support biventricular repair. *LA* left atrium, *LV* left ventricle, *RA* right atrium. (Courtesy of Prof K. Dimopoulos)

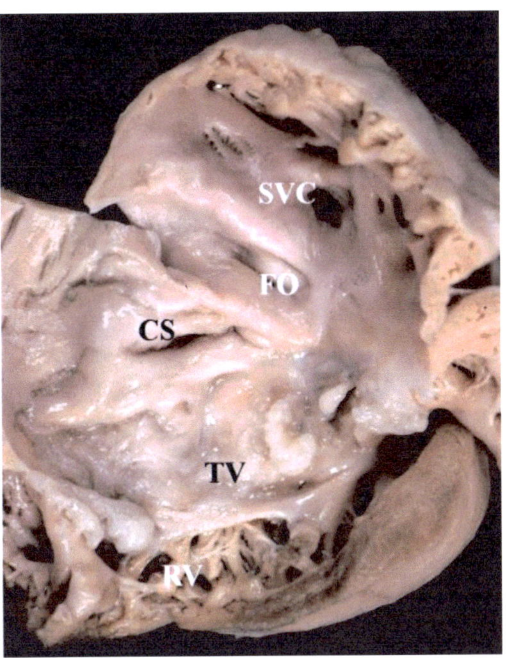

Fig. 2.21 Severe Ebstein anomaly: right atrial and ventricular (RV) chambers opened anteriorly to highlight the huge dilated atrium the plastered septal and posterior leaflet of the tricuspid valve (TV) into the ventricle, dysplasia of the leaflets themselves. The residual right ventricle is at the apex. *CS* coronary sinus, *FO* fossa ovalis, *SVC* superior vena cava

displaced orifice of the tricuspid valve tends to dilate (mainly at its outflow component), but may be anatomically and functionally inadequate to sustain the pulmonary circulation, hence cannot be used for biventricular repair: functional univentricular heart variant (Figs. 2.20 and 2.21).

- Other hearts with one big and one small ventricle achieve this feature because of atresia or critical stenosis of an arterial valve, usually in the setting of an intact ventricular septum.
- Hearts in which there is straddling and/or overriding of an atrioventricular valve may not be amenable to biventricular repair.
- In complete atrioventricular septal defects, a common atrioventricular junction is usually guarded by a common atrioventricular valve [39]. The common valve and junction can be predominantly connected to one or the other ventricle (unbalanced atrioventricular septal defect), causing a significant disproportion between the two ventricular cavities; this results in one of the ventricles (right or left) being too small to support the pulmonary or systemic circulation, hence precluding biventricular repair [40–45] (Fig. 2.22). In extreme cases, the left ventricle may be quite hypoplastic.
- Hearts with an extremely large ventricular septal defect expanding to the apex, may be considered functional univentricular.

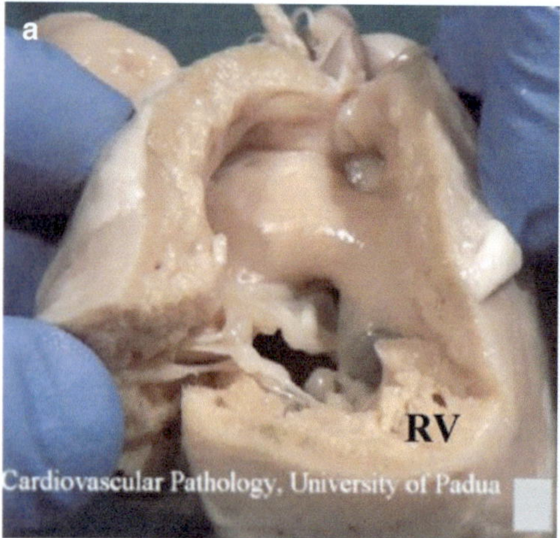

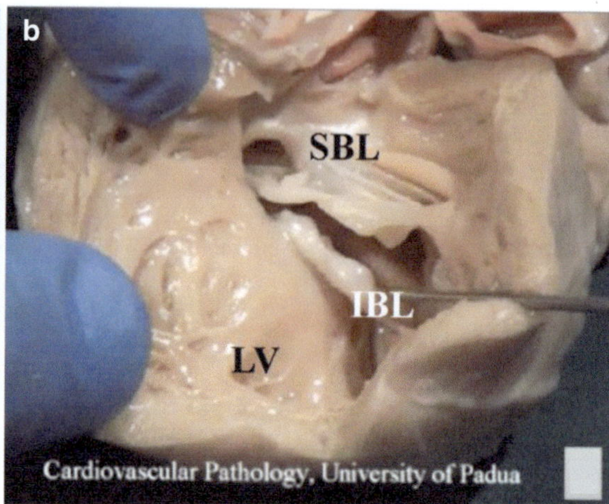

Fig. 2.22 Unbalanced atrioventricular septal defect, with dominant left ventricle (LV). In (**a**) the right ventricle (RV) has been opened according to the blood flow along the acute margin of the heart and the outflow tract. Note the right ventricular hypertrophy. In (**b**) the large left ventricle with the superior and inferior bridging leaflets (IBL)

Heterotaxy (Isomerism) Syndromes

In the normal body, there is an asymmetry of internal organs. If this asymmetry is lost during development, an unusual degree of symmetry of the thoracic and abdominal organs is retained and visceral heterotaxy is present.

Heterotaxy syndrome is defined as an abnormal arrangement of the internal thoracoabdominal organs along the left-right axis of the body.

Isomerism is present when there is development of paired structures along the left-right axis of the body, being both morphologically of left or right type.

The morphology of the atrial appendages is almost always in harmony with the arrangements of the thoracic and abdominal organs. Thus, by examining the atrial appendages, we can identify the hallmarks of two types of heterotaxy syndrome:

- Right atrial isomerism, with asplenia and right laterality on both sides of the body along its long axis
- Left atrial isomerism, with polysplenia and left laterality.

Left and right atrial isomerism are associated with any combination of cardiac and extracardiac abnormalities (see Table 2.1).

In atrial isomerism, the connection of the two atria of the same (right or left) morphology to the ventricles can be defined as:

- "Ambiguous" biventricular atrioventricular connection, when the two morphologically similar atria are connected to two separate ventricles
- "Univentricular" atrioventricular connection when the atria are connected to one ventricle. In this case, the ventricles are usually of different sizes, with the smaller ventricle not connected to an atrium. The morphology of the ventricular cavity can be of dominant left type (with a rudimentary right ventricle), dominant right type (with a rudimentary left ventricle) or, more, rarely a solitary or indeterminate ventricle [46]. Hence, there are 3 types of univentricular atrioventricular connection:

  - Double inlet ventricle,
  - Absent left, or
  - Absent right.

Table 2.1 Morphologic features of right and left atrial isomerism

Cardiac morphology	Right atrial isomerism	Left atrial isomerism
Position of the heart in the chest	Dextrocardia (50%), levocardia 50%	Typically levocardia, dextrocardia (20%), mesocardia (10%)
Situs abdominis (position of the abdominal great vessels)	Aorta and IVC on the same side of the spine, with IVC anterior to the aorta	Azygos continuation of IVC Azygos vein posterior and to the left of the aorta
Atrial appendages and atrial morphology	Two morphologically right atrial appendages A common atrium (50%) An ostium secundum defect (30%)	Two morphologically left atrial appendages A common atrium in 40% A secundum atrial septal defect in 30%

Atrioventricular connection	Biventricular atrioventricular connection (60%)
	Univentricular connection:
	• Absent right
	• Absent left
	• Double inlet:
	  • To the right ventricle (55%)
	  • To the left ventricle (45%).
		Biventricular atrioventricular connection (60%),
		Univentricular connection (40%):
		• Double inlet right ventricle
		• Absent right
		• Absent left

Atrioventricular (AV) junction	Common AV valve (90%)	Common AV valve (40%) two separate valves (35%)
Ventricular morphology	Right ventricle dominant with left ventricular hypoplasia in up to 40%: • L-loop (60%) • D-loop in (40%)	D-loop morphology (80%)
Ventriculo-arterial connections	DORV (40%) TGA with pulmonary atresia (30%) and RVOTO	RVOTO (40%) Aortic obstruction (25%)
Systemic veins	Bilateral superior vena cava (50%) Left superior vena cava to left-sided atrium (50%) Absent coronary sinus Hepatic veins to IVC Inferior vena cava to left sided atrium (30%)	Bilateral superior vena cava (70%) Interrupted IVC and azygos continuation Absent coronary sinus (70%) Anomalous hepatic veins directly to the atrium (30%)
Pulmonary veins (PVs)	Total anomalous pulmonary venous connection (intracardiac or extracardiac)	Bilateral return: 2 PVs into the left sided and 2 PVs to the right sided atrium (50%) All PVs to the left sided atrium (35%) All PVs to the right sided atrium (15%)
Conduction system	Bilateral sinus nodes A sling of specialized tissue connects the two atrioventricular nodes	The sinus node is hypoplastic, abnormally positioned and present in only half of the cases Discontinuation between the AV node and the ventricular conduction tissue. With AV block in up to 30%

Any type of ventriculoarterial connection may coexist in atrial isomerism:

- In right atrial isomerism, the most frequent ventriculoarterial connection is discordant or double outlet connections
- In left atrial isomerism the most common is a concordant ventriculoarterial connection.

Venoatrial connection abnormalities are almost the rule in patients with atrial isomerism and influence clinical presentation, management and outcome:

- In right atrial isomerism, there is often a total anomalous pulmonary venous connection of the extracardiac type, mainly in the superior vena cava and only seldom in the inferior vena cava or portal system. In only one third, the connection is intra-cardiac. The coronary sinus is usually absent.

- In left atrial isomerism, the inferior vena cava is interrupted and there is azygos continuation to the superior vena cava, with the hepatic veins draining directly to one or both atria.

Intracardiac anomalies are present in 100% of patients with right atrial isomerism and are usually more complex than those seen in left atrial isomerism, which are present in 85% of patients.

Cardiovascular anomalies associated with right and/or left atrial isomerism include: secundum atrial septal defect, muscular ventricular septal defects, right ventricular outflow tract obstruction, pulmonary valve dysplasia, right aortic arch, double outlet right ventricle and TGA, patent arterial duct and, rarely, coronary arteries anomalies.

Pulmonary Atresia

Pulmonary valve atresia or critical pulmonary valve stenosis with intact ventricular septum usually develops progressively during pregnancy as a consequence of a hypoplastic right ventricle outflow, supporting the blood flow theory, i.e. that blood flow during fetal life contributes to the development of the ventricles and great vessels. This represents the base for the development of intrauterine cardiac intervention therapeutic approach [47–50], i.e. that intervention during fetal life can restore blood flow and favour the growth of cardiovascular structures.

Pulmonary atresia with intact ventricular septum is characterized by the absence of communication between the right ventricular outflow tract and the pulmonary trunk in the setting of single aortic outlet from the left ventricle [51–53] (Fig. 2.23). As in HLHS, the size of the right ventricle can vary considerably:

- Normal size cavity with an imperforate pulmonary valve.
- Severely hypoplastic cavity, no outflow tract, massive hypertrophy of the parietal wall and right ventricular coronary artery fistulae [51, 54, 55].; the associated anomalies can influence the management and outcome of these patients [49, 52].
- dilated right ventricle with thinning of the parietal wall in the setting of tricuspid regurgitation. The tricuspid valve can be dysplastic

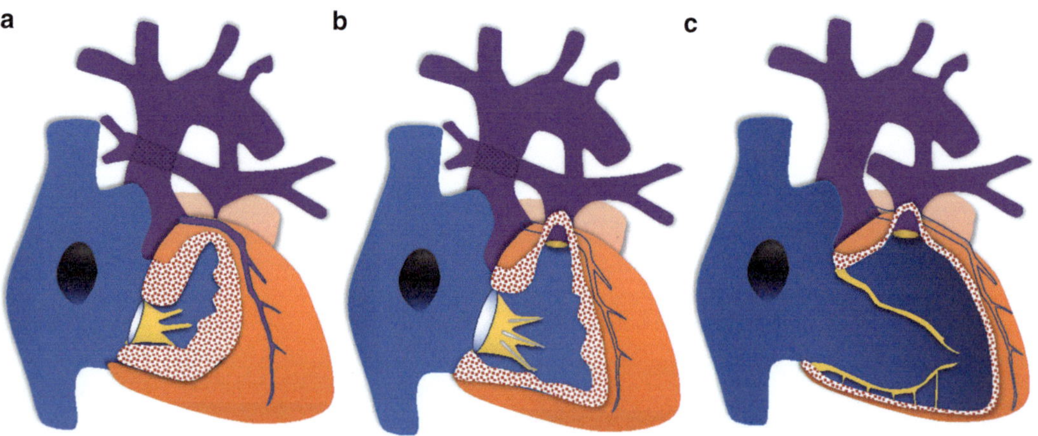

Fig. 2.23 Diagram of the pulmonary atresia with intact septum: in (**a**) The right ventricular chamber is small and the atresia of the pulmonary valve is associated with subpulmonary stenosis due to hypertrophic parietal wall; In (**b**) the pulmonary valve has been formed but imperforate and the size of the ventricle is only mildly hypoplastic. In (**c**) the pulmonary atresia is associated to tricuspid valve Ebstein anomaly with thinning parietal wall

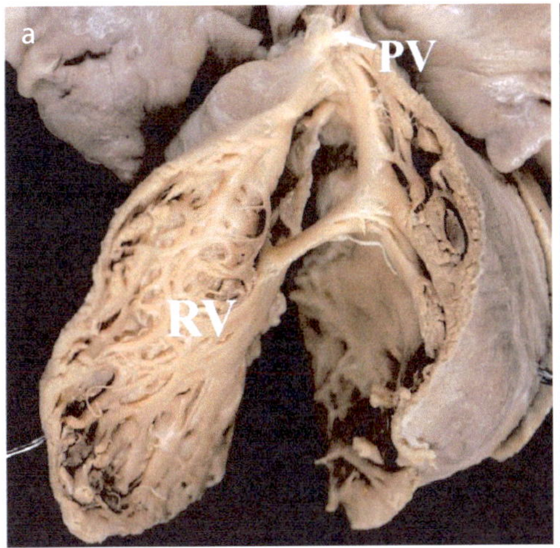
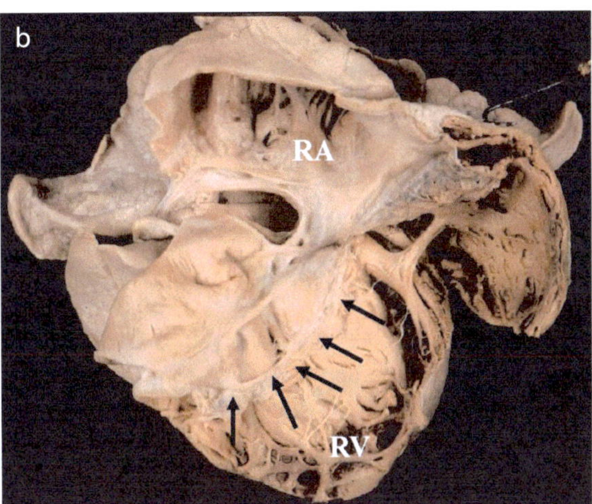

Fig. 2.24 Pulmonary atresia with imperforate valve and dilated right ventricle with thinning of the parietal wall (**a**). In (**b**) view of the right chambers with dilated right atrium, and displacement into the right ventricle of the tricuspid valve annulus. *PV* pulmonary valve, *RV* right ventricle, *RA* right atrium

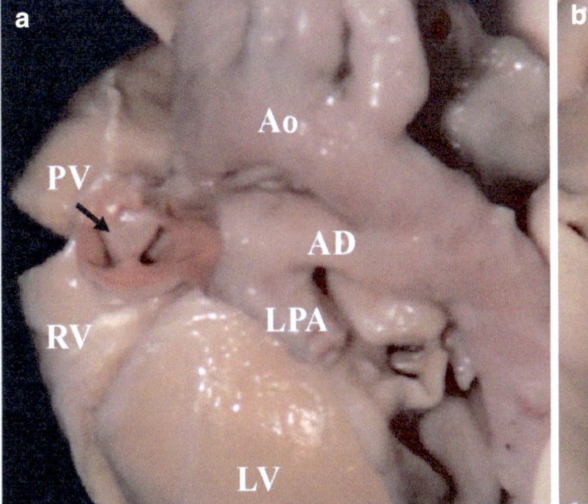
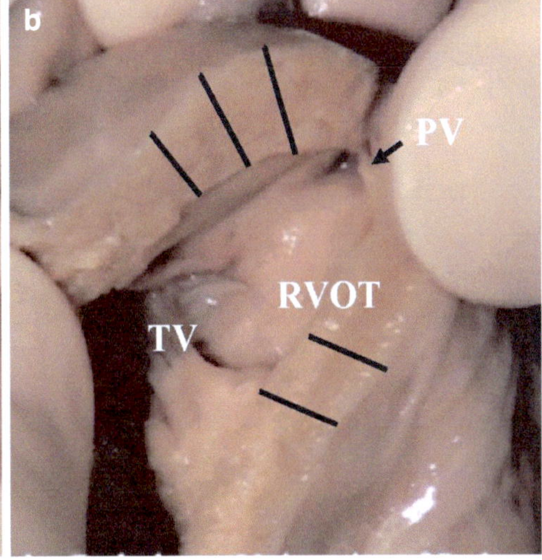

Fig. 2.25 Pulmonary atresia with intact septum. In (**a**) left anterior view from above showing the imperforate pulmonary valve and in (**b**) the right outflow tract with severe hypertrophy of the parietal wall

and cause volume overload, potentially promoting right ventricular growth (Fig. 2.24). It can be also with normal cusps but of diminutive size.

The tricuspid valve dimensions are directly proportional to the size of the right ventricular cavity [56–58] (Fig. 2.23). The presence of all three components of the morphologically right ventricle (inlet, trabecular/apical and outlet) is not synonymous with an adequate cavity size, since an important role is played by the secondary right ventricular hypertrophy (Fig. 2.25) which can be confined to only the apical and or the outlet components [59].

Pulmonary arteries are usually of normal size when retrogradely supplied by the ductus arteriosus. The presence of a restricted foramen ovale can reduce right-to-left shunting and favor tricuspid valve and right ventricular growth.

Fistulae or RV-coronary artery connections are present in between 20% to 50% of the cases of pulmonary atresia with an intact ventricular septum in morphology series [50, 51, 60, 61].

Three types of valves can be identified in the right ventricular outflow tract of patients with pulmonary valve atresia/critical valve stenosis and an intact ventricular septum:

- Imperforate valve, dome-shaped, with 2–4 raphes or three identifiable cusps and well-formed commissures (as if the 3 cusps had fused after differentiation). There is usually continuity between the right ventricle and the pulmonary trunk (Fig. 2.25). Only seldom is there muscular pulmonary atresia with no continuity between the outflow and the pulmonary trunk.
- Three dysplastic thick leaflets (10–20% of patients with critical pulmonary valve stenosis), with a pinhole central orifice allowing very limited blood flow through the valve. The central orifice can vary in size, but what appears to be constant is the hypoplasia of the pulmonary annulus and dilatation of the pulmonary trunk and pulmonary branches.
- Bicuspid or unicuspid valve and hypoplasia of the annulus, with critical pulmonary valve stenosis. The cusps of a bicuspid valve are well-formed and thin, with or without a raphe, but with two well-formed commissures. The annulus is still smaller than with a tricuspid pulmonary valve. The unicuspid valve is characterised by a curtain like cusp, with only one commissure and an eccentrically displaced orifice. One or two raphes can be present as remnants of a commissure. The cusps can be dysplastic.

The right ventricle is variable in size but is usually small in ~50% of cases, moderately hypoplastic in 25%, and normal in only 10–15% of cases. The right infundibulum is also hypoplastic, with a hypertrophic parietal wall and subvalvular stenosis. The tricuspid valve is underdeveloped and dysplastic, with a small tricuspid annulus and short chordae. In some cases, the septo-marginal trabeculation can be prominent, producing a bipartitioned right ventricle. Sinusoidal communications between the right ventricle and the coronary arteries may develop as a mechanism of decompression of blood/pressure from the right ventricle. In some cases endocardial fibroelastosis can be detected in the right ventricle [50, 55].

The right atrium is usually enlarged and hypertrophied, and the foramen ovale is usually patent. The arterial duct is not as hypoplastic as one would expect since it is essential for ensuring adequate pulmonary arterial blood flow. The pulmonary arteries are usually normal in size, and only in about 10% of the cases they may be hypoplastic.

Associated anomalies can be summarised as: hypoplastic tricuspid valve (60%), atrial septal defect (40%), patent foramen ovale (60%) and dysplastic tricuspid valve (30%), Fibroelastosis of the right ventricle (30%), Ebstein tricuspid valve (15%). Infrequently, there may be aortic valve dysplasia and supravalvular aortic stenosis that impacts on management [62–64].

References

1. Barlow A, Pawade A, Wilkinson JL, Anderson RH. Cardiac anatomy in patients undergoing the fontan procedure. Ann Thorac Surg. 1995;60(5):1324–30.
2. Jacobs ML, Anderson RH. Nomenclature of the functionally univentricular heart. Cardiol Young. 2006;16(Suppl. 1):3–8.
3. Guidelines for the Management of Congenital Heart Diseases in childhood and adolescence. Cardiol Young. 2017;27(S3):S1–S105.
4. Franklin RCG, et al. Nomenclature for congenital and paediatric cardiac disease: the international Paediatric and congenital cardiac code (IPCCC) and the eleventh iteration of the international classification of diseases (ICD-11). Cardiol Young. 2017;27(10):1872–938.
5. van Praagh R, David I, Wright GB, van Praagh S. Large RV plus small LV is not single RV. Circulation. 1980;61, no. 5. Circulation:1057–9.
6. Anderson RH, Cook AC. Morphology of the functionally univentricular heart. Cardiol Young. 2004;14(S1):3–12.
7. Cook AC, Anderson RH. The functionally univentricular circulation: anatomic substrates as related to function. Cardiol Young. 2005;15(SUPPL. 3):7–16.
8. Van Praagh R, David I, Van Praagh S. What is a ventricle? - the single-ventricle trap. Pediatr Cardiol. 1982;2(1):79–84.
9. Anderson RH, Mohun TJ, Moorman AFM. What is a ventricle? Cardiol Young. 2011;21(SUPPL. 2):14–22.

10. Jacobs JP, Maruszewski B. Functionally Univentricular heart and the Fontan operation: lessons learned about patterns of practice and outcomes from the congenital heart surgery databases of the European Association for Cardio-Thoracic Surgery and the Society of Thoracic Surgeons. World J Pediatr Congenit Hear Surg. 2013;4(4):349–55.

11. James H. Moller, Julien I. E. Hoffman. Pediatric cardiovascular medicine. Google Libri.

12. Anderson RH, Ho SY. Sequential segmental analysis - description and categorization for the millennium. Cardiol Young. 1997;7(1):98–116.

13. Thiene G, Frescura C. Anatomical and pathophysiological classification of congenital heart disease. Cardiovasc Pathol. 2010;19(5):259–74.

14. Bellsham-Revell H, Masani N. Educational series in congenital heart disease: The sequential segmental approach to assessment. Echo Res Pract. 2019;6(1):R1–8.

15. Anderson RH, Wilkinson JL, Gerlis LM, Smith A, Becker AE. Atresia of the right atrioventricular orifice. Br Heart J. 1977;39(4):414–28.

16. Soto B, Bertranou EG, Bream PR, Souza A, Bargeron LM. Angiographic study of univentricular heart of right ventricular type. Circulation. 1979;60(6):1325–34.

17. Martinez RM, Anderson RH. Echo-morphological correlates in atrioventricular valvar atresia. Cardiol Young. 2006;16(Suppl. 1):27–34.

18. Alphonso N, et al. Guidelines for the management of neonates and infants with hypoplastic left heart syndrome: the European Association for Cardio-Thoracic Surgery (EACTS) and the Association for European Paediatric and Congenital Cardiology (AEPC) Hypoplastic left heart Sy. Eur J Cardiothorac Surg. 2020;58(3):416–99.

19. Tchervenkov CI, Jacobs ML, Tahta SA. Congenital heart surgery nomenclature and database project: Hypoplastic left heart syndrome. Ann Thorac Surg. 2000;69(4 Suppl):170–9.

20. Sharland G, Rollings S, Simpson J, Anderson D. Hypoplastic left-heart syndrome. Lancet. 2001;357(9257):722.

21. Elliott MJ. A European perspective on the management of hypoplastic left heart syndrome. Cardiol Young. 2004;14(Suppl 1):41–6.

22. Murtuza B, Elliott MJ. Changing attitudes to the management of hypoplastic left heart syndrome: a European perspective. Cardiol Young. 2011;21(SUPPL. 2):148–58.

23. Tchervenkov CI, et al. The nomenclature, definition and classification of hypoplastic left heart syndrome. Cardiol Young. 2006;16(4):339–68.

24. Barron DJ, Kilby MD, Davies B, Wright JG, Jones TJ, Brawn WJ. Hypoplastic left heart syndrome. Lancet. 2009;374(9689):551–64.

25. Karamlou T, Diggs BS, Ungerleider RM, Welke KF. Evolution of treatment options and outcomes for hypoplastic left heart syndrome over an 18-year period. J Thorac Cardiovasc Surg. 2010;139(1):119–27.

26. Angelini A, Fedrigo M, Frescura C, Thiene G. Fetal anatomy: The interatrial septum in the fetus with congenital heart disease. In: Butera G, Cheatham J, Pedra C, Schranz D, Tulzer G, editors. Fetal and hybrid procedures in congenital heart diseases. Cham: Springer; 2016. p. 111–5.

27. Roeleveld PP, et al. Hypoplastic left heart syndrome: from fetus to fontan. Cardiol Young. 2018;28:1275–88.

28. Crucean A, et al. Re-evaluation of hypoplastic left heart syndrome from a developmental and morphological perspective. Orphanet J Rare Dis. 2017;12(1):138.

29. Thiene G, Daliento L, Frescura C, De Tommasi M, Macartney FJ, Anderson RH. Atresia of left atrioventricular orifice. Anatomical investigation in 62 cases. Br Heart J. 1981;45(4):393–401.

30. Rajendra T, Becker AE, Moller JH, Edwards JE. Double inlet left ventricle straddling tricuspid valve. Heart. 1974;36(8):747–59.

31. de la Cruz MV, Miller BL. Double-inlet left ventricle. Circulation. 1968;37(2):249–60.

32. Frescura C, Thiene G. The new concept of Univentricular heart. Front Pediatr. 2014;2:62.

33. Keeton BR, et al. Univentricular heart of right ventricular type with double or common inlet. Circulation. 1979;59(2):403–11.

34. Anderson RH, Wilcox BR. The surgical anatomy of ventricular septal defect. J Card Surg. 1992;7(1):17–35.

35. Dobell ARC, Van Praagh R. The Holmes heart: historic associations and pathologic anatomy. Am Heart J. 1996;132(2 Pt 1):437–45.

36. Anderson RH, Anderson C, Zuberbuhler JR. Further morphologic studies on hearts with pulmonary atresia and intact ventricular septum. Cardiol Young. 1991;1(2):105–13.

37. Jost CHA, Connolly HM, Dearani JA, Edwards WD, Danielson GK. Ebstein's anomaly. Circulation. 2007;115(2):277–85.

38. Holst KA, et al. Surgical management and outcomes of Ebstein anomaly in neonates and infants: a Society of Thoracic Surgeons congenital heart surgery database analysis. Ann Thorac Surg. 2018;106(3):785–91.

39. Angelini A, et al. Autopsy in adults with congenital heart disease (ACHD). Virchows Arch. 2020;476(6):797–820.

40. Cohen MS, Jacobs ML, Weinberg PM, Rychik J. Morphometric analysis of unbalanced common atrioventricular canal using two-dimensional echocardiography. J Am Coll Cardiol. 1996;28(4):1017–23.

41. Jegatheeswaran A, et al. Echocardiographic definition and surgical decision-making in unbalanced atrioventricular septal defect: a congenital heart surgeons' society multiinstitutional study. Circulation. 2010;122(11 SUPPL):1.

42. Cohen MS, et al. Echocardiographic features defining right dominant unbalanced atrioventricular septal defect: a multi-institutional congenital heart surgeons' society study. Circ Cardiovasc Imaging. 2013;6(4):508–13.

43. Meza JM, et al. The congenital heart Surgeon's society complete atrioventricular septal defect cohort: baseline, Preintervention echocardiographic characteristics. Semin Thorac Cardiovasc Surg. 2019;31(1):80–6.

44. Calkoen EE, et al. Atrioventricular septal defect: from embryonic development to long-term follow-up. Int J Cardiol. 2016;202:784–95.

45. Overman DM, et al. Unbalanced atrioventricular septal defect: definition and decision making. World J Pediatr Congenit Hear Surg. 2010;1(1):91–6.

46. Mahle WT, Silverman NH, Marx GR, Anderson RH. Echo-morphological correlates concerning the functionally univentricular heart in the setting of isomeric atrial appendages. Cardiol Young. 2006;16(SUPPL. 1):35–42.

47. Schidlow DN, Tworetzky W, Wilkins-Haug LE. Percutaneous fetal cardiac interventions for structural heart disease. Am J Perinatol. 2014;31(7):629–36.

48. Van Aerschot I, Rosenblatt J, Boudjemline Y. Fetal cardiac interventions: Myths and facts. Arch Cardiovasc Dis. 2012;105(6–7):366–72.

49. Gardiner HM, et al. Morphologic and functional predictors of eventual circulation in the fetus with pulmonary atresia or critical pulmonary stenosis with intact septum. J Am Coll Cardiol. 2008;51(13):1299–308.

50. Guleserian KJ, Armsby LB, Thiagarajan RR, del Nido PJ, Mayer JE. Natural history of pulmonary atresia with intact ventricular septum and right-ventricle-dependent coronary circulation managed by the single-ventricle approach. Ann Thorac Surg. 2006;81(6):2250–8.

51. Gittenberger-deGroot A C, Tennsted C, Chaoui R, Lie-Venema H, Sauer U, Poelmann R E. Ventriculo coronary arterial communications (VCAC) and myocardial sinusoids in hearts with pulmonary atresia with intact ventricular septum:two different diseases. Progress in Pediatric Cardiology 2001;13(3): 157–64.

52. Freedom RM, Wilson G, Trusler GA, Williams WG, Rowe RD. Pulmonary atresia and intact ventricular septum: a review of the anatomy, myocardium, and factors influencing right ventricular growth and guidelines for surgical intervention. Scand Cardiovasc J. 1983;17(1):1–28.

53. Anderson RH, Spicer D. Fistulous communications with the coronary arteries in the setting of hypoplastic ventricles. Cardiol Young. 2010;20(Suppl 3):86–91.

54. Lewis AB, et al. Right ventricular growth potential in neonates with pulmonary atresia and intact ventricular septum. J Thorac Cardiovasc Surg. 1986;91(6):835–40.

55. Angelini A, Fedrigo M, Frescura C, Thiene G. Fetal anatomy: the pulmonary valve in fetal pulmonary valve disease. Springer; 2016.

56. Yoshimura N, et al. Pulmonary atresia with intact ventricular septum: strategy based on right ventricular morphology. J Thorac Cardiovasc Surg. 2003;126(5):1417–26.

57. Salvin JW, et al. Fetal tricuspid valve size and growth as predictors of outcome in pulmonary atresia with intact ventricular septum. Pediatrics. 2006;118(2):e415–20.

58. Yuan S-M. Fetal cardiac interventions: an update of therapeutic options. Rev Bras Cir Cardiovasc. 2014;29(3):388–95; Accessed 20 Sep 2020 from https://www.ncbi.nlm.nih.gov/pmc/articles/PMC4412330/.

59. Hawkins JA, et al. Early and late results in pulmonary atresia and intact ventricular septum. J Thorac Cardiovasc Surg. 1990;100(4):492–7; Accessed 20 Sep 2020 from https://pubmed.ncbi.nlm.nih.gov/1699087/.

60. Daubeney PEF, et al. Pulmonary atresia with intact ventricular septum: predictors of early and medium-term outcome in a population-based study. J Thorac Cardiovasc Surg. 2005;130(4):1071.e1–9.

61. Kipps AK, Powell AJ, Levine JC. Muscular infundibular atresia is associated with coronary ostial atresia in pulmonary atresia with intact ventricular septum. Congenit Heart Dis. 2011;6(5):444–50.

62. Liava'a M, Brooks P, Konstantinov I, Brizard C, D'Udekem Y. Changing trends in the management of pulmonary atresia with intact ventricular septum: the Melbourne experience. Eur J Cardiothorac Surg. 2011;40(6):1406–11.

63. Wright L, Kochilas L, Knight J, Thomas A. Long-term outcomes after intervention for pulmonary atresia with intact ventricular septum: a study from the pediatric cardiac care consortium. J Am Coll Cardiol. 2018;71(11):A2675.

64. LaPar DJ, Bacha E. Pulmonary atresia with intact ventricular septum with borderline tricuspid valve: how small is too small. Semin Thorac Cardiovasc Surg Pediatr Card Surg Annu. 2019;22:27–31.

Epidemiology of Univentricular Hearts

3

Andrew Constantine and Paul Clift

Abbreviations

CHD   Congenital heart disease
HLHS Hypoplastic left heart syndrome
UVH   Univentricular heart

Patients with a univentricular heart (UVH) represent 5–10% of all congenital heart disease (CHD), with a male preponderance of 1.2 to 2:1 depending on the underlying anatomy [1–3]. The overall prevalence of UVH in Quebec, Canada in 2010 was 0.24 per 1000 children [4]. Hypoplastic left heart syndrome (HLHS) represents the most common underlying anatomy, followed by tricuspid atresia, double inlet left ventricle and pulmonary atresia with an intact interventricular septum (Table 3.1). Reporting the epidemiology of functionally univentricular hearts (UVH) must account for group heterogeneity, the lack of a uniform nomenclature and the limitations and

Table 3.1 Major types of functionally univentricular heart

Diagnostic category (% of total[a])
Hypoplastic left heart syndrome (38)
Tricuspid atresia (15)
Double-inlet left ventricle (14)
Pulmonary atresia with intact IVS (10)
Other UVH (22)

[a]Data from the Danish Register of Congenital Heart Disease from 1977–2009 [3]. "Other UVH "includes UVH in association with mitral atresia, unbalanced atrio-ventricular canal defects, double outlet right ventricle, Ebstein anomaly, straddling atrio-ventricular valve, and other variants. IVS, inter-ventricular septum; UVH, uni-ventricular heart.

methodological inconsistencies of population-based studies (Table 3.2).

The most recent estimates of the overall annual incidence of UVH include terminations of pregnancy in fetuses with UVH; in Denmark, the mean annual incidence from 1977 to 2009 was 0.39 per 1000 cases with a four-fold reduction in the number of UVH live births from 0.34 to 0.08 per 1000 live births (Fig. 3.1) [3]. Earlier prenatal diagnosis and an increase in terminations of pregnancy have contributed to the reduction in live births. Nonetheless, the prevalence of UVH has continued to rise thanks to improvements in the survival of children with UVH, which is influenced by multiple factors: widely available and more accurate prenatal screening, advances in fetal interventions, the development and refinement of surgical techniques (including the Fontan

A. Constantine
Adult Congenital Heart Centre and National Centre for Pulmonary Hypertension, Royal Brompton Hospital, London, UK

The National Heart and Lung Institute, Imperial College London, London, UK

P. Clift (✉)
Adult Congenital Heart Disease Unit, Queen Elizabeth Hospital, Birmingham, UK
e-mail: pclift@nhs.net

© The Author(s), under exclusive license to Springer Nature Switzerland AG 2023
P. Clift et al. (eds.), *Univentricular Congenital Heart Defects and the Fontan Circulation*,
https://doi.org/10.1007/978-3-031-36208-8_3

Table 3.2 Challenges faced in the accurate reporting of the epidemiology of functionally univentricular hearts

Heterogeneous population	UVH consists of a broad range of CHD, including valve atresia, double inlet ventricles, unbalanced atrio-ventricular septal defects, and other anatomical variants (see **Chaps. 1–5**)
Definition of UVH	Definitions centring around the inability to perform a biventricular repair are "intervention-centric", but capture the diversity of underlying morphologies included Current usage of the term UVH usually includes functionally univentricular circulations i.e. cardiac anatomies consisting of 4 chambers with 1 functionally adequate ventricle e.g. HLHS and PA-IVS.
Inconsistencies in reporting	CHD prevalence or incidence may be reported by lesion e.g. HLHS, complexity e.g. CHD of great complexity as per the 32nd Bethesda conference document [5], or by functional anatomy e.g. functionally univentricular heart
Incidence and birth prevalence	Birth prevalence (number of cases per 1000 live births) is often used in place of the incidence (rate of new cases e.g. per annum, *in utero*)

CHD congenital heart disease, *HLHS* hypoplastic left heart syndrome, *PA-IVS* pulmonary atresia with intact inter-ventricular septum, *UVH* univentricular heart

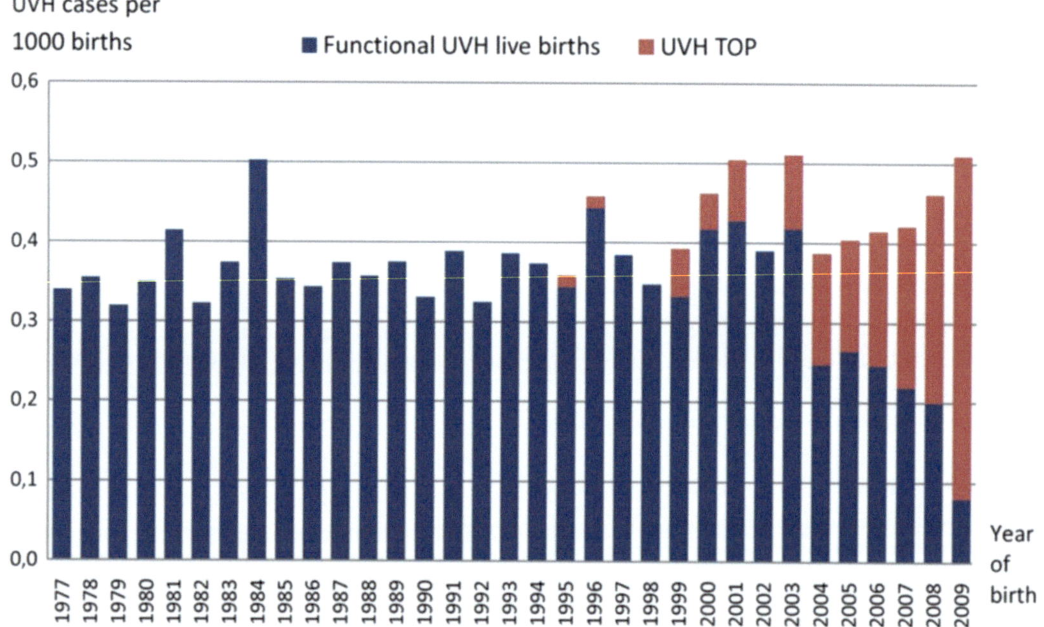

Fig. 3.1 Incidence of functional univentricular hearts (UVH) and termination of pregnancy due to a fetus with functional UVH (UVH TOP) by birth rate per year in Denmark from 1977 to 2009. (Reprinted from Idorn et al. [3] with permission from Elsevier)

and Norwood repairs), and better supportive medical and intensive care support. A recent German national registry study of 15,703 CHD patients between 1996 and 2015 found that UVH was the fourth most common diagnosis, with an overall increase in the proportion of complex CHD since 2008 [6]. Even in HLHS, the UVH group with the worst survival rate, survival with HLHS has improved from 3% at 1 year in the 1970's [7] to 39% at 3-years due to the innovations of the Norwood Procedure [3].

UVH still carries significant morbidity and mortality, explaining the lower overall prevalence in adult compared to paediatric CHD cohorts. Nonetheless, the prevalence of adults with UVH is increasing in developed countries, estimated at 0.08 per 1000 patients in 2010, and accounts for 1.3% of adults with CHD [4]. Patients with more complex defects, such as HLHS and heterotaxy syndromes, are deriving the greatest benefit from modern surgical techniques, and many of these patients are now reaching adulthood but are at greater risk of late adverse events and early mortality compared to other forms of UVH [8, 9]. Overall, CHD practitioners face an expanding, ageing and more complex CHD population, including UVH survivors who pose major challenges in terms of management and resource allocation. Understanding the contribution of genetics, and the interplay of genes and environmental factors in the development of UVH, will allow better characterisation of this relatively new population and will form the basis for the personalised medicine of the coming decades.

References

1. Sittiwangkul R, Azakie A, Arsdell GSV, Williams WG, McCrindle BW. Outcomes of tricuspid atresia in the Fontan era. Ann Thorac Surg. 2004;77(3):889–94.
2. Hansen JH, Petko C, Bauer G, Voges I, Kramer H-H, Scheewe J. Fifteen-year single-center experience with the Norwood operation for complex lesions with single-ventricle physiology compared with hypoplastic left heart syndrome. J Thorac Cardiovasc Surg. 2012;144(1):166–72.
3. Idorn L, Olsen M, Jensen AS, Juul K, Reimers JI, Sørensen K, et al. Univentricular hearts in Denmark 1977 to 2009: incidence and survival. Int J Cardiol. 2013;167(4):1311–6.
4. Marelli AJ, Raluca I-I, Mackie AS, Liming G, Nandini D, Mohammed K. Lifetime prevalence of congenital heart disease in the general population from 2000 to 2010. Circulation. 2014;130(9):749–56.
5. Webb GD, Williams RG. 32nd Bethesda conference: "care of the adult with congenital heart disease". J Am Coll Cardiol. 2001;37(5):1162–5.
6. Pfitzer C, Helm PC, Ferentzi H, Rosenthal L-M, Bauer UMM, Berger F, et al. Changing prevalence of severe congenital heart disease: results from the National Register for congenital heart defects in Germany. Congenit Heart Dis. 2017;12(6):787–93.
7. Fyler DC. Report of the New England regional infant cardiac program. Pediatrics. 1980;65(2):377–461.
8. Iyengar AJ, Winlaw DS, Galati JC, Wheaton GR, Gentles TL, Grigg LE, et al. The extracardiac conduit Fontan procedure in Australia and New Zealand: hypoplastic left heart syndrome predicts worse early and late outcomes. Eur J Cardiothorac Surg. 2014;46(3):465–73; discussion 473.
9. Ohuchi H, Negishi J, Noritake K, Hayama Y, Sakaguchi H, Miyazaki A, et al. Prognostic value of exercise variables in 335 patients after the Fontan operation: a 23-year single-center experience of cardiopulmonary exercise testing. Congenit Heart Dis. 2015;10(2):105–16.

Part II

Management of the Fetus and Neonate with a Univentricular Heart

Prenatal Diagnosis of the Functionally Univentricular Heart

4

Anna Seale and Lindsey Hunter

Introduction

First trimester screening ultrasound scans are performed in early pregnancy, between 11 and 13 weeks, to confirm the presence of a fetal heartbeat, identify multiple pregnancies and estimate the date of delivery. They also aid screening for chromosomal and cardiac anomalies by measuring the nuchal translucency (NT), i.e. the ultrasound appearance of the fluid filled space at the back of the fetal neck. An increased NT can be associated with genetic abnormalities and/or congenital heart disease (CHD) [1]. In centres with expertise, fetuses with an increased NT are offered an early fetal echocardiogram to assess the cardiac structures in detail.

Technological advances have improved the ability to detect CHD earlier in gestation, either by a transabdominal or transvaginal approach, however this is still technically challenging due to fetal movement and reduced image resolution. Therefore, first trimester fetal echocardiography is reserved for women considered "high risk" of having a baby with CHD, e.g. fetuses with increased NT or a strong family history of CHD. Despite the above challenges, single ventricle hearts are the lesions most commonly detected in early pregnancy, seen as an "abnormal four chamber view".

Prenatal cardiac screening was introduced in the mid-1980's when a French group proposed that the four-chamber view of the heart should be incorporated into the routine obstetric scan between 18 and 22 weeks of gestation (second trimester). Since that time, second trimester screening programmes have progressed and now incorporate views to assess the outflow tracts and blood vessels in the upper mediastinum [2]. Currently, in the United Kingdom, 50% of all major CHD is diagnosed prenatally, with 80% of hypoplastic left heart syndrome (HLHS) cases receiving a prenatal diagnosis. Lesions that can be detected as abnormalities of the four chamber view are, indeed, the most common defects diagnosed prenatally: in the normal heart, the right and left heart chambers are balanced in size, therefore significant ventricular disproportion is relatively easy to detect on fetal scans (Fig. 4.1).

There are limitations to prenatal screening, particularly a raised maternal body mass index, anterior placenta, reduced liquor volume, difficult fetal position or multiple fetuses (e.g. twin pregnancy). The optimal time for assessment of the fetal heart is, usually, between 18 and 28 weeks of gestation, when the ventricles are generally "balanced". As gestation progresses into the third trimester, right

A. Seale (✉)
Department of Paediatric Cardiology, Birmingham Children's Hospital, Birmingham, UK
e-mail: annaseale@nhs.net

L. Hunter
Department of Paediatric Cardiology, Royal Hospital for Children, Glasgow, UK
e-mail: Lindsey.Hunter@ggc.scot.nhs.uk

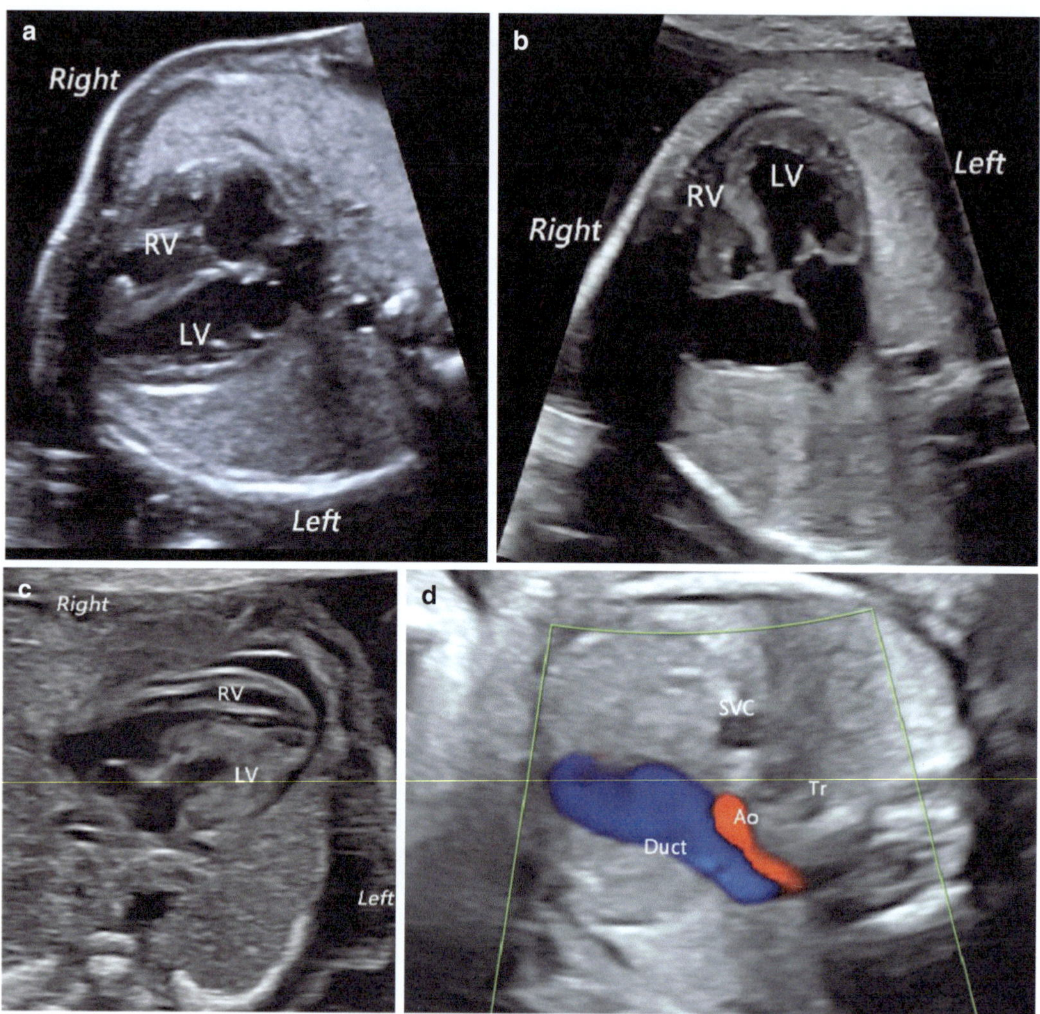

Fig. 4.1 (**a**) Normal four chamber view at second trimester screening; (**b**) small unipartite right ventricle in pulmonary atresia intact ventricular septum; (**c**) hypoplastic left heart syndrome, 4 chamber view and the three vessel tracheal view (**d**) showing retrograde flow in a small aortic arch. *LV* left ventricle, *RV* right ventricle, *Ao* Aorta, *Tr* Trachea, *SVC* Superior vena cava

heart dominance is the normal physiological feature, making assessment of the heart in the latter stages of pregnancy more challenging. In addition, the third trimester scans may suffer from limited echocardiographic windows, while some cases of CHD may be progressive in later gestation.

Prenatal Assessment

When congenital heart disease (CHD) is suspected during the screening scan, referral is made to a fetal cardiologist for assessment and a defini-tive diagnosis. The fetal cardiologist undertakes a detailed fetal echocardiogram to ascertain the exact morphology of the heart in a bid to determine potential management plans and the longer term prognosis. In a fetus diagnosed with a uni-ventricular heart, features identified prenatally that are known to reduce the likelihood of a well-functioning Fontan circulation, include: heart block; abnormal systemic venous return (left atrial isomerism); atrioventricular valve regurgitation; hypoplastic pulmonary arteries ± multiple aorto-pulmonary collaterals; risk of high pulmonary artery pressure (restrictive atrial septum in

HLHS); poor ventricular function/hydrops and genetic abnormalities.

In addition to the cardiologist, it is vital that the fetus is thoroughly assessed by a fetal medicine specialist, to identify extra-cardiac or genetic/chromosomal abnormalities. Babies with a single ventricle circulation can have associated genetic or chromosomal abnormalities, which can profoundly affect their prognosis, for example Turner's syndrome [3], trisomy 18 or 13. The exact risk depends upon the morphological subtype of the univentricular CHD. Therefore women are offered invasive genetic testing by amniocentesis or chorionic villous sampling, if CHD is detected. These procedures carry a small risk, approximately 1%, of miscarriage or premature delivery. Detail of extra-cardiac and genetic abnormalities will therefore guide the counselling (see below).

Morphological Subtypes

HLHS and Variants

During the fetal scan, it is possible to differentiate between different types of classical HLHS (aortic atresia/ mitral atresia; aortic atresia/ mitral stenosis; aortic stenosis/mitral stenosis) as well as HLHS variants, e.g. unbalanced atrioventricular septal defects (AVSD), or double outlet right ventricle with left ventricular hypoplasia. This morphological detail is important for counselling, as some anatomical subtypes have a poorer prognosis, such as the unbalanced AVSD [4].

Critical Aortic Stenosis

Although sometimes a challenging diagnosis, critical aortic stenosis (AS) can be detected at 18–22 weeks gestation and some fetuses progress to HLHS by term. Critical AS often presents with a dilated left ventricle (LV); poor LV systolic function; a dysplastic aortic valve with limited antegrade flow and retrograde filling of the transverse arch via the arterial duct. In the presence of these morphological features, most of these fetuses will progress to anatomy akin to HLHS (aortic stenosis/mitral stenosis) by term (Fig. 4.2). Therefore to provide accurate counselling, the fetal cardiologist needs to "predict" which fetuses

will progress to HLHS and those who are likely to achieve a biventricular repair. Scoring systems, based on ultrasound findings, have been developed to help predict which fetuses presenting with critical aortic stenosis at the mid trimester scan, will indeed progress to HLHS. Risk factors for progression include: left to right flow at the level of the atrial septum; evidence of left ventricular dysfunction; retrograde filling of the transverse aortic arch, bidirectional flow in the pulmonary veins and a monophasic mitral valve inflow Doppler [5].

Further scoring systems, in the form of the threshold scoring system, are employed to identify those who may benefit from fetal intervention [6, 7]. The rationale for fetal intervention is that, relieving the obstruction to the left ventricular outflow will promote growth of the left heart structures and increase the chance of a biventricular repair after birth. Although technically feasible it is not clear whether intervention alters the natural history of the disease and the risk of miscarriage/early delivery is approximately 10%. Freud et al. presented the postnatal outcomes of 100 patients undergoing fetal aortic valvuloplasty: 43% ($n = 38$) of all live-born patients were managed with a biventricular circulation [8].

However, Gardiner et al. have challenged the scoring systems used to identify cases of evolving HLHS, showing that a substantial proportion of fetuses meeting the criteria for emerging HLHS had sustained a biventricular circulation without fetal intervention [9]. Although a biven-

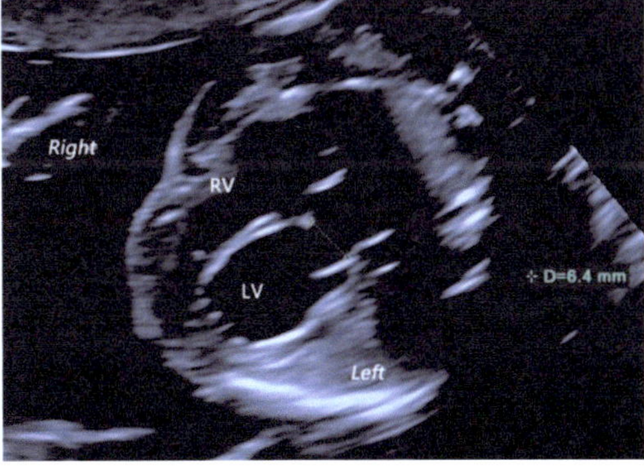

Fig. 4.2 Critical aortic stenosis at 20 weeks gestation, when diagnosed at this stage, the lesion usually progresses to hypoplastic left heart syndrome. In this case, pregnancy was discontinued. *LV* left ventricle, *RV* right ventricle

tricular repair may be achieved in a highly selected population with fetal critical aortic stenosis, many survivors have evidence of persistent diastolic dysfunction; pulmonary hypertension and right heart failure in teenage years [10]. Perhaps, intervention at 20 weeks of gestation is too late. Fetuses with evolving stenosis may be better candidates, but there is evidence that fetuses with critical aortic stenosis presenting in the third trimester are more likely to achieve a biventricular circulation in the absence of intervention [11]. Hence, the role of fetal intervention in this group is still debated.

Restrictive Atrial Septum

Up to 10% of fetuses with classical HLHS will have a restrictive atrial septum. These babies have a particularly poor prognosis and require urgent decompression of the left atrium after birth. Predicting atrial restriction allows for prenatal discussion and planning, ensuring the most appropriate and experienced personnel are present at delivery.

Prenatal pulmonary venous Doppler waveforms are assessed in a bid to demonstrate evidence of severe atrial restriction (Fig. 4.3). Echocardiographic indices of prenatal restriction include: absent diastolic forward flow, a 'to-and-fro' pattern in the pulmonary venous waveform; or ratio of the velocity time integrals of antegrade pulmonary venous flow against retrograde flow from the left atrium, 3:1 being the upper limit of normal [12, 13].

Although immediate intervention provides a short term solution for left atrial restriction, there is increasing evidence that prolonged exposure to left atrial hypertension in fetal life results in irreversible

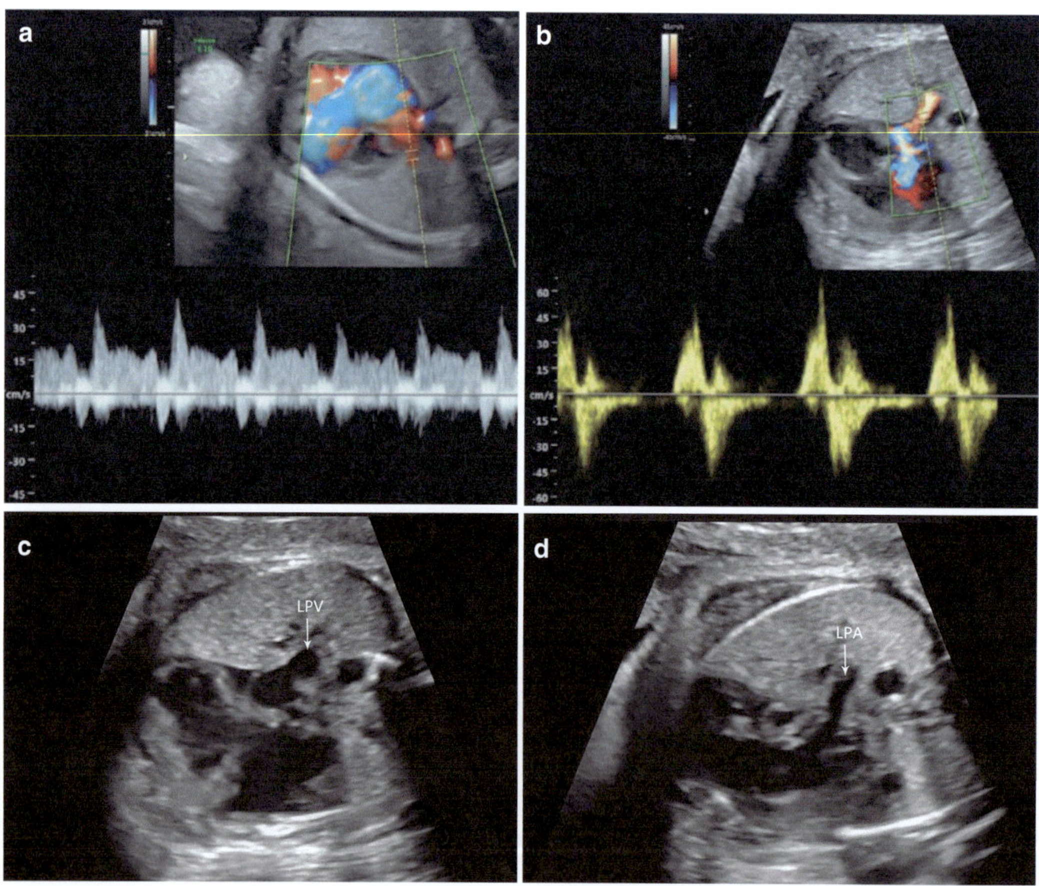

Fig. 4.3 Hypoplastic left heart syndrome—normal pulmonary venous Doppler wave forms (**a**) and abnormal waveform found when there is a restrictive atrial septum (**b**). The pulmonary veins in this case were dilated (**c**) and could be mistaken for branch pulmonary arteries (**d**). *LA* left atrium, *LPV* left pulmonary vein, *LPA* left pulmonary artery, *PV* pulmonary valve, *RA* right atrium, *RV* right ventricle

damage to the pulmonary microvasculature, evident on fetal MRI, the so-called "nutmeg lung" [14]. In the longer term, these microvasculature changes limit the success of the Fontan circulation. In-utero balloon septostomy and stenting has been described, [15, 16] however, stenting in the context of HLHS has not been proven to benefit long-term survival.

Other Morphological Features

Other important morphological features, which may influence the outcome of HLHS include:

- Pulmonary venous connections: anomalous venous connections are associated with poor outcome.
- Associated right heart anomalies: poor prognostic factors include tricuspid valve regurgitation, impaired right ventricular function, fetal hydrops and pulmonary valve anomalies. Table 4.1

Pulmonary Atresia with Intact Ventricular Septum

Unlike other univentricular lesions, pulmonary atresia with intact ventricular septum (PA/IVS) is rarely associated with genetic or chromosomal abnormalities.

Like most forms of CHD, PA/IVS has a morphological spectrum. At the milder end of the spectrum fetuses present with a well-proportioned, tripartite right ventricular cavity which is amenable to a biventricular circulation. Conversely a presentation with a diminutive, monopartite right ventricle will undeniably follow a univentricular pathway (Fig. 4.1b).

It is well recognised that progression can occur in utero, for example at 20 weeks of gestation there may pulmonary stenosis with a relatively well developed right ventricle, but progression during pregnancy results in pulmonary valve atresia with associated ventricular hypertrophy and in some cases a biventricular circulation is unachievable. It is, therefore, the role of the fetal cardiologist to monitor and, if possible, predict which patients are at risk of progression. Lowenthal et al. [17] suggest that a fetal tricuspid valve:mitral valve ratio greater than 0.63 predicted favourable tricuspid valve size (z-score) at birth; antegrade pulmonary valve flow and more than moderate tricuspid valve regurgitation conferred a favourable outcome postnatally. In addition, Cao et al. [18] found that a tricuspid valve z-score $> = -3$ was associated with a 2-ventricle postnatal strategy.

PA/IVS can be associated with fistulae communicating between the right ventricle and coronary arteries. Colour flow Doppler is a useful prenatal modality to detect such communications. Furthermore fetuses with fistulae are at risk of developing coronary artery stenoses, which is a poor prognostic factor. Although stenoses are undetectable prenatally, the presence of fistulae alone increases the likelihood of a univentricular pathway. [18] Table 4.2.

Table 4.1 Prenatal risk factors in hypoplastic left heart syndrome

Prenatal risk factors for poor outcome in hypoplastic left heart syndrome
• Restrictive atrial septum
• Tricuspid valve regurgitation
• Right ventricular dysfunction
• Fetal hydrops
• Pulmonary valve anomaly
• Small ascending aorta (<2mm), aortic atresia
• Total anomalous pulmonary venous connection
• For "hypoplastic left heart variants": unbalanced AVSD; complete heart block (isomerism), small/discontinuous branch pulmonary arteries/ multiple aorto-pulmonary collateral arteries.
• Genetic abnormalities and extra-cardiac problems

Table 4.2 Prenatal risk factors in pulmonary atresia/critical pulmonary stenosis with intact ventricular septum

Prenatal risk factors for poor outcome in pulmonary atresia/ critical pulmonary stenosis with intact ventricular septum
• Small tricuspid valve annulus (z score <3)
• Absence of forward flow across the pulmonary valve
• Unipartite ventricle
• Coronary fistulae
• Low-velocity tricuspid valve regurgitation (failing right ventricle)
• Severe Ebstein malformation with severe tricuspid valve regurgitation
• Fetal Hydrops
• Small/discontinuous branch pulmonary arteries/ multiple aorto-pulmonary collateral arteries (rare)
• Genetic abnormalities and extra-cardiac problems

In the presence of critical pulmonary stenosis, prenatal intervention in the form of pulmonary valvuloplasty has been performed in selected centres, [19] but this approach remains controversial and has not been universally adopted.

Tricuspid Atresia and Double Inlet Left Ventricle

Tricuspid Atresia

Tricuspid atresia exists when the tricuspid valve is either absent or imperforate. It can be associated with either concordant or discordant ventricular-arterial connections (Fig. 4.4). There can be associated pulmonary stenosis and, in the presence of concordant ventricular-arterial connections, subpulmonary stenosis at the level of the ventricular septal defect (VSD). There can be associated aortic coarctation in the presence of discordant ventricular-arterial connection.

Progression of pulmonary or sub-pulmonary valve stenosis may occur during pregnancy, therefore, serial assessments are made by the fetal cardiologist to formulate an appropriate postnatal management plan, for example, the need for prostaglandin E infusion. The need and timing of postnatal intervention, to augment or restrict pulmonary blood flow, depends on the morphology of the pulmonary valve and VSD.

In tricuspid atresia, the right ventricle is typically hypoplastic, and a positive outcome is reliant upon a morphologically normal and well-functioning left ventricle. Poor prognostic factors (that are rare) include mitral valve regurgitation, impaired left ventricular function and fetal hydrops.

No acute intervention is required postnatally in babies with a balanced circulation, who will progress to a cavo-pulmonary anastomosis at a few months of age. In some cases an atrial septostomy is required to ensure that blood flows unrestricted from the right to left atrium.

Double Inlet Left Ventricle

Double inlet left ventricle (DILV) exists when two atrioventricular valves open into a morphological left ventricle. The hypoplastic morphological right ventricle may be either to the left or right (Fig. 4.5). Like tricuspid atresia, DILV can be associated with concordant or discordant ventricular-arterial connections. In the presence of discordant ventricular-arterial connection, the communication between the right and left ventricles can become restrictive and this is frequently associated with coarctation of the aorta.

Pulmonary stenosis can occur in the presence of either concordant or discordant VA connections, but is more prevalent in concordant VA

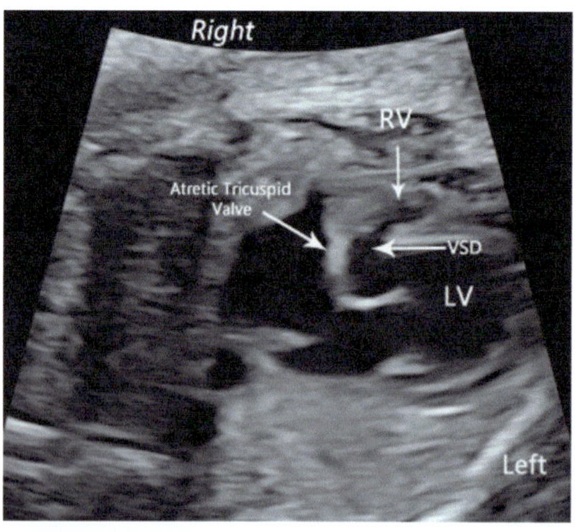

Fig. 4.4 Four chamber view of tricuspid atresia in the second trimester. *LV* left ventricle, *RV* right ventricle, *MV* mitral valve

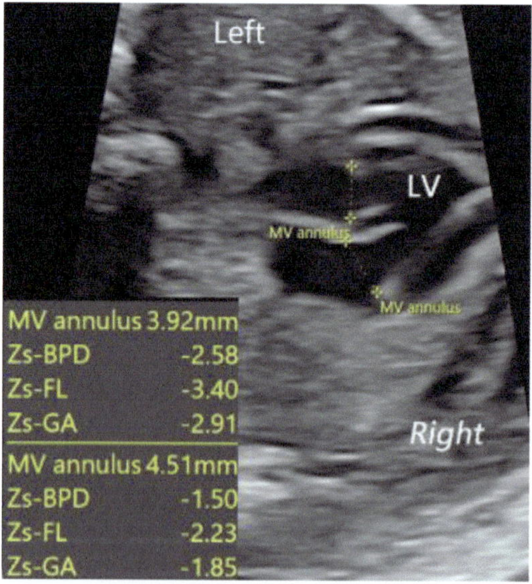

Fig. 4.5 Four chamber view of double inlet left ventricle in the second trimester. *LV* left ventricle

connections. Some fetuses have no obstruction to either outlet and, in this situation, a pulmonary artery (PA) band may be required within the first few weeks of life, as the pulmonary vascular resistance drops, to prevent pulmonary over circulation and the development of pulmonary vascular disease.

Some fetuses with DILV present with a stenotic atrioventricular valve and a balloon atrial septostomy may be required. Furthermore the development of in utero complete heart block is a risk and a poor prognostic factor.

Individualised Management Plan

The heterogeneity in both tricuspid atresia and DILV requires a bespoke management plan and will alter the timing and intervention required in each case. There can be progression in the degree of pulmonary stenosis or VSD narrowing throughout pregnancy, so serial assessments are required to formulate an appropriate postnatal management plan. Positively, in some cases, the neonatal circulation is well balanced and no acute intervention is required, indeed some patients with DILV can have a balanced circulation into adult life.

Isomerism of the Right and Left Atrial Appendages

Isomerism (heterotaxy) is frequently associated with complex congenital cardiac lesions including a functionally univentricular heart, AVSD, outflow tract obstruction and systemic and pulmonary venous malformations (Figs. 4.6 and 4.7). There may be mesocardia or dextrocardia, as well as laterality abnormalities of the abdominal organs. The fetal cardiologist needs to complete a sequential segmental analysis of the cardiac structures. However, it is often very challenging to delineate anomalous and obstructed pulmonary veins (Fig. 4.6), or non-confluent branch pulmonary arteries in the fetus, both of which are poor prognostic markers in the presence of right atrial isomerism.

Isomerism of the left atrial appendages (left atrial isomerism) can be associated with polysplenia, malrotation of the gut, and biliary atresia. Right atrial isomerism is associated with asplenia and, therefore, immune dysfunction. Careful assessment of the extra-cardiac structures of the fetus is, thus, imperative. However the aforementioned abnormalities cannot be detected by prenatal ultrasound and it is important to emphasise the potential effects of such abnormalities on prognosis during parental counselling.

Most fetuses with a univentricular heart survive to birth, however fetuses with left atrial isomerism are at risk of in-utero demise [20]. This is likely due to the development of complete heart block (CHB), myocardial dysfunction and fetal hydrops. Those fetuses who develop CHB are at risk of developing a spongiform, non-

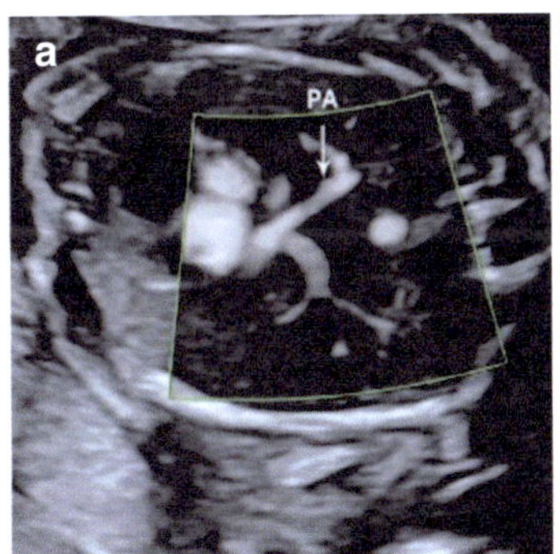
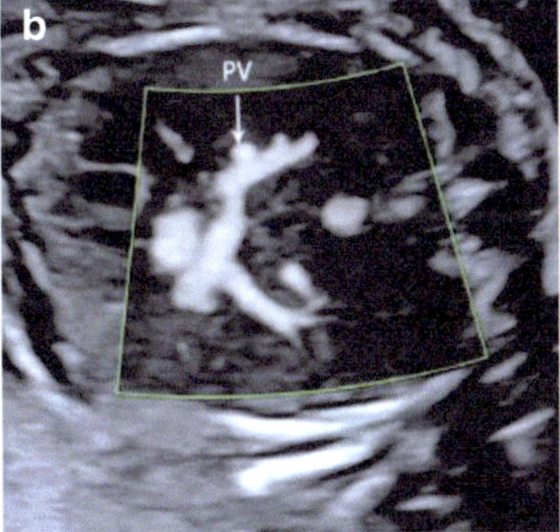
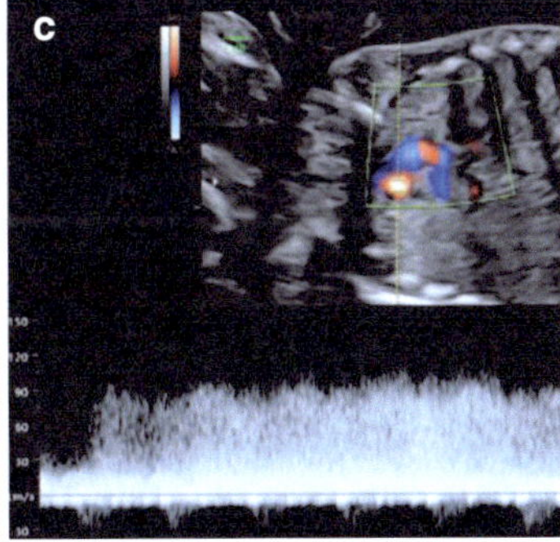

Fig. 4.6 The pulmonary arteries (**a**) and pulmonary veins (**b**) in a case of right atrial isomerism with unbalanced atrioventricular septal defect and pulmonary atresia in the second trimester. The pulmonary veins form a confluence which is connected to the superior vena cava, the connection is obstructed (**c**), resulting in a continuous pulmonary venous Doppler trace. *PA* pulmonary arteries, *PV* pulmonary venous confluence

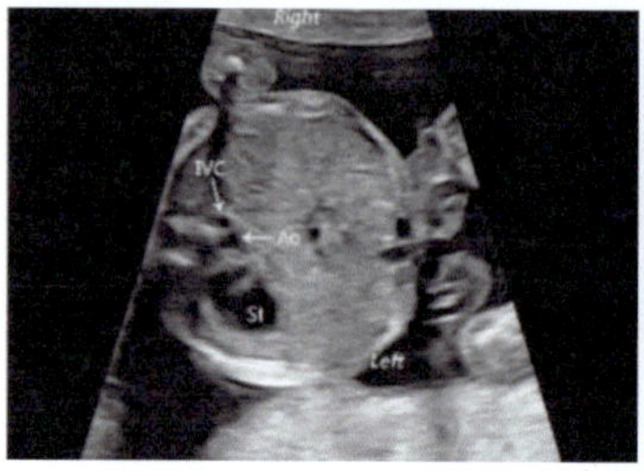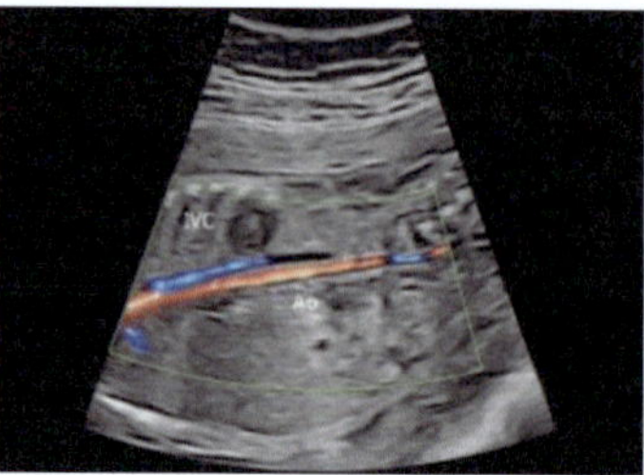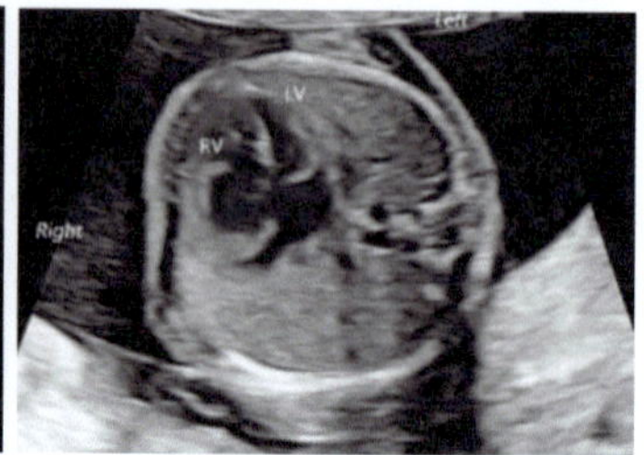

Fig. 4.7 A fetus with left atrial isomerism and an unbalanced atrioventricular septal defect. Situs view shows the IVC posterior to the aorta (**a**), the sagittal view shows the aorta and IVC running in parallel (**b**), four chamber view shows absence of the atrial septum (common atrium), a small left ventricle and loss of off-setting of the atrioventricular valves (**c**). *Ao* aorta, *IVC* inferior vena cava, *LV* left ventricle, *RV* right ventricle, *St* stomach.

compacted appearance of the ventricles, and appear to do particularly poorly after birth, even if the only intervention required is ventricular pacing [21].

When Septation of the Heart and a Biventricular Circulation cannot be achieved

Some patients with adequately-sized right and left ventricles may follow the univentricular pathway postnatally, as the surgeon is unable to perform a satisfactory biventricular repair (e.g. in double outlet right ventricle (DORV) with a non-committed VSD). It can be particularly difficult to identify these fetuses prenatally with certainty, but serial echocardiography can help in the assessment. Management decisions are often difficult even after birth, and a final management plan may not be achieved until the child is bigger. It is important to discuss this uncertainty with the parents.

Effect of Prenatal Diagnosis on Outcome

Some studies have suggested that a prenatal diagnosis of a univentricular circulation does not impact upon the long term outcome. [22, 23] Individuals have argued that patients with a prenatal diagnosis have more complex cardiac lesions and extra-cardiac anomalies, but this has not been reported in larger prenatal series [24, 25]. Prenatal published data tends to group all univentricular morphologies together [24–26]. Tworetzky et al. reported that a postnatal HLHS diagnosis was the only risk factor for early mortality and the prenatally diagnosed patients were likely to have reduced pre-operative morbidity [27]. This has been supported by other groups, [22, 25] and, importantly, there is emerging evidence that prenatally diagnosed patients have a lower propensity to pre-operative brain injury [28].

Prenatal diagnosis does provide the parents with the option of discontinuing pregnancy. Rates of termination vary depending upon cultural beliefs and other demographic factors. Birmingham, UK, reported that the termination rate in the 1990's for HLHS was 44% [29], but this dropped to 25% in the early part of the twenty-first century - likely due to improved surgical results [30]. In Sweden, Ohman et al. recently reported that, since prenatal diagnosis and surgery were introduced in 1993, there has been a decline in live births of HLHS (rate of termination of pregnancy 56%, 2001–2010). However, of those born, the vast majority undergo surgical intervention [31].

When assessing the longer term outcome of HLHS, it has been suggested that a prenatal diagnosis may be associated with poorer outcome [32]. This reflects the Birmingham experience; which hypothesizes that the prenatal group has a higher rate of co-morbidities; premature spontaneous deliveries and a higher number with aortic atresia. Lui et al. have reported their outcome to Fontan completion in the prenatally diagnosed group: when including all morphological sub-

Table 4.3 Benefits of prenatal diagnosis

Advantages of prenatal diagnosis of a functionally univentricular heart
• Allows time for parental choice : active management; comfort care or TOP
• Opportunity for genetic testing and assessment of extra-cardiac problems
• Guides counselling in the presence of poor prognostic factors
• Enables parents and families to receive psychological support
• Gives opportunity for parental psychological interventions
• Plan timing and place of delivery, with appropriate personnel in attendance
• Allows immediate initiation of prostaglandin E; emergency BAS or pacing
• Is associated with lower pre-operative morbidity and neurological injury

BAS balloon atrial septostomy, *TOP* termination of pregnancy

types ($n = 502$), 67% survived at least 6 months post-Fontan completion [26]. The prenatal multivariable risk factors for death included fetal hydrops, right ventricular dominance and extra-cardiac abnormalities. Table 4.3.

Counselling

Prenatal diagnosis allows for bespoke, informative prenatal counselling, parental choice and engagement with the multi-disciplinary team (MDT): fetal and maternal medicine specialists; midwives; cardiac nurse specialists; neonatologists and geneticists. Involvement of the MDT ensures accurate and early identification of additional extra-cardiac and genetic abnormalities, which will tailor the prenatal counselling and inform the delivery and postnatal management plan.

Explaining complex cardiac anatomy can be difficult and should be presented appropriately, while ensuring the important messages are communicated. Counselling must cover the following aspects:

1. The cardiac lesion, using diagrams and models where possible
2. Additional extra-cardiac anomalies
3. Uncertainties about the scan/ assessment
4. Association of cardiac abnormalities and genetic/ chromosomal abnormalities.; where appropriate, invasive or non-invasive prenatal testing (NIPT) should be offered and the risk/ benefits discussed. Association with neurodevelopmental differences.
5. Potential cardiac interventions and surgery involved in the univentricular pathway
6. The natural history of the disease and the option of a comfort care pathway, when appropriate
7. The option of termination of pregnancy.

These are life-changing and distressing discussions for parents. Compassion and empathy is required, as the family takes time to consider their options. Assimilating complex information during one meeting is often not possible, and follow-up meetings and ongoing support from specialist cardiac nursing teams and midwifes are crucial. Ideally, information should be given over several meetings to ensure all aspects are covered and understood; appropriate reading material, sign-posting to parent support groups, and engagement with psychological support services should be offered.

In the current era, patients and parents often use social media as a source of information and support; it is important to advise caution. Views on social media may not represent established facts and figures in relation to outcomes, and health systems may vary around the world in their approach and management of CHD.

Initial counselling usually takes place at approximately 20 weeks of gestation. As this is a significant period of time before the baby reaches term, parents need to be aware of the risks of in-utero death, prematurity, small for gestational age baby and neonatal death, which may all occur before surgery can be performed. Quoting risks/ outcomes from postnatal series may be misleading, as they fail to take into account the aforementioned prenatal and pre-operative neonatal risks.

Risks associated with the proposed catheter or surgical procedures should be discussed, as well as longer-term outcomes and morbidity associated with a Fontan circulation. Ideally, centre-specific mortality and morbidity should be quoted. When discussing surgical interventions, it is important to include the potential length of hospital stay, which may be months in some situations; the need for frequent outpatient visits; home monitoring programmes; feeding difficulties, which include home naso-gastric feeding; and the longer term neurodevelopmental outcomes.

Finally, it is important to emphasise that not all babies that set out on the Fontan pathway reach Fontan completion. Some patients are not able to progress through the stages due to poor haemodynamics and/or ventricular function. Options of transplantation are often limited.

Families who decide upon a pathway of comfort care postnatally should meet with the neonatal and paediatric palliative care teams prenatally to ensure their expectations and wishes are met. In this situation, a decision to deliver closer to home with no or minimal fetal monitoring during labour may be appropriate. Excellent communication between the parents and medical/ midwife teams is essential to ensure this pathway meets the needs of the family, particularly as some babies can survive for weeks, months and even a few years without intervention, even with a duct-dependent circulation. Some families prefer their baby to be stabilised after delivery and assessed, before making a decision to proceed with surgical intervention or comfort care.

Prenatal Diagnosis and Neurodevelopmental Outcomes

It is increasingly evident that the neurodevelopment prognosis for children with CHD is multifactorial and accumulative from fetal life to adulthood. It is influenced by:

- Genetic and epigenetic factors, which account for around 30% of the neurodevelopmental outcomes in CHD [33]
- Fetal haemodynamics and the fetal circulation
- Gestational age at delivery

- The complexity of CHD
- Exposure to cardiopulmonary bypass
- Parent-child relationships, and
- Parents' perception of their child's illness.

At term, the brain of an infant with CHD is known to be developmentally immature and smaller when compared to a term baby unaffected by CHD [34, 35]. Prolonged exposure of the fetal brain to an abnormal circulatory environment results in abnormal maturation and white matter injury, more akin to a preterm infant. Therefore, timing of delivery is critical, particularly if the already fragile neonatal brain is subsequently exposed to the rigors of cardiopulmonary bypass. [34, 36–38]

A 'brain sparing' phenomenon has been observed in fetuses with placental insufficiency, with a reduction in the middle cerebral artery (MCA) pulsatility index. This 'brain sparing' effect has also been witnessed in fetuses with CHD but, despite this potentially protective phenomenon, some infants with CHD demonstrate impaired brain growth and development, secondary to lower cerebral oxygenation and lower nutritional content of the cerebral blood [39, 40].

There is emerging evidence that patients with a functionally univentricular circulation are more affected [39]. Those with absence of antegrade aortic arch flow are particularly at risk [37]. Sethi et al. demonstrated that a smaller ascending aortic diameter and aortic atresia were particularly associated with abnormalities in cerebral blood flow [41]. This has been supported by recent data, showing that ascending aortic size at birth relates to the white matter microstructure in adolescence post-Fontan palliation [42].

Long-term follow-up studies have demonstrated that children with CHD have a lower than average outcome in several neurodevelopmental domains: executive function; psychomotor; literacy; numeracy and processing [43, 44]. McCusker et al. found no statistical difference in verbal reasoning scores or general IQ, however Singh et al. reported that in single ventricle adolescents more than a decade from their last surgical procedure, there are widespread anomalies in autonomic, mood and cognitive regulatory areas of the brain [45]. Hence, patients undergoing the Fontan pathway may be particularly susceptible to neurodevelopmental problems.

Conversely, children with CHD have been shown to have increased resilience. Maternal perceptions of the severity of the child's condition has a greater influence on psychological outcomes than the medical personnel's perception of the severity of the disease [43].

Thus, there are modifiable variables that, with early intervention, can improve the long-term neurodevelopmental outcome of children with CHD [43, 46].

Delivery and Immediate Postnatal Care

The fetus with a univentricular circulation should be monitored throughout pregnancy, with further fetal cardiac assessment at 28 weeks and 34 weeks of gestation. During this time, fetal medicine input is required to assess fetal growth and well-being.

Delivery should happen in a tertiary level neonatal unit, ideally within or in proximity to a surgical centre. There is evidence that delivery of a baby with HLHS <10 min from a cardiac centre is associated with reduced pre-transport mortality compared to those born >90 min away [47]. In the presence of some morphologies, for example HLHS with restrictive atrial septum or CHB, it is imperative that delivery is in close proximity to interventional cardiologists and a surgical team to provide early or immediate intervention.

In the vast majority of cases, babies can be delivered normally by vaginal delivery, unless there are maternal or obstetric contraindications. In some instances, a caesarean section is necessary, for example when there is complete heart block (CHB) and the fetal heart rate cannot be monitored to detect evidence of fetal distress.

There is increasing evidence that, not only the location, but the timing of delivery is important. Previously, there was a tendency for babies with a prenatal diagnosis of CHD to be delivered

between 37–38 weeks of gestation, i.e. "early-term" [25]. However, recent evidence suggests that those born early-term have an increased risk of neurological morbidity compared to those born at full term, at >39 weeks of gestation, [48] possibly due to the developmental immaturity of the CHD brain.

The prenatal management plan should state whether a prostaglandin infusion is required immediately after birth for those with suspected aortic arch obstruction or a duct-dependent pulmonary circulation. The baby should be stabilised on the neonatal unit and managed by neonatologists trained in the care of babies with complex CHD. A thorough neonatal examination should look for extra-cardiac anomalies, and a detailed cardiological assessment will confirm the CHD and guide further management.

Emotional support should be provided to parents, as a continuation of the prenatal support by the specialist cardiac nursing teams and psychologists.

References

1. Ghi T, Huggon IC, Zosmer N, Nicolaides KH. Incidence of major structural cardiac defects associated with increased nuchal translucency but normal karyotype. Ultrasound Obstet Gynecol. 2001;18(6):610–4.
2. Yagel S, Cohen SM, Achiron R. Examination of the fetal heart by five short-axis views: a proposed screening method for comprehensive cardiac evaluation. Ultrasound Obstet Gynecol. 2001;17(5):367–9.
3. Patel A, Hickey E, Mavroudis C, Jacobs JP, Jacobs ML, Backer CL, et al. Impact of noncardiac congenital and genetic abnormalities on outcomes in hypoplastic left heart syndrome. Ann Thorac Surg. 2010;89(6):1805–13; discussion 13–4.
4. Lee TM, Aiyagari R, Hirsch JC, Ohye RG, Bove EL, Devaney EJ. Risk factor analysis for second-stage palliation of single ventricle anatomy. Ann Thorac Surg. 2012;93(2):614–8; discussion 9.
5. McElhinney DB, Tworetzky W, Lock JE. Current status of fetal cardiac intervention. Circulation. 2010;121(10):1256–63.
6. McElhinney DB, Marshall AC, Wilkins-Haug LE, Brown DW, Benson CB, Silva V, et al. Predictors of technical success and postnatal biventricular outcome after in utero aortic valvuloplasty for aortic stenosis with evolving hypoplastic left heart syndrome. Circulation. 2009;120(15):1482–90.

7. Hunter LE, Chubb H, Miller O, Sharland G, Simpson JM. Fetal aortic valve stenosis: a critique of case selection criteria for fetal intervention. Prenat Diagn. 2015;35(12):1176–81.

8. Freud LR, McElhinney DB, Marshall AC, Marx GR, Friedman KG, del Nido PJ, et al. Fetal aortic valvuloplasty for evolving hypoplastic left heart syndrome: postnatal outcomes of the first 100 patients. Circulation. 2014;130(8):638–45.

9. Gardiner HM, Kovacevic A, Tulzer G, Sarkola T, Herberg U, Dangel J, et al. Natural history of 107 cases of fetal aortic stenosis from a European multicenter retrospective study. Ultrasound Obstet Gynecol. 2016;48(3):373–81.

10. Burch M, Kaufman L, Archer N, Sullivan I. Persistent pulmonary hypertension late after neonatal aortic valvotomy: a consequence of an expanded surgical cohort. Heart. 2004;90(8):918–20.

11. Freud LR, Moon-Grady A, Escobar-Diaz MC, Gotteiner NL, Young LT, McElhinney DB, et al. Low rate of prenatal diagnosis among neonates with critical aortic stenosis: insight into the natural history in utero. Ultrasound Obstet Gynecol. 2015;45(3):326–32.

12. Better DJ, Apfel HD, Zidere V, Allan LD. Pattern of pulmonary venous blood flow in the hypoplastic left heart syndrome in the fetus. Heart. 1999;81(6):646–9.

13. Divanovic A, Hor K, Cnota J, Hirsch R, Kinsel-Ziter M, Michelfelder E. Prediction and perinatal management of severely restrictive atrial septum in fetuses with critical left heart obstruction: clinical experience using pulmonary venous Doppler analysis. J Thorac Cardiovasc Surg. 2011;141(4):988–94.

14. Saul D, Degenhardt K, Iyoob SD, Surrey LF, Johnson AM, Johnson MP, et al. Hypoplastic left heart syndrome and the nutmeg lung pattern in utero: a cause and effect relationship or prognostic indicator? Pediatr Radiol. 2016;46(4):483–9.

15. Marshall AC, Levine J, Morash D, Silva V, Lock JE, Benson CB, et al. Results of in utero atrial septoplasty in fetuses with hypoplastic left heart syndrome. Prenat Diagn. 2008;28(11):1023–8.

16. Chaturvedi RR, Ryan G, Seed M, van Arsdell G, Jaeggi ET. Fetal stenting of the atrial septum: technique and initial results in cardiac lesions with left atrial hypertension. Int J Cardiol. 2013;168(3):2029–36.

17. Lowenthal A, Lemley B, Kipps AK, Brook MM, Moon-Grady AJ. Prenatal tricuspid valve size as a predictor of postnatal outcome in patients with severe pulmonary stenosis or pulmonary atresia with intact ventricular septum. Fetal Diagn Ther. 2014;35(2):101–7.

18. Cao L, Tian Z, Rychik J. Prenatal echocardiographic predictors of postnatal management strategy in the fetus with right ventricle hypoplasia and pulmonary atresia or stenosis. Pediatr Cardiol. 2017;38(8):1562–8.

19. Tulzer A, Arzt W, Gitter R, Prandstetter C, Grohmann E, Mair R, et al. Immediate effects and outcome of in-utero pulmonary valvuloplasty in fetuses with pulmonary atresia with intact ventricular septum or critical pulmonary stenosis. Ultrasound Obstet Gynecol. 2018;52(2):230–7.

20. Pepes S, Zidere V, Allan LD. Prenatal diagnosis of left atrial isomerism. Heart. 2009;95(24):1974–7.

21. Friedberg MK, Ursell PC, Silverman NH. Isomerism of the left atrial appendage associated with ventricular noncompaction. Am J Cardiol. 2005;96(7):985–90.

22. Mahle WT, Clancy RR, McGaurn SP, Goin JE, Clark BJ. Impact of prenatal diagnosis on survival and early neurologic morbidity in neonates with the hypoplastic left heart syndrome. Pediatrics. 2001;107(6):1277–82.

23. Feinstein JA, Benson DW, Dubin AM, Cohen MS, Maxey DM, Mahle WT, et al. Hypoplastic left heart syndrome: current considerations and expectations. J Am Coll Cardiol. 2012;59(1 Suppl):S1–42.

24. Weber RW, Stiasny B, Ruecker B, Fasnacht M, Cavigelli-Brunner A, Valsangiacomo Buechel ER. Prenatal diagnosis of single ventricle physiology impacts on cardiac morbidity and mortality. Pediatr Cardiol. 2019;40(1):61–70.

25. Brown DW, Cohen KE, O'Brien P, Gauvreau K, Klitzner TS, Beekman RH 3rd, et al. Impact of prenatal diagnosis in survivors of initial palliation of single ventricle heart disease: analysis of the National Pediatric Cardiology Quality Improvement Collaborative database. Pediatr Cardiol. 2015;36(2):314–21.

26. Liu MY, Zielonka B, Snarr BS, Zhang X, Gaynor JW, Rychik J. Longitudinal assessment of outcome from prenatal diagnosis through Fontan operation for over 500 fetuses with single ventricle-type congenital heart disease: the Philadelphia fetus-to-Fontan cohort study. J Am Heart Assoc. 2018;7(19):e009145.

27. Tworetzky W, McElhinney DB, Reddy VM, Brook MM, Hanley FL, Silverman NH. Improved surgical outcome after fetal diagnosis of hypoplastic left heart syndrome. Circulation. 2001;103(9):1269–73.

28. Peyvandi S, De Santiago V, Chakkarapani E, Chau V, Campbell A, Poskitt KJ, et al. Association of Prenatal Diagnosis of critical congenital heart disease with postnatal brain development and the risk of brain injury. JAMA Pediatr. 2016;170(4):e154450.

29. Brackley KJ, Kilby MD, Wright JG, Brawn WJ, Sethia B, Stumper O, et al. Outcome after prenatal diagnosis of hypoplastic left-heart syndrome: a case series. Lancet. 2000;356(9236):1143–7.

30. Rasiah SV, Ewer AK, Miller P, Wright JG, Barron DJ, Brawn WJ, et al. Antenatal perspective of hypoplastic left heart syndrome: 5 years on. Arch Dis Child Fetal Neonatal Ed. 2008;93(3):F192–7.

31. Ohman A, El-Segaier M, Bergman G, Hanseus K, Malm T, Nilsson B, et al. Changing epidemiology of Hypoplastic left heart syndrome: results of a National Swedish Cohort Study. J Am Heart Assoc. 2019;8(2):e010893.

32. Rogers L, Pagel C, Sullivan ID, Mustafa M, Tsang V, Utley M, et al. Interventional treatments and risk

factors in patients born with hypoplastic left heart syndrome in England and Wales from 2000 to 2015. Heart. 2018;104(18):1500–7.

33. Marelli A, Miller SP, Marino BS, Jefferson AL, Newburger JW. Brain in congenital heart disease across the lifespan: the cumulative burden of injury. Circulation. 2016;133(20):1951–62.

34. Andropoulos DB, Hunter JV, Nelson DP, Stayer SA, Stark AR, McKenzie ED, et al. Brain immaturity is associated with brain injury before and after neonatal cardiac surgery with high-flow bypass and cerebral oxygenation monitoring. J Thorac Cardiovasc Surg. 2010;139(3):543–56.

35. Miller SP, McQuillen PS, Hamrick S, Xu D, Glidden DV, Charlton N, et al. Abnormal brain development in newborns with congenital heart disease. N Engl J Med. 2007;357(19):1928–38.

36. McQuillen PS, Goff DA, Licht DJ. Effects of congenital heart disease on brain development. Prog Pediatr Cardiol. 2010;29(2):79–85.

37. Limperopoulos C, Tworetzky W, McElhinney DB, Newburger JW, Brown DW, Robertson RL Jr, et al. Brain volume and metabolism in fetuses with congenital heart disease: evaluation with quantitative magnetic resonance imaging and spectroscopy. Circulation. 2010;121(1):26–33.

38. Dimitropoulos A, McQuillen PS, Sethi V, Moosa A, Chau V, Xu D, et al. Brain injury and development in newborns with critical congenital heart disease. Neurology. 2013;81(3):241–8.

39. Donofrio MT, Bremer YA, Schieken RM, Gennings C, Morton LD, Eidem BW, et al. Autoregulation of cerebral blood flow in fetuses with congenital heart disease: the brain sparing effect. Pediatr Cardiol. 2003;24(5):436–43.

40. Sun L, Macgowan CK, Sled JG, Yoo SJ, Manlhiot C, Porayette P, et al. Reduced fetal cerebral oxygen consumption is associated with smaller brain size in fetuses with congenital heart disease. Circulation. 2015;131(15):1313–23.

41. Sethi V, Tabbutt S, Dimitropoulos A, Harris KC, Chau V, Poskitt K, et al. Single-ventricle anatomy predicts delayed microstructural brain development. Pediatr Res. 2013;73(5):661–7.

42. Zaidi AH, Newburger JW, Wypij D, Stopp C, Watson CG, Friedman KG, et al. Ascending aorta size at birth predicts white matter microstructure in adolescents who underwent Fontan palliation. J Am Heart Assoc. 2018;7(24):e010395.

43. McCusker CG, Armstrong MP, Mullen M, Doherty NN, Casey FA. A sibling-controlled, prospective study of outcomes at home and school in children with severe congenital heart disease. Cardiol Young. 2013;23(4):507–16.

44. McCusker CG, Doherty NN, Molloy B, Casey F, Rooney N, Mulholland C, et al. Determinants of neuropsychological and behavioural outcomes in early childhood survivors of congenital heart disease. Arch Dis Child. 2007;92(2):137–41.

45. Singh S, Roy B, Pike N, Daniel E, Ehlert L, Lewis AB, et al. Altered brain diffusion tensor imaging indices in adolescents with the Fontan palliation. Neuroradiology. 2019;61(7):811–24.

46. McCusker CG, Doherty NN, Molloy B, Rooney N, Mulholland C, Sands A, et al. A controlled trial of early interventions to promote maternal adjustment and development in infants born with severe congenital heart disease. Child Care Health Dev. 2010;36(1):110–7.

47. Morris SA, Ethen MK, Penny DJ, Canfield MA, Minard CG, Fixler DE, et al. Prenatal diagnosis, birth location, surgical center, and neonatal mortality in infants with hypoplastic left heart syndrome. Circulation. 2014;129(3):285–92.

48. Calderon J, Stopp C, Wypij D, DeMaso DR, Rivkin M, Newburger JW, et al. Early-term birth in single-ventricle congenital heart disease after the Fontan procedure: neurodevelopmental and psychiatric outcomes. J Pediatr. 2016;179:96–103.

Postnatal Management and Pre-Operative Assessment of the Univentricular Patient

Shree Vishna Rasiah and Michael John Harris

Postnatal Management

- **Delivery**
  - Once an antenatal diagnosis of a univentricular heart condition is made, the plan would be to deliver the baby in a neonatal intensive care unit (NICU), preferably in one with close proximity to paediatric cardiology services [1, 2].
  - As with all other congenital heart conditions, babies born with univentricular hearts are commonly not growth restricted at birth, but they can experience a tailing off in the growth velocity in the latter parts of pregnancy [3, 4].
  - The underlying cardiac condition does not seem to impact on their fetal development.
  - Growth restriction can be a poor prognosis in these groups of babies [5].
  - The majority of them are delivered at term by normal vaginal delivery unless there were concerns about fetal distress or maternal wellbeing [6].
  - The neonatal team should be informed about all babies due to deliver with a univentricular heart and they should be present at the delivery. Although the majority of these babies do not require resuscitation at birth [6], those with poor mixing are likely to be hypoxic following delivery and may need ventilatory support.
  - The need for ventilatory support should be assessed on an individual basis. Oxygen saturations in the 80%'s should be expected following delivery and routine use of oxygen supplementation should be discouraged unless clinically indicated.
  - If the babies are born in a good condition, routine obstetric management should be carried out. This includes delayed cord clamping and, before transfer to the neonatal intensive care unit, skin to skin contact with the mother to help with the early bonding process.
  - There is little urgency to take these clinically stable babies to the neonatal intensive care unit, and this can be an important time for the parents to be with and enjoy their new baby.
- **Neonatal Unit Management**
  - Once on the NICU, the baby's vital signs need to be continuously monitored. This includes regular blood gas monitoring to ensure cardiorespiratory stability during post-natal adaptation.
  - The monitoring of lactate levels is crucial in cardiac babies as a marker of adequate perfusion and oxygenation and as an indicator for possible intervention.

S. V. Rasiah · M. J. Harris (✉)
Birmingham Women's and Children's NHS
Foundation Trust, Birmingham, UK
e-mail: michael.harris2@nhs.net

- Those babies with duct dependent lesions will need an intravenous Prostaglandin infusion. A dose of 5 nanograms/kg/min is usually more than sufficient to maintain ductal patency [7] and circulatory stability prior to transfer for further assessment and/or intervention. At this dose of prostaglandin infusion, it is very rare for babies to experience side effects [8, 9], which are primarily apnoeic episodes.
- Those babies without a duct dependent lesion should be monitored closely initially to ensure appropriate physiological adaptation. Any deviations from haemodynamic stability should be identified and rectified.
- It is important to encourage mothers to express their breast milk regularly if they are wishing to breastfeed. The babies can be given the initial colostrum whilst on the prostaglandin infusion.
- Postnatal echocardiogram will confirm the antenatal findings, the adequacy of circulatory mixing and the patency of the ductus arteriosus in duct dependent conditions. Cardiac function should also be assessed and if inadequate, inotropic support should be provided to support cardiac output.
- **Genetic testing**
  - All babies with a univentricular heart diagnosis should be offered genetic testing [10]. If this has not been performed antenatally, this should be carried out postnatally with the parents' consent.
  - Some genetic conditions are so severe and life-limiting in and of themselves that cardiac surgery is not indicated, for example trisomies 13 and 18.
  - Trisomy 21 is a relative contraindication to univentricular palliation, as is Turner Syndrome (XO).
  - Other genetic conditions exist that may influence the postnatal management of these babies.
- **Heterotaxy**
  - Babies with heterotaxy syndromes will need further investigations to identify associated conditions.

- These investigations will include abdominal ultrasonography to assess the abdominal viscera and their orientation, and the presence or absence of the spleen, the bile ducts and the gallbladder, particularly in left atrial isomerism. The kidneys and any abnormalities thereof should be identified.
- Those babies with abdominal situs abnormalities or other laterality abnormalities may require an upper gastrointestinal contrast study to ensure that there is no evidence of malrotation.
- These investigations can be carried out electively in the postnatal period to guide on-going management of these babies.

Issues Encountered in Postnatal Period

Babies with univentricular heart conditions can encounter certain problems which will need to be addressed accordingly.

- **Respiratory distress syndrome**
  - If babies with univentricular heart conditions are born prematurely, they might develop respiratory distress syndrome (RDS).
  - If these babies are hypoxic due to a respiratory cause, then their ventilation should be supported and oxygen supplementation provided.
  - Varying degrees of ventilatory support are available, including non-invasive forms with high flow air or oxygen, or CPAP, or full ventilation via an endotracheal tube.
  - Ventilated babies might need surfactant to treat potential surfactant deficiency.
- **Pulmonary over-circulation syndrome**
  - This condition is encountered in babies with a duct dependent condition e.g. Hypoplastic Left Heart Syndrome (HLHS) who have persistently high oxygen saturation and a rising lactic acidosis.
  - The pathophysiology of this phenomenon is the result of increased pulmonary circu-

lation due to falling pulmonary vascular resistance.

- This causes 'steal' from the systemic circulation, resulting in reduced systemic perfusion. If not managed appropriately, this is detrimental to the baby.
- Babies in this state generally require intubation. Manipulation of the ventilator to produce hypoventilation results in an increase in pulmonary vascular resistance and improves systemic circulation by reducing the left to right shunt at the ductal level.
- Such babies may require relatively early surgical intervention.

- **Poor saturations suggesting poor mixing (restrictive atrial septum)**
  - A handful of babies will have very poor oxygenation and saturation after delivery despite all efforts to support them.
  - In cases of HLHS, this is likely to suggest poor mixing because of a restrictive or intact atrial septum.
  - Some cases might have been identified antenatally but this is not always possible or predictable.
  - **This is a time critical emergency.**

    The prognosis for these babies is dire if there is no effective mixing at the atrial level [11].

    Most babies with this condition will need to be intubated and ventilated and transferred to the paediatric cardiology unit urgently to undergo procedures to relieve the restriction to atrial mixing.

    Depending on the centre, this may involve percutaneous septostomy or surgical septectomy with the contemporaneous application of bilateral pulmonary artery bands.

    Alternatively, this variant of HLHS is known to be associated with a dismal prognosis and it may be more appropriate [1, 12], following thorough assessment and discussion, to redirect care along the palliative route.

- **Intrauterine growth restriction**
  - If babies are born very small or early, then they need to be stabilised and managed on a prostaglandin infusion whilst they grow.
  - The aim would be to grow the babies to a suitable size and gestation so that they are of sufficient weight and maturity to more safely undergo surgical or other intervention.
  - Ideally, these babies should have a corrected gestational age equivalent to term and should be more than 2500 g in weight, but the thresholds for intervention in operating units are variable.

Paediatric Cardiology Management

- Once the baby is stable on the NICU on the Prostaglandin infusion, they may be transferred to the Paediatric Cardiology Unit, if not co-located with the NICU, for further assessment and plans for surgical or other intervention.
  - Those babies who need ventilatory support will normally be transferred to the Paediatric Intensive Care Unit. Again, practice varies on a centre-specific basis.

Pre-Operative Assessment

- The time between the delivery of a baby with a univentricular heart condition and the initial intervention is crucial. The aim of this time is to present a baby in optimal condition for surgery or other further management or intervention. This time should be used to confirm the anatomy, identify any extra-cardiac anomalies, including genetic differences, and allow time for education of parents and the wider family.
- In countries with established and largely effective prenatal screening programmes, prenatal diagnosis rates in excess of 50% for complex congenital heart defects are possible [13, 14].

- This means that many babies with these conditions are born in controlled, planned circumstances, when stability can be achieved at an early stage and pre-operative morbidity can largely be avoided [15, 16].
- There is still a proportion of babies who are born and present with symptoms of haemodynamic compromise secondary to a previously undiagnosed cardiac condition.
  - In whatever manner these babies present, it is imperative those born with univentricular heart conditions are stabilised early by all necessary means [17].

Confirm the Diagnosis

- It is essential to make, confirm or expand the diagnosis of a univentricular heart condition.
  - The primary means of diagnosis is transthoracic echocardiography (TTE). TTE can reliably distinguish all forms of univentricular disease, and provides a road map for further investigations to clarify areas of uncertainty.
- Univentricular disease comes in many forms including: HLHS and other right ventricle-dependent circulations, those which are left ventricle-dependent, and those that lie somewhere in between [18].

Haemodynamic category	Example univentricular heart conditions
Reduced systemic perfusion	Hypoplastic left heart syndrome
Reduced pulmonary blood flow	Variants of double inlet ventricle (DILV), tricuspid Atresia (TA), pulmonary atresia/intact ventricular septum (PA/IVS)
Excessive pulmonary blood flow	Variants of DILV, TA, double outlet right ventricle (DORV)
Balanced systemic and pulmonary circulations	Variants of DILV, TA, DORV

- This categorisation is helpful to assist in determining management.

- For example, depending on the variant of univentricular heart disease, some babies may require high risk surgery at an early stage, and others may require little or no intervention until the time of superior cavopulmonary connection.

Confirm the Diagnosis—Is it Truly a Univentricular heart Condition?

- On most occasions, the diagnosis of a univentricular heart condition is clear. Occasionally, there may be some debate as to the adequacy of the pumping chambers and the inlet valves.
  - This is especially true of borderline left ventricle conditions, some cases of pulmonary atresia/intact ventricular septum and some cases of double outlet right ventricle.
  - Decision making then becomes a combination of accurate imaging and consideration of extra-cardiac factors, the judicious application of prognostic data from the literature, and the clinical experience and expertise of the multi-disciplinary team.
  - It is true that some babies proceed down an initial univentricular pathway, but are subsequently able to undergo septation [19, 20].

Identify Additional Cardiac Lesions

- It is possible for babies with univentricular heart conditions to have multiple additional cardiac diagnoses over and above the underlying main lesion. For this reason, a sequential approach to excluding abnormalities should be followed.
  - All of the anatomical and functional features should be examined as they either have a bearing on the technical aspects of surgery or on prognosis.

- Some associated cardiac lesions add sufficiently to the complexity of the lesion that the risk:benefit analysis is such that intervention is not offered, and comfort care is recommended.
- The threshold of different units for offering or declining intervention is highly variable and dependent on local expertise and experience [21].

Important Anatomical Features to Consider Include

- Atrial arrangements
  - Laterality defects immediately add a level of complexity and added morbidity and mortality to any univentricular heart conditions [22]
- Pulmonary and systemic venous drainage [23]
- Adequacy of the atrial communication
  - This is especially important in HLHS, but also other UVH. The special case of intact or restrictive atrial septum in HLHS carries an exceedingly poor prognosis [12, 24].
- Presence of atrioventricular valve regurgitation
- Function of the dominant ventricular chamber
- Presence or absence of ventricular septal defects and accurate description thereof
- Subarterial stenoses
- Morphology and characteristics of the arterial valves, the presence of any dysplasia, stenosis or regurgitation, particularly for the valve that is or will become the systemic outflow valve
- Presence, characteristics and adequacy of the arterial duct, if present and if necessary to maintain systemic or pulmonary blood flow
- The relative sizes of the great arteries and any important stenoses, which may be of prognostic value
  - e.g. size of the ascending aorta in HLHS
  - the presence of a hypoplastic arch and/or coarctation in various forms of UVH
  - branch PA stenoses

Further Investigations to Aid in Diagnosis

- The use of Computed Tomography (CT) and Magnetic Resonance Imaging (MRI) is now common place in complex univentricular lesions, especially those with laterality defects or where there are concerns about the arterial, systemic venous or pulmonary venous anatomy.
- Cross sectional imaging is very useful for extra-cardiac lesions that may have a bearing on prognosis; for example, evidence of lung pathology (nutmeg lung) in cases of restrictive/intact interatrial septum in HLHS [25, 26].

Interventions

- Establishing accurately the diagnosis and any associated cardiac and non-cardiac lesions will determine which of the available interventions will be best in terms of both immediate and longer term outcome.
- The choice of procedure, which may be surgical, interventional or some combination of the two, is often centre-specific.
- The basic strategy of any procedure is to provide balanced systemic and pulmonary perfusion. There are a number of means to achieve this in the multiple univentricular conditions that exist.
  - For example, the treatment for HLHS involves some form of Norwood type procedure or an initial hybrid procedure.
- Primary transplant has been undertaken occasionally in these situations, but this is vanishingly rare [21, 27].
- **Risks of intervention**
  - Interventions for univentricular heart conditions are some of the riskiest in terms of short and longer term mortality [17, 18], with emerging evidence of longer-term neurological morbidity, amongst others.
  - Establishing the diagnosis, and any associated cardiac and extra-cardiac lesions,

helps with assessing the individual risk of any intervention for a patient.

- Communicating such risks meaningfully to the family can be very difficult [28].
- Both multi- and single centre studies have demonstrated multiple pre-operative risk factors that affect the outcome of the Norwood operation [21, 29, 30].
- Some of these are centre-specific, but there are some common themes.

These risk factors may be [31, 32]:

Patient-related	Lower birth weight Prematurity Genetic abnormality Extra-cardiac abnormalities • Airway • Brain • Kidney • Spinal • Respiratory abnormalities
Anatomical	Mitral stenosis/aortic atresia variant of HLHS Smaller ascending aorta size Restrictive atrial septum Significant i.e. moderate or more AV valve regurgitation
Pre-operative	Shock ECMO use
Operative	See later chapters
Post-operative	See later chapters

- Interestingly, many studies show a convergence of survival at >1 year regardless of the risk factors [30].
- Particular risk factors for other univentricular heart conditions are less well defined due to the relative rarity and heterogeneity of these conditions [18, 22]. Studies are usually blighted by confounding variables that make drawing strong conclusions difficult.

Communication with Parents and Families

- The final key element for the time between delivery and intervention is for communication with the parents.

- In many cases, the cardiac condition has been diagnosed in fetal life. This is usually possible with a high degree of accuracy and detail, and so many parents will have been thoroughly counselled and will be well prepared for the arduous road ahead even prior to delivery [33, 34].
- However, not all nuances of cardiac lesions can be established prior to birth, and a proportion of extra-cardiac anomalies will also only be discovered after delivery.
- Invasive prenatal karyotyping is often declined, and so there may be new and sometimes rather unusual genetic diagnoses to consider following postnatal genetic testing [10].
- Furthermore, many patients are clearly 'syndromic' but have no identifiable genetic marker underlying the constellation of anomalies.
- Therefore, the time after delivery and before surgery is crucial for accurate information to be given in regard to all of these factors, but also with regard to the short and longer term risk of any interventions. Parents can be very different in their approach to information, with some wanting minute detail, and others content with minimal information. Striking this balance remains the art of medicine.
  - This is the time for discussions regarding the merits of intervention versus palliative care, although many parents will have decided antenatally that they wish to pursue all surgical options for their child.
  - Very few in this day and age pursue comfort care as the primary management [21].
  - It is crucial that discussions are documented, and if possible, parents should be provided with written records of the discussions.
- Access by parents to appropriately trained specialist nurses can be very helpful for further explanation and counselling.
  - This relationship has often begun prenatally and can carry on quite naturally following delivery [33].

Summary

- The mode of delivery for babies with univentricular heart conditions is seldom affected by the underlying cardiac lesion, if known.
- Many babies with complex univentricular heart conditions progress through pregnancy remarkably well, and are born with minimal requirement for post-natal resuscitation.
- Some babies only present at some hours, or even days, of age and require emergency stabilisation, rather than that which can be planned following fetal diagnosis.
- The aim of the time between delivery and intervention is to present a patient in a stable, optimised haemodynamic and nutritional state, with the diagnosis firmly established.
- Any significant risk factors should have been identified and incorporated into pre-operative counselling and consent.
- Co-morbidities should have been identified, as much as possible, and measures put in place to mitigate their effects.
- Any chromosomal and/or genetic anomalies should have been identified. Full discussions should have been had amongst the multi-disciplinary team to decide the optimum management strategy.
- The parents should have been fully and adequately counselled with the options available to them, including the option of comfort care.
- They should be in possession of all of the facts about their baby and the short, medium and long term risks to their baby's health and the particular risks associated with surgery or intervention.

References

1. Sathanandam SK, Philip R, Gamboa D, Van Bergen A, Ilbawi MN, Knott-Craig C, et al. Management of hypoplastic left heart syndrome with intact atrial septum: a two-Centre experience. Cardiol Young. 2016;26(6):1072–81.
2. Morris SA, Ethen MK, Penny DJ, Canfield MA, Minard CG, Fixler DE, et al. Prenatal diagnosis, birth location, surgical center, and neonatal mortality in infants with hypoplastic left heart syndrome. Circulation. 2014;129(3):285–92.
3. Cnota JF, Hangge PT, Wang Y, Woo JG, Hinton AC, Divanovic AA, et al. Somatic growth trajectory in the fetus with hypoplastic left heart syndrome. Pediatr Res. 2013;74(3):284–9.
4. Triebwasser JE, Treadwell MC. In utero evidence of impaired somatic growth in Hypoplastic left heart syndrome. Pediatr Cardiol. 2017;38(7):1400–4.
5. Miller TA, Ghanayem NS, Newburger JW, McCrindle BW, Hu C, DeWitt AG, et al. Gestational age, birth weight, and outcomes six years after the Norwood procedure. Pediatrics. 2019;143(5):e20182577.
6. Peterson AL, Quartermain MD, Ades A, Khalek N, Johnson MP, Rychik J. Impact of mode of delivery on markers of perinatal hemodynamics in infants with hypoplastic left heart syndrome. J Pediatr. 2011;159(1):64–9.
7. Yucel IK, Cevik A, Bulut MO, Dedeoglu R, Demir IH, Erdem A, et al. Efficacy of very low-dose prostaglandin E1 in duct-dependent congenital heart disease. Cardiol Young. 2015;25(1):56–62.
8. Saxena A, Sharma M, Kothari SS, Juneja R, Reddy SC, Sharma R, et al. Prostaglandin E1 in infants with congenital heart disease: Indian experience. Indian Pediatr. 1998;35(11):1063–9.
9. Heymann MA, Clyman RI. Evaluation of alprostadil (prostaglandin E1) in the management of congenital heart disease in infancy. Pharmacotherapy. 1982;2(3):148–55.
10. Hopkins MK, Dugoff L, Kuller JA. Congenital heart disease: prenatal diagnosis and genetic associations. Obstet Gynecol Surv. 2019;74(8):497–503.
11. Lowenthal A, Kipps AK, Brook MM, Meadows J, Azakie A, Moon-Grady AJ. Prenatal diagnosis of atrial restriction in hypoplastic left heart syndrome is associated with decreased 2-year survival. Prenat Diagn. 2012;32(5):485–90.
12. Arai S, Fujii Y, Kotani Y, Kuroko Y, Kasahara S, Sano S. Surgical outcome of hypoplastic left heart syndrome with intact atrial septum. Asian Cardiovasc Thorac Ann. 2015;23(9):1034–8.
13. Bakker MK, Bergman JEH, Krikov S, Amar E, Cocchi G, Cragan J, et al. Prenatal diagnosis and prevalence of critical congenital heart defects: an international retrospective cohort study. BMJ Open. 2019;9(7):e028139.
14. Chakraborty A, Gorla SR, Swaminathan S. Impact of prenatal diagnosis of complex congenital heart disease on neonatal and infant morbidity and mortality. Prenat Diagn. 2018;38(12):958–63.
15. Levey A, Glickstein JS, Kleinman CS, Levasseur SM, Chen J, Gersony WM, et al. The impact of prenatal diagnosis of complex congenital heart disease on neonatal outcomes. Pediatr Cardiol. 2010;31(5):587–97.
16. Landis BJ, Levey A, Levasseur SM, Glickstein JS, Kleinman CS, Simpson LL, et al. Prenatal diagnosis of congenital heart disease and birth outcomes. Pediatr Cardiol. 2013;34(3):597–605.
17. Feinstein JA, Benson DW, Dubin AM, Cohen MS, Maxey DM, Mahle WT, et al. Hypoplastic left heart

syndrome: current considerations and expectations. J Am Coll Cardiol. 2012;59(1 Suppl):S1–42.

18. Alsoufi B, Slesnick T, McCracken C, Ehrlich A, Kanter K, Schlosser B, et al. Current outcomes of the Norwood operation in patients with single-ventricle malformations other than hypoplastic left heart syndrome. World J Pediatr Congenit Heart Surg. 2015;6(1):46–52.

19. Emani SM, McElhinney DB, Tworetzky W, Myers PO, Schroeder B, Zurakowski D, et al. Staged left ventricular recruitment after single-ventricle palliation in patients with borderline left heart hypoplasia. J Am Coll Cardiol. 2012;60(19):1966–74.

20. Oladunjoye OO, Piekarski B, Banka P, Marx G, Breitbart RE, Del Nido PJ, et al. Staged ventricular recruitment in patients with borderline ventricles and large ventricular septal defects. J Thorac Cardiovasc Surg. 2018;156(1):254–64.

21. Greenleaf CE, Urencio JM, Salazar JD, Dodge-Khatami A. Hypoplastic left heart syndrome: current perspectives. Transl Pediatr. 2016;5(3):142–7.

22. Buca DIP, Khalil A, Rizzo G, Familiari A, Di Giovanni S, Liberati M, et al. Outcome of prenatally diagnosed fetal heterotaxy: systematic review and meta-analysis. Ultrasound Obstet Gynecol. 2018;51(3):323–30.

23. Hancock HS, Romano JC, Armstrong A, Yu S, Lowery R, Gelehrter S. Single ventricle and Total anomalous pulmonary venous connection: implications of prenatal diagnosis. World J Pediatr Congenit Heart Surg. 2018;9(4):434–9.

24. Tanem J, Rudd N, Rauscher J, Scott A, Frommelt MA, Hill GD. Survival after Norwood procedure in high risk patients. Ann Thorac Surg. 2019;144:339.

25. Goltz D, Lunkenheimer JM, Abedini M, Herberg U, Berg C, Gembruch U, et al. Left ventricular obstruction with restrictive inter-atrial communication leads to retardation in fetal lung maturation. Prenat Diagn. 2015;35(5):463–70.

26. Saul D, Degenhardt K, Iyoob SD, Surrey LF, Johnson AM, Johnson MP, et al. Hypoplastic left heart syndrome and the nutmeg lung pattern in utero: a cause and effect relationship or prognostic indicator? Pediatr Radiol. 2016;46(4):483–9.

27. John MM, Razzouk AJ, Chinnock RE, Bock MJ, Kuhn MA, Martens TP, et al. Primary transplantation for congenital heart disease in the neonatal period: long-term outcomes. Ann Thorac Surg. 2019;108:1857–64.

28. Ahmed H, Naik G, Willoughby H, Edwards AG. Communicating risk. BMJ. 2012;344:e3996.

29. Rogers L, Pagel C, Sullivan ID, Mustafa M, Tsang V, Utley M, et al. Interventional treatments and risk factors in patients born with hypoplastic left heart syndrome in England and Wales from 2000 to 2015. Heart. 2018;104(18):1500–7.

30. Alsoufi B, Mori M, Gillespie S, Schlosser B, Slesnick T, Kogon B, et al. Impact of patient characteristics and anatomy on results of Norwood operation for Hypoplastic left heart syndrome. Ann Thorac Surg. 2015;100(2):591–8.

31. Tabbutt S, Ghanayem N, Ravishankar C, Sleeper LA, Cooper DS, Frank DU, et al. Risk factors for hospital morbidity and mortality after the Norwood procedure: a report from the pediatric heart network single ventricle reconstruction trial. J Thorac Cardiovasc Surg. 2012;144(4):882–95.

32. Shamszad P, Gospin TA, Hong BJ, McKenzie ED, Petit CJ. Impact of preoperative risk factors on outcomes after Norwood palliation for hypoplastic left heart syndrome. J Thorac Cardiovasc Surg. 2014;147(3):897–901.

33. Bratt EL, Jarvholm S, Ekman-Joelsson BM, Mattson LA, Mellander M. Parent's experiences of counselling and their need for support following a prenatal diagnosis of congenital heart disease--a qualitative study in a Swedish context. BMC Pregnancy Childbirth. 2015;15:171.

34. Marokakis S, Kasparian NA, Kennedy SE. Prenatal counselling for congenital anomalies: a systematic review. Prenat Diagn. 2016;36(7):662–71.

Imaging to Aid Decision Making in the Neonate

Hannah Bellsham-Revell

Introduction

Echocardiography is the mainstay of initial imaging in the neonate. If a patient has had a fetal diagnosis it is important to review the fetal data (including any fetal MRI) prior to seeing the patient. If important questions still exist after echocardiography, then further modalities such as cardiac CT, MRI or angiography may be required. [1] These methods are particularly good at looking at systemic or pulmonary venous anomalies and complex great vessel and arch anatomy.

Morphological Diagnosis

The exact morphological diagnosis should be obtained using a standard sequential segmental approach [2, 3]. Once the diagnosis is ascertained, it is important to then look at in more detail life-maintaining structures, procedure defining structures and prognostic structures.

Life-maintaining Structures (Fig. 6.1)

These are structures that are essential for the circulation to support life and without which the child would become critically unwell.

- **Arterial Duct:** For many single ventricle conditions patency of the arterial duct is essential to provide either the systemic or pulmonary blood flow. In some conditions more than one duct can be seen or the duct may be absent. The position, geometry and course of the arterial duct should be documented as this may be important particularly if stenting of the arterial duct is to be considered. [4]
- **Atrial Communication:** The atrial communication is important where either mixing is obligatory or where there is a severely stenotic or atretic atrioventricular connection. The size and position of the defect should be assessed with the transatrial Doppler gradient, as well as evidence of restriction:
  - *Left inflow obstruction*: Dilation of pulmonary veins and pulmonary vein Doppler looking for significant A wave reversal
  - *Right inflow obstruction*: Dilatation of the inferior caval vein and hepatic veins with flow reversal

H. Bellsham-Revell (✉)
Evelina London Children's Hospital, London, UK
e-mail: hannah.bellsham-revell@gstt.nhs.uk

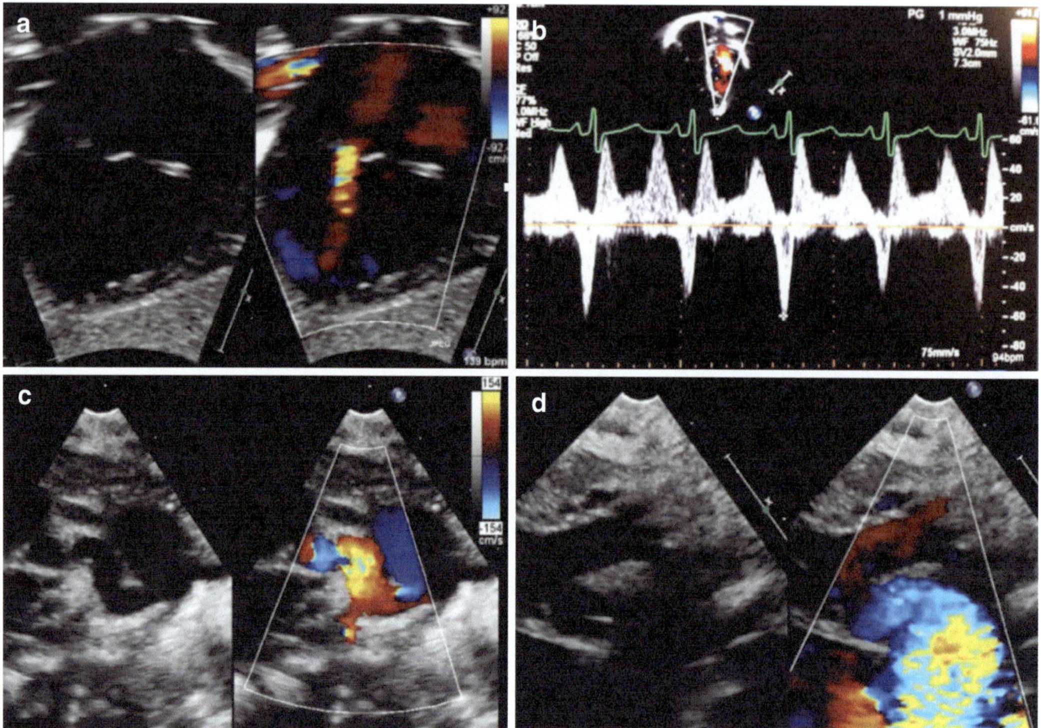

Fig. 6.1 Life-maintaining structures. (**a**) Restrictive atrial septum with (**b**) significant A wave reversal (**c**) Tortuous arterial duct and (**d**) large arterial duct in interrupted arch

- Atrial restriction in left heart obstruction can be of great importance prognostically as congestion in utero can damage the lungs leading to lymphangiectasia [5, 6].
- Echocardiographic parameters should be used in conjunction with the clinical picture for example desaturation and congested chest x-ray in left inflow obstruction and hepatomegaly in right inflow obstruction.

Procedure-defining Structures

Single ventricle conditions can be divided into:

- *Inadequate systemic blood flow* (e.g. critical left heart obstruction)
- *Inadequate pulmonary blood flow* (e.g. critical right heart obstruction)
- *Too much pulmonary blood flow* (e.g. single ventricle conditions with neither significant right nor left outflow obstruction)

- *Balanced blood flow* (e.g. single ventricle conditions with adequate systemic flow and restriction to pulmonary blood flow from pulmonary stenosis etc)

Assessing systemic and pulmonary blood flow: the pathway of blood to the systemic and pulmonary circulation should be assessed at each step. Potential restriction can occur at the atrial septum, inflow valve, ventricle, outflow and arch. The decision on the method of palliation will depend on the level and extent of obstruction.

- **Atrial septum:** see above
- **Inflow** (Fig. 6.2)**:**
  - The size, morphology and function of the inflow needs to be assessed.
  - Measurements should be performed and z-scores obtained. [2]
  - The assessment will vary depending on whether the inflow is an atrioventricular valve or a mitral/tricupsid valve.

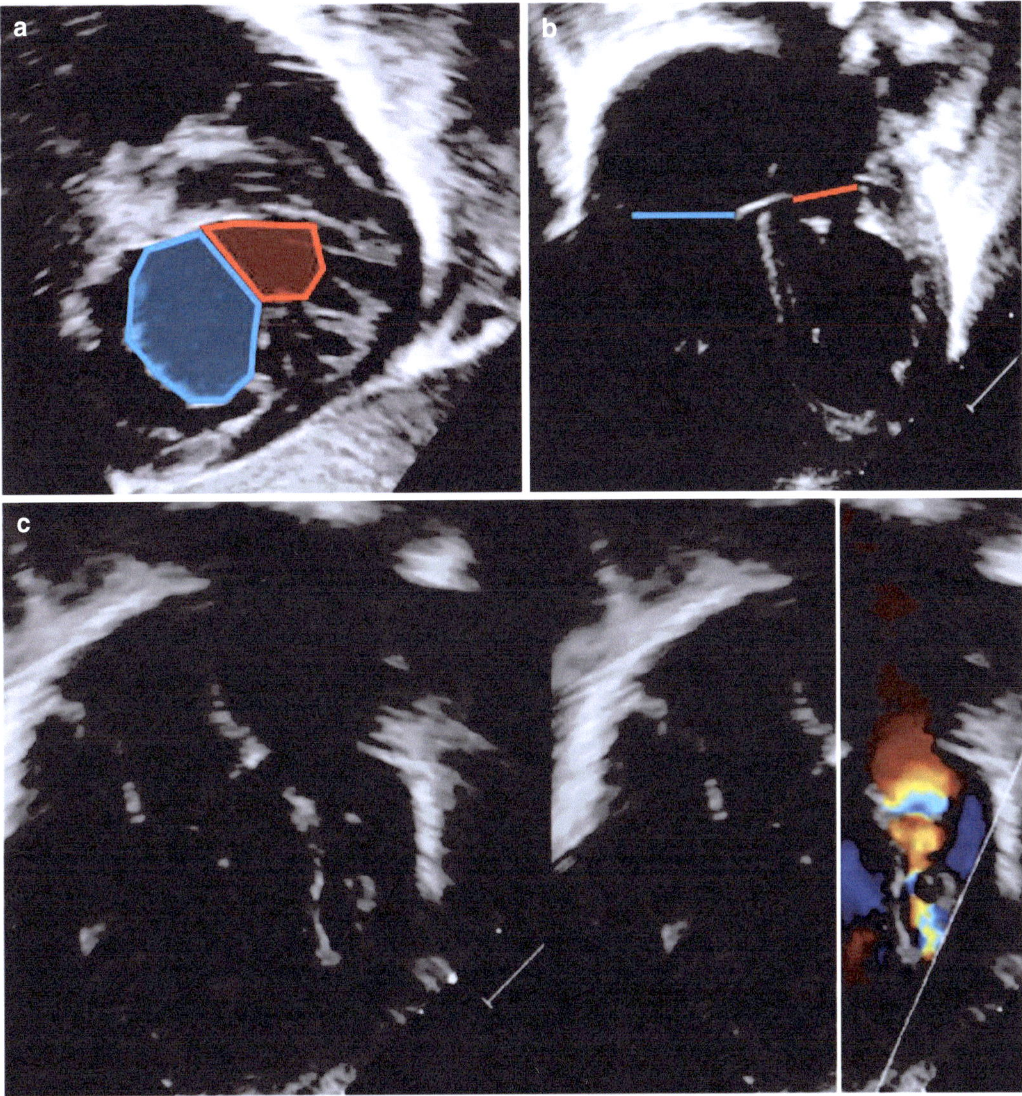

Fig. 6.2 Atrioventricular valves. (**a**) Unbalanced atrioventricular septal defect with left and right atrioventricular valve areas traced (**b**) Tricuspid and mitral valves measured for z-scoring (**c**) Dysplastic and stenotic mitral valve on 2D and colour

- The number of papillary muscles, the length of cords and leaflet motion should be described and can be assessed using 2D and 3D echocardiography [7, 8].
- Inflow Doppler can give an estimate of gradient, but this can be challenging in the presence of downstream obstruction (due to high ventricular end diastolic pressure) and also in the newborn where the pulmonary pressures are high and therefore pulmonary flow is not at usual post-natal levels.
- In unbalanced atrioventricular septal defects scores have been developed to aid decision making looking at angulation of the valves and predicted valve area. [9–11]

In some children with a large atrial component there may be streaming across the left atrioventricular valve which may then be underestimated.

- **Ventricle:**
  - The size, compliance and systolic function of the ventricle is important. The size of the ventricle is dependent on loading conditions and cannot be used in isolation, e.g. in the presence of a large atrial septal defect or for the left ventricle if pulmonary venous drainage is anomalous or on the initial newborn scan.
  - Diastology can be difficult to assess on the newborn scan, particularly in the face of obstruction. With critical obstruction there is likely to be a later effect on the compliance of the ventricle
  - In the left ventricle endocardial fibroelastosis is an important finding to note.
- **Outflow:**
  - The size, morphology and function of the outflow tract needs to be assessed.
  - Measurements should be performed and z-scores obtained. [2]
  - The number of valve leaflets and function of the outflow valve should be assessed with presence of stenosis or regurgitation noted as well as any sub-valvar obstruction.
  - For those with critical aortic stenosis scores to predict successful short-term biventricular repair have been proposed [12–14], although the longer term remains uncertain given ongoing obstruction or LV diastolic impairment can lead to multiple re-interventions and pulmonary hypertension.
- **Ventricular septal defect** (Fig. 6.3):
  - In some patients, their systemic or pulmonary flow may be dependent on a ventricular septal defect. The Doppler gradient may give an indication of whether there is any restriction.
  - The size and position can be assessed on 2D echocardiography, but as defects are seldom round, the size can be over or underestimated.
- Three dimensional echocardiography allows visualisation en face to assess the true extent of the defect [7, 8]. This can also help the surgeon in understanding whether the VSD can be safely enlarged without the risk of heart block, or whether another method of augmenting systemic or pulmonary flow is required.
  - It is also important to note that over time ventricular septal defects can become restrictive.
- **Aorta** (Fig. 6.4):
  - The size of the ascending aorta, transverse arch and any coarctation should be noted in order to define whether, and what type of arch augmentation is required.
  - The sidedness and branching pattern will also potentially affect the type of operation performed.
  - Retrograd e flow in the aortic arch suggests that the heart cannot support the systemic circulation as there is not enough aortic forward flow and therefore the duct is supplying the head and neck vessels as well as the lower body.
- **Branch pulmonary arteries** (Fig. 6.4):
  - The anatomy and continuity of the branch pulmonary arteries should be defined as this may affect the mode of augmentation of pulmonary blood flow as well as being prognostically important.
  - Note should also be made of any additional sources of pulmonary blood flow e.g. major aortopulmonary collaterals.

Prognostic Structures

If a patient is planned to go down the Fontan pathway, attention also needs to be paid to features which are known to be risk factors for mortality and morbidity.

- **Ventricular Function:**
  - Antenatal ventricular dysfunction is worrying as the fetal heart is relatively unloaded. If post-natally systolic function is moder-

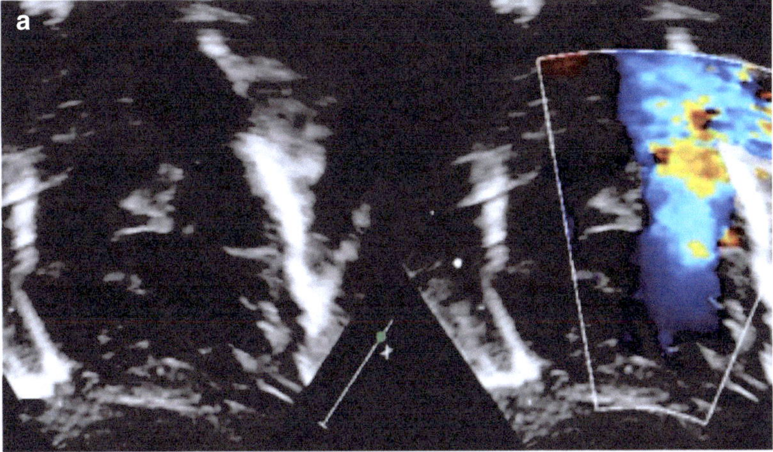

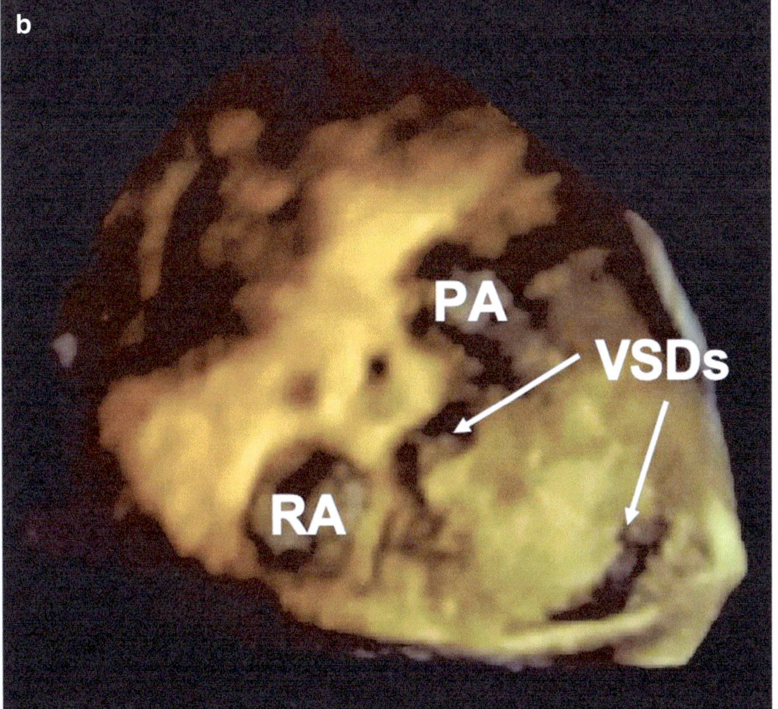

Fig. 6.3 Ventricular septal defect. (**a**) Subcostal view in double inlet left ventricle showing flow from left ventricle through an unrestricted ventricular septal defect to the outlet chamber and aorta (**b**) En face 3D echocardiography view of ventricular septal defects [pulmonary artery (PA), right atrium (RA)]

ately or severely reduced this is a risk factor for mortality [15, 16].

- Diastolic function of the ventricle and the ventriculo-ventricular interaction should also be considered, for example in those with critical aortic stenosis and a very large left ventricle with impaired function [17].
- The assessment of ventricular function can be challenging in the single ventricle setting as most tools are designed for the left ventricle or sub-pulmonary right ventricle in the biventricular setting. The mainstay tends to be subjective assessment which has limited accuracy even in those with experience [18].
- Attempts should be made to use objective measures where possible ranging from the simple e.g. m-mode, tricuspid annular planar systolic excursion and fractional area change to tissue Doppler, speckle tracking and 3D volumetric assessment [19–26].

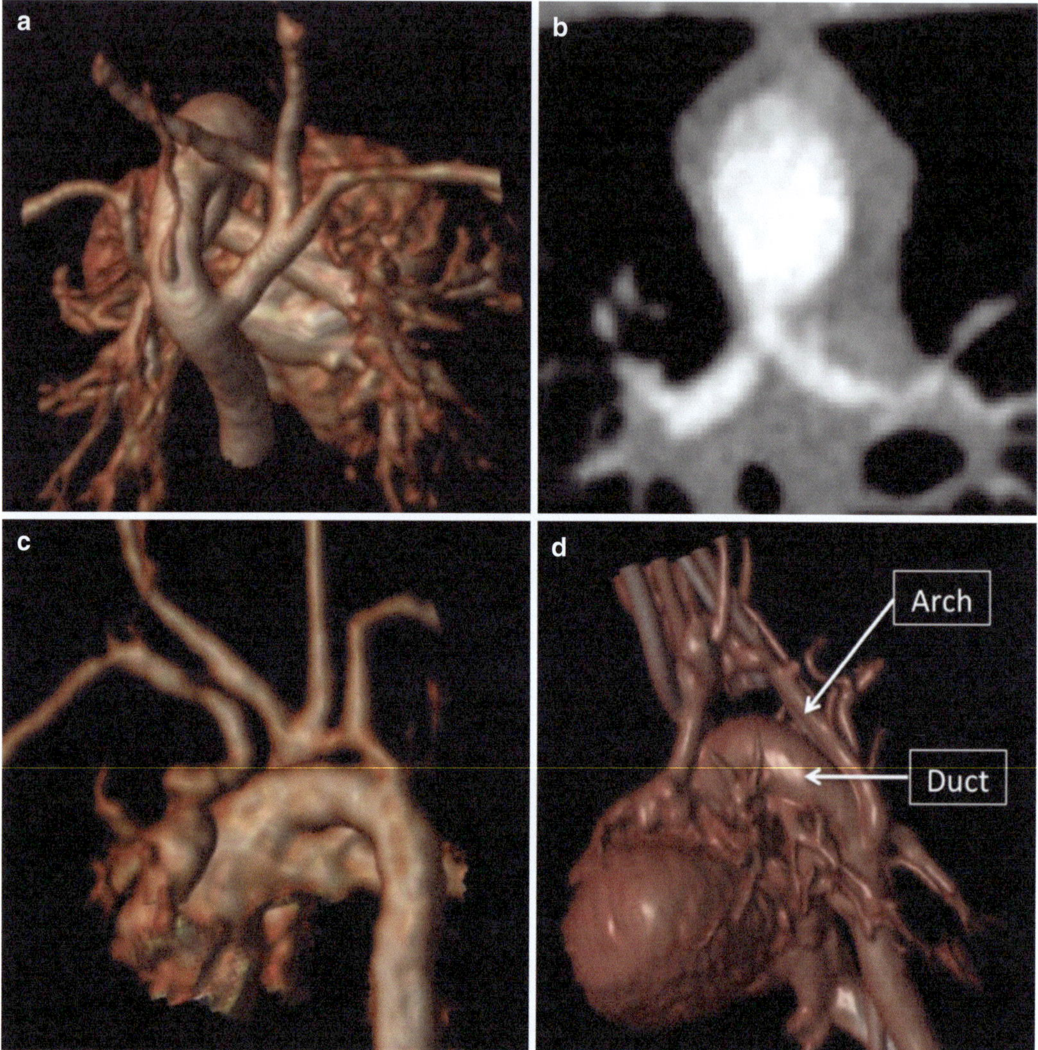

Fig. 6.4 CT and MRI imaging. (**a**) MRI showing right aortic arch with aberrant subclavian artery in a patient with hypoplastic left heart syndrome (**b**) CT scan showing hypoplastic branch pulmonary arteries (**c**) MRI showing complex aortic anatomy with coarctation and isolated left subclavian artery (**d**) CT showing extremely abnormal and tortuous aortic arch

- **Atrioventricular Valve Function:**
  - Antenatal more than mild atrioventricular regurgitation is equally worrying, and usually implies either systolic impairment or an intrinsically abnormal valve [27] and applies on the initial post-natal scan also.
  - Valve repair in the neonatal period is technically challenging, and atrioventricular valve regurgitation is associated with worse short and longer term outcome [28, 29].

- **Coronary Arteries** (Fig. 6.5)**:**
  - In ventricles with a patent inflow but obstructed outflow (e.g. pulmonary atresia with an intact ventricular septum and the mitral stenosis/aortic atresia HLHS sub-type) fistulous connections can be seen from the coronary arteries to the ventricular cavity.
  - In the most extreme form in pulmonary atresia with an intact ventricular septum

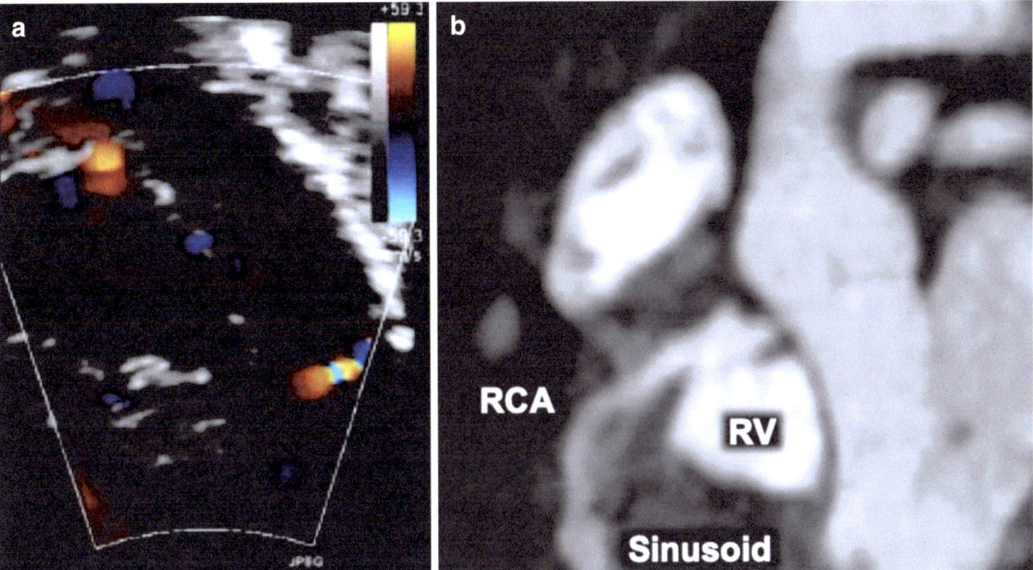

Fig. 6.5 Coronary artery abnormalities. (**a**) Coronary artery fistulae in hypoplastic left heart syndrome (**b**) Coronary atresia with right ventricular dependent coro-nary circulation in a patient with pulmonary atresia with an intact ventricular septum

there is complete coronary ostial atresia and there is a right ventricle dependent coronary circulation [30]. In this situation, coronary flow is dependent on increased right ventricular pressures, and therefore decompression of the RV can result in profound ischaemia. Even without decompression the prognosis remains poor.

- In the HLHS group the origins are usually normal [31] and the significance of fistulae is still debated. [32–34]

- **Branch Pulmonary Arteries:**
  - The Fontan circulation is dependent on passive flow through an unobstructed circuit, and therefore any intrinsic branch pulmonary artery stenosis could herald problems in the future [35].
- **Pulmonary Vascular Resistance:**
  - As well as an unobstructed circuit, low downstream pressures are required for the Fontan circuit to work [35].
  - In children who have had obstructed pulmonary venous return in utero (e.g.

obstructed TAPVD or an intact or highly restrictive atrial septum in HLHS) there may already be significant damage to the pulmonary vascular bed.
- Echocardiogram can look for signs of obstruction, but the clinical picture is also important to assess.
- Additionally, it is important to protect the pulmonary vascular bed from too much pulmonary blood flow so assessment of not only if there is not enough, but whether there is too much pulmonary blood flow is essential.

References

1. Chaosuwannakit N, Makarawate P. Diagnostic accuracy of low-dose dual-source cardiac computed tomography as compared to surgery in univentricular heart patients. J Cardiothorac Surg. 2018;13:39.
2. Lopez L, Colan SD, Frommelt PC, Ensing GJ, Kendall K, Younoszai AK, Lai WW, Geva T. Recommendations for quantification methods during the performance of a pediatric echocardiogram: a report from the pediatric measurements writing

Group of the American Society of echocardiography pediatric and congenital heart disease council. J Am Soc Echocardiogr. 2010;23:465–95.

3. Bellsham-Revell H, Masani N. Educational series in congenital heart disease: the sequential segmental approach to assessment. Echo Res Pract. 2018;6:R1–8.

4. Qureshi AM, Goldstein BH, Glatz AC, Agrawal H, Aggarwal V, Ligon RA, McCracken C, McDonnell A, Buckey TM, Whiteside W, Metcalf CM, Petit CJ. Classification scheme for ductal morphology in cyanotic patients with ductal dependent pulmonary blood flow and association with outcomes of patent ductus arteriosus stenting. Catheter Cardiovasc Interv. 2019;93:933–43.

5. Glatz JA, Tabbutt S, Gaynor JW, Rome JJ, Montenegro L, Spray TL, Rychik J. Hypoplastic left heart syndrome with atrial level restriction in the era of prenatal diagnosis. Ann Thorac Surg. 2007;84:1633–8.

6. Hosein RBM, Clarke AJB, McGuirk SP, Griselli M, Stumper O, De Giovanni JV, Barron DJ, Brawn WJ. Factors influencing early and late outcome following the Fontan procedure in the current era. The 'two commandments'?☆. Eur J Cardiothorac Surg. 2007;31:344–53.

7. Simpson JM, Miller O. Three-dimensional echocardiography in congenital heart disease. Arch Cardiovasc Dis. 2011;104:45–56.

8. Charakida M, Pushparajah K, Simpson J. 3D echocardiography in congenital heart disease: a valuable tool for the surgeon. Futur Cardiol. 2014;10:497–509.

9. Overman DM, Baffa JM, Cohen MS, Mertens L, Gremmels DB, Jegatheeswaran A, McCrindle BW, Blackstone EH, Morell VO, Caldarone C, Williams WG, Pizarro C. Unbalanced atrioventricular septal defect: definition and decision making. World J Pediatr Congenit Heart Surg. 2010;1:91–6.

10. Jegatheeswaran A, Pizarro C, Caldarone CA, Cohen MS, Baffa JM, Gremmels DB, Mertens L, Morell VO, Williams WG, Blackstone EH, McCrindle BW, Overman DM. Echocardiographic definition and surgical decision-making in unbalanced atrioventricular septal defect: a congenital heart Surgeons' Society multiinstitutional study. Circulation. 2010;122:S209–15.

11. Cohen MS, Jegatheeswaran A, Baffa JM, Gremmels DB, Overman DM, Caldarone CA, McCrindle BW, Mertens L. Echocardiographic features defining right dominant unbalanced atrioventricular septal defect: a multi-institutional congenital heart Surgeons' Society study. Circ Cardiovascular Imaging. 2013;6:508–13.

12. Rhodes LA, Colan SD, Perry SB, Jonas RA, Sanders SP. Predictors of survival in neonates with critical aortic stenosis. Circulation. 1991;84:2325–35.

13. Lofland GK, McCrindle BW, Williams WG, Blackstone EH, Tchervenkov CI, Sittiwangkul R, Jonas RA. Critical aortic stenosis in the neonate: a multi-institutional study of management, outcomes, and risk factors. Congenital heart surgeons society. J Thorac Cardiovasc Surg. 2001;121:10–27.

14. Hickey EJ, Caldarone CA, Blackstone EH, Lofland GK, Yeh T Jr, Pizarro C, Tchervenkov CI, Pigula F, Overman DM, Jacobs ML, McCrindle BW. Critical left ventricular outflow tract obstruction: the disproportionate impact of biventricular repair in borderline cases. J Thorac Cardiovasc Surg. 2007;134:1429–1437.e7.

15. Altmann K, Printz BF, Solowiejczky DE, Gersony WM, Quaegebeur J, Apfel HD. Two-dimensional echocardiographic assessment of right ventricular function as a predictor of outcome in hypoplastic left heart syndrome. Am J Cardiol. 2000;86:964–8.

16. Kulkarni A, Neugebauer R, Lo Y, Gao Q, Lamour JM, Weinstein S, Hsu DT. Outcomes and risk factors for listing for heart transplantation after the Norwood procedure: an analysis of the single ventricle reconstruction trial. J Heart Lung Transplant. 2016;35:306–11.

17. Forsha D, Li L, Joseph N, Kutty S, Friedberg MK. Association of left ventricular size with regional right ventricular mechanics in Hypoplastic left heart syndrome. Int J Cardiol. 2019;298:66–71.

18. Bellsham-Revell HR, Simpson JM, Miller OI, Bell AJ. Subjective evaluation of right ventricular systolic function in hypoplastic left heart syndrome: how accurate is it? J Am Soc Echocardiogr. 2013;26:52–6.

19. Mertens LL, Friedberg MK. Imaging the right ventricle—current state of the art. Nat Rev Cardiol. 2010;7:551–63.

20. Petko C, Möller P, Hoffmann U, Kramer H-H, Uebing A. Comprehensive evaluation of right ventricular function in children with different anatomical subtypes of hypoplastic left heart syndrome after Fontan surgery. Int J Cardiol. 2010;150:1–5.

21. Ruotsalainen HK, Bellsham-Revell HR, Bell AJ, Pihkala JI, Ojala TH, Simpson JM. Right ventricular systolic function in hypoplastic left heart syndrome: a comparison of manual and automated software to measure fractional area change. Echocardiography. 2017;34:587–93.

22. Bellsham-Revell HR, Tibby SM, Bell AJ, Miller OI, Razavi R, Greil GF, Simpson JM. Tissue Doppler time intervals and derived indices in hypoplastic left heart syndrome. Eur Heart J Cardiovasc Imaging. 2012;13:400–7.

23. Mahle WT, Coon PD, Wernovsky G, Rychik J. Quantitative echocardiographic assessment of the performance of the functionally single right ventricle after the Fontan operation. CTY. 2001;11:399–406.

24. Friedberg MK, Dragulescu A. Serial assessment of right ventricular strain in Hypoplastic left heart syndrome: deformation imaging in deformed hearts. J Am Soc Echocardiogr. 2019;32:651–4.

25. Kutty S, Graney BA, Khoo NS, Li L, Polak A, Gribben P, Hammel JM, Smallhorn JF, Danford DA. Serial assessment of right ventricular volume and function in surgically palliated hypoplastic left heart syndrome using real-time transthoracic

three-dimensional echocardiography. J Am Soc Echocardiogr. 2012;25:682–9.

26. Petko C, Hoffmann U, Möller P, Scheewe J, Kramer H-H, Uebing A. Assessment of ventricular function and Dyssynchrony before and after stage 2 palliation of Hypoplastic left heart syndrome using two-dimensional speckle tracking. Pediatr Cardiol. 2010;31:1037–42.

27. Stamm C, Anderson RH, Ho SY. The morphologically tricuspid valve in hypoplastic left heart syndrome. Eur J Cardiothorac Surg. 1997;12:587–92.

28. Mahle WT, Spray TL, Wernovsky G, Gaynor JW, Clark BJ. Survival after reconstructive surgery for Hypoplastic left heart syndrome : a 15-year experience from a single institution. Circulation. 2000;102(3):I136–41.

29. King G, Ayer J, Celermajer D, Zentner D, Justo R, Disney P, Zannino D, d'Udekem Y. Atrioventricular valve failure in Fontan palliation. J Am Coll Cardiol. 2019;73:810–22.

30. Chikkabyrappa SM, Loomba RS, Tretter JT. Pulmonary atresia with an intact ventricular septum: preoperative physiology, imaging, and management. Semin Cardiothorac Vasc Anesth. 2018;22:245–55.

31. Lloyd TR, Evans TC, Marvin WJ. Morphologic determinants of coronary blood flow in the hypoplastic left heart syndrome. Am Heart J. 1986;112:666–71.

32. O'Connor WN, Cash JB, Cottrill CM, Johnson GL, Noonan JA. Ventriculocoronary connections in hypoplastic left hearts: an autopsy microscopic study. Circulation. 1982;66:1078–86.

33. Salih C, McCarthy KP, Ho SY. The fibrous matrix of ventricular myocardium in hypoplastic left heart syndrome: a quantitative and qualitative analysis. Ann Thorac Surg. 2004;77:36–40.

34. Glatz JA, Fedderly RT, Ghanayem NS, Tweddell JS. Impact of mitral stenosis and aortic atresia on survival in Hypoplastic left heart syndrome. Ann Thorac Surg. 2008;85:2057–62.

35. Gewillig M, Brown SC. The Fontan circulation after 45 years: update in physiology. Heart. 2016;102:1081–6.

Univentricular Heart: Decision Making in the Management of the Neonate

Alvise Tosoni

Single Ventricle Physiology

The concept of single ventricle physiology differs from single ventricle anatomy, as it can apply also to some congenital lesions with 2 well-formed ventricles suitable for a biventricular repair (e.g. truncus arteriosus, interrupted aortic arch).

Conceptually single ventricle physiology is characterized by:

- Mixing of pulmonary and systemic venous returns
- One pump serving two circulations (pulmonary and systemic) in parallel
- Equal oxygen saturation in pulmonary arteries and aorta

In this model of circulation the cardiac output is the sum of pulmonary blood flow (Qp) and systemic blood flow (Qs). If there are not significant anatomic restrictions to limit flow to either circulation, what is determining the partition of cardiac output between Qp and Qs is the balance between pulmonary and systemic vascular resistance (PVR and SVR). The ideal Qp/Qs is close to 1 (i.e. Qp = Qs). This means that the single ventricle, in the best conditions, is pumping twice as much as a systemic ventricle would normally do [1] (Fig. 7.1).

During the neonatal period the hemodynamic system goes through significant adaptive changes. In the first 6–8 weeks of life, there is a fast decline in PVR [2], which leads to a change in Qp/Qs and a cascade of hemodynamic changes (Fig. 7.2):

1. As PVR drops, more flow will distribute to the pulmonary circulation, increasing Qp/Qs;
2. Total cardiac output (CO) increases in order to maintain an adequate Qs and oxygen delivery (DO_2), hence:
   (a) Net Qp increases even more, eventually leading to congestion of the lungs;
   (b) The congested lungs become less compliant, and the patient develops tachypnea and dyspnea, leading to increased oxygen consumption (VO_2);
   (c) Gas exchange can be impaired in congested lungs, leading to a decrease in $SpvO_2$;
3. The increase in total CO is achieved at the expense of ventricular volume overload and increased wall stress, which increases the workload and oxygen consumption for the single ventricle.
4. The increased workload of the single ventricle may occur in the face of an impaired coronary perfusion. In fact, the ventricular volume load increases end-diastolic pressure, while a patent ductus arteriosus (when present) may

A. Tosoni (✉)
Pediatric Intensive Care Unit, Department of Women's and Children's Health, University Hospital of Padua, Padua, Italy
e-mail: alvise.tosoni@aopd.veneto.it

P. Clift et al. (eds.), *Univentricular Congenital Heart Defects and the Fontan Circulation*,
https://doi.org/10.1007/978-3-031-36208-8_7

Normal physiology	Single-ventricle physiology
$CO \cong Qp \cong Qs$	$CO = Qp + Qs$
$SatO_2 > SpaO_2$	$SatO_2 = SpaO_2$
$SmvO_2 = SpaO_2$	$SmvO_2 < SpaO_2$
$SpvO_2 \cong SatO_2$	$SpvO_2 > SatO_2$

Fig. 7.1 Normal physiology compared to single-ventricle physiology. [*CO* cardiac output, *Qp* pulmonary blood flow, *Qs* Systemic blood flow, *SatO₂* systemic arterial oxygen saturation, *SpaO₂* oxygen saturation in the pulmonary artery, *SmvO₂* mixed venous oxygen saturation, *SpvO₂* oxygen saturation in the pulmonary veins]

result in a low systemic diastolic blood pressure, and, hence, low coronary perfusion pressure.

Arterial Oxygen Saturation in Single Ventricle Physiology

> The single ventricle physiology, in the absence of any anatomic factor limiting pulmonary blood flow, has a fragile period of compensation, which evolves to congestive heart failure and eventually shock if no actions are taken [3].

In univentricular hearts, arterial oxygen saturation (SatO₂) is not just determined by gas exchange in the lungs and ventilation/perfusion (V/Q) matching, but it is greatly influenced by the proportional admixture of pulmonary (SpvO₂) and systemic venous saturations (SvO₂) (Fig. 7.3):

$$SatO_2 = \left\{ \left[(Qp / Qs) \times SpvO_2 \right] + SvO_2 \right\} / (Qp / Qs + 1)$$

Qp/Qs at the Bedside

Since a real mixed venous saturation (SmvO₂) is not measurable, SvO₂ can be taken as a surro-gate whenever there is a central venous line (CVL) in superior vena cava proximal to any venous "mixing".

Applying Fick's principle (discounting the aliquot of dissolved oxygen):

$$Qp = VO_2 / \left[\left(SpvO_2 - SpaO_2 \right) \times \left(1.36 \times Hb \right) \right]$$

$$Qs = VO_2 / \left[\left(SatO_2 - SvO_2 \right) \times \left(1.36 \times Hb \right) \right]$$

$$Qp / Qs = \left(SatO_2 - SvO_2 \right) / \left(SpvO_2 - SpaO_2 \right)$$

Since in single ventricle physiology $SatO_2 = SpaO_2$

$$Qp / Qs = \left(SatO_2 - SvO_2 \right) / \left(\mathbf{SpvO_2} - SatO_2 \right)$$

> It is important to note that high Qp/Qs can yield higher SatO₂ despite a poor DO₂. SatO₂ alone is not a good indicator of Qp/Qs or DO₂.

While SatO₂ and SvO₂ can be measured at the bedside, SpvO₂ can only be assumed (i.e. 95%) but not measured. Calculating Qp/Qs can be clinically useful, but we need to be aware that imputing the wrong SpvO₂ value can produce a significant error in the Qp/Qs estimation [4, 5].

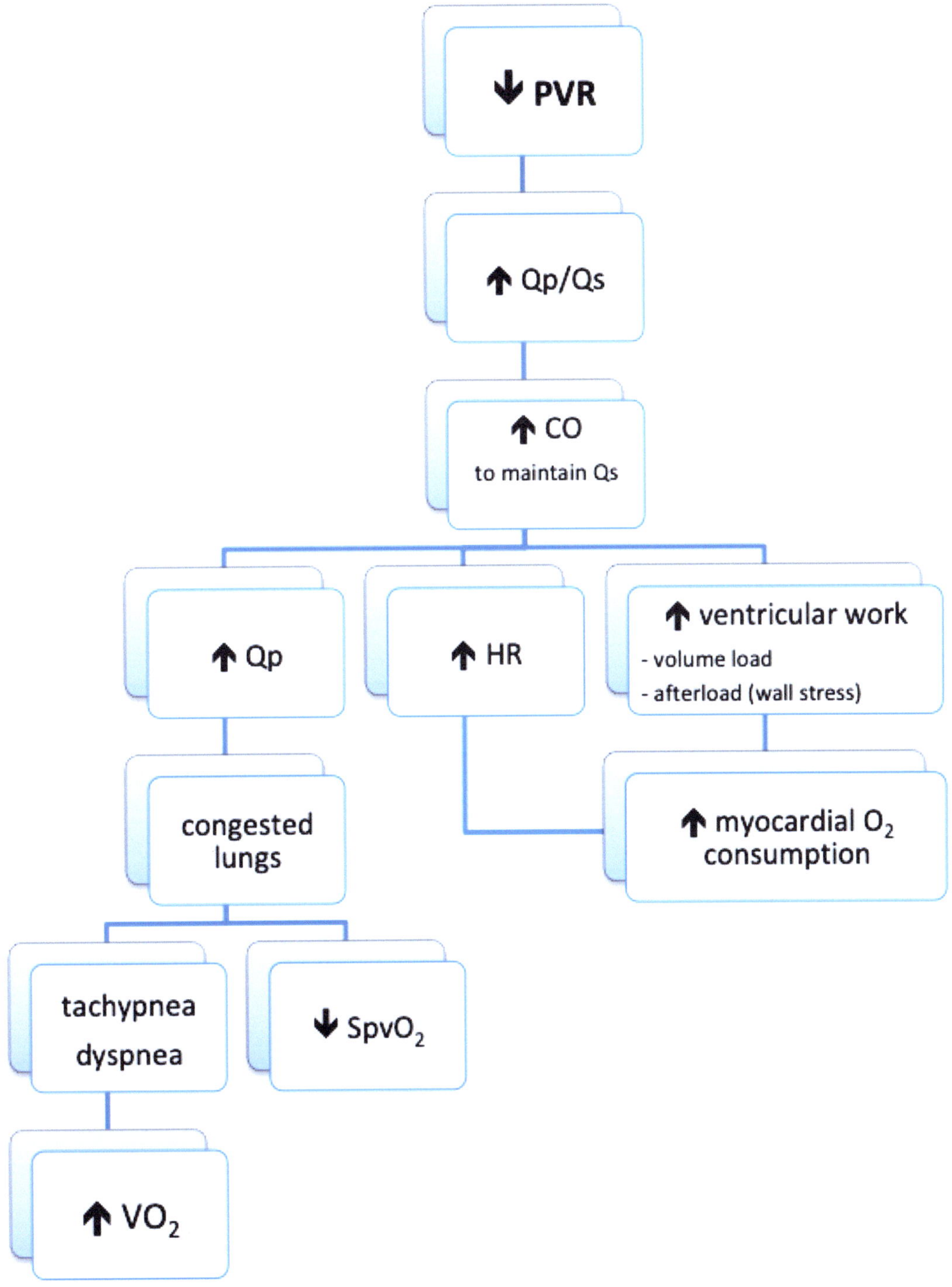

Fig. 7.2 Effects induced by PVR drop on single-ventricle hemodynamics. [*PVR* pulmonary vascular resistance, *Qp* pulmonary blood flow, *Qs* Systemic blood flow, *HR* heart rate, *SpvO₂* oxygen saturation in pulmonary veins, *VO₂* oxygen consumption]

O$_2$ saturation	determinants
SpvO$_2$	V/Q diffusion
SvO$_2$	ERO$_2$ = VO$_2$/DO$_2$ SatO$_2$
SatO$_2$	SpvO$_2$ SvO$_2$ Qp/Qs

Fig. 7.3 determinants of hemoglobin oxygen saturation. [*SpvO$_2$* oxygen saturation in the pulmonary veins, *SvO$_2$* venous oxygen saturation, *SatO$_2$* systemic arterial oxygen saturation, *ERO$_2$* oxygen extraction ratio, *DO$_2$* delivery of oxygen, *VO$_2$* oxygen consumption]

Single Ventricle Anatomy

Functionally single ventricle refers to a group of cardiac malformations where only one cardiac ventricle is available to support the circulation. Most such patients used to be described as having single ventricles, or univentricular hearts, even though almost all possess two ventricular chambers, with one being small and/or incomplete [6].

Categorization of Functionally Single Ventricle:

- Univentricular atrioventricular (AV) connections:
    (a) Double-inlet ventricle
    (b) Absent AV connection
- Biventricular AV connection with hypoplasia of one ventricle

The newborn may have either pulmonary or aortic obstruction, or bilaterally unobstructed outflows. Either the systemic or pulmonary venous return may also be abnormally connected (Fig. 7.4).

Key determinants in the first anatomic assessment are:

- Obstruction to outflows
- Obstruction to inflows
- Flow across the atrial septum
- Systemic and pulmonary venous returns
- Atrioventricular valve regurgitation

Pre-operative Management

When a prenatal diagnosis of a single ventricle malformation is present, the delivery should be carried out in a tertiary hospital with a congenital heart disease program. The newborn should be rapidly moved to the CICU or a NICU with expertise in cardiac intensive care.

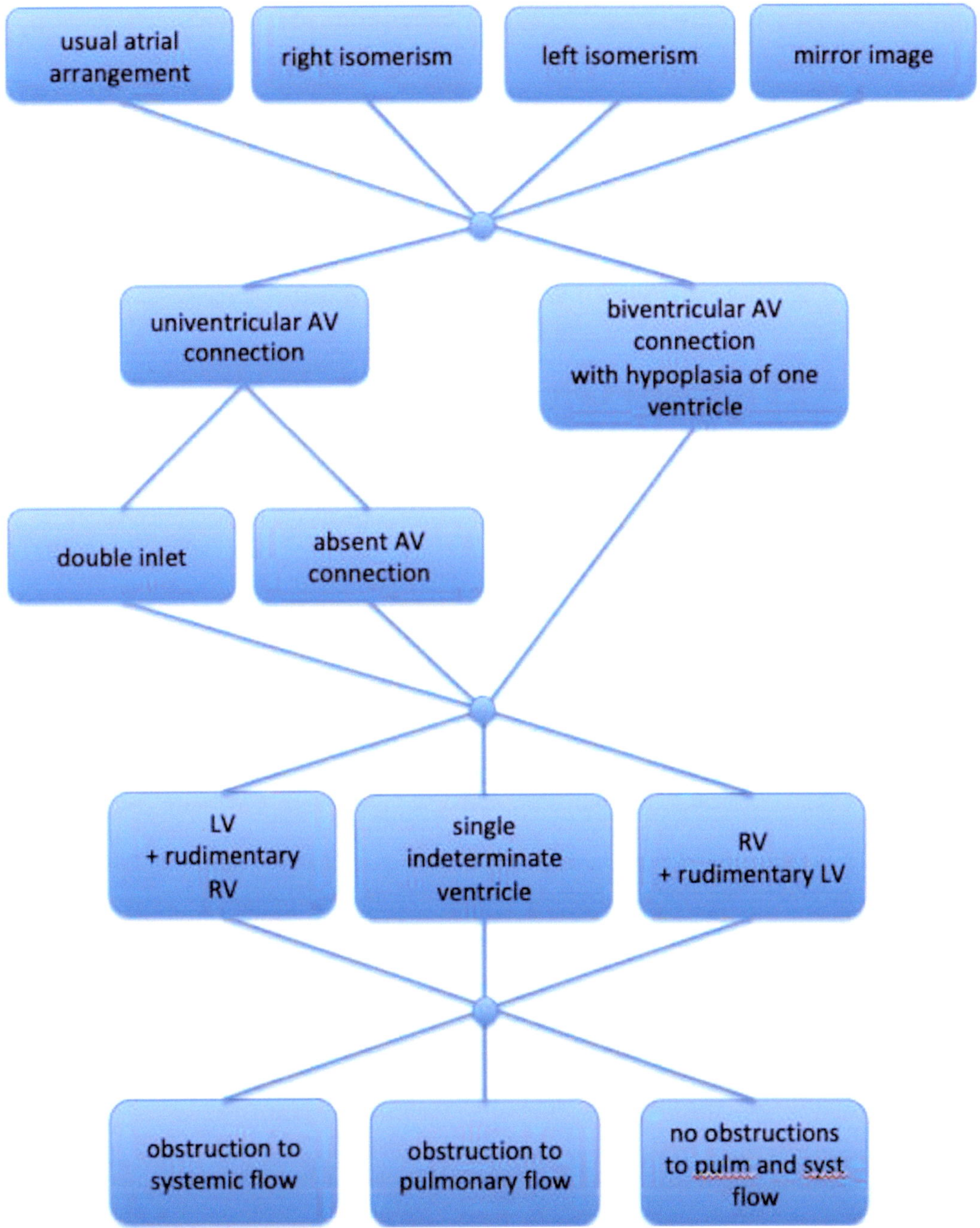

Fig. 7.4 functionally single ventricles arrangements. (Adapted from: Anderson RH, Ho SY. *Which Hearts Are Unsuitable for Biventricular Correction? Ann Thorac Surg* 66:621–6, 1998 [7])

Immediate Postnatal Care and Management

1. Place the newborn in a radiant warmer bed
2. Begin cardiac monitoring: pulse oximetry, ECG, heart rate (HR), non invasive blood pressure, respiratory rate
3. Cardiology consultation for identification of the anatomical features, which may constitute an immediate risk to the patient:
   (a) Is there a reliable source of systemic blood flow?
      - If NO: start prostaglandin E1 (PGE1) infusion
   (b) Is there a reliable source of pulmonary blood flow?
      - If NO: start PGE1 infusion
   (c) Is there any impediment to pulmonary venous return?
      - If absent left AV connection and restrictive foramen ovale: emergency atrial balloon atrioseptostomy

Non-invasive echocardiography is usually able to provide these answers; cardiac catheterization or computed tomography are rarely required.

PGE1 infusion at 5–50 ng/kg/min is usually sufficient to maintain ductus arteriosus patency. Once patency of the ductus arteriosus has been established, the dose may be titrated to the lowest effective dose to minimize side effects, including fever (14%), apnoea (12%), peripheral vasodilatation (10%), bradycardia (7%) and hypotension (4%) [8].

4. Placement of a reliable venous access: umbilical venous line (UVL) or CVL. The tip should be positioned at the atrio-caval junction to allow the measurement of SvO_2.

Pre-operative Care and Management

Primary goals are:

1. Maximization of oxygen delivery to the tissues
2. Nutrition

Maximization of Oxygen Delivery to the Tissues

Attention should be paid to the delicate and dynamic balance between PVR and SVR, requiring ongoing monitoring.

In the absence of obstructions, the relative blood flow to each circulatory component depends predominantly on the relative balance between PVR and SVR. This balance is made even more precarious when the ductus arteriosus remains patent, allowing a continuous diastolic runoff away from the systemic into the pulmonary circulation.

The presence of certain anatomic lesions, e.g. AV valve regurgitation (worsening the ventricular volume overload) and systemic outflow tract obstruction (with unobstructed pulmonary blood flow) can accelerate the progression to high Qp/Qs congestive heart failure.

Close monitoring and clinical reassessments are important to detect when the Qp/Qs balance is shifting. Initially, an increase in Qp/Qs will manifest as higher $SatO_2$ and mild tachypnea and tachycardia. As Qp/Qs keeps rising at the expense of Qs, the neonate will present signs and symptoms of congestive heart failure: tachypnea, increased work of breathing (WOB), tachycardia, poor peripheral perfusion, hepatomegaly, decreased urine output, diaphoresis, increased ERO_2 (decreased SvO_2, $SatO_2$-$SvO_2 > 30\%$) and blood lactate concentration [1, 8–10].

When these clinical signs appear, medical intervention is required (Fig. 7.5) in order to:

- Limit volume load
- Rebalance Qp/Qs acting on PVR and SVR
- Maximize DO_2 and reduce VO_2

Diuretics

An elevated Qp causes an increase in extravascular lung water (EVLW), thus reducing lung compliance and impairing gas exchange.

The use of loop-diuretics (i.e. furosemide) can relieve congestion while also helping to reduce the volume load to the single ventricle [11].

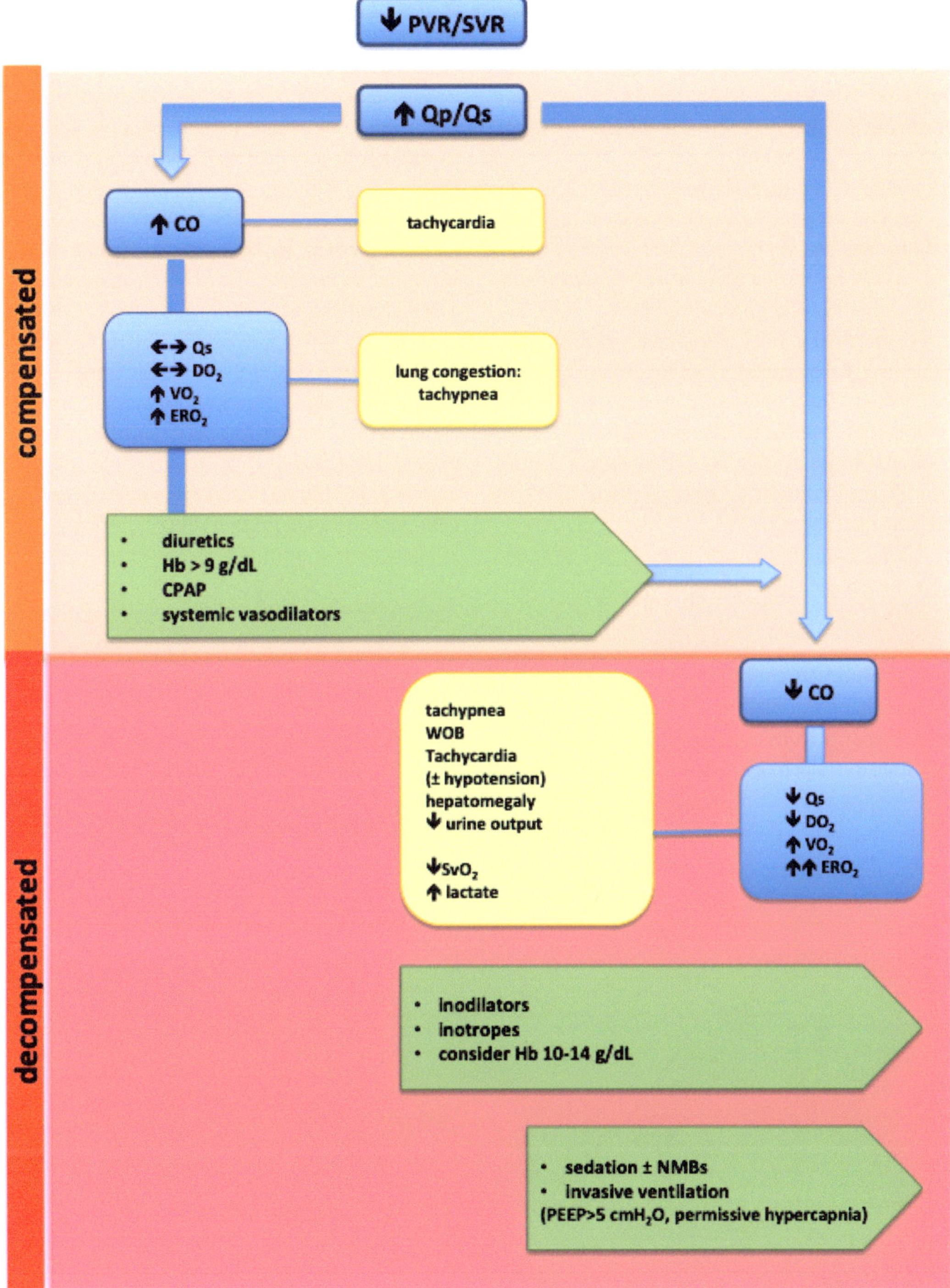

Fig. 7.5 medical interventions for high Qp/Qs

Continuous Positive Airways Pressure (CPAP)

Applying a continuous positive air pressure may improve congestive heart failure by different mechanisms [12]:

- It induces a fluid shift from the alveoli and the interstitial space to the pulmonary circulation, consequently:
  - Decreasing the amount of intrapulmonary shunting and improving $SpvO_2$;
  - Improving lung compliance and reducing tachypnea and work of breathing;
- PVR is characterized by a U-shaped relation to lung volume (the lowest PVR being at functional residual capacity, FRC) (see Fig. 7.6). CPAP could reduce Qp by pushing lung volume over the FRC [13].
- CPAP reduces the afterload of the systemic ventricle, by decreasing the transmural pressure [13].

Hemoglobin Threshold for Transfusion

The common rationale for red blood cells (RBC) transfusion is to increase DO_2. Hemoglobin is a key element of DO_2, and, potentially, the easiest to manipulate, but optimization of the other components is essential. Decision to transfuse RBC should not be taken solely based upon hemoglobin concentration.

For newborns with single ventricle physiology, who have stable hemodynamics, adequate oxygenation and normal end-organ function, RBC transfusion is not recommended if the hemoglobin concentration is >9.0 g/dL. Clinical judgment needs to be used for setting higher hemoglobin targets, e.g. in case of myocardial dysfunction and high ERO_2 [14–16].

Inotropes and Vasoactive Medications

Inotropic agents may be warranted if signs of poor cardiac output and hypoperfusion persist despite adequate evaluation of ductal patency, intracardiac mixing, intravascular volume and hemoglobin concentration [8] (Fig. 7.7).

If there is a normal/high mean arterial pressure, the best strategy is to combine inotropic support (to increase CO = Qp + Qs) and systemic vasodilatation (to favor Qs). Inodilators, e.g. milrinone and dobutamine, can achieve both these goals. Milrinone (0.35–0.75 mcg/kg/min) is preferable because it induces less sinus tachycardia than dobutamine.

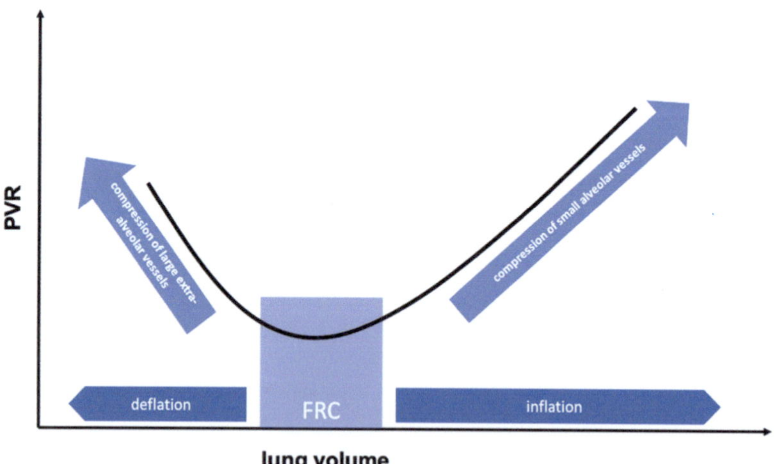

Fig. 7.6 Relationship between pulmonary vascular resistance (PVR) and lung volume. PVR is at the lowest when lung volume is at functional residual capacity (FRC). At low lung volumes, PVR rises due to the progressive compression of large extra-alveolar vessels. At high lung volumes, PVR increases due to the progressive compression of small alveolar vessels by the distending alveoli

Drug	Contractility	SVR	PVR
Adrenaline	↑	↑ - ↑↑↑	0 - ↑
Noradrenaline	0	↑↑↑	0 - ↑
Dobutamine	↑	↓	↓
Dopamine	↑	↑	0 - ↑
Milrinone	↑	↓	↓
Nitroprusside	0	↓↓	↓

Fig. 7.7 the effects of various inotropic agents on contractility, SVR and PVR

In case of hypotension, low-dose Epinephrine infusion (0.01–0.05 mcg/kg/min) should be considered in order to increase CO while maintaining an adequate organ and coronary perfusion pressure.

Sedation, Muscle Paralysis and Invasive Ventilation

In some cases, signs of inadequate DO_2 may persist despite all the aforementioned interventions, or might be precipitated by an intercurrent event (e.g. sepsis, necrotizing enterocolitis).

In these cases, a more invasive medical intervention is required: sedation and invasive mechanical ventilation. Paralysis may be used to further reduce VO_2 and take full control of the ventilation. In fact, maintaining PEEP above physiologic values and inducing a permissive hypercapnia increase PVR, favoring Qs over Qp [8].

Nutrition

Necrotizing enterocolitis (NEC) is a rare condition in term newborns, but more common in newborns with CHD, with an estimated incidence ranging from 1.6% to 9%. NEC has not been associated with increased mortality rates in infants with CHD [17].

An earlier surgical palliation may be required when non-surgical manipulations are inadequate to overcome the imbalance or prevent the need for a prolonged administration of PGE1 and the potential adverse effects and consequences associated with it.

The risk of NEC is higher in newborns with cyanotic heart defects, duct-dependent lesions, truncus arteriosus, aortopulmonary window and single ventricle physiology. Other risk factors are premature birth (<36 weeks), episodes of poor systemic perfusion, and a maximum dose of PGE1 > 50 ng/kg/minute. The pathophysiology behind NEC may be mesenteric ischemia caused by altered mesenteric blood flow and retrograde diastolic flow in the descending aorta [18].

A proper preoperative nutrition is important, as malnutrition has significant impacts on morbidity, mortality, and neurologic outcome. Nutritional goals should be a caloric intake of 110–120 kcal/kg/day, ensuring a protein intake of at least 1.5 g/kg/day to prevent negative protein balance. These goals need to be met starting enteral nutrition and/or parenteral nutrition (PN) in the first 24 h of life [17, 19–22].

Nevertheless, many clinicians are uneasy feeding patients with single ventricle physiology because of the concern for feeding intolerance and NEC. Conversely, minimal enteral nutrition (MEN, 10–20 mL/kg/day), aids in intestinal mucosa trophism and has been associated with a decreased incidence of NEC. A very recent position statement by the ESPNIC strongly supports the provision of enteral nutrition in term neonates with CHD, even with an umbilical arterial line (UAC) in place and during PGE1 infusion, with a close monitoring for clinical signs of feeding intolerance [21].

There are few published data regarding nutritional guidelines and feeding protocols in neonates with CHD. Standardized feeding protocols that include clear definitions for feeding intolerance, acceptable criteria for withholding of feeds, minimization of interruptions for routine procedures, and clear caloric goals with frequent growth assessment are likely to improve overall care [19, 21, 22].

Surgery

The goal of all initial palliative procedures is to establish [10, 23] (Fig. 7.8):

- Unobstructed pulmonary and systemic venous return
- Unobstructed systemic outflow
- Limit blood flow to the lungs, with normal pulmonary arterial pressures.

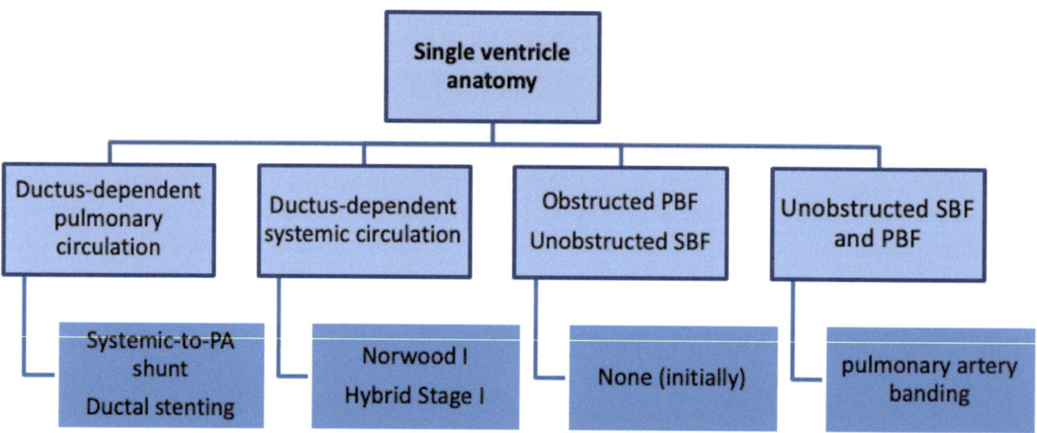

Fig. 7.8 surgical management of newborns with single ventricle anatomy. [*PBF* pulmonary blood flow, *SBF* systemic blood flow, *PA* pulmonary artery]. (Adapted from: V Yarlagadda, M Almodovar. "Perioperative care of the infant with single ventricle physiology" Current Treatment Options in Cardiovascular Medicine (2011) 13:444–455)

Bibliography

1. Mastropietro CW, Tourner SP. Parallel circulations: managing single-ventricle physiology. http://neoreviews.aappublications.org/.
2. Rudolph AM. The changes in the circulation after birth their importance in congenital heart disease. http://ahajournals.org.
3. Khairy P, Poirier N, Mercier LA. Univentricular heart. Circulation. 2007;115:800–12.
4. Nelson DP, Schwartz SM, AC C. Neonatal physiology of the functionally univentricular heart. Cardiol Young. 2004;4 Suppl 1:52–60.
5. Schwartz SM, Dent CL, Musa NL, Nelson DP. Single-ventricle physiology. Crit Care Clin. 2003;19:393–411.
6. Wilkinson JL, Anderson RH. Anatomy of functionally single ventricle. World J Pediatr Congenit Heart Surg. 2012;3:159–64. https://doi.org/10.1177/2150135111421508.
7. Anderson RH, Ho SY. Which hearts are unsuitable for biventricular correction? Ann Thorac Surg. 1998;66:621–6.
8. Graham EM, Bradley SM, Atz AM. Preoperative management of hypoplastic left heart syndrome. Expert Opin Pharmacother. 2005;6:687–93.
9. Davies R. Decision-making for surgery in the management of patients with univentricular heart. Front Pediatr. 2015;3:61. https://doi.org/10.3389/fped.2015.00061.
10. Yarlagadda V, v., Almodovar MC. Perioperative care of the infant with single ventricle physiology. Curr Treat Options Cardiovasc Med. 2011;13:444–55. https://doi.org/10.1007/s11936-011-0134-9.
11. Rossouw B. Balancing the heart and the lungs in children with large cardiac shunts emergencies in children with large cardiac shunts. CME. 2013;31:16–20.
12. Kato T. Positive airway pressure therapy for heart failure. World J Cardiol. 2014;6:1175–91. https://doi.org/10.4330/wjc.v6.i11.1175.
13. Shekerdemian L, Bohn D. Cardiovascular effects of mechanical ventilation. Arch Dis Child. 1999;80:475–80. https://doi.org/10.1136/adc.80.5.475.
14. Cholette JM, Willems A, Valentine SL, Bateman ST, Schwartz SM. Recommendations on RBC transfusion in infants and children with acquired and congenital heart disease from the pediatric critical care transfusion and anemia expertise initiative. Pediatr Crit Care Med. 2018;19:S137–48. https://doi.org/10.1097/PCC.0000000000001603.
15. Doctor A, Cholette JM, Remy KE, Argent A, Carson JL, Valentine SL, Bateman ST, Lacroix J. Recommendations on RBC transfusion in general critically ill children based on hemoglobin and/or physiologic thresholds from the pediatric critical care transfusion and anemia expertise initiative. Pediatr Crit Care Med. 2018;19:S98–S113. https://doi.org/10.1097/PCC.0000000000001590.
16. Valentine SL, Bembea MM, Muszynski JA, Cholette JM, Doctor A, Spinella PC, Steiner ME, Tucci M, Hassan NE, Parker RI, Lacroix J, Argent A, Carson JL, Remy KE, Demaret P, Emeriaud G, Kneyber MCJ, Guzzetta N, Hall MW, Macrae D, Karam O, Russell RT, Stricker PA, Vogel AM, Tasker RC, Turgeon AF, Schwartz SM, Willems A, Josephson CD, Luban NLC, Lehmann LE, Stanworth SJ, Zantek ND, Bunchman TE, Cheifetz IM, Fortenberry JD, Delaney M, van de Watering L, Robinson KA, Malone S, Steffen KM, Bateman ST. Consensus recommendations for rbc transfusion practice in critically ill children from the pediatric critical care transfusion and anemia expertise initiative. Pediatr Crit Care Med. 2018;19:884–98. https://doi.org/10.1097/PCC.0000000000001613.
17. Martini S, Beghetti I, Annunziata M, Aceti A, Galletti S, Ragni L, Donti A, Corvaglia L. Enteral nutrition in term infants with congenital heart disease: Knowledge gaps and future directions to improve clinical practice. Nutrients. 2021;13(3):932.
18. Mcelhinney DB, Hedrick HL, Bush DM, Pereira GR, Stafford PW, William GJ, Spray TL, Wernovsky G. Necrotizing enterocolitis in neonates with congenital heart disease: risk factors and outcomes. Pediatrics. 2000;106(5):1080–7.
19. Marino LV, Johnson MJ, Davies NJ, Kidd CS, Fienberg J, Richens T, Bharucha T, Beattie RM, ASE D. Improving growth of infants with congenital heart disease using a consensus-based nutritional pathway. Clin Nutr. 2020;39:2455–62. https://doi.org/10.1016/j.clnu.2019.10.031.
20. Marino LV, Johnson MJ, Hall NJ, Davies NJ, Kidd CS, Daniels ML, Robinson JE, Richens T, Bharucha T, ASE D. The development of a consensus-based nutritional pathway for infants with CHD before surgery using a modified Delphi process. Cardiol Young. 2018;28:938–48. https://doi.org/10.1017/S1047951118000549.
21. Tume LN, Valla FV, Joosten K, Jotterand Chaparro C, Latten L, Marino LV, Macleod I, Moullet C, Pathan N, Rooze S, van Rosmalen J, SCAT V. Nutritional support for children during critical illness: European Society of Pediatric and Neonatal Intensive Care (ESPNIC) metabolism, endocrine and nutrition section position statement and clinical recommendations. Intensive Care Med. 2020;46:411–25. https://doi.org/10.1007/s00134-019-05922-5.
22. Karpen HE. Nutrition in the cardiac newborns. Evidence-based nutrition guidelines for cardiac newborns. Clin Perinatol. 2016;43:131–45.
23. O'Brien P, Boisvert JT. Current management of infants and children with single ventricle anatomy. J Pediatr Nurs. 2001;16:338–50. https://doi.org/10.1053/jpdn.2001.26573.

Catheter Interventions in the Initial Palliation of Univentricular Hearts

Chetan Mehta and Oliver Stumper

Introduction

The majority of children born with univentricular hearts (UVH) depend on the ductus arteriosus to provide adequate pulmonary or systemic blood flow. Maintaining ductal patency by prostaglandin infusion is crucial for survival to intervention. Furthermore, there is the importance of complete mixing of the systemic and pulmonary venous return without obstructions.

The challenge of catheter and surgical interventions in the initial palliation of children with UVH is to bridge them over the first 3–4 months of age, until the pulmonary vascular resistance is low enough to allow the creation of a bidirectional cavopulmonary shunt. Interventional catheter techniques are increasingly being used to avoid cardio-pulmonary bypass [1].

Balloon Atrial Septostomy

An adequate atrial communication is crucial in UVH patients such as tricuspid or mitral atresia, or children with HLHS with a restrictive atrial septum [2]. Though the atrial communication may not be restrictive at birth, there is a risk that it may become so with growth of the patient. Thus, catheter balloon septostomy (Rashkind) should be performed routinely in cases with tricuspid or mitral atresia, pulmonary atresia with intact ventricular septum unsuitable for opening pulmonary valve and cases of HLHS with intact septum, which present in extremis.

Access should be via the femoral vein or umbilical vein using a 6 or 7 French sheath. Any other approach is very difficult [3]. For more than 50 years this procedure was performed with a silicone balloon catheter, which however very occasionally could rupture and thus were withdrawn from the market in early 2019. Rashkind balloon septostomy used to be a bed-side emergency procedure under ultrasound guidance, modern practice has moved towards life saving septostomy being performed in the cath-lab.

The restrictive atrial septum is crossed from the right atrium with a 4 French endhole catheter to enter the left sided pulmonary veins. The septostomy balloon is passed over a 0.018 in. guidewire and inflated within the left atrium with recommended volume of dilute contrast. Balloon inflation should be monitored on ultrasound and fluoroscopy to ensure that it is free from the mitral valve and left atrial appendage. The balloon is then pulled quickly across the atrial septum. The fibrous portion of the atrial

C. Mehta (✉) · O. Stumper
Heart Unit, Birmingham Children's Hospital, BWCH NHS Trust, Birmingham, UK
e-mail: Chetan.Mehta1@nhs.net;
Oliver.Stumper@nhs.net

© The Author(s), under exclusive license to Springer Nature Switzerland AG 2023
P. Clift et al. (eds.), *Univentricular Congenital Heart Defects and the Fontan Circulation*,
https://doi.org/10.1007/978-3-031-36208-8_8

septum is essentially torn—giving feedback to the operator and being evident on repeat ultrasound. In cases with HLHS, the left atrial cavity may be too small to accommodate a fully inflated balloon, in this scenario static balloon dilation of the atrial septum may be a better choice. In cases where the atrial septum is intact or thickened, the septum may be impossible to cross, and blade or needle septostomy may be indicated [4].

Balloon septostomy can only tear the fibrous portion of the interatrial septum. The muscular portion of the atrial septum may temporarily dilate but eventually will recoil—needing repeat intervention.

Atrial Septal Stenting

In cases with a failed septostomy or recurrent restriction across the atrial septum, there must be consideration to implant a large stent across the atrial septum providing a communication of some 7–8 mm. Such stents can be implanted via a 2 mm (6 French) sheath from the femoral vein or with a hybrid approach Fig. 8.1. It is important to centre the stent in the middle of the atrial septum to prevent embolisation. Equally, the risk of embolisation of the stent is higher in cases that have just undergone failed adequate balloon septostomy, particularly those with a large static balloon rather than a pull-back septostomy.

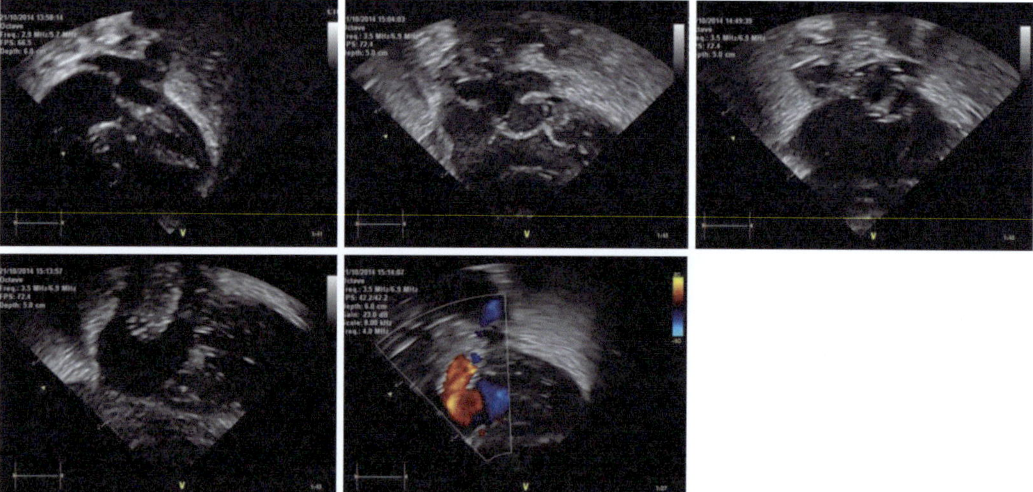

Fig. 8.1 Hybrid atrial septal stenting in hypoplastic left heart syndrome with intact atrial septum under echo guidance

Ductal stenting for Duct Dependent Pulmonary Blood Flow

In babies with tricuspid atresia and pulmonary atresia, the sole source of blood supply is via the patent ductus arteriosus. Some 80% of babies born with tricuspid atresia usually need intervention in the neonatal period. This can either be a surgical shunt or catheter ductal stenting [5].

A surgical systemic-to-pulmonary artery shunt (SPS), has provided effective palliative treatment for duct-dependent lesions for some 70 years. There have been numerous technical and post-operative management changes for shunts over the years. Nonetheless, the early and late mortality is around 10%, and morbidity after surgery is significant—even in the current era [6].

Since the mid 1990s transcatheter stenting of the ductus arteriosus in duct dependent pulmonary circulation has been performed. Initially with mixed and at times poor results [7]. Recent published series however show excellent results such that ductal stenting in a duct dependent pulmonary circulation has become an acceptable alternative, if not the treatment of first choice [8].

Detailed pre-procedural imaging involving a CT angiogram will inform about ductal anatomy and tortuosity to guide patient selection and best vascular access route. Patient selection and procedural planning is key to success. Most cases can be managed with a 1.3 mm sheath inserted into either a vein or artery, without opening the chest or the need for cardiac surgical intervention on cardiopulmonary bypass. It is important to cover the entire ductal length from the aorta to the left pulmonary artery to prevent development of stenosis on stopping the Prostaglandin infusion. In this respect, it is important to have a large enough landing zone for the pulmonary artery end of the stent. If this area is small, then significant branch pulmonary artery stenosis, and at times occlusion, may develop over time, which needs avoiding in patients on a univentricular care pathway. Alwi and colleagues reported an early mortality of 5.4% after ductal stenting with freedom from reintervention of 89% at 6 months and 55% at 12 months [9]. For patients on a univentricular care pathway, ductal patency is required for 4–6 months until conversion to a superior cavo-pulmonary anastomosis can be achieved with low risk. In a recent study on ductal stenting in univentricular hearts, 63% of patients reached stage II with no reintervention and 15.1% required catheter re-interventions [10].

Recent comparative studies between surgical shunts and catheter stenting of the ductus have been supportive of ductal stenting, with a reported reduction in hospital stay, overall mortality and morbidity and better pulmonary arterial growth [11, 12].

However, it has also become clear that the length of palliation for ductal stenting, using small diameter coronary stents, is strictly limited due to very significant tissue ingrowth. This is despite the universal use of dual-antiplatelet medications after the stent implantation. Effective palliation, without re-intervention, beyond 3–4 months remains the exception. Newer stent designs, including drug eluting stents, may address this problem.

With increasing evidence of better results of ductal stenting over a surgical shunt, the surgical approach has been adapted to create a ventricle to pulmonary artery non-valved tube to secure pulmonary blood flow. Even though this is open surgery on bypass in the neonatal period, current outcomes are promising and appear to provide longer term palliation and allow the option of addressing branch pulmonary artery stenosis at the same time [5].

Ductal stenting for Duct Dependent Systemic Blood Flow

In children with hypoplastic left heart syndrome, systemic perfusion is dependent on the adequate size of the ductus arteriosus to provide blood flow to the aorta, the head and neck vessels and the coronary arteries. At the same time the amount of blood flow to the lungs, in the setting of rapidly dropping pulmonary vascular resistance after birth, has to be limited. These requirements led to

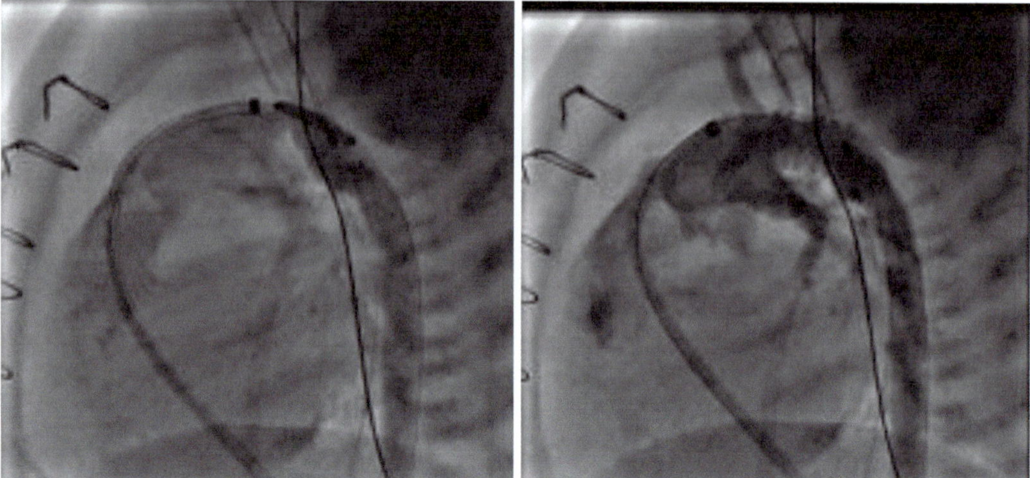

Fig. 8.2 Stenting of patent ductus arteriosus in hypoplastic left heart syndrome post bilateral PA bands

a joint surgical and catheter approach, which, in its many variations, has been termed the hybrid approach to HLHS [13, 14].

It is currently not possible to reliably limit branch pulmonary artery blood flow by transcatheter techniques. Thus, through a midline sternotomy, the surgeon places restrictive bilateral pulmonary artery bands. Ductal patency, and thus perfusion of the body, is maintained by prostaglandin infusion throughout. In some centres the systemic duct is then stented during the same procedure via a 5 French sheath inserted into the main pulmonary artery through the midline sternotomy. In other centres, bilateral pulmonary artery banding is performed as an isolated surgical procedure and the child is simply maintained on prostaglandin infusion. Balloon atrial septostomy (above) or stenting of the systemic arterial duct is then performed at a later stage. The systemic duct requires a larger stent (typically 6–8 mm) Fig. 8.2 and care must be taken not to produce severe obstruction for retrograde cerebral and coronary perfusion. If that occurs a second stent may have to be implanted to resolve the issue [15].

Only a few centres worldwide routinely perform this so-called first stage hybrid palliation for HLHS and they report excellent results. Others, who have established a high quality surgical Norwood program, have reserved the hybrid approach for extremely sick or premature babies, but have not been able to replicate these results [16].

Furthermore, despite the development of bespoke self-expandable stent systems, there remains concern about the suitability of some patients due to their aortic arch anatomy and the potential for severe retrograde aortic arch obstruction.

Management of Pulmonary Atresia with Intact Septum

Pulmonary atresia with intact ventricular septum is a common univentricular cardiac lesion, which is particularly prevalent in Eastern Asia. If the right ventricle and the tricuspid valve are of reasonable size, and there is absence of coronary sinusoids, then there is good evidence that the catheter perforation of the pulmonary valve together with sequential ballooning and possibly stenting of the arterial duct is the technique of choice to achieve best outcomes, with the majority of children eventually achieving 1.5 or biventricular repair [17].

The atretic pulmonary valve is normally perforated with either the use of a dedicated radiofrequency wire, a coronary wire used for chronic coronary vessel occlusion or with the inner core wire of a standard 0.021″ guidewire. The pulmonary valve is then dilated sequentially. Depending on the size of the right ventricle and the resultant systemic saturations after perforation and ballooning of the pulmonary valve, the arterial duct is then stented during the same procedure. A balloon septostomy is normally avoided, so as to ensure increased filling pressure to the hypertrophied right ventricle. Right ventricular growth is achieved by increasing forward flow together with the commonly observed pulmonary regurgitation.

Catheter Interventions to Augment Pulmonary Blood Flow in Fallot-Type Lesions with Univentricular Physiology

A further subset of patients suffer from functionally univentricular hearts with severely limited blood flow due to the presence of multilevel subpulmonary stenosis in the setting of unbalanced atrioventricular septal defects, ventricular imbalance, straddling atrioventricular valves or similar lesions which would make complete septation/biventricular repair a very high risk procedure with uncertain long-term outcome.

In such cases transcatheter stenting of the right ventricular outflow tract may provide excellent medium to long-term palliation at minimal risk [18]. The use of peripheral vascular stents for this indication has to be preferred above using coronary stents, due to their ability to be further dilated over time [19]. It is important to exclude patients with transposition physiology from this approach, because it could lead to a situation whereby pulmonary venous blood increasingly returns to the lungs without achieving adequate mixing and no overall rise in systemic saturations.

Catheter Interventions After Primary Surgical Palliation

Cardiac surgical palliation of univentricular hearts is well established (Chap. 4.19) but may run into difficulties before conversion to a cavo pulmonary shunt. Gore-Tex tubes (either used for systemic-to-pulmonary shunts or ventricle-to-pulmonary artery non-valved conduits) may get stenosed or simply will get too small for a growing infant. These tubes can be stented and upsized to a larger diameter [20] and branch pulmonary artery stenoses can be addressed by balloon angioplasty with good effect.

Aortic arch obstruction after surgical reconstruction is a major contributor to progressive ventricular dysfunction in the univentricular heart. Balloon angioplasty has been shown to be highly effective in addressing this problem, with a very low need for re-intervention [21].

Summary

Cardiac catheter interventions are an integral part in the acute management of the critically ill neonate with a univentricular circulation. A vast range of procedures and techniques have been developed over the past three decades, frequently replacing surgery and providing excellent low risk palliation in the staged management of univentricular hearts.

The next frontiers for catheter interventions in UVH will be the catheter creation of cavopulmonary shunts and transcatheter Fontan completion [22, 23].

References

1. Jacobs JP, Maruszewski B. Functionally Univentricular heart and the Fontan operation: lessons learned about patterns of practice and outcomes from the congenital heart surgery databases of the EACTS and STS. World J Pediatr Congenital Heart Surg. 2013;4(4):349–55.

2. Vlahos AP, Lock JE, et al. Hypoplastic left heart syndrome with intact or highly restrictive atrial septum: outcome after neonatal transcatheter atrial septostomy. Circulation. 2004;109(19):2326–30.

3. Mackie SA, Aiyagari R, Zampi JD. Balloon atrial septostomy by a right internal jugular venous approach in a newborn with hypoplastic left heart syndrome with a restrictive atrial septum. Congenit Heart Dis. 2014;9(5):E140–2.

4. Pedra CAC. Atrial septostomies. In: Urgent interventional therapies. Hoboken, NJ: Wiley; 2014. p. 253–64.

5. Rao PS. Management of congenital heart disease: state of the art—part II—cyanotic heart defects. Child Aust. 2019;6(4):54.

6. Petrucci O, O'Brien S, et al. Risk factors for mortality and morbidity after the neonatal Blalock-Taussig shunt procedure. Ann Thorac Surg. 2011;92:642–52.

7. Gibbs JL, Wren C, et al. Stenting of the arterial duct combined with banding of the pulmonary arteries and atrial septectomy or septostomy: a new approach to palliation for the hypoplastic left heart syndrome. Br Heart J. 1993;69:551–5.

8. Alwi M. Stenting the ductus arteriosus: case selection, technique and possible complications. Ann Pediatr Cardiol. 2008;1(1):38–45.

9. Alwi M, Choo KK, et al. Initial results and medium-term follow-up of stent implantation of patent ductus arteriosus in duct-dependent pulmonary circulation. J Am Coll Cardiol. 2004;44(2):438–45.

10. Celebi A, Yucel IK, et al. Stenting of the ductus arteriosus in infants with functionally univentricular heart disease and ductal-dependent pulmonary blood flow: a single-center experience. Catheter Cardiovasc Interv. 2017;89(4):699–708.

11. Bentham JR, Zava N, et al. Duct stenting versus modified Blalock Taussig shunt in neonates with duct-dependent pulmonary blood flow. Associations with clinical outcomes in a multicenter national study. Circulation. 2018;137(6):581–8.

12. Glatz A, et al. Comparison between patent ductus arteriosus stent and modified Blalock-Taussig shunt as palliation for infants with ductal-dependent pulmonary blood flow: insights from the congenital catheterization research collaborative. Circulation. 2018;137:589–601.

13. Schranz D, Bauer A, et al. Fifteen-year single center experience with the Giessen hybrid approach for hypoplastic left heart and variants: current strategies and outcomes. Pediatr Cardiol. 2015;36:365–73.

14. Galantowicz M, Cheatham JP. Lessons learned from the development of a new hybrid strategy for the management of hypoplastic left heart syndrome. Pediatr Cardiol. 2005;26:190–9.

15. Stoica SC, Philips AB, et al. The retrograde aortic arch in the hybrid approach to hypoplastic left heart syndrome. Ann Thorac Surg. 2009;88:1939–47.

16. Ohye RG, Schranz D, D'Udekem Y. Current therapy for hypoplastic left heart syndrome and related single ventricle lesions. Circulation. 2016;134:1265–79.

17. Alwi M, et al. Concomitant stenting of the patent ductus arteriosus and radiofrequency valvotomy in pulmonary atresia with intact ventricular septum and intermediate right ventricle: early in-hospital and medium-term outcomes. J Thorac Cardiovasc Surg. 2011;141:1355–61.

18. Stumper O, Ramchandani B, et al. Stenting of the right ventricular outflow tract. Heart. 2013;99:1603–8.

19. Quandt D, Ramchandani B, et al. Initial experience with the cook formula balloon expandable stent in congenital heart disease. Catheter Cardiovasc Interv. 2015;85:259–66.

20. Penford G, Quandt D, et al. Stenting and over-dilating small Gore-Tex vascular grafts in complex congenital heart disease. Catheter Cardiovasc Interv. 2018;91:71–80.

21. Chessa M, Dindar A, et al. Balloon angioplasty in infants with aortic obstruction after the modified stage I Norwood procedure. Am Heart J. 2000;140(2):227–31.

22. Sizarov A, Raimondi F, et al. Vascular anatomy in children with univentricular hearts regarding transcatheter bidirectional Glenn anastomosis. Arch Cardiovasc Dis. 2017;110:223–33.

23. Prabhu S, Anderson B, et al. A simplified technique for interventional Extracardiac Fontan. World J Pediatr Congenit Heart Surg. 2017;8(1):92–8.

Comfort Care in Patients with a Single Ventricle

9

Carolina Perez, Joanna Laddie, and Hannah Bellsham Revell

What Is Paediatric Palliative Care?

The term "palliative" is derived from the Latin word *pallium* meaning a cloak. Palliative care aims to cloak the patient's symptoms and provide comfort even when treatments aimed at cure are no longer possible. For many years palliative care has been synonymous with end of life care and in adult medicine this is generally true. However, paediatric palliative care encompasses more. The Association for Children's Palliative Care gives a definition of palliative care for children and young people with life-limiting conditions as "an active and total approach to care, embracing physical, emotional, social and spiritual elements. It focuses on enhancement of quality of life for the child and support for the family and includes the management of distressing symptoms, provision of respite and care through death and bereavement" [1].

C. Perez (✉)
Consultant in Paediatric Palliative Medicine,
Cambridge University Hospitals NHS Foundation
Trust, Cambridge, UK
e-mail: carolina.perez@nhs.net

J. Laddie
Consultant in Paediatric Palliative Medicine, Evelina
London Children Hospital, London, UK
e-mail: joanna.laddie@gstt.nhs.uk

H. B. Revell
Paediatric Cardiologist Consultant, Evelina London
Children Hospital, London, UK
e-mail: hannah.bellsham-revell@gstt.nhs.uk

Why Palliative Care Should Be Offered to Parents of Neonates with a Functional Single Ventricle?

Palliative care involvement in congenital heart disease is still relatively uncommon. In the last few decades, there has been ongoing innovation and improvement of surgical and percutaneous interventions matched with better outcomes.

In the current era, management options for HLHS include staged palliative surgery, cardiac transplantation (which is not a cure as it holds significant risk and may require secondary transplant, compassionate care without surgery and termination of pregnancy after prenatal diagnosis.

Over the last 40 years, surgical technique has evolved and these significant strides have reduced mortality. Current results show long-term survival best estimates range from 70% to 80% for 10 year survival for reconstructive surgery for HLHS in expert centres [2]. For those infants who receive a heart, the 5-year survival is approximately 70% [3].

Despite the recent NHS England Congenital Heart Disease (CHD) consultation which recommended that clinicians should use nationally approved paediatric palliative care from the point of diagnosis (including the antenatal period) for very severe forms of CHD [4], the reality is that the optimum timing for involvement of paediatric palliative care alongside other treatments with children with severe CHD is still a matter of discussion among professionals.

When making life and death decisions for an infant, parents and health professionals must consider primarily the infant's best interests [5]. When we consider a child's best interests, we tend to focus solely on the potential benefits and burdens of the proposed interventions but it is also important to consider the potential benefits and burdens of the alternatives, including the option to forgo life-prolonging interventions. Different parents and different providers, may judge the same situation very differently. To some, the benefits of prolonging life, even for a short time in the face of significant morbidity, outweigh the burdens of even significant suffering. For others, suffering is a more important goal than prolonging life. In such cases, there is often no single right answer [6].

The American Academy of Pediatrics recognises that most such decisions fall into a grey area in which several goals of care may be ethically permissible. The Academy recommends that providers seek to overrule parents only when parents make decisions that are clearly contrary to the infant's best interests. Merely disagreeing with parents' values and preferences is insufficient [7, 8].

To ensure honest communication, parents should be told of all their options in a factually accurate and non-coercive manner to make an informed decision regarding the care of their child.

It is important for families to understand that the surgery for single ventricle physiology remains palliative and not reparative and it is inevitably associated with increasing long term morbidity and mortality [9]. Indeed, all functional single ventricles have a similar long-term burden of intensive surgical and medical therapies and face uncertainty beyond the second decade of life. The overall reduced life expectancy should be addressed honestly in order to avoid false expectations.

The majority of these children will have 3 surgeries in the first 5 years of life (and some of them will not go home until the second surgery has been done). They may undergo cardiac catheterisation and interventions that might be frightening and painful for the child and may need lifelong monitoring and treatment of complications including progressive ventricular dysfunction, arrhythmia, thromboembolic disease, liver disease, renal dysfunction, protein losing enteropathy, potential need for heart transplantation and premature death [6]. Late research also highlights that there is significant risk of neurological problems, including motor delays, behavioural abnormalities, learning disabilities and other problems among survivors [10–13].

In light of the above parents must weigh the benefits and burdens of medical interventions using their own life experiences, values, and beliefs to help them choose between less than ideal options.

The need for accurate information regarding the role of palliative care requires true understanding and proficient communication skills to ensure that preconceived ideas regarding paediatric palliative care can be addressed.

A discussion of palliative treatment includes a full discussion of what parents can expect if this is the choice they make, an explanation of the therapies that can be employed to minimise their baby's suffering to ensure that they have no pain or discomfort through the dying process and to explore what is the preferred place of care/death for these families [8]. In the UK the newborn may remain in the hospital or parents may opt to take their baby home or to the hospice, depending on where they live and local services availability. Paediatric palliative care services may also help parents to talk to their other children about the current situation of the baby and will support the family after the infant passes away.

Finally, even if parents choose active treatment for their infants, the involvement of paediatric palliative care can be beneficial to ensure parallel planning. Ideally, the parallel planning process should begin at diagnosis of a life-limiting or life-threatening condition to discuss a range of potential outcome options for care when prognostication is uncertain [14].

Due to the uncertainty in the prognosis, the risk of sudden death and the long-term morbidities that these children may develop, paediatric palliative care would offer a holistic approach to care (physically, emotionally, socially and spiritually), facilitating improved symptom control and better informed decision-making, as well as allowing families to accept, plan and prepare for the possibility of death [15]. Planning for the future at times of great uncertainty has been shown to be comforting for parents and children [16].

Comfort Care Without Surgery

Paediatric palliative care teams support and manage many symptoms associated with the infant's condition in collaboration with other specialists. Paediatric palliative care teams give practical advice regarding symptoms and can provide symptom management plans (SMP) which are a step by step guide for parents and/or professionals to manage the baby's symptoms in the home or hospice.

Due to the fact that children with HLHS do not survive long once the ductus arteriosus closes, children who are not treated with surgery or medications to maintain the patency of the ductus (ie, prostaglandin) will generally pass away within the first few weeks of life. If the closure of the duct is within the first days of life, the baby may not need any medications to relieve their symptoms. However, if the infant lives longer, we may see more symptoms secondary to the low output.

Symptoms which may need to be treated are:

- Dyspnoea:
  - Dyspnoea is defined as the sense that breathing has become unpleasant. The baby may develop breathing difficulties as they weaken at the end of life or secondary to fluid accumulation in the lungs.
  - Firstly, non-pharmacological interventions should be explored. Sometimes having a fan in the room to gently blow air across the infant's face may be helpful. Repositioning the baby, in a more straight and upright position, can help to reduce "splinting" from the diaphragm.
  - Oxygen is a potent dilator of the pulmonary circulation. High concentrations of oxygen for patients with single ventricle conditions with unrestricted pulmonary blood (such as HLHS) can cause an increase in pulmonary blood flow leading to pulmonary overcirculation. This in turn leads to further pulmonary congestion and also steals from the systemic circulation leading to systemic underperfusion (e.g. gut ischaemia) and also potentially myocardial ischaemia from coronary steal. Therefore, the need for oxygen should be considered very carefully and should be discontinued if there is no apparent symptomatic benefit.
  - The most common pharmacological measures used to manage dyspnoea are (see Table 9.1):
- Benzodiazepines:
  - Benzodiazepines act on receptors in higher centres to relieve anxiety, and on receptors in the respiratory centre.
  - Buccal midazolam is particularly useful for intervening in acute episodes of dyspnoea.

Table 9.1 Symptoms more common found in infants with HLH and medications used to relieve these symptoms (Reference: Oxford Specialist Handbook in Paediatrics. Pediatric Palliative Medicine. Second edition. Richard D. W. Hain. Satbir Singh Jassal)

Drug	Symptom	Dose and route
Midazolam	Dyspnoea/agitation	Buccal 25 μg/kg/dose Enteral 50 μg/kg/dose Sc or iv 0.5–1 mg/24 h
Morphine	Dyspnoea	30–50% of the dose used for pain
Furosemide	Dyspnoea secondary to pulmonary oedema	Enteral 0.5–2 mg/kg/dose
Chloral hydrate	Agitation	Enteral 30 mg/kg/dose
Paracetamol	Pain	Enteral 10–15 mg/kg/dose
Morphine	Pain	Enteral 50 μg/kg/dose Sc or iv 5 μg/kg/h

- Opioids:
  - There are opioid receptors in the respiratory and cough centres of the brain.
  - Morphine is well established as a first-line strong opioid. Morphine is believed to reduce air hunger and reduce respiratory rate.
  - Morphine is commonly used as background treatment for dyspnoea.
  - Doses of opioid effective for dyspnoea are 30–50% of those required for pain.
  - A single-dose trial of low dose morphine can be very effective in assessing and treating potential dyspnea when the situation is unclear.
- Agitation:
  - The baby may become agitated due to their breathing or other reasons for which babies become irritable. Treatable causes should be addressed (such as constipation, pain, or hunger). The infant may respond to consoling measures such as rocking, patting and cuddling. If however, the baby cannot be settled, they might benefit from a short acting benzodiazepine such as buccal midazolam.
- Oedema/Swelling of body tissues:
  - The baby may have generalised soft tissue swelling of their face and body due to accumulation of fluid. This in itself does not require treatment unless it causes them distress or discomfort.
  - If the fluid accumulates within their lungs it may worsen their breathing. In this scenario the infant may benefit from diuretics such as furosemide. However, diuretics should be considered carefully as they may worsen renal impairment due to decreased cardiac output.
- Feeding intolerance:
  - Infants are given comfort through oral feeding. However, if the baby is breathless or has episodes of intestinal ischemia, they may have difficulties tolerating their feeds, which may cause them to vomit or be in pain. If this is the case, reducing the feed volume, rate or frequency, switching to rehydration solution or having a period of gut rest should be considered.
- Ischaemic pain:
  - Secondary to steal from the systemic circulation and low cardiac output the infant may have episodes of cardiac and/or intestinal ischaemic pain (see feeding intolerance).
  - Mild pain is often effectively managed with paracetamol or ibuprofen.
  - As pain becomes more severe and these medications become less effective, opioids such as morphine become the standard therapy.

Should the baby have difficulty tolerating medications or should his/her symptoms become more challenging to treat enterally, a continuous subcutaneous (SC) or intravenous (IV) infusion should be considered.

Conclusion

Advances in the diagnosis and treatment of patients with single ventricle conditions have increased survival into childhood. However, these treatments are still deemed to be palliative. Due to uncertainty about outcomes, discussion with parents should be open. Parents must be fully supported throughout the decision-making process, and this support must continue regardless of the choices they make. Paediatric palliative care works holistically by offering support with complex symptom management, advance care planning and end of life care. This support is best given in the context of early referral to explore parallel planning and to be able to make plans with the family to encompass hoping for the best and planning for the worst.

References

1. Chambers L, Dodd W, McCulloch R, et al. A guide to the development of Children's palliative care services. 3rd ed. Bristol: Association for Children's Palliative Care; 2009.

2. Pundi KN, Johnson JN, Dearani JA, et al. 40-year follow-up after the Fontan operation: long-term outcomes of 1,052 patients. J Am Coll Cardiol. 2015;66(15):1700–10.

3. Chrisant MRK, Naftel DC, Drummond-Webb J, et al. Fate of infants with hypoplastic left heart syndrome listed for cardiac transplantation: a multi-center study. J Heart Lung Transplant. 2005;24(5):576–82.

4. NHS England. Proposed congenital heart disease standards and service specifications: a consultation. Leeds: NHS England; 2014. https://www.engage.england.nhs.uk/consultation/congenital-heart-disease-standards/user_uploads/chd-consultation-doc-fin.pdf.

5. American Academy of Pediatrics Committee on Bioethics. Guidelines on foregoing life-sustaining medical treatment. Pediatrics. 1994;93(3):532–6.

6. Kon AA, et al. Parental refusal of surgery in an infant with tricuspid atresia. Pediatrics. 2016;138(5):e20161730. https://doi.org/10.1542/peds.2016-1730.

7. Mercurio MR, Maxwell MA, Mears BJ, Ross LF, Silber TJ. American Academy of Pediatrics policy statements on bioethics: summaries and commentaries: part 2. Pediatr Rev. 2008;29(3):e15–22.

8. Kon AA. Healthcare providers must offer palliative treatment to parents of neonates with hypoplastic left heart syndrome. Arch Pediatr Adolesc Med. 2008;162(9):844–8.

9. Kempny A, et al. Single-ventricle physiology in the UK: an ongoing challenge of growing numbers and of growing complexity of congenital heart disease. Heart. 2014;100(17):1315–6.

10. Hangge PT, Cnota JF, Woo JG, et al. Microcephaly is associated with early adverse neurologic outcomes in hypoplastic left heart syndrome. Pediatr Res. 2013;74(1):61–7.

11. Sarajuuri A, Jokinen E, Puosi R, et al. Neurodevelopment in children with hypoplastic left heart syndrome. J Pediatr. 2010;157(3):414–420.e4.

12. Tabbutt S, Nord AS, Jarvik GP, et al. Neurodevelopmental outcomes after staged palliation for hypoplastic left heart syndrome. Pediatrics. 2008;121(3):476–83.

13. Bordacova L, Docolomanska D, Masura J. Neuropsychological outcome in children with hypoplastic left heart syndrome. Bratisl Lek Listy (Tlacene Vyd). 2007;108(4–5):203–6.

14. Sidgwick P, et al. Parallel planning and the paediatric critical care patient. Arch Dis Child. 2019;104:994–7.

15. Bertaud S, et al. The importance of early involvement of paediatric palliative care for patients with severe congenital heart disease. Arch Dis Child. 2016;101:984–7.

16. Widdas D, McNamara K, Edwards F. A core care pathway for children with life-limiting and life-threatening conditions. 3rd ed. Bristol: Together for Short Lives; 2013.

Part III

Surgical Management

History of the Fontan Surgical Procedure

10

Paul Clift

Congenital heart disease has long been recognised as a cause of infant mortality. Historical accounts of postmortem studies in the eighteenth and nineteenth centuries give detailed anatomical descriptions of cardiac anomalies. Whilst the cause of cyanosis remained a subject of debate, in many of these individuals it was accepted that it was related to a cardiac malformation.

In the 1850s, Peacock published a series of cases of children with cardiac malformations, in which there was in effect a single ventricle [1]. He speculated that there was cessation of cardiac development at certain stages of embryological life, with the right or left heart structures failing to develop. In other cases, he describes normal atrial and atrioventricular development but failure of normal ventricular septation and arterial development. We recognise his descriptions as cases of pulmonary atresia with intact septum, hypoplastic left heart, and double inlet left ventricle with transposition and pulmonary stenosis.

Several case series up to the early 1900s described the various types of single ventricle anatomy, including a chapter in the 1936 Maude Abbotts' Atlas of Congenital Heart Disease [2]. All recognised the lack of treatment options and dire prognosis, with survival to adult life very rarely reported. The importance of the degree of

pulmonary stenosis was recognised around this time, focusing on the fact that additional blood flow to the lungs may improve the degree of cyanosis and lead to improved survival.

Blalock's shunt operation was pivotal in the development of surgical palliation of the single ventricle. The recognition that certain forms of cyanotic heart disease were associated with poor pulmonary circulation and that the formation of the subclavian to pulmonary artery shunt was effective and safe [3] opened the road for the development of congenital cardiac surgery. Whilst the concept of cardiopulmonary bypass was described by several authors [4–6], it was not until 1953 when John Gibbons successfully closed an atrial septal defect using cardiopulmonary bypass, demonstrating that intra-cardiac repair was feasible [7]. A modified version of his technique was used by John Kirklin and colleagues, who developed the cardiac surgical programme at the Mayo clinic [8].

Investigators used animal models to understand whether the right ventricle was essential for driving the pulmonary circulation. Cautery of the right ventricular free wall in dogs rendered it non-functional, with minimal incremental increases in venous pressure, demonstrating that survival without a right ventricular impulse was possible [9, 10]. Anastomosis of the right atrial appendage to the main pulmonary artery in dogs proved feasible [11] and complete bypass of the right heart by means of a superior caval

P. Clift (✉)
Adult Congenital Heart Disease Unit, Queen Elizabeth Hospital, Birmingham, UK
e-mail: pclift@nhs.net

anastomosis to the right pulmonary artery [12] and inferior caval anastomosis to the left atrium was shown to be survivable, both acutely and with a long-term survival of several years in dogs [13–16]. Glenn described the successful anastomosis of the superior vena cava to the disconnected right pulmonary in dogs [17] and, later, in a 7 year old with a univentricular heart [18]. Following this publication, the procedure became widely known as the Glenn procedure. Subsequent publications testified to its safety and durability in the palliation of single ventricle circulations [19–21].

Fontan had attempted complete right heart bypass unsuccessfully in animals prior to performing the procedure that bears his name in a young woman with tricuspid atresia. Following a second successful procedure performed in 1970, he published his cases in Thorax in 1971 [22], and the era of the Fontan palliation of the single ventricle circulation had begun. Rapidly, the concept of right heart bypass became adopted and modified, evolving into the staged palliation that is performed today, i.e. the lateral tunnel [23] or extra cardiac conduit total cavopulmonary anastomosis [24]. Nowadays, most patients undergoing Fontan palliation are expected to survive to adult life.

The Fontan circulation is the unnatural evolution of the single ventricle anatomy, developed through physiological experimentation and surgical innovation, driven by the poor prognosis of this condition and the desire to improve the lives of these patients. It has created a new physiology that challenges us to develop innovative therapies to overcome complications, prolong life and improve the quality of life of our patients.

References

1. Peacock TB. Malformations consisting in arrest of development ocurring at an early period of foetal life. In: On malformations of the human heart, etc: with original cases and illustrations. London: John Churchill and Sons; 1866. p. 14–32.
2. Abbott M. Atlas of congenital heart disease. New York Heart Association, New York; 1936.
3. Taussig H, Blalock A. Surgery of congenital heart disease. Br Med J. 1947;2(4524):462.
4. Gibbon JH Jr, et al. The closure of interventricular septal defects in dogs during open cardiotomy with the maintenance of the cardiorespiratory functions by a pump-oxygenator. J Thorac Surg. 1954;28(3):235–40.
5. Amosov NM, et al. Preliminary experience with the use of artificial circulation in cardiac surgery. Vestn Khir Im I I Grek. 1961;86:10–20.
6. Senning A. Extracorporeal circulation combined with hypothermia. Acta Chir Scand. 1954;107(5):516–24.
7. Kurusz M. May 6, 1953: the untold story. ASAIO J. 2012;58(1):2–5.
8. Kirklin JW, et al. Studies in extracorporeal circulation. I. Applicability of Gibbon-type pump-oxygenator to human intracardiac surgery: 40 cases. Ann Surg. 1956;144(1):2–8.
9. Starr I, Jeffers W, Meade R. The absence of conspicuous increments of venous pressure after severe damage to the right ventricle of the dog, with a discussion of the relation between clinical congestive failure and heart disease. Am Heart J. 1943;26(3):291–301.
10. Bakos ACP. The question of the function of the right ventricular myocardium: an experimental study. Circulation. 1950;1(4):724–32.
11. Rodbard S, Wagner D. By-passing the right ventricle. Proc Soc Exp Biol Med. 1949;71:69–70.
12. Carlon CA, Mondini PG, De Marchi R. Surgical treatment of some cardiovascular diseases. J Int Coll Surg. 1951;16(1):1–11.
13. Robicsek F, et al. New surgical method in the therapy of congenital cardiac defects with decreased pulmonary circulation (pulmonary circulation with evasion of the right side of the heart). Magy Tud. 1957;8(1–2):79–82.
14. Robicsek F, et al. Complete bypass of the right heart. Am Heart J. 1963;66(6):792–7.
15. Robicsek F, Sanger PW, Gallucci V. Long term complete circulatory exclusion of the right side of the heart: hemodynamic observations. Am J Cardiol. 1966;18(6):867–75.
16. Robicsek F, et al. Observations following four years of complete circulatory exclusion of the right heart. Ann Thorac Surg. 1969;8(6):530–6.
17. Glenn W, Patino J. Circulatory by-pass of the right heart. 1. Preliminary observations on the direct delivery of vena caval blood into the pulmonary arterial circulation. Azygous vein-pulmonary artery shunt. Yale J Biol Med. 1954;27:147–51.
18. Glenn WWL. Circulatory bypass of the right side of the heart. N Engl J Med. 1958;259(3):117–20.
19. Azzolina G, Eufrate S, Pensa P. Tricuspid atresia: experience in surgical management with a modified cavopulmonary anastomosis. Thorax. 1972;27(1):111–5.
20. di Carlo D, et al. The role of cava-pulmonary (Glenn) anastomosis in the palliative treatment of congenital heart disease. J Thorac Cardiovasc Surg. 1982;83(3):437–42.

21. Kopf GS, et al. Thirty-year follow-up of superior vena cava-pulmonary artery (Glenn) shunts. J Thorac Cardiovasc Surg. 1990;100(5):662–71.
22. Fontan F, Baudet E. Surgical repair of tricuspid atresia. Thorax. 1971;26(3):240–8.
23. de Leval MR, et al. Total cavopulmonary connection: a logical alternative to atriopulmonary connection for complex Fontan operations. Experimental studies and early clinical experience. J Thorac Cardiovasc Surg. 1988;96(5):682–95.
24. Marcelletti C, et al. Inferior vena cava-pulmonary artery extracardiac conduit. A new form of right heart bypass. J Thorac Cardiovasc Surg. 1990;100(2):228–32.

Early Modifications of Fontan Surgery and Evolution of the Total Cavo-Pulmonary Connection (TCPC)

11

Phil Botha

Although the initial report by Fontan and Baudet described a "Surgical repair of tricuspid atresia", the limitations of the atriopulmonary connection soon became apparent to both the authors and others adopting this technique [1]. This led to a refinement of indications and exclusion criteria, the so-called "ten commandments" of the Fontan circulation [2]. Although the original concept was for the right atrium to become the pump driving pulmonary blood flow, it became clear that the circulation could not only function without a pump, but that the distending atrium becomes non-functional and served as a nidus for arrhythmia and thrombosis. The procedure therefore underwent successive refinements to reduce energy loss and as a result, saw improvements not only in short- and long-term outcomes but also in applicability to different anatomic substrates.

Problems and Modifications of the Atriopulmonary Fontan

In the report by Fontan, homograft valves were placed at both the inferior caval/right atrial junction and to connect the atrial appendage to the proximal right pulmonary artery in two of three patients. This approach was adopted as a result of unsuccessful experiments in dogs, which were thought to be the result of inadequate contractility of the non-hypertrophied normal right atrium, and in the absence of a valve, reflux of blood into the inferior vena cava with atrial contraction. Several problems with this approach became apparent, most notably the availability of suitable homografts, and their tendency to obstruction and thrombosis. Kreutzer reported in 1973 the direct anastomosis of the right atrium to the pulmonary artery and with no valve placed at the IVC, completely avoided the need for a homograft (Fig. 11.1a) [3]. Bjork described an alternative of patch or conduit connection of the right atrium to the right ventricle. By 1980, the indication for the Fontan operation had expanded to several variants of single functional ventricle anatomy beyond tricuspid atresia using these techniques [9].

Comparing the results of 100 patients that underwent repair of tricuspid atresia in 1983 Fontan and colleagues found a greater proportion of asymptomatic patients and higher postoperative exercise capacity in patients repaired using an aortic valve homograft [10]. In some patients in the series, a Dacron non valved conduit was interposed between the right atrium and right ventricular outlet chamber in VA concordance. Catheterisation of patients following AP Fontan however failed to show a significant step-up from systemic venous pressure to the pulmonary

P. Botha (✉)
Department of Cardiac Surgery, Birmingham Children's Hospital, Birmingham, UK
e-mail: p.botha@nhs.net

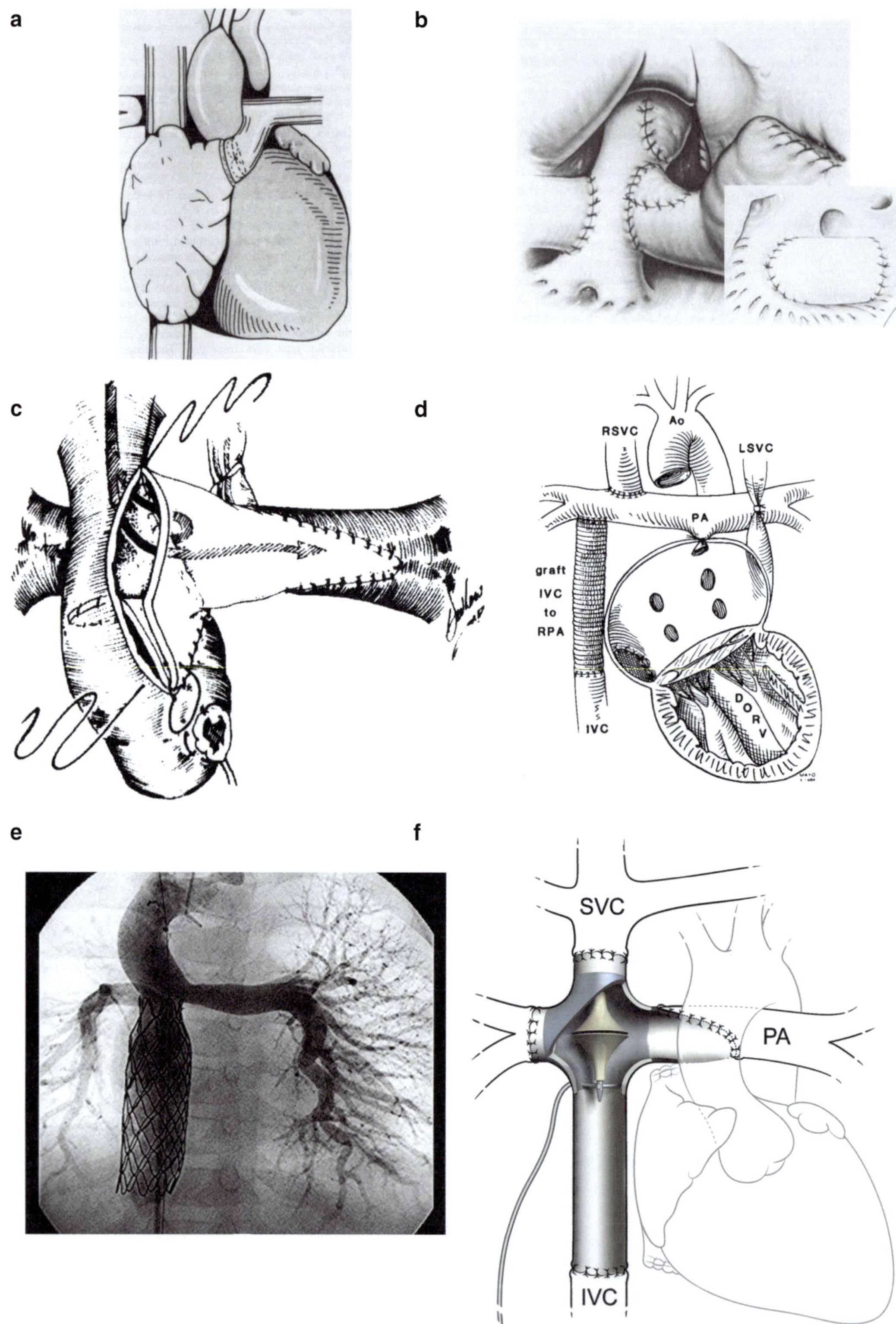

Fig. 11.1 Fontan modifications and evolution. (**a**) Kreutzer modification of the Atriopulmonary Fontan [3]. (**b**) Lateral tunnel TCPC—inset shows tubular baffle joining IVC to SVC orifice within RA [4]. (**c**) Hemi-Fontan [5]. (**d**) Extracardiac conduit TCPC [6]. (**e**) Transcatheter Fontan completion using covered stent [7]. (**f**) Mechanically assisted cavopulmonary connection (conceptual) [8]. Images reproduced with permission from original publications as referenced

arteries in the long term, calling to question the utility of the right atrium as a pump. Dilation of the atrium led to arrhythmia and thrombus formation with detrimental impact on long term pulmonary vascular resistance as a result of thrombo-embolism.

Lateral tunnel Fontan

The total cavopulmonary connection (TCPC) was popularised by a report from De Leval and colleagues, showing reduced energy loss through a lateral atrial baffle connecting the IVC directly to the RPA, excluding most of the right atrium [4]. Although this approach had been reported earlier by Puga and colleagues to achieve TCPC in complex venous anatomy [11], the sound physiological reasoning by De Leval inspired a rapid transition away from the atriopulmonary connection internationally (Fig. 11.2).

In De Leval's description, the lateral tunnel TCPC was achieved by dividing the SVC above the junction to the right atrium and anastomosing it end-to-side to the superior aspect of the Right pulmonary artery (Fig. 11.1b). The residual SVC attached to the right atrium is anastomosed to the inferior aspect of the RPA, with patch enlargement to the same size as the IVC. A popular alternative technique has been the hemi-Fontan, in which the SVC is anastomosed side-to side to the RPA, and the entire cavo-atrial junction roofed over with an allograft patch, closing off the opening to the right atrium [5] (Fig. 11.1c). This facilitates staged completion of the TCPC, at which time the patch is partially removed and the IVC joined to the SVC within the right atrium using a tubularised baffle of expanded polytetrafluoroethylene (PTFE) or pericardium. This lateral tunnel thus forms the Fontan pathway partially of the lateral/posterior wall of the right atrium, and partially of baffle material. This excludes the majority of the atrium from the effects of pulmonary arterial pressure. As the tunnel is constructed partially of autologous tissue that can grow with the child, Fontan completion can theoretically be undertaken earlier in life, reducing the duration of cardiac volume loading and desaturation. In

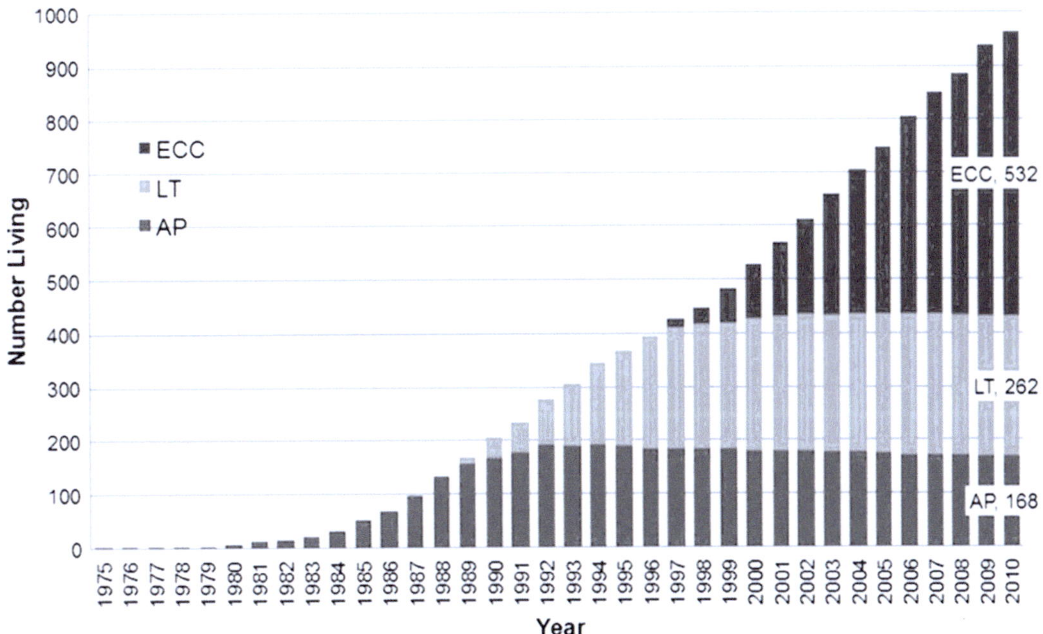

Fig. 11.2 Distribution of the techniques used in the growing population of Fontan patients alive in Australia and New Zealand. AP indicates atriopulmonary connection; ECC, extracardiac conduit; and LT, lateral tunnel. Reproduced with permission from d'Udekem et al., Circulation 2014 [12]

the Australia and New Zealand Fontan registry, the median time of Lateral tunnel Fontan completion has been 3.8 years as opposed to 4.8 years for the extracardiac Fontan [12], although several reports have demonstrated the feasibility of earlier Fontan completion with extracardiac conduits [13].

One disadvantage of the lateral tunnel approach is the requirement for both cardiopulmonary bypass and aortic cross-clamping. Although superior to the atrio-pulmonary Fontan in respect of energy loss, concerns have been raised that the intra-cardiac suture lines and dilation of the right atrial wall forming part of the pathway may predispose to a higher incidence of arrhythmia in the long term. Several large single-centre and registry publications have found this not to be the case [14, 15].

Extracardiac Conduit Fontan

Most registries now demonstrate the prevalent approach to creating a TCPC to be the extracardiac conduit [12, 16]. First described by Humes and colleagues to facilitate the creation of a Fontan circulation in patients with Heterotaxy [6], the technique was further popularised by Marcelletti and colleagues for other indications [17] (Fig. 11.1d). PTFE has replaced Dacron as the most widely used conduit for this purpose, due to a lower rate of thrombotic/obstructive complications and re-intervention [18]. The procedure can be completed using CPB and without aortic cross-clamping, but also without the use of CPB. The degree of offset between the junction of the superior vena cava and the conduit anastomosis to the RPA has been studied extensively in computational fluid dynamics models and also in vivo using MRI [19, 20]. To date, these studies have suggested that maximal energetic efficiency and hepatic flow distribution could be achieved by individualising the design of the pathway in a patient-specific manner, although this remains to be proven in the clinical setting. Modifications of the extracardiac conduit pathway may be required

in patients with heterotaxy and abnormal venous connections. These include a partially intracardiac conduit pathway, conduit placement to the left of the atrium, or alternatively, a left-sided lateral tunnel [21, 22].

Fenestration

The relative merits of a fenestration decompressing the Fontan pathway into the atrium has remained the topic of considerable debate. Laks described the use of an adjustable snare to regulate the fenestration flow in the early postoperative period, and the so-called partial Fontan [23]. The associated reduction in central venous pressure and increase in preload (at the expense of desaturation), can increase cardiac output early post procedure and has been reported to reduce the duration of pleural drainage in some series and a randomised controlled trial in low risk Fontan candidates [24]. Several institutions have however abandoned routine fenestration, choosing only to fenestrate if the early haemodynamics show a trans-pulmonary gradient greater than 12 mmHg or PA pressure greater than 18 mmHg [25]. The presence of a fenestration has been correlated with an increased need for post-operative intervention, typically transcatheter device closure, and due to a risk of paradoxical embolisation, most would recommend anticoagulation with Warfarin or Aspirin.

Cardiopulmonary Bypass

Several institutions have demonstrated the feasibility of Fontan completion without the need for CPB [25]. The use of a direct shunt during anastomosis and judicious use of volume expansion and inotropy allow the procedure to be undertaken safely without the need for extracorporeal circulation. Duration of chest tube drainage and other early post-operative outcomes were similar in patients without CPB [26].

Transcatheter Fontan

A further approach to avoid the need for CPB (and surgery altogether), is transcatheter Fontan completion. Although this has not gained widespread use, the connection at the second stage palliation can be created such that a covered stent can be placed from the IVC to the RPA/SVC connection [7] (Fig. 11.1e), or a large fenestration closed using an occluder device. This requires more extensive surgical preparation at the time of the superior cavopulmonary connection. As only small numbers of this procedure have been reported, feasibility in a wider population of anatomical substrates and superiority over conventional surgical approaches remain unproven.

Y-graft Fontan

As the nearest clinically applicable approximation of the Optiflo configuration [27], Y-graft Fontan connection has been pursued by some institutions to optimise energetics and hepatic flow distribution. It appears that a custom-made area-preserving graft is required [28], as commercially available bifurcating grafts have not shown energetic benefits in vivo [29]. Although hepatic flow distribution appears to be improved with the Y-graft, concerns remain over a greater potential for thrombotic complications in the smaller limbs of a bifurcating graft.

Powered TCPC

Ultimately the use of mechanical assistance in the cavo-pulmonary circuit seems like the necessary next step to improve energetics and reduce the incidence of the long-term complications of the Fontan circulation. A pulsatile ventricular assist device has been used successfully in a single reported case to bridge a patient with failing Fontan physiology to transplantation by supporting the right side [30]. Rodefeld and colleagues have demonstrated the feasibility in vitro of an impeller within the circuit that remains non-

obstructive to flow when non-functional [8] (Fig. 11.1f). Although existing continuous flow assist devices have proven feasible in fluid dynamics models, until recently, the absence of suitable animal models for testing these modalities have been a major impediment to the progress of their development [31].

References

1. Fontan F, Baudet E. Surgical repair of tricuspid atresia. Thorax. 1971;26:240–8.
2. Choussat A, Fontan F, Besse P. Selection criteria for Fontan's procedure. In: Anderson RH, Shinebourne EA, editors. Pediatric cardiology. Churchill Livingstone; 1978. p. 559–5.
3. Kreutzer G, Galíndez E, Bono H, De Palma C, Laura JP. An operation for the correction of tricuspid atresia. J Thorac Cardiovasc Surg. 1973;66:613–21.
4. de Leval MR, Kilner P, Gewillig M, Bull C. Total cavopulmonary connection: a logical alternative to atriopulmonary connection for complex Fontan operations. Experimental studies and early clinical experience. J Thorac Cardiovasc Surg. 1988;96:682–95.
5. Norwood WI, Jacobs ML, Murphy JD. Fontan procedure for hypoplastic left heart syndrome. Ann Thorac Surg. 1992;54:1025–30.
6. Humes RA, Feldt RH, Porter CJ, Julsrud PR, Puga FJ, Danielson GK. The modified Fontan operation for asplenia and polysplenia syndromes. J Thorac Cardiovasc Surg. 1988;96:212–8.
7. Galantowicz M, Cheatham JP. Fontan completion without surgery. Semin Thorac Cardiovasc Surg Pediatr Card Surg Annu. 2004;7:48–55.
8. Rodefeld MD, Marsden A, Figliola R, Jonas T, Neary M, Giridharan GA. Cavopulmonary assist: long-term reversal of the Fontan paradox. J Thorac Cardiovasc Surg. 2019;158:1627–36.
9. Marcelletti C, Mazzera E, Olthof H, Sebel PS, Düren DR, Losekoot TG, Becker AE. Fontan's operation: an expanded horizon. J Thorac Cardiovasc Surg. 1980;80:764–9.
10. Fontan F, Deville C, Quaegebeur J, Ottenkamp J, Sourdille N, Choussat A, Brom GA. Repair of tricuspid atresia in 100 patients. J Thorac Cardiovasc Surg. 1983;85:647–60.
11. Puga FJ, Chiavarelli M, Hagler DJ. Modifications of the Fontan operation applicable to patients with left atrioventricular valve atresia or single atrioventricular valve. Circulation. 1987;76:III53–60.
12. d'Udekem Y, Iyengar AJ, Galati JC, et al. Redefining expectations of long-term survival after the Fontan procedure: twenty-five years of follow-up from the entire population of Australia and New Zealand. Circulation. 2014;130:S32–8.

13. Ota N, Fujimoto Y, Murata M, Tosaka Y, Ide Y, Tachi M, Ito H, Sugimoto A, Sakamoto K. Impact of postoperative hemodynamics in patients with functional single ventricle undergoing Fontan completion before weighing 10 kg. Ann Thorac Surg. 2012;94:1570–7.
14. Lasa JJ, Glatz AC, Daga A, Shah M. Prevalence of arrhythmias late after the Fontan operation. Am J Cardiol. 2014;113:1184–8.
15. Balaji S, Daga A, Bradley DJ, et al. An international multicenter study comparing arrhythmia prevalence between the intracardiac lateral tunnel and the extracardiac conduit type of Fontan operations. J Thorac Cardiovasc Surg. 2014;148:576–81.
16. Jacobs JP, Maruszewski B. Functionally univentricular heart and the fontan operation: lessons learned about patterns of practice and outcomes from the congenital heart surgery databases of the European association for cardio-thoracic surgery and the society of thoracic surgeons. World J Pediatr Congenit Heart Surg. 2013;4:349–55.
17. Marcelletti C, Corno A, Giannico S, Marino B. Inferior vena cava-pulmonary artery extracardiac conduit. A new form of right heart bypass. J Thorac Cardiovasc Surg. 1990;100:228–32.
18. van Brakel TJ, Schoof PH, de Roo F, Nikkels PGJ, Evens FCM, Haas F. High incidence of Dacron conduit stenosis for extracardiac Fontan procedure. J Thorac Cardiovasc Surg. 2014;147:1568–72.
19. Masters JC, Ketner M, Bleiweis MS, Mill M, Yoganathan A, Lucas CL. The effect of incorporating vessel compliance in a computational model of blood flow in a total cavopulmonary connection (TCPC) with caval centerline offset. J Biomech Eng. 2004;126:709–13.
20. Tang E, Restrepo M, Haggerty CM, Mirabella L, Bethel J, Whitehead KK, Fogel MA, Yoganathan AP. Geometric characterization of patient-specific total cavopulmonary connections and its relationship to hemodynamics. JACC Cardiovasc Imaging. 2014;7:215–24.
21. Michielon G, Gharagozloo F, Julsrud PR, Danielson GK, Puga FJ. Modified Fontan operation in the presence of anomalies of systemic and pulmonary venous connection. Circulation. 1993;88:II141–8.
22. Kanter KR. Alternative techniques for the Fontan operation, vol. 19. Operative Techniques; 2014. p. 64–79.
23. Laks H, Pearl JM, Haas GS, Drinkwater DC, Milgalter E, Jarmakani JM, Isabel-Jones J, George BL, Williams RG. Partial Fontan: advantages of an adjustable interatrial communication. Ann Thorac Surg. 1991;52(5):1084–95.
24. Lemler MS, Scott WA, Leonard SR, Stromberg D, Ramaciotti C. Fenestration improves clinical outcome of the fontan procedure: a prospective, randomized study. Circulation. 2002;105:207–12.
25. Petrossian E, Reddy VM, Collins KK, et al. The extracardiac conduit Fontan operation using minimal approach extracorporeal circulation: early and midterm outcomes. J Thorac Cardiovasc Surg. 2006;132:1054–63.
26. McCammond AN, Kuo K, Parikh VN, Abdullah K, Balise R, Hanley FL, Roth SJ. Early outcomes after extracardiac conduit Fontan operation without cardiopulmonary bypass. Pediatr Cardiol. 2012;33:1078–85.
27. Soerensen DD, Pekkan K, de Zelicourt D, Sharma S, Kanter K, Fogel M, Yoganathan AP. Introduction of a new optimized total cavopulmonary connection. Ann Thorac Surg. 2007;83:2182–90.
28. Yang W, Chan FP, Reddy VM, Marsden AL, Feinstein JA. Flow simulations and validation for the first cohort of patients undergoing the Y-graft Fontan procedure. J Thorac Cardiovasc Surg. 2015;149:247–55.
29. Trusty PM, Wei Z, Sales M, Kanter KR, Fogel MA, Yoganathan AP, Slesnick TC. Y-graft modification to the Fontan procedure: increasingly balanced flow over time. J Thorac Cardiovasc Surg. 2019;159:652–61. https://doi.org/10.1016/j.jtcvs.2019.06.063.
30. Prêtre R, Häussler A, Bettex D, Genoni M. Right-sided Univentricular cardiac assistance in a failing Fontan circulation. Ann Thorac Surg. 2008;86:1018–20.
31. Van Puyvelde J, Rega F, Minami T, Claus P, Cools B, Gewillig M, Meyns B. Creation of the Fontan circulation in sheep: a survival model. Interact Cardiovasc Thorac Surg. 2019;29:15–21.

Staged Approach to Total Cavo-Pulmonary Connection

12

Matteo Ponzoni and Massimo A. Padalino

Introduction

The cavo-pulmonary connection, commonly known as Fontan circulation, was first reported in 1972 by Fontan and Baudet [1]. Fontan later stated in the so-called "ten commandments" [2], two fundamental requirements to achieve the Fontan circulation are a preserved ventricular function and a low pulmonary vascular resistance (<4 WU*m^2). In the absence of a subpulmonary ventricle, the only propulsive force to ensure pulmonary blood flow is the "Fontan paradox", i.e. an unphysiological pressure gradient between the caval district and the pulmonary arteries [3].

Neonatal pulmonary vascular bed immaturity is the main reason why a one-stage early completion of the Fontan circulation is not feasible. Since months are required for the pulmonary vascular resistance to gradually decrease [4], intermediate surgical steps are usually necessary to achieve a balanced circulation in newborns with a functionally single-ventricle. This is the concept of a staged Fontan completion [5], that has the following objectives:

1. Balance the systemic and pulmonary circulation, in order to achieve a satisfactory systemic oxygenation and organ perfusion.
2. Correct any obstruction to systemic outflow, protecting the single ventricle from pressure overload.
3. Avoid pulmonary overcirculation and progressive vascular disease, allowing physiological maturation of the pulmonary vascular bed.
4. Guarantee adequate mixing of systemic and pulmonary venous blood at atrial level.
5. Lessen the impact of preload mismatch at each stage of the palliation, minimizing acute changes in ventricular volume and diastolic dysfunction.

Since its adoption, the staged approach allowed a significant reduction in operative mortality from 16% to 7% [5], which nowadays has further improved, reaching values <2% in recent series [6, 7].

First Stage of Palliation

The first stage of palliation is usually carried out in the first days or weeks of life, and the surgical strategy depends on the physiopathological profile of the patient, according to their underlying cardiac defect:

M. Ponzoni · M. A. Padalino (✉)
Pediatric and Congenital Cardiac Surgery Unit, Department of Cardio-thoracic and Vascular Sciences, and Public Health, University of Padua, Padua, Italy
e-mail: massimo.padalino@unipd.it

- **Pulmonary under circulation** (Qp/Qs <1): systemic-to-pulmonary artery shunt.
- **Pulmonary over circulation** (Qp/Qs >1): pulmonary artery banding.
- **Systemic outflow obstruction**: Damus-Kaye-Stansel (DKS) or Norwood operations.

Systemic-to-Pulmonary Artery Shunt

In case of inadequate (low) pulmonary blood flow, or a ductal-dependent pulmonary flow, infusion of prostaglandin E1 is indicated. Common side-effects include hypotension, apneas, hyperthermia, seizures and the persistent risk of ductal occlusion [8] or necrotizing enterocolitis [9], factors that limit the long-term use of prostaglandins. Ductal stenting with a pre-mounted coronary stent is currently commonly used as an alternative, avoiding intravenous prostaglandin E infusion over several weeks [10]. Since the first report in 1992 by Gibbs et al. [11], this technique has been refined, proving its non-inferiority to surgery [12]. However, the anatomical complexity of ductal morphologies may complicate this procedure, which still has a relatively long learning-curve. Thus, a durable surgical systemic-to-pulmonary artery shunt is often considered the definitive palliative treatment of this condition. Many techniques have been implemented through the decades:

- **Classic Blalock-Taussig-Thomas shunt** (1945): termino-lateral anastomosis between the divided left subclavian artery and the left pulmonary artery (Fig. 12.1a) [13].
- **Central shunts**: anastomosis between the descending aorta and the left pulmonary artery

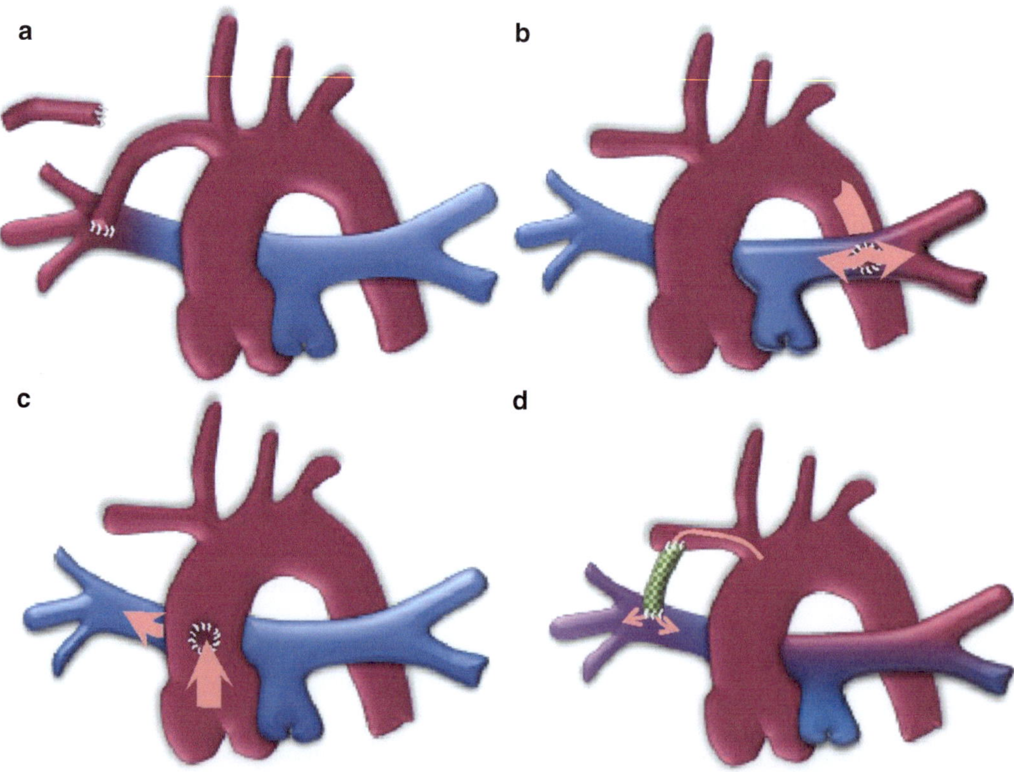

Fig. 12.1 Shunts for augmenting pulmonary blood flow. (**a**) the original Blalock Taussig shunt, with division of the subclavian artery and end-to-side anastomosis to the pulmonary artery. (**b**) descending aorta to left pulmonary artery (Potts) shunt. (**c**) Ascending aorta to right pulmonary artery shunt. (**d**) modified Blalock-Taussig shunt, using a PTFE tube

(Potts shunt, 1946, Fig. 12.1b) or between the ascending aorta and the right pulmonary artery (Waterston shunt, 1962, Fig. 12.1c) [14, 15].

- **Modified Blalock-Taussig-Thomas shunt** (1962): interposition of a PTFE conduit 3–3.5 mm diameter (according to newborn's weight) between the right or left subclavian artery and the ipsilateral pulmonary artery (Fig. 12.1d) [16].

Due to reported low incidence of early shunt complications, low in-hospital mortality [17] and relatively low surgical complexity, the modified Blalock-Taussig-Thomas shunt is the most adopted worldwide. It can be accomplished through either a lateral thoracotomy or median sternotomy, without the need of cardio-pulmonary bypass.

Pulmonary Artery Banding

Firstly described by Muller and Danimann in 1951 in a infant with a large ventricular septal defect [18], this technique consists in the placement of a Teflon or other synthetic material tape around the main pulmonary trunk, which is tightened in order to achieve a pulmonary artery pressure of about 50% or less of the systemic pressure, an increase of 5–10 mmHg in systolic blood pressure and a reduction in systemic oxygenation to 80–85% [19]. The Trusler formula (22 mm + 1 mm/kg for single-ventricle lesions) has classically been adopted to guide the optimal band length determination [20].

The procedure is usually accomplished through a median sternotomy (although a thoracotomy approach is feasible), without cardio-pulmonary bypass, often under trans-esophageal echocardiographic guidance. Care must be taken in:

- Positioning the band, which must not be too proximal, in order to avoid pulmonary valve distortion;

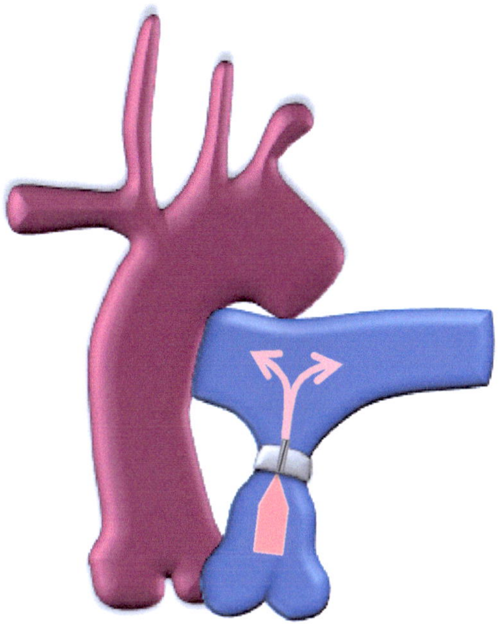

Fig. 12.2 Pulmonary artery band. A pulmonary artery band is used to restrict blood flow to the lungs and protect the pulmonary circulation from developing pulmonary vascular disease

- Fixing the band to the adventitia of the pulmonary artery to prevent distal migration of the band, that may cause distortion of the pulmonary artery branches (Fig. 12.2).

Damus-Kaye-Stansel and Norwood Operations

When a systemic outflow tract obstruction is present, pulmonary artery banding for prevention of pulmonary over circulation is contraindicated, because of the consistent risk of pressure overload for the single-ventricle, which will inexorably result in hypertrophic myocardial response and systemic outflow tract obstruction, leading to diastolic dysfunction and congestive heart failure.

Thus, the Damus-Kaye-Stanseel [21–23] and Norwood operations [24] have been proposed to palliate this clinical scenario in the neonatal period. Common aspects of these techniques are:

- Division of main pulmonary trunk, with distal portion closed using a patch.
- Latero-lateral anastomosis of the ascending aorta to the proximal pulmonary artery.
- Atrial septostomy, to achieve complete blood mixing at atrial level.
- Controlled pulmonary antegrade flow through a modified Blalock-Taussig-Thomas shunt or a right ventricle-to-pulmonary artery PTFE shunt ("Sano modified shunt") [25], of 4–6 mm of diameter.

The main difference between the Damus-Kaye-Stansel and Norwood operations is the extensive aortic arch reconstruction and augmentation by means of a homograft patch in the Norwood operation, originally described as a physiologic repair for hypoplastic left heart syndrome with aortic atresia [24].

The physiological basis of these two techniques is to allow flow into the systemic circulation bypassing the systemic flow obstruction, and to create a novel and modulated source of pulmonary flow through a systemic-to-pulmonary artery shunt. These procedures are carried out through a median sternotomy approach, on cardiopulmonary bypass, and require a period of deep hypothermic systemic circulatory arrest or antegrade selective cerebral perfusion for the Norwood operation.

The perioperative period after the first stage palliation is usually characterized by unstable hemodynamics, and the clinical goal is to achieve a crucial balance between the systemic and pulmonary circulations. Infusion of inotropic drugs is often necessary to support the function of the single ventricle, while mechanical ventilation is carefully adjusted to modulate pulmonary vascular resistance, which may vary acutely and dramatically in the postoperative period. Adequate anticoagulation is warranted to prevent shunt thrombosis and ensure adequate flow through the shunt. The ideal arterial blood gas analysis after this first stage of palliation includes a CO_2 concentration of about 40–45 mmHg, O_2 concentration of about 35–40 mmHg, O_2 saturation of 75–80%, a normal lactate concentration (that reflects satisfactory organ perfusion), and a blood pH close to 7.4. If the patient is hyper-ventilated, pulmonary vascular resistance may fall acutely and pulmonary overflow with systemic low flow will occur; in this case, the neonate has typically good oxygenation parameters but a progressive circulatory collapse. On the other hand, if the patient is under-ventilated, pulmonary vascular resistance increases, leading to pulmonary low flow and systemic overflow; this clinical scenario presents with initial hemodynamic stability in a desaturated patient. Judicious postoperative management of mechanical ventilation is thus mandatory, together with pharmacological modulation of systemic vascular resistance by means of vasoconstrictor or vasodilator drugs [26–28].

Second Stage of Palliation

Critical drawbacks of the first stage of palliation are:

- A state of chronic desaturation, because of complete mixing of pulmonary and systemic venous return;
- Chronic volume overload of the single-ventricle, which supports both the pulmonary and systemic circulation.

The second stage of palliation is usually performed in early infancy, at 3–9 months of age, according to the clinical settings (i.e. body weight, arterial oxygen saturation, hemodynamics), after pulmonary vascular resistances have fallen to normal levels. Its basic principle is to divert half of the systemic venous drainage, i.e. superior vena cava return, directly to the pulmonary vascular bed [29]. This produces two main effects:

- Improved systemic oxygenation, by reducing the amount of desaturated blood that mixes with oxygenated blood at atrial level;
- Reduced overload of the single-ventricle, by draining one half of the systemic venous return into the pulmonary bed, bypassing the single-ventricle and improving ventricular energetics [30].

This concept was originally described by Glenn et al. in 1958 [29], who performed a direct termino-terminal anastomosis between the transected superior vena cava and the divided right pulmonary artery, also known as the Classic Glenn shunt (Fig. 12.3a). This procedure includes the separation of the right and left pulmonary arterial branches, which receive different amounts of blood, predisposing to asymmetrical development of the arterial pulmonary vasculature. To minimize this problem, refinements were made to the original technique, resulting in the **bidirectional cavo-pulmonary connection,** also known as **Bidirectional Glenn Shunt** (BDG), in which the superior vena cava is anastomosed terminal-laterally to the right pulmonary artery, without interruption of the main pulmonary branches (Fig. 12.3b) [31].

Another variant is the **Hemi-Fontan procedure**, first described by Norwood and Jacobs in 1988 [5], in which the superior vena cava-right atrium continuity is kept intact, while superior systemic venous drainage is baffled to the pulmonary arteries through an ingenious anastomosis, which involves the inferior-lateral aspect of the superior vena cava, the roof of the right atrium, the inferior border of the right pulmonary artery, and a prosthetic patch (Fig. 12.3c).

All these procedures are usually performed through a median sternotomy, on cardiopulmonary bypass with bicaval venous cannulation, and usually on a beating heart. An exception to this is the Hemi-Fontan procedure, which requires aortic cross-clamping and cardioplegic arrest. However, most surgeons prefer to adopt the BDG procedure for the second stage of palliation, because of a reported similar medium-term survival, lower surgical complexity and postoperative complication rates compared to the Hemi-Fontan procedure [32].

The debate is still open regarding the ligation (or not) of a previous systemic-to-pulmonary artery shunt at the time of the second stage palliation. Not ligating the shunt may guarantee better growth of pulmonary vasculature, providing an antegrade and pulsatile pulmonary blood flow [33]. Despite comparable medium-term outcomes, a patent systemic-to-pulmonary artery shunt may prolong hospital stay and pleural effusions [34]. However, a final decision can be made intraoperatively, based on:

- invasively assessed superior vena cava and atrial pressures,
- whether pulmonary arteries growth need to be promoted, or
- whether post-procedural O_2 saturations remain low despite a satisfactory technical result and preoperative hemodynamics.

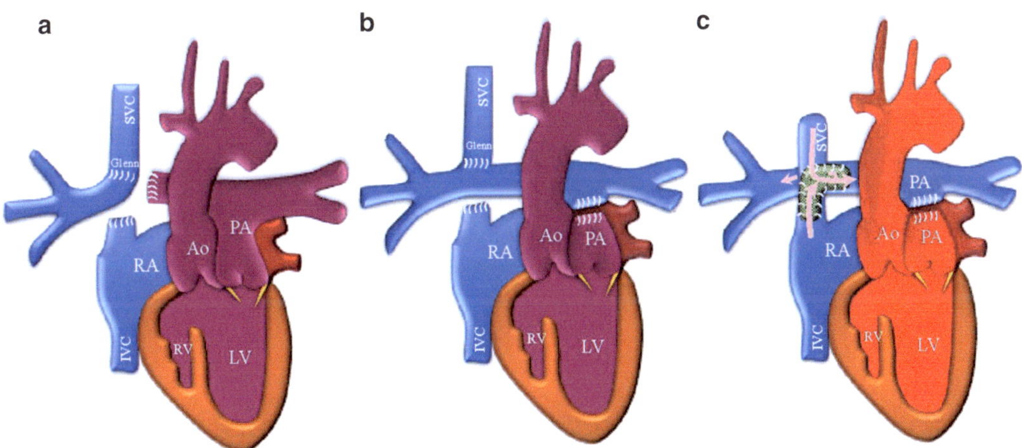

Fig. 12.3 (**a**) classical Glenn shunt, with the superior vena cava (SVC) connected to a divided right pulmonary artery, and antegrade flow to the left pulmonary artery from the ventricle. (**b**), bidirectional Glenn shunt, with termino-lateral anastomosis of the SVC to the right pulmonary artery, which is connected to the left pulmonary artery. For this shunt to work efficiently, the pulmonary arteries should not receive antegrade flow from the systemic ventricle, which would compete with the Glenn shunt. (**c**) a baffle is used to connect the superior vena cava to the right pulmonary artery

The appropriate timing of second stage palliation is still a matter of debate [35]. Preoperative imaging (2-dimensional echocardiography, cardiac catheterization, cardiac magnetic resonance and/or CT) is applied to evaluate whether the patient who has survived first stage of palliation fulfills required hemodynamic criteria for further palliation, i.e.:

– Preserved single-ventricle function;
– Appropriately-sized pulmonary arteries;
– Low pulmonary vascular resistance;
– Adequate atrioventricular valve function, or need for concomitant surgical repair;
– In case of aortic arch reconstruction or DKS surgery, patch distortion or residual systemic outflow obstruction, that should be known prior to surgery.

Physiologically, pulmonary vascular resistance falls to a level similar to the mature circulation of the adult at the age of 3–6 months [4]. Some authors advocate the advantages of an earlier accomplishment of the second stage, in order to mitigate the effects of chronic single-ventricular volume overload and prolonged systemic hypoxia [36, 37]. However, results from larger series demonstrated that an early second stage palliation did not improve outcomes and a timing of 3–6 months after the Norwood procedure was associated with the highest transplant-free survival [38]. Regardless of timing, performing the superior cavo-pulmonary anastomosis as an intermediate step before Fontan completion has been proven to reduce morbidity and mortality at the time of the last stage of palliation [39, 40].

Third Stage of Palliation

After the second stage of palliation, the infant enters a period of relative clinical stability, which usually enables adequate growth/physical development. However, as time goes by, the severity of systemic O_2 desaturation tends to increase, together with its consequences, i.e. secondary erythrocytosis (a rise in hemoglobin concentration and hematocrit), and the risk of thrombosis and embolism. Underlying factors that affect arterial oxygenation are:

• Growth of the inferior part of the body, which now contributes more than half to the systemic venous drainage;
• Development of arterio-venous collaterals or fistulas at pulmonary level, which create an arterio-venous intrapulmonary shunt that aggravates desaturation; these fistulas are caused by the absence of hepatic venous blood reaching the pulmonary circulation [41];
• Development of venous-venous collaterals from the superior to the inferior vena cava, in an attempt to decompress the bidirectional cavo-pulmonary connection at the expense of cyanosis.

When saturation falls constantly below 75%, a further surgical step should be considered. Assessment of the growth and status of the pulmonary vasculature, usually by means of a preoperative cardiac catheterization, is mandatory. Important measurements are:

• Pulmonary arterial pressure and pulmonary vascular resistance;
• Single-ventricle function and, in particular, end-diastolic ventricular pressure;
• Atrio-ventricular valve function;
• Pulmonary vascular bed development (using the Nakata index calculation);
• Presence of systemic-to-pulmonary collaterals, which can be closed by coil embolization;
• Residual obstruction to the systemic output.

The original Fontan technique (Fig. 12.4a) [1], and its early modifications by Kreutzer's (Fig. 12.4b) [42] and Doty (Fig. 12.4c) [43] for Fontan circulation completion, redirect inferior vena cava drainage into the pulmonary bed through the right atrium, since it was originally (erroneously) thought the atrial systole could effectively contribute to forward blood flow. For this reason, these procedures are commonly referred to as "atrio-pulmonary" Fontan connection.

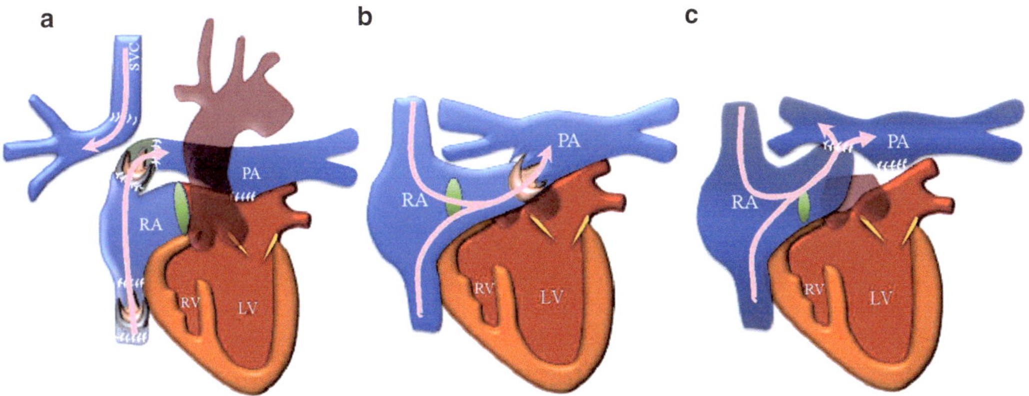

Fig. 12.4 Types of atriopulmonary Fontan. (**a**) the original Fontan technique with a classical Glenn shunt (superior vena cava, SVC, to divided right pulmonary artery) and use of homografts in the inferior vena cava and the anastomosis between the right atrium (RA) and left pulmonary artery (PA) in a patient with tricuspid atresia. The atrial septal defect is closed. (**b**) Kreutzer's modification with RA (appendage) to pulmonary artery anastomosis, preserving the pulmonary valve and closing the atrial septal defect. (**c**) Doty's modification with a divided pulmonary artery and RA to right PA anastomosis with closure of the atrial septal defect

However, de Leval et al. demonstrated that the atrial contraction was hemodynamically not relevant for the Fontan circulation, and implemented a novel technique [44], introducing the concept of the total cavo-pulmonary connection (TCPC). In this variant, the inferior vena cava blood flow is rerouted towards the right pulmonary artery (which has been previously anastomosed termino-laterally with the superior vena cava, by means of a BDG or a Hemi Fontan procedure), utilizing a prosthetic baffle which excludes most of the right atrium (the so-called intra-atrial "lateral tunnel", Fig. 12.5a). Major concerns about this technique are:

- Incomplete exclusion of the right atrium from the Fontan circulation, which results in a persistent risk for atrial dilatation and arrhythmia;
- Extensive suture lines in the right atrium, which may contribute to the creation of aberrant conduction circuits and predispose to supraventricular arrhythmias;
- The relative surgical complexity of creating a not stenotic, but also not redundant baffle/pathway, and the risks of inferior vena cava/TCPC stenosis, blood stasis and thrombosis.

Later, in 1990, Marcelletti et al. proposed a completely extra-cardiac prosthetic conduit to redirect the inferior vena cava drainage directly into the right pulmonary artery [45]. In detail, a PTFE conduit (16–20 mm diameter) is interposed between the inferior vena cava (which is transected from the right atrium at the atrio-caval junction), and termino-laterally with the inferior aspect of the right pulmonary artery (Fig. 12.5b). This procedure usually occurs after the bidirectional Glenn shunt.

The extracardiac conduit procedure presents with some technical advantages, such as:

- A simpler surgical technique, which does not require cardioplegic arrest, or even cardiopulmonary bypass in some cases [46];
- Absence of intra-atrial suture lines, which reduces the long-term risk of atrial arrhythmias, and hence reduces morbidity and mortality [47].

However, a major drawback is the dimension of the conduit, which must ensure adequate venous drainage throughout the patient's life.

It is clear that these two different techniques of TCPC entail significant implications in the timing of operation, which is variable among sur-

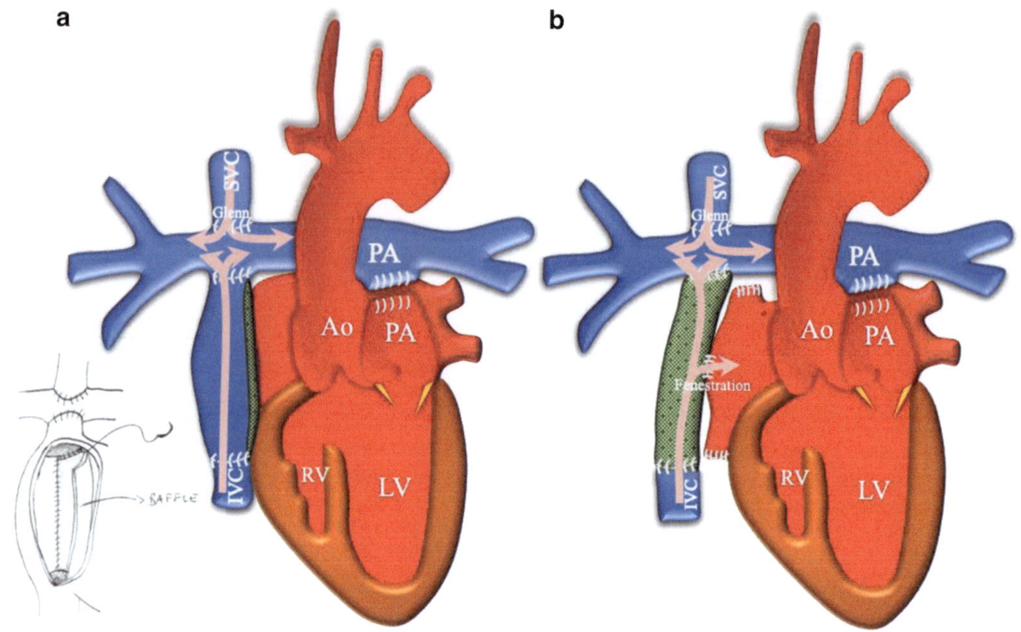

Fig. 12.5 Types of total cavopulmonary connection. (**a**) bidirectional Glenn anastomosis and lateral tunnel. (**b**) bidirectional Glenn anastomosis and extracardiac conduit with fenestration

gical centers, and usually ranges from 2 to 6 years of age:

- In the extracardiac conduit technique, a later timing is preferred, to ensure the greatest growth of the child before surgery, allowing a larger and possibly more durable conduit implantation;
- In The lateral-tunnel procedure, an earlier timing could be pursued, avoiding a prolonged exposure of the child to chronic hypoxia.

This tendency was confirmed by reports from the Australia and New Zealand Fontan registry, with the lateral tunnel Fontan completed 1 year earlier, on average, when compared to the extracardiac Fontan (3.8 years old vs 4.8 years) [48]. However, a recent review [7] demonstrated a global trend towards earlier palliation (age range 4.6–9.8 years until 1990 vs 2.0–5.6 years in the latest era), with growing evidence of good postoperative outcomes and long-term functional status with an earlier Fontan completion [49–51], even with an extracardiac conduit technique.

After the third stage completion, the entire systemic venous drainage is redirected into the pulmonary bed, bypassing the single-ventricle completely (i.e. TCPC). This results in:

- Elimination of systemic and pulmonary venous blood mixing, with potential resolution of systemic desaturation (depending on the presence of a fenestration or additional collaterals);
- Drastic reduction of single-ventricle preload, predisposing to acute decompensation and circulatory failure.

Key points of perioperative management after Fontan completion are:

- Preservation of single ventricle function, through inotropic drugs infusion and surgical correction of atrio-ventricular valve regurgitation;
- Providing adequate ventricular preload through volume expanders, especially in the early postoperative period;

- Consider performing a Fontan circuit-atrial fenestration at time of surgery.

The fenestration of the Fontan circuit has the rationale of:

- Decompressing the inferior vena cava system and mitigate the effects of an acute increase of systemic venous pressure on abdominal organs;
- Augment the single-ventricle preload by right-to-left shunting, preserving systemic cardiac output at the expense of cyanosis.

A randomized controlled trial demonstrated the efficacy of a fenestration in reducing postoperative effusions, hospital stay and need for additional procedures [52]. However, this is accomplished at the expense of systemic desaturation (about 5%) and the risk of fenestration thrombosis and/or paradoxical embolism, hence requires a period of anticoagulation (at least 6 months postoperatively).

Fontan Conversion Surgery

The outcomes of the Fontan operation have improved over recent decades, with current early mortality rates as low as 0.5%, and 15-year survival which reaches 95% in some series [7]. As prognosis has improved, the inevitable drawbacks of the palliative nature of this unnatural circulation have emerged, creating a novel and emerging population of "failing Fontan" patients [53, 54]. In particular, classic atrio-pulmonary variants of Fontan have proven to be particularly susceptible to failure due to right atrial dilatation and subsequent arrhythmias and blood stasis/thrombosis, stimulating the concept of surgery for conversion of an atriopulmonary Fontan to the more efficient TCPC. Introduced by Mavroudis et al. [55] and adopted by several centers worldwide [55–59], the Fontan conversion surgery includes a take-down of the previous atrio-pulmonary connection, reestablishment of the Fontan circuit through a lateral-tunnel or extracardiac conduit, with additional right atrial reduction plasty, atrial ablation and a DDD pacemaker and epicardial lead implantation (when necessary), Despite its technical complexity, this procedure can have a low early mortality and satisfactory long-term outcomes in optimal candidates, with a 10-year survival that can reach 83% [56].

References

1. Fontan F, Baudet E. Surgical repair of tricuspid atresia. Thorax. 1971;26:240–8.
2. Choussat A, Fontan F, Besse P. Selection criteria for Fontan's procedure. In: Anderson RH, Shinebourne EA, editors. Pediatric cardiology. London: Churchill Livingstone; 1978. p. 559–5.
3. Rychik J. The relentless effects of the Fontan paradox. Semin Thorac Cardiovasc Surg Pediatr Card Surg Annu. 2016;19(1):37–43.
4. Lucas RV, JWS G, Anderson RC, Adams P, Ferguson DJ. Maturation of the pulmonary vascular bed: a physiologic and anatomic correlation in infants and children. Am J Dis Child. 1961;101(4):467–75.
5. Norwood WI, Jacobs ML. Fontan's procedure in two stages. Am J Surg. 1993;166(5):548–51.
6. Jacobs JP, Mayer JE Jr, Mavroudis C, et al. The Society of Thoracic Surgeons congenital heart surgery database: 2017 update on outcomes and quality. Ann Thorac Surg. 2017;103(3):699–709.
7. Kverneland LS, Kramer P, Ovroutski S. Five decades of the Fontan operation: a systematic review of international reports on outcomes after univentricular palliation. Congenit Heart Dis. 2018;13(2):181–93.
8. Reddy SC, Saxena A. Prostaglandin E1: first stage palliation in neonates with congenital cardiac defects. Indian J Pediatr. 1998;65(2):211–6.
9. Becker KC, Hornik CP, Cotten CM, Clark RH, Hill KD, Smith PB, Lenfestey RW. Necrotizing enterocolitis in infants with ductal-dependent congenital heart disease. Am J Perinatol. 2015;32(7):633–8.
10. Eilers L, Qureshi AM. Advances in pediatric ductal intervention: an open or shut case? Curr Cardiol Rep. 2020;22(3):14.
11. Gibbs JL, Rothman MT, Rees MR, Parsons JM, Blackburn ME, Ruiz CE. Stenting of the arterial duct: a new approach to palliation for pulmonary atresia. Br Heart J. 1992;67:240–5.
12. Glatz AC, Petit CJ, Goldstein BH, et al. Comparison between patent ductus arteriosus stent and modified Blalock-Taussig shunt as palliation for infants with ductal-dependent pulmonary blood flow: insights from the congenital catheterization research collaborative. Circulation. 2018;137(6):589–601.

13. Blalock A, Taussig HG. The surgical treatment of malformations of the heart in which there is pulmonary stenosis or pulmonary atresia. JAMA. 1945;128:189.

14. Potts WT, Sumter S, Gibson S. Anastomosis of the aorta to a pulmonary artery: certain types in congenital heart disease. JAMA. 1946;132:631.

15. Waterston DH. Treatment of Fallot's tetralogy in children under one year of age. Rozhl Chir. 1962;41:181–3.

16. Klinner W, Pasini M, Schaudig A. Anastomosis between systemic and pulmonary arteries with the aid of plastic prostheses in cyanotic heart diseases. Thoraxchirurgie. 1962;10:68–75.

17. Woolf PK, Stephenson LW, Meijboom E, Bavinck JH, Gardner TJ, Donahoo JS, Edie RN, Edmunds LH Jr. A comparison of Blalock-Taussig, Waterston, and polytetrafluoroethylene shunts in children less than two weeks of age. Ann Thorac Surg. 1984;38(1):26–30.

18. Muller WH, Danimann JF. The treatment of certain congenital malformations of the heart by the creation of pulmonic stenosis to reduce pulmonary hypertension and excessive pulmonary blood flow; a preliminary report. Surg Gynecol Obstet. 1952;95(2):213–9.

19. Agasthi P, Graziano JN. Pulmonary artery banding. In: StatPearls [internet]. Treasure Island (FL): StatPearls Publishing; 2020. p. 2020.

20. Trusler GA, Mustard WT. A method of banding the pulmonary artery for large isolated ventricular septal defect with and without transposition of the great arteries. Ann Thorac Surg. 1972;13(4):351–5.

21. Damus PS. Ann Thorac Surg. 1975;20:724–5.

22. Kaye MP. Anatomic correction of transposition of great arteries. Mayo Clin Proc. 1975;50:638–40.

23. Stansel HC. A new operation for D-loop transposition of the great vessels. Ann Thorac Surg. 1975;19:565–7.

24. Norwood WI, Lang P, Hansen DD. Physiologic repair of aortic atresia-hypoplastic left heart syndrome. N Engl J Med. 1983;308(1):23–6.

25. Sano S, Ishino K, Kawada M, Arai S, et al. Right ventricle-pulmonary artery shunt in first-stage palliation of hypoplastic left heart syndrome. J Thorac Cardiovasc Surg. 2003;126(2):504–9.

26. Jonas RA. Comprehensive surgical management of congenital heart disease. Boca Raton: CRC Press; 2004.

27. Rudolph A. Congenital diseases of the heart. 2009.

28. Shillingford M, Ceithaml E, Bleiweis M. Surgical considerations in the management of hypoplastic left heart syndrome. Semin Cardiothorac Vasc Anesth. 2013;17(2):128–36.

29. Glenn WW. Circulatory bypass of the right side of the heart. IV. Shunt between superior vena cava and distal right pulmonary artery; report of clinical application. N Engl J Med. 1958;259(3):117–20.

30. Tanoue Y, Sese A, Ueno Y, Joh K, Hijii T. Bidirectional Glenn procedure improves the mechanical efficiency of a total cavopulmonary connection in high-risk fontan candidates. Circulation. 2001;103(17):2176–80.

31. Bridges ND, Jonas RA, Mayer JE, Flanagan MF, Keane JF, Castaneda AR. Bidirectional cavopulmonary anastomosis as interim palliation for high-risk Fontan candidates. Early results. Circulation. 1990;82(5 Suppl):IV170–6.

32. Edelson JB, Ravishankar C, Griffis H, Zhang X, Faerber J, Gardner MM, Naim MY, Macsio CE, Glatz AC, Goldberg DJ. A comparison of bidirectional Glenn vs. hemi-Fontan procedure: an analysis of the single ventricle reconstruction trial public use dataset. Pediatr Cardiol. 2020;41(6):1166–72.

33. Turner ME, Richmond ME, Quaegebeur JM, et al. Intact right ventricle-pulmonary artery shunt after stage 2 palliation in hypoplastic left heart syndrome improves pulmonary artery growth. Pediatr Cardiol. 2013;34(4):924–30.

34. Yan T, Tong G, Zhang B, Yan F, Zhou X, Wang X, Lu H, Ma T, Wang X, Yu H, Sun Z, Zhang W. The effect of antegrade pulmonary blood flow following a late bidirectional Glenn procedure. Interact Cardiovasc Thorac Surg. 2018;26(3):454–9.

35. Jonas RA. Indications and timing for the bidirectional Glenn shunt versus the fenestrated Fontan circulation. J Thorac Cardiovasc Surg. 1994;108:522–4.

36. Chang AC, Hanley FL, Wernovsky G, Rosenfeld HM, Wessel DL, Jonas RA, Mayer JE, Lock JE, Castaneda AR. Early bidirectional cavopulmonary shunt in young infants. Postoperative course and early results. Circulation. 1993;88(5 pt 2):II149–58.

37. Reddy VM, Liddicoat JR, Hanley FL. Primary bidirectional superior cavopulmonary shunt in infants between 1 and 4 months of age. Ann Thorac Surg. 1995;59(5):1120–6.

38. Meza JM, Hickey EJ, Blackstone EH, et al. The optimal timing of stage 2 palliation for hypoplastic left heart syndrome. Circulation. 2017;136:1737–48.

39. Pridjian AK, Mendelsohn AM, Lupinetti FM, et al. Usefulness of the bidirectional Glenn procedure as staged reconstruction for the functional single ventricle. Am J Cardiol. 1993;71:959–62.

40. Alejos JC, Williams RG, Jarmakani JM, et al. Factors influencing survival in patients undergoing the bidirectional Glenn anastomosis. Am J Cardiol. 1995;75:1048–50.

41. Duncan BW, Kneebone JM, Chi EY, et al. A detailed histologic analysis of pulmonary arteriovenous malformations in children with cyanotic congenital heart disease. J Thorac Cardiovasc Surg. 1999;117:931–8.

42. Kreutzer G, Galíndez E, Bono H, De Palma C, Laura JP. An operation for the correction of tricuspid atresia. J Thorac Cardiovasc Surg. 1973;66(4):613–21.

43. Doty D, Marvin W Jr, Lauer R. Modified Fontan procedure. Methods to achieve direct anastomosis of right atrium to pulmonary artery. J Thorac Cardiovasc Surg. 1981;81(3):470–5.

44. de Leval MR, Kilner P, Gewillig M, Bull C. Total cavopulmonary connection: a logical alternative to atriopulmonary connection for complex Fontan operations. Experimental studies and early clinical experience. J Thorac Cardiovasc Surg. 1988;96(5):682–95.

45. Marcelletti C, Corno A, Giannico S, Marino B. Inferior vena cava-pulmonary artery extracardiac conduit. A new form of right heart bypass. J Thorac Cardiovasc Surg. 1990;100(2):228–32.

46. Petrossian E, Reddy VM, Collins KK, Culbertson CB, MacDonald MJ, Lamberti JJ, Reinhartz O, Mainwaring RD, Francis PD, Malhotra SP, Gremmels DB, Suleman S, Hanley FL. The extracardiac conduit Fontan operation using minimal approach extracorporeal circulation: early and midterm outcomes. J Thorac Cardiovasc Surg. 2006;132(5):1054–63.

47. Ben Ali W, Bouhout I, Khairy P, Bouchard D, Poirier N. Extracardiac versus lateral tunnel Fontan: a meta-analysis of long-term results. Ann Thorac Surg. 2019;107(3):837–43.

48. d'Udekem Y, Iyengar AJ, Galati JC, Forsdick V, Weintraub RG, Wheaton GR, Bullock A, Justo RN, Grigg LE, Sholler GF, Hope S, Radford DJ, Gentles TL, Celermajer DS, Winlaw DS. Redefining expectations of long-term survival after the Fontan procedure: twenty-five years of follow-up from the entire population of Australia and New Zealand. Circulation. 2014;130(11 Suppl 1):S32–8.

49. Shiraishi S, Yagihara T, Kagisaki K, Hagino I, Ohuchi H, Kobayashi J, Kitamura S. Impact of age at Fontan completion on postoperative hemodynamics and long-term aerobic exercise capacity in patients with dominant left ventricle. Ann Thorac Surg. 2009;87(2):555–61.

50. Madan P, Stout KK, Fitzpatrick AL. Age at Fontan procedure impacts exercise performance in adolescents: results from the pediatric heart network multicenter study. Am Heart J. 2013;166(2):365–72.

51. Bezuska L, Lebetkevicius V, Lankutis K, Sudikiene R, Sirvydis VJ, Tarutis V. Fontan completion for younger than 3 years of age: outcome in patients with functional single ventricle. Pediatr Cardiol. 2015;36(8):1680–4.

52. Lemler MS, Scott WA, Leonard SR, Stromberg D, Ramaciotti C. Fenestration improves clinical outcome of the fontan procedure: a prospective, randomized study. Circulation. 2002;105:207–12.

53. Deal BJ, Jacobs ML. Management of the failing Fontan circulation. Heart. 2012;98(14):1098–104.

54. Elder RW, Wu FM. Clinical approaches to the patient with a failing Fontan procedure. Curr Cardiol Rep. 2016;18(5):44.

55. Mavroudis C, Backer CL, Deal BJ, Johnsrude CL. Fontan conversion to cavopulmonary connection and arrhythmia circuit cryoblation. J Thorac Cardiovasc Surg. 1998;115(3):547–56.

56. Park HK, Shin HJ, Park YH. Outcomes of Fontan conversion for failing Fontan circulation: mid-term results. Interact Cardiovasc Thorac Surg. 2016;23(1):14–7.

57. Van Melle JP, Wolff D, Hörer J, Belli E, Meyns B, Padalino M, et al. Surgical options after Fontan failure. Heart. 2016;102(14):1127–33.

58. Hoashi T, Shimada M, Imai K, Komori M, Kurosaki K, Ohuchi H, Ichikawa H. Long-term therapeutic effect of Fontan conversion with an extracardiac conduit. Eur J Cardiothorac Surg. 2020;57(5):951–7.

59. Padalino MA, Ponzoni M, Castaldi B, Leoni L, Chemello L, Toscano G, Gerosa G, Di Salvo G, Vida VL. Surgical management of failing Fontan circulation: results from 30 cases with 285 patient-years follow-up. Eur J Cardiothorac Surg. 2022;61:338–45.

Classical Norwood Stage I and Modifications

13

Phil Botha

Classical Stage I Norwood

The first description in 1980 of a successful palliative procedure for Hypoplastic Left Heart Syndrome (HLHS) by Norwood and colleagues ushered in a new era in the management of this previously universally fatal congenital cardiac lesion [1]. In the same year Doty and colleagues described a success using a tubular interposition prosthesis between the proximal main pulmonary artery and the aortic arch [2]. From these initial experiences, the high rate of early mortality made transplantation a viable alternative, as many children born with HLHS are otherwise good candidates. The inadequate supply of suitable donors and improving results with refinements of staged palliation resulted in transplantation playing a progressively smaller role in the neonatal period. In the 40 years since inception, use of the Norwood procedure has expanded to other complex single ventricle pathologies, with successive technical modifications resulting in steadily improving results.

Early Modifications

In 1983 Norwood and colleagues reported a series of 10 cases, in which the first four patients had systemic blood flow established using a conduit from the right ventricular free wall or main pulmonary artery to the thoracic aorta. Pulmonary blood flow was limited by pulmonary artery banding but none of these four patients survived. The subsequent six patients had aorto-pulmonary amalgamation and a Blalock-Taussig-Thomas (BTT) or central shunt, and this was successful in palliating five patients to Fontan completion [3]. Doty and colleagues reported 54 autopsy specimens of aortic atresia in 1984, highlighting the high incidence of co-existing coarctation (80%) and therefore the need for concomitant arch repair [4]. This was further emphasised by the publication of a series of 25 neonates by Jonas and colleagues in 1986 [5]. With an early mortality of 24%, this report highlighted several important considerations in successful palliation. The authors stressed the importance of the creation of a wide septectomy to prevent recurrent atrial level restriction and complete arch repair to avoid a residual gradient. Similarly, careful reconstruction of the central pulmonary arteries and selection of shunt size were considered paramount in balancing the circulation and ensuring well developed pulmonary arteries for success at the second stage of palliation.

P. Botha (✉)
Department of Cardiac Surgery, Birmingham
Children's Hospital, Birmingham, UK
e-mail: p.botha@nhs.net

© The Author(s), under exclusive license to Springer Nature Switzerland AG 2023
P. Clift et al. (eds.), *Univentricular Congenital Heart Defects and the Fontan Circulation*,
https://doi.org/10.1007/978-3-031-36208-8_13

The first report studying more than 100 Norwood stage 1 procedures demonstrated an evolution in several aspects of the operation [6]. The use of a homograft patch to facilitate aortic arch repair and side-to-side amalgamation of the aorta and distal pulmonary artery stump was highlighted for its impact on improved haemostasis. In addition to patching of the arch, resection of the posterior coarctation shelf was also advocated as an additional measure to reduce recoarctation. The latter part of this experience demonstrated improved pulmonary blood flow with a 4 mm central interposition shunt originating from the distal arch patch. This series also showed a widening of the inclusion criteria to other anatomical variants, including unbalanced atrioventricular septal defect in 10 patients, and double-outlet right ventricle with aortic and mitral atresia in 12. Despite this expansion of indication to other complex anatomies, early mortality in this series was 29%.

Alternative strategies aimed at avoiding cardiopulmonary bypass utilising Norwood's early concept of MPA to descending aorta interposition graft and pulmonary artery band remained popular in some centres until the early '90s [7]. At the same time, separating the second and third stages into a bidirectional cavopulmonary shunt at stage 2 and subsequent Fontan completion gained popularity [8–10]. Concurrently, it was also becoming apparent that prolonged periods of circulatory arrest during stage 1 palliation were associated with poor outcomes [11]. Techniques for avoiding prolonged circulatory arrest through the use of regional cerebral perfusion became prevalent as a result [12], and methods followed for continuous perfusion of the body and/or heart throughout the procedure [13]. Results steadily improved with the first reports emerging of early survival exceeding 90% for stage I palliation if undertaken within the first month of life [14], and similar success of the procedure demonstrated in other anatomic anomalies [15, 16].

Modifications of Aortic Arch Repair

Early series demonstrated that the aortic arch repair could be an Achilles' heel of the first stage Norwood palliation, and can contribute significantly to morbidity and mortality [3, 17]. The incidence of aortic arch obstruction after the Norwood procedure has been reported to be as high as 36–46% [18, 19]. Balloon angioplasty of residual/re-coarctation has been shown to be effective in relieving obstruction in the majority of patients, with around 2–4% of patients requiring surgical redo aortic arch repair [18, 20–22]. Several modifications of the aortic arch repair have been proposed to minimise the incidence of this complication. The original description of the procedure involved the amalgamation of the aorta and proximal pulmonary artery/duct without the excision of the coarctation segment, and without the use of additional patch material in the reconstruction. This approach evolved to include an incision across the coarctation segment, and patch augmentation using allograft material to reduce residual or recurrent arch obstruction. This remains a common approach in some institutions. Many however feel that leaving a prominent posterior shelf of coarctation tissue within the arch creates a significant risk for recoarctation. Excision of the posterior shelf together with reconstruction using no additional patch material was first described by two groups in the same year [23, 24], and was subsequently shown to reduce the incidence of recurrent arch obstruction in non-randomised consecutive series from 12/26 (46%) to 3/20 (15%) [25]. The hope that the use of only autologous materials would facilitate normal growth of the arch has been questioned by more recent reports [26], incorporating a more radical approach to arch reconstruction, necessitating the use of patch material in the majority of anatomical substrates. Xenograft pericardial or jugular vein patches have been proposed as an alternative to allografts, with an 18% incidence of recurrent arch obstruction reported with the former [27]. No long-term follow-up studies have reported the comparative durability of bovine jugular vein patches. The potential benefits of reducing allosensitization and viral transmission has been highlighted and have resulted in the introduction of curved patches of bovine pericardium to facilitate neonatal aortic arch reconstruction in recent years.

The interdigitating technique of arch reconstruction has been put forward as a further modification to potentially reduce the incidence of recurrent obstruction by a number of groups over the past 15 years. This involves complete excision of the coarctation and ductal tissue within the arch, with longitudinal incisions made in the anterior and posterior aspect of the descending aorta. The proximal posterior transverse arch is then interdigitated into the posterior incision in the descending aorta, and the anterior arch augmented using an allograft patch. The report of Burkhart and colleagues found in consecutive patients that this modification further reduced the incidence of recurrent obstruction form 15% to 0 of 33 (*p* <0.001) [25] Similarly, in a larger consecutive series, Lamers and colleagues found a reduction in the rate of arch reintervention from 22/79 (28%) with coarctectomy and posterior anastomosis, to 1/63 (2%) with the interdigitating technique [28]. The standard approach to aorto-pulmonary amalgamation has been a side-to-side anastomosis with augmentation in many institutions. An alternative method has been described with end-to-side anastomosis of the MPA to the arch patch, with rates of arch reintervention of 25% in keeping with other reports without coarctectomy [21]. The report did highlight a higher rate of re-intervention in patients with ascending aortic diameter of less than 2.5 mm, not demonstrated consistently with the standard technique [22].

Norwood stage I—Common technical modifications
- Aorto-pulmonary amalgamation
  - side-to-side / "double-barrel"
  - end-to-side
- Atrial septectomy
(restrictive ASD in staged LV recruitment)
- Aortic arch repair
  - patch augmentation only
  - Autologous tissue only
  - Coarctectomy, anastomosis and patch augmentation
  - Interdigitating repair
- Pulmonary conduit
  - Modified BTT shunt
  - RVPA shunt
    Distal anastomosis to left/ right of aorta
    Valved conduit
      Transmural RV implantation
      "Dunk technique"

Shunt Modifications

From the earliest reported experience, the careful balance of the pulmonary and systemic blood flow was identified as critical, and initial use of 4 mm Polytetrafluoroethylene (PTFE) central shunts evolved into 3.5 or 3 mm modified Blalock Taussig Thomas shunt in the majority of patients. With smaller calibre shunts, thrombosis remained a significant concern, but alternatives to PTFE including saphenous vein homograft have not achieved widespread popularity [29]. Early attempts to improve control of pulmonary blood flow via the modified BTT shunt included adjustable snares and the application of clips [30, 31]. In 2003, Sano and colleagues reported a series of 19 consecutive patients that underwent stage one palliation with a right ventricle to pulmonary artery (RVPA) shunt to the distal stump of the pulmonary artery [32]. The reduction in systemic and coronary steal phenomena resulted in improved postoperative haemodynamic stability. Some institutions have advocated for RVPA shunt placement to the Right of the aorta, as having a survival advantage, at the cost of central PA hypoplasia [33]. Analysis of this variable in a propensity-matched multicentre cohort (67 patients per group) found a reduced rate of surgical shunt revisions (17.9% vs 0%, $p < 0.001$), fewer serious adverse events (84 vs 46/100, $p = 0.01$), and improved transplant-free survival at 3 years (61% vs 80%, $p = 0.04$) with the shunt distal anastomosis created to the right pulmonary artery [34].

Valved RVPA conduits have been proposed as a method to reduce regurgitation and resultant right ventricular volume load. The largest published series in this regard demonstrated good early outcomes in terms of mortality, and a 20% rate of early re-intervention on the conduit [35]. The rate was particularly high in recipients of composite conduits constructed from PTFE and aortic homografts. This group also demonstrated a higher incidence of late death, for unclear reasons, compared to composite conduits using small pulmonary homografts and a small number of cryopreserved veins. The use of a ring-reinforced PTFE conduit implanted trans-murally into the right ventricle (the "dunk" technique) has been lauded as reducing the rate of conduit re-intervention, and improving pulmonary artery growth [36, 37]. More recently, applying surgical clips to reduce the RVPA shunt diameter and subsequent removal by balloon dilatation has been demonstrated as a method of improving circulatory balance and possibly late pulmonary artery growth [38, 39] (Yasukawa et al. EJCTS). Considerable controversy has however persisted regarding the relative merits of BTT and RVPA shunts in the setting of the stage 1 palliation, resulting in the inception of the landmark randomised SVR trial.

Single Ventricle Reconstruction Trial

The single ventricle reconstruction trial randomised 549 neonates across 15 North American institutions to a Norwood procedure with either a modified BTT shunt or an RVPA shunt. This landmark study demonstrated non-proportional hazards in the two groups, with greater early transplant-free survival in the RVPA group prior to second-stage palliation, and no difference between the two groups thereafter. Important results from the resultant publications are summarised in Table 13.1.

Table 13.1 Summary of results from single ventricle reconstruction trial and resulting publications

Date	Author	Journal	Duration of follow-up	Key findings (BTTS vs RVPA)
2010	Ohye et al. [40]	NEJM	12 months	Transplant-free survival 64% vs 74%, $0 = 0.01$ More unintended interventions ($p = 0.003$) and complications in RVPA group ($p = 0.002$)
2012	Newburger et al. [41]	Circulation	14 months	Neurodevelopmental outcomes at 14 months lower than normative means (PDI 74 ± 19, MDI 89 ± 18) related to innate patient factors and overall morbidity in the first year
2013	Hill et al. [22]	Circulation	12 months	18% incidence of procedure for re-coarctation (92 balloon, 39 surgical) No decrease in 1 year transplant-free survival
2014	Newburger et al. [42]	Circulation	4.8 ± 1.1 year	Transplant-free survival 61% vs 67% ($p = 0.15$) Pre-Fontan RVEF 44.7 ± 6.0% vs 41.7 ± 5.1% ($p = 0.007$)
2016	Oster et al. [43]	J am heart Assoc	First interstage	Interstage mortality in patients discharged home on digoxin 2.9% vs 12.3% (HR 3.5, 95% CI, 1.1–11.7, $p = 0.04$)
2017	Andersen et al. [34]	JTCVS	12 months	Fewer surgical shunt revisions in RVPA shunts placed to the right of the neo-aorta (8.3 vs 1.9 events per 100 infants, $p = 0.05$)
2018	Mahle et al. [44]	JHLT	6 years	14% met criteria for heart failure, not associated with shunt type
2018	Newburger et al. [45]	Circulation	7.1 ± 1.6 yr	Transplant-free survival 59% vs 64% $p = 0.25$ Catheter interventions 0.23 vs 0.38/patient-year $p < 0.001$

NEJM New England Journal of Medicine, *PDI* Psychomotor development Index, *MDI* Mental Development Index, *JTVCVS* Journal of Thoracic and Cardiovascular Surgery, *JHLT* Journal of Heart and Lung Transplantation.
BTTS Blalock Taussig Thomas shunt, *RVPA* Right ventricle to pulmonary artery shunt, *RVEF* Right ventricular ejection fraction

References

1. Norwood WI, Kirklin JK, Sanders SP. Hypoplastic left heart syndrome: experience with palliative surgery. Am J Cardiol. 1980;45:87–91.
2. Doty DB, Marvin WJ, Schieken RM, Lauer RM. Hypoplastic left heart syndrome: successful palliation with a new operation. J Thorac Cardiovasc Surg. 1980;80:148–52.
3. Norwood WI, Lang P, Hansen DD. Physiologic repair of aortic atresia-hypoplastic left heart syndrome. N Engl J Med. 1983;308:23–6.
4. Hawkins JA, Doty DB. Aortic atresia: morphologic characteristics affecting survival and operative palliation. J Thorac Cardiovasc Surg. 1984;88:620–6.
5. Jonas RA, Lang P, Hansen D, Hickey P, Castaneda AR. First-stage palliation of hypoplastic left heart syndrome. The importance of coarctation and shunt size. J Thorac Cardiovasc Surg. 1986;92:6–13.
6. Pigott JD, Murphy JD, Barber G, Norwood WI. Palliative reconstructive surgery for hypoplastic left heart syndrome. Ann Thorac Surg. 1988;45:122–8.
7. Tucker WY, McKone RC, Weesner KM, Kon ND. Hypoplastic left heart syndrome: palliation without cardiopulmonary bypass. J Thorac Cardiovasc Surg. 1990;99:885–8.
8. Lamberti JJ, Spicer RL, Waldman JD, Grehl TM, Thomson D, George L, Kirkpatrick SE, Mathewson JW. The bidirectional cavopulmonary shunt. J Thorac Cardiovasc Surg. 1990;100:22–30.
9. Norwood WI, Jacobs ML, Murphy JD. Fontan procedure for hypoplastic left heart syndrome. Ann Thorac Surg. 1992;54:1025–30.
10. Pridjian AK, Mendelsohn AM, Lupinetti FM, Beekman RH, Dick M, Serwer G, Bove EL. Usefulness of the bidirectional Glenn procedure as staged reconstruction for the functional single ventricle. Am J Cardiol. 1993;71:959–62.
11. Starnes VA, Griffin ML, Pitlick PT, Bernstein D, Baum D, Ivens K, Shumway NE. Current approach to hypoplastic left heart syndrome. Palliation, transplantation, or both? J Thorac Cardiovasc Surg. 1992;104:189–95.
12. Pigula FA, Siewers RD, Nemoto EM. Regional perfusion of the brain during neonatal aortic arch reconstruction. J Thorac Cardiovasc Surg. 1999;117s:1023–4.
13. Kishimoto H, Kawahira Y, Kawata H, Miura T, Iwai S, Mori T. The modified Norwood palliation on a beating heart. J Thorac Cardiovasc Surg. 1999;118:1130–2.
14. Iannettoni MD, Bove EL, Mosca RS, Lupinetti FM, Dorostkar PC, Ludomirsky A, Crowley DC, Kulik TJ, Rosenthal A. Improving results with first-stage palliation for hypoplastic left heart syndrome. J Thorac Cardiovasc Surg. 1994;107:934–40.
15. Kanter KR, Miller BE, Cuadrado AG, Vincent RN. Successful application of the Norwood procedure for infants without hypoplastic left heart syndrome. Ann Thorac Surg. 1995;59:301–4.
16. Jacobs ML, Rychik J, Murphy JD, Nicolson SC, Steven JM, Norwood WI. Results of Norwood's operation for lesions other than hypoplastic left heart syndrome. J Thorac Cardiovasc Surg. 1995;110:1555–62.
17. Bartram U, Grünenfelder J, Van Praagh R. Causes of death after the modified Norwood procedure: a study of 122 postmortem cases. Ann Thorac Surg. 1997;64:1795–802.
18. Zellers TM. Balloon angioplasty for recurrent coarctation of the aorta in patients following staged palliation for hypoplastic left heart syndrome. Am J Cardiol. 1999;84:231–3.
19. Ashcraft TM, Jones K, Border WL, Eghtesady P, Pearl JM, Khoury PR, Manning PB. Factors affecting long-term risk of aortic arch recoarctation after the Norwood procedure. Ann Thorac Surg. 2008;85:1397–402.
20. Tworetzky W, McElhinney DB, Burch GH, Teitel DF, Moore P. Balloon arterioplasty of recurrent coarctation after the modified Norwood procedure in infants. Catheter Cardiovasc Interv. 2000;50:54–8.
21. Sakurai T, Rogers V, Stickley J, Khan N, Jones TJ, Barron DJ, Brawn WJ. Single-center experience of arch reconstruction in the setting of Norwood operation. Ann Thorac Surg. 2012;94:1534–9.
22. Hill KD, Rhodes JF, Aiyagari R, et al. Intervention for recoarctation in the single ventricle reconstruction trial: incidence, risk, and outcomes. Circulation. 2013;128:954–61.
23. Bu'Lock FA, Stumper O, Jagtap R, Silove ED, De Giovanni JV, Wright JG, Sethia B, Brawn WJ. Surgery for infants with a hypoplastic systemic ventricle and severe outflow obstruction: early results with a modified Norwood procedure. Br Heart J. 1995;73:456–61.
24. Fraser CD, Mee RB. Modified Norwood procedure for hypoplastic left heart syndrome. Ann Thorac Surg. 1995;60:S546–9.
25. Burkhart HM, Ashburn DA, Konstantinov IE, De Oliveira NC, De Oliviera NC, Benson L, Williams WG, Van Arsdell GS. Interdigitating arch reconstruction eliminates recurrent coarctation after the Norwood procedure. J Thorac Cardiovasc Surg. 2005;130:61–5.
26. Devlin PJ, McCrindle BW, Kirklin JK, et al. Intervention for arch obstruction after the Norwood procedure: prevalence, associated factors, and practice variability. J Thorac Cardiovasc Surg. 2019;157:684–695.e8.
27. Morell VO, Wearden PA. Experience with bovine pericardium for the reconstruction of the aortic arch in patients undergoing a Norwood procedure. Ann Thorac Surg. 2007;84:1312–5.
28. Lamers LJ, Frommelt PC, Mussatto KA, Jaquiss RDB, Mitchell ME, Tweddell JS. Coarctectomy combined with an interdigitating arch reconstruction results in a lower incidence of recurrent arch obstruction after the Norwood procedure than coarctectomy alone. J Thorac Cardiovasc Surg. 2012;143:1098–102.

29. Tam VK, Murphy K, Parks WJ, Raviele AA, Vincent RN, Strieper M, Cuadrado AR. Saphenous vein homograft: a superior conduit for the systemic arterial shunt in the Norwood operation. Ann Thorac Surg. 2001;71:1537–40.

30. Schmid FX, Kampmann C, Kuroczynski W, Choi YH, Knuf M, Tzanova I, Oelert H. Adjustable tourniquet to manipulate pulmonary blood flow after Norwood operations. Ann Thorac Surg. 1999;68:2306–9.

31. Kuduvalli M, McLaughlin KE, Trivedi DB, Pozzi M. Norwood-type operation with adjustable systemic-pulmonary shunt using hemostatic clip. Ann Thorac Surg. 2001;72:634–5.

32. Sano S, Ishino K, Kawada M, Arai S, Kasahara S, Asai T, Masuda Z-I, Takeuchi M, Ohtsuki S-I. Right ventricle-pulmonary artery shunt in first-stage palliation of hypoplastic left heart syndrome. J Thorac Cardiovasc Surg. 2003;126:504–9.

33. Barron DJ, Brooks A, Stickley J, Woolley SM, Stumper O, Jones TJ, Brawn WJ. The Norwood procedure using a right ventricle-pulmonary artery conduit: comparison of the right-sided versus left-sided conduit position. J Thorac Cardiovasc Surg. 2009;138:528–37.

34. Andersen ND, Meza JM, Byler MR, Lodge AJ, Hill KD, Hornik CP, Jaquiss RDB. Comparison of right ventricle-pulmonary artery shunt position in the single ventricle reconstruction trial. J Thorac Cardiovasc Surg. 2017;153:1490–1500.e1.

35. Reinhartz O. Homograft Valved right ventricle to pulmonary artery conduit as a modification of the Norwood procedure. Circulation. 2006;114:I594–9.

36. Schreiber C, Kasnar-Samprec J, Hörer J, Eicken A, Cleuziou J, Prodan Z, Lange R. Ring-enforced right ventricle-to-pulmonary artery conduit in Norwood stage I reduces proximal conduit stenosis. Ann Thorac Surg. 2009;88:1541–5.

37. Baird CW, Myers PO, Borisuk M, Pigula FA, Emani SM. Ring-reinforced Sano conduit at Norwood stage I reduces proximal conduit obstruction. Ann Thorac Surg. 2015;99:171–9.

38. Murtuza B, Jones TJ, Barron DJ, Brawn WJ. Temporary restriction of right ventricle-pulmonary artery conduit flow using haemostatic clips following Norwood I reconstruction: potential for improved outcomes. Interact Cardiovasc Thorac Surg. 2012;14:327–9.

39. Yasukawa T, Hoashi T, Kitano M, Shimada M, Imai K, Kurosaki K, Ichikawa H. Interstage management of pulmonary blood flow after the Norwood procedure with right ventricle-to-pulmonary artery conduit. Eur J Cardiothorac Surg. 2020;58(3):551–8.

40. Ohye RG, Sleeper LA, Mahony L, et al. Comparison of shunt types in the Norwood procedure for single-ventricle lesions. N Engl J Med. 2010;362:1980–92.

41. Newburger JW, Sleeper LA, Bellinger DC, et al. Early developmental outcome in children with hypoplastic left heart syndrome and related anomalies: the single ventricle reconstruction trial. Circulation. 2012;125:2081–91.

42. Newburger JW, Sleeper LA, Frommelt PC, et al. Transplantation-free survival and interventions at 3 years in the single ventricle reconstruction trial. Circulation. 2014;129:2013–20.

43. Oster ME, Kelleman M, McCracken C, Ohye RG, Mahle WT. Association of Digoxin with Interstage Mortality: results from the pediatric heart network single ventricle reconstruction trial public use dataset. J Am Heart Assoc. 2016;5:I82.

44. Mahle WT, Hu C, Trachtenberg F, et al. Heart failure after the Norwood procedure: an analysis of the single ventricle reconstruction trial. J Heart Lung Transplant. 2018;37:879–85.

45. Newburger JW, Sleeper LA, Gaynor JW, et al. Transplant-free survival and interventions at 6 years in the SVR trial. Circulation. 2018;137:2246–53.

Hybrid Strategies for Hypoplastic Left Heart Syndrome and Comprehensive Stage II Repair

14

Alvise Guariento and Vladimiro L. Vida

Introduction

Definitions

The spectrum of disease defined as "hypoplastic left heart syndrome" (HLHS) includes patients with a wide variety of possible combinations of hypoplasia or obstruction of left-sided structures. However, all these lesions result in single ventricular physiology with various degrees of hypoplasia of the systemic ventricle and obstruction of the systemic outflow tract.

Common surgical strategies for this group of patients are:

- Stage I Norwood Operation
- Heart transplantation
- Palliative care

The outcomes of the stage I Norwood operation have significantly improved over time [1], but there continues to be significant morbidity and mortality [2].

More recently, stenting of a patent ductus arteriosus (PDA) combined with banding of the pulmonary arteries (PAs) and balloon atrial septostomy or septectomy ("Hybrid stage I repair") has been proposed as a new approach for HLHS (Fig. 14.1) [3–5]. This is then followed by a second stage at 4–6 months of age, consisting of reconstruction of the aortic arch, aortopulmonary connection, and cavo-pulmonary connection ("Comprehensive stage II repair"). Finally, a Stage III Fontan operation is achieved.

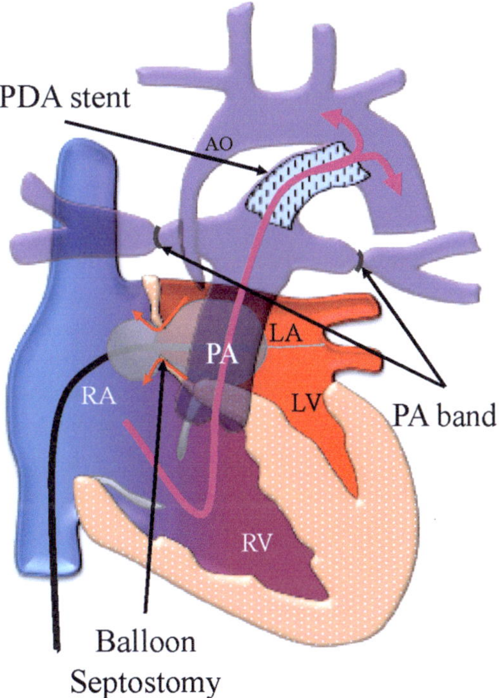

Fig. 14.1 Graphic representation of the hybrid stage I procedure in hypoplastic left heart syndrome

A. Guariento · V. L. Vida (✉)
Pediatric and Congenital Cardiac Surgery Unit, Department of Cardiac, Thoracic and Vascular Sciences and Public Health, University of Padua, Padua, Italy
e-mail: alvise.guariento@unipd.it;
vladimiro.vida@unipd.it

History

In 1980, Bill Norwood was the first to propose banding of the PAs as a palliative approach for HLHS patients [3]. However, what we know today as the "hybrid procedure" was first reported by Gibbs et al. in 1993, after early studies with implantable stents for maintaining PDA patency in a PDA-dependent systemic circulation, albeit with limited success [3]. After this initial report, other groups continued to develop this strategy, with the first effective series of patients reported in 2002 [4]. The Giessen Pediatric Heart Center (Justus-Liebig University, Giessen, Germany) took the lead in promoting this procedure, with these techniques now often referred to as "the Giessen approach" [5, 6].

Surgical Technique

Hybrid Stage I Repair

Pulmonary Artery Banding

- This procedure is usually performed in a catheterization laboratory or hybrid procedure room, under general anesthesia and elective ventilation. Surgical access is obtained by median sternotomy, without the institution of cardiopulmonary bypass ("off-pump").
- The main branch PAs are banded using Dacron or PTFE (Polytetrafluoroethylene, Goretex) conduits. When a PTFE conduit is chosen, a 3.5 mm tube is cut in the center along its longitudinal axis, and half the length of the theoretical band that would have been used to band the main PA (according to Trusler's rule [7]) is used to band the PA branches.
- Direct measurement of the branch PA pressure can be performed by introducing a catheter into each artery [8]. The bands are tightened in order to obtain a reduction of the pressure to one-third of the systemic pressure. The efficacy of the banding is then verified by echocardiographic assessment. If this is confirmed to be successful, the PAs bands are secured to the arteries with additional sutures [5].

Ductus Arteriosus Stenting and Atrial Septostomy

- PDA stenting is usually performed immediately after the PA banding, to avoid displacement of the stent. However, this has also been performed at the initial stages of the procedure.
- Vascular access can be achieved through the femoral vessels or with a purse-string between the main PA and the PDA. Pre-mounted balloon-expandable stents of appropriate diameter and length are used for the PDA stent. At this point, the prostaglandin infusion is stopped.
- In the event of a restrictive atrial septal defect, balloon septostomy is performed. Alternatively, atrial septectomy has been described in the initial experience by Gibbs et al. under cardiopulmonary bypass and circulatory arrest [3].
- The entire procedure is performed under radiographic control with final angiographic confirmation of the position of the PDA stent (Fig. 14.2). Care is taken to avoid any left PA obstruction. Again, echocardiographic assessment is performed to check the PAs and the flow in the ascending aorta [5].
- The anticoagulant strategy is generally a bolus of 50–100 IU/kg of heparin administered as a single bolus prior to stent insertion and 300 IU/kg/Day as a continuous infusion for the next 24 h. Subsequently, when feeding is started, prophylactic anti-aggregation is initiated with a 3–5 mg/kg/day of acetylsalicylic acid.

Comprehensive Stage II Repair

- The procedure begins with a redo sternotomy and central cannulation. This is usually achieved by arterial cannulation into the innominate artery (typically with a Dacron graft anastomosed to the artery in order to avoid post-cannulation stenosis) or in the main PA, and bicaval cannulations.
- The previously placed PA bands are carefully removed while lowering the temperature to

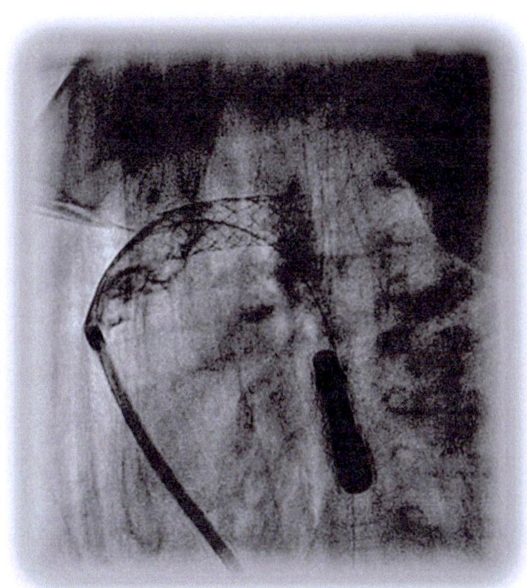

Fig. 14.2 Angiography obtained at the end of the procedure showing the PDA stenting

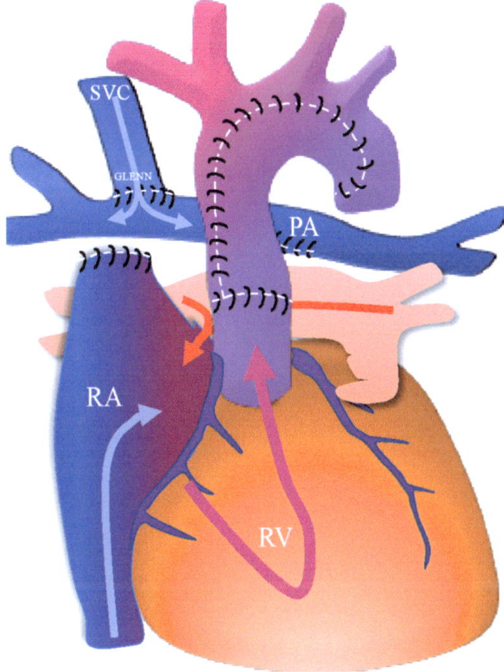

Fig. 14.3 Graphic representation of the comprehensive stage II procedure in hypoplastic left heart syndrome

18–20 °C. A cardioplegic arrest with antegrade cardioplegia is then obtained. Deep hypothermic cardiac arrest (DHCA) is initiated and an atrial septectomy is performed to ensure adequate interatrial shunting. The PDA is ligated and divided, with particular care to the proximal left PA. The distal part of the aortic arch is then reconstructed with a pulmonary homograft patch and regional cerebral perfusion is started. Once the entire arch has been shaped, a Damus-Kaye-Stansel anastomosis is performed, creating an aortopulmonary connection.

- The PAs are bilaterally enlarged with a patch of autologous pericardium in most patients. The patient is rewarmed, and a bidirectional cavopulmonary shunt is performed on an on-pump beating heart, in the standard fashion (see Fig. 14.3).

Outcomes

Almost three decades have elapsed since the first description of the hybrid approach for HLHS forms. Since then, efforts have been made to promote this technique, and medium and long-term results are now available. To date, nearly 15% of North American institutions are performing this technique (but with different indications), which represents a relatively small proportion of centres despite the initial enthusiasm for this new approach [9].

Initial experiences have reported high morbidity and mortality due to the inherent learning curve [10]. Recent studies have shown promising early survival after a hybrid approach, with a 30-day mortality as low as 4% [11]. However, at longer follow-up, survival appears to be comparable to the standard Norwood approach (1-year survival ~45%) [2].

Interstage mortality (5%) and reoperation rates (36%) have also been shown to be similar to those reported for the Norwood procedure [11]. Minimising inter-stage mortality is important in the management of these patients. The main features that should be routinely assessed during this phase are:

- Adequate retrograde perfusion in the ascending aorta
- Adequate atrial shunting
- Right ventricular function
- Atrioventricular valve regurgitation

The presence of aortic atresia and a birth weight of 2.0 kg or less have been shown to be significant predictors of operative mortality [12]. Hybrid patients weighing <2.6 kg and premature patients had the higher overall mortality in another report (83% vs 25% and 70% vs 0%, respectively) [2]. A multicenter analysis by the Congenital Heart Surgeons' Society seemed to suggest that the negative impact of lower birth weight (<2 kg) on survival may be the cause of increased mortality with a hybrid approach [9]. The Giessen group reported exceptional results after hybrid palliation, with a survival of 84% at 1 year, 78% at 2 years, 77.8% at 10 years, and 77% at 15 years [13]. The outcomes and potential of the hybrid procedure are, therefore, still debated.

Controversies

One of the most controversial concepts of hybrid physiology is the dependence of the supra aortic branches and coronary arteries on retrograde perfusion from the aortic isthmus [12]. This has been shown to have a negative impact on survival, particularly during the interstage period [14]. As mentioned, careful monitoring is needed to detect retrograde arch obstruction, particularly in cases with aortic atresia [14].

Furthermore, retrograde perfusion of the aortic arch has been associated with impaired cerebral perfusion in patients soon after hybrid palliation or during the interstage period [15]. Data on the neurodevelopmental outcomes of these patients have been inconsistent. While some studies supported benefits related to the avoidance of cardiopulmonary bypass and deep hypothermic arrest in neonates, others showed neurodevelopmental delay similar to Norwood patients [16].

Finally, another concept that has been extensively investigated is the potential lack of PA growth due to the restriction induced by the bands placed at Stage I [17]. Indeed, previous studies have shown an increase in the need for PA interventions in this group of patients, on their Fontan pathway. Long-term follow-up studies are needed to assess whether this impacts on the likelihood of Fontan failure [18].

Future Perspectives

Current guidelines for a hybrid palliation of HLHS are still unclear, with different center advocating multiple indications, ranging from:

- First stage palliation in all patients
- Selective use in particular anatomical variations
- Initial palliation in high-risk patients

There is no doubt that the main advantage of these strategies is the deferral of an extensive surgical repair, like the Norwood procedure, with the avoidance of cardiopulmonary bypass and deep hypothermic cardiocirculatory arrest in a neonate.

The most recent data seem to show a trend towards more specific indications, like:

- Premature patients
- Birth weight <2.5 kg
- Potential biventricular conversion at II stage

However, only long-term studies or randomized control investigations will give a definitive answer in the near future.

References

1. Stasik CN, Goldberg CS, Bove EL, Devaney EJ, Ohye RG. Current outcomes and risk factors for the Norwood procedure. J Thorac Cardiovasc Surg. 2006;131:412–7.
2. Sower CT, Romano JC, Yu S, Lowery R, Pasquali SK, Zampi JD. Early and midterm outcomes in high-risk

single-ventricle patients: hybrid vs norwood palliation. Ann Thorac Surg. 2019;108:1849–55.

3. Gibbs JL, Wren C, Watterson KG, Hunter S, Hamilton JRL. Stenting of the arterial duct combined with banding of the pulmonary arteries and atrial septectomy or septostomy: a new approach to palliation for the hypoplastic left heart syndrome. Br Heart J. 1993;69:551–5.

4. Akintuerk H, Michel-Behnke I, Valeske K, Mueller M, Thul J, Bauer J, et al. Stenting of the arterial duct and banding of the pulmonary arteries: basis for combined Norwood stage I and II repair in hypoplastic left heart. Circulation. 2002;105:1099–103.

5. Akintürk H, Michel-Behnke I, Valeske K, Mueller M, Thul J, Bauer J, et al. Hybrid transcatheter-surgical palliation–basis for univentricular or biventricular repair: the Giessen experience. Pediatr Cardiol. 2007;28:79–87.

6. Yerebakan C, Murray J, Valeske K, Thul J, Elmontaser H, Mueller M, et al. Long-term results of biventricular repair after initial Giessen hybrid approach for hypoplastic left heart variants. J Thorac Cardiovasc Surg. 2015;149:1112–22.

7. Trusler GA, Mustard WT. A method of banding the pulmonary artery for large isolated ventricular septal defect with and without transposition of the great arteries. Ann Thorac Surg. 1972;13:351–5.

8. Zampi JD, Hirsch JC, Goldstein BH, Armstrong AK. Use of a pressure guidewire to assess pulmonary artery band adequacy in the hybrid stage I procedure for high-risk neonates with Hypoplastic left heart syndrome and variants. Congenit Heart Dis. 2013;8:149–58.

9. Karamlou T, Overman D, Hill KD, Wallace A, Pasquali SK, Jacobs JP, et al. Stage 1 hybrid palliation for hypoplastic left heart syndrome-assessment of contemporary patterns of use: an analysis of the Society of Thoracic Surgeons congenital heart surgery database. J Thorac Cardiovasc Surg. 2015;149:195–202.

10. Galantowicz M, Cheatham JP, Phillips A, Cua CL, Hoffman TM, Hill SL, et al. Hybrid approach for Hypoplastic left heart syndrome: intermediate results after the learning curve. Ann Thorac Surg. 2008;85:2063–71.

11. Nwankwo UT, Morell EM, Trucco SM, Morell VO, Kreutzer J. Hybrid strategy for neonates with ductal-dependent systemic circulation at high risk for Norwood. Ann Thorac Surg. 2018;106:595–601.

12. Pizarro C, Davies RR, Woodford E, Radtke WA. Improving early outcomes following hybrid procedure for patients with single ventricle and systemic outflow obstruction: defining risk factors. Eur J Cardio-Thoracic Surg. 2014;47:995–1001.

13. Yerebakan C, Valeske K, Elmontaser H, Yörüker U, Mueller M, Thul J, et al. Hybrid therapy for hypoplastic left heart syndrome: myth, alternative, or standard? J Thorac Cardiovasc Surg. 2016;151:1112–23.

14. Stoica SC, Philips AB, Egan M, Rodeman R, Chisolm J, Hill S, et al. The retrograde aortic arch in the hybrid approach to Hypoplastic left heart syndrome. Ann Thorac Surg. 2009;88:1939–47.

15. Haller C, Caldarone CA. The evolution of therapeutic strategies: niche apportionment for hybrid palliation. Ann Thorac Surg. 2018;106:1873–80.

16. Knirsch W, Liamlahi R, Hug MI, Hoop R, von Rhein M, Prêtre R, et al. Mortality and neurodevelopmental outcome at 1 year of age comparing hybrid and Norwood procedures. Eur J Cardio-Thoracic Surg. 2012;42:33–9.

17. Davies RR. Stage 1 hybrid palliation for hypoplastic left heart syndrome-assessment of contemporary patterns of use: an analysis of the Society of Thoracic Surgeons congenital heart surgery database. J Thorac Cardiovasc Surg. 2015;149:203–4.

18. Baba K, Kotani Y, Chetan D, Chaturvedi RR, Lee KJ, Benson LN, et al. Hybrid versus Norwood strategies for single-ventricle palliation. Circulation. 2012;126:S123–31.

Part IV

The Fontan Physiology

Determinants of Cardiac Output and Exercise Tolerance in the Fontan Circulation

Pradeepkumar Charla, Adam W. Powell, and Gruschen R. Veldtman

Introduction

Cardiac output in the Fontan circulation is often preserved or slightly diminished at rest. Characteristically however it is distinctly inadequate for the exercising muscles during incremental exertion. This is an important contributor to the observation that more than 90% of Fontan patients have moderate or severely reduced exercise tolerance as compared to age and gender matched controls [1].

The underlying causes for this diminished cardiovascular performance are multifactorial and are summarized in this chapter [2].

Hemodynamic Responses

There are marked hemodynamic and anatomic differences between individuals with single ventricular physiology and a Fontan circulation, and those with a biventricular circulation and a sub-pulmonary right ventricle. Key hemodynamic findings for individuals a **normal** circulation are:

– Central and peripheral venous pressures are kept low by right ventricle (RV) action
– Pulsatile, high energy flow is pushed into the pulmonary circulation and beyond, causing shear stresses that optimize endothelial mediated vasodilation and pulmonary arterial compliance relative to the RV stroke volume

In the Fontan circulation by contrast, there is no sub-pulmonary ventricle and the resultant haemodynamic and neurohormonal adjustments are quite profound:

– There is obligatory elevation in resting central and peripheral venous pressures. These pressures are usually around 10–15 mmHg in an optimal Fontan circulation but can be significantly higher [3].
– The pressure gradient that normally exists between the venous capillary bed and the right atrium (RA) when a RV is present, is abolished in the Fontan circulation.
– A profound shift in the "venous" gradient occurs such that it is generated between the peripheral venous capillary bed and the left atrium. In this new circulation the dominant resistor is the pulmonary capillary bed [4] (Fig. 15.1).

P. Charla
University of Rochester School of Medicine, Rochester, NY, USA

A. W. Powell
Department of Pediatrics, University of Cincinnati College of Medicine, Cincinnati, OH, USA

The Heart Institute, Cincinnati, OH, USA
e-mail: Adam.powell@cchmc.org

G. R. Veldtman (✉)
Scottish Adult Congenital Heart Cardiac Service, Golden Jubilee National University Hospital, Glasgow, Scotland
e-mail: gruschen.veldtman@gjnh.scot.nhs.uk

© The Author(s), under exclusive license to Springer Nature Switzerland AG 2023
P. Clift et al. (eds.), *Univentricular Congenital Heart Defects and the Fontan Circulation*,
https://doi.org/10.1007/978-3-031-36208-8_15

- Blood volume increases predominantly in the venous compartment as angiotensin II and aldosterone is upregulated
- These adaptive cardiovascular responses obligate greater lymphatic flow and lymphatic neovascularization [5, 6].
- Lymphatic overflow and subsequent dysfunction is common as larger proportions of the blood volume depends on lymphatic drainage for its central return (Fig. 15.2)

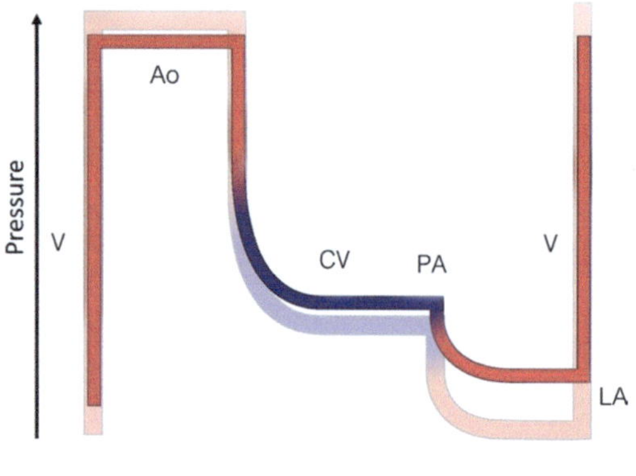

Fig. 15.1 Flow/pressure/saturation diagram of the Fontan circulation: changes over time. Fontan haemodynamics late (full colour) superimposed on Fontan early (transparent): with time the ventricular end-diastolic pressure and pulmonary vascular resistance increase, resulting in overall decreased flow and increased caval vein pressure/congestion. A downward progressive spiral ensues. *Ao* aorta, *CV* caval veins, *LA* left atrium, *PA* pulmonary artery, *V* single ventricle

- Non-pulsatile blood flow that is also subject to gravitational forces, exacerbates pulmonary endothelial dysfunction and contributes to a relatively fixed pulmonary vascular resistance
- Venous vessel walls become "arterialized" and significantly dilated, increasingly lacking the ability to adjust their "tone" physiologically, i.e. venous capacitance and compliance becomes decreased
- Splanchnic blood volume and splanchnic venous tone loses its ability to change tone in response to dynamic demands as is evidenced by lack of change with Valsalva and postural change
- Preload to the systemic ventricle is critical to performance and is vulnerable to minor changes in the circulations: relatively minor pulmonary vascular resistance (PVR) alterations: PVR values of greater than 2 WU with associated cardiac index (CI) < 2.5 L/min/m^2 has been associated with a high risk of Fontan failure
- Ventricular diastolic performance, with end-diastolic pressure (EDP) $\geq$ 12 mmHg, and occult diastolic dysfunction [defined as a post 15 mL/kg fluid challenge increase in ventricular EDP $\geq$ 15 mmHg] being highly associated Fontan failure and/or mortality outcomes [7].
- The size and capacitance of the pulmonary venous vasculature [8]

Fig. 15.2 (**a**) Lower limb and pelvic lymphatics in a normal individual. (**b**) Lower limb and pelvic lymphatics in an individual with a Fontan. Courtesy: Prof Vibeke Hjortdal

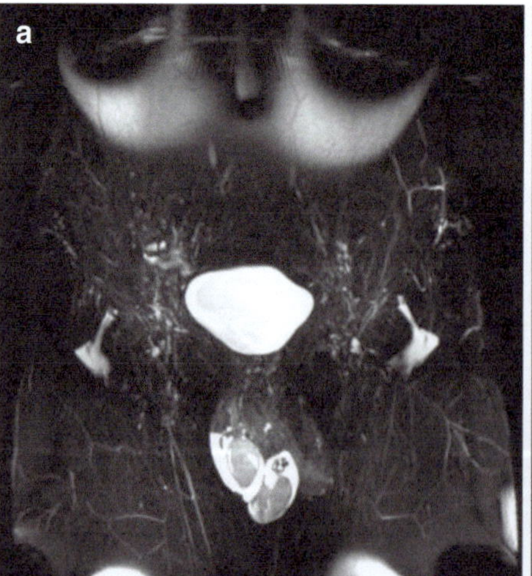

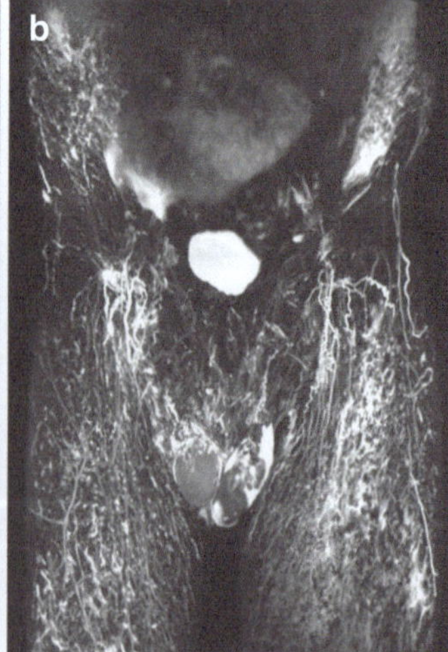

– The peripheral muscle pump and pulmonary mechanics which may contribute as much as 30% to cardiac output [9]

Ventricular structural alterations are common due to altered fiber orientation and arrangement, fibrosis and myocardial energetics resulting in disturbed systolic and diastolic function as well as possible intraventricular dyssynchrony [10, 11].

There is profound neurohormonal activation akin to that seen in heart failure including BNP, ET-1, NE, hsCRP, sTNF-RI, and IL-6 among other markers [12].

Ventricular-vascular coupling is abnormal, specifically arterial elastance is usually abnormally elevated [13].

Maladaptive Cardiovascular Responses During Exercise

The response to exercise is abnormally and typically cardiac index usually cannot augment more than 50% above baseline as opposed to the 200–300% rise seen in normal biventricular circulations. Most of the limitation in cardiac output response occurs due to lack in ventricular stroke volume augmentation (Fig. 15.3) consequent upon contractile and diastolic properties outlined below [14].

There is an inability to augment ventricular stroke volume secondary to:

– A progressive decline in end-systolic elastance (Ees, end systolic elastance), MSW

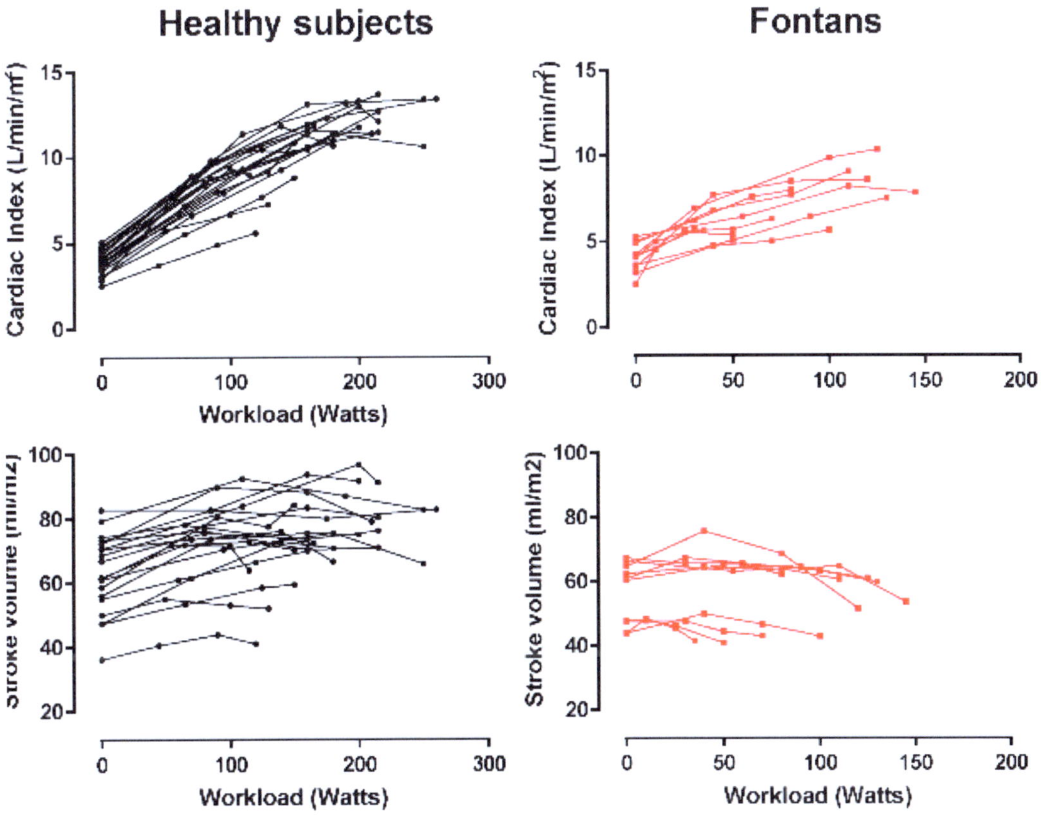

Fig. 15.3 Changes in cardiac index and stroke volume from rest to peak exercise in controls (left panels) and Fontan patients (right panels)

[slope of the preload recruitable stroke work], PWR [maximal ventricular power] max/indexed end-diastolic area (EDAI) and peak rate of ventricular pressure rise (dP/dTmax, peak rate of ventricular pressure rise)) and EDAI during exercise

- A significant decrease in Tau [isovolumic constant of ventricular relaxation] sa heart rate increases [15]
- A decline in indexed end-diastolic volume as exercise progresses consistent with ventricular preload deprivation during exercise [16].

Venous pressures rise profoundly during exercise usually augmenting by as much as 88% above baseline [17]. Flow efficiency reduces, energy losses increase during exercise, and is more marked in the presence of smaller Fontan conduits. Similarly, smaller pulmonary vascular beds are associated with reduced exercise capacity.

Chronotropic and heart rate reserves are both reduced during peak exercise and other parameters of autonomic function are also deranged [14]. Maldistribution of pulmonary blood flow has also been shown to be negatively associated with exercise function [18].

The Role of Skeletal Muscle Mass

Skeletal muscle mass and respiratory muscle mass often are reduced in Fontan patients. This reduced muscle mass is highly correlated with reduced exercise performance [19]. Muscle perfusion is also reduced during exercise and is likely to be a key mechanism for limitation in exercise performance.

Fontan patients have slower skeletal muscle oxygenation kinetics with the resultant altered skeletal muscle metabolism possibly being a factor in the reduced aerobic capacity in these patients [20].

The High Functioning Fontan

Despite these observations there exists a group of Fontan patients that have normal or near normal functional capacity, i.e. >80% of predicted peak

VO_2 [21]. They comprise up to 20% of asymptomatic Fontan patients. High functioning Fontans characteristically have higher VO_2 during the submaximal exercise phase despite similar heart rates and exercise workload, suggesting a preserved Starling mechanism leading to better stroke volume and/or better peripheral extraction as compared to the lesser functioning peers.

High functioning Fontan patients tend to have had a shorter, less complicated postoperative course, normal systolic function on resting echocardiogram and higher self-reported physical activity.

Potential Therapeutic Strategies

Subclinical hemodynamic abnormalities should be sought through routine surveillance: Early recognition of hemodynamic and other culprit lesions through regular surveillance monitoring may allow prompt treatment with the possibility of better available treatment options and more favourable treatment responses. Possible abnormalities that are identifiable on routine screening include: occult Fontan pathway obstruction, thrombo-embolic disease, obstructive sleep apnoea, elevated pulmonary vascular resistance [22].

Cardiopulmonary exercise test (CPET) with peripheral venous pressure monitoring as a screening tool may be helpful in identifying adverse haemodynamics. Abnormal venous pressures at rest or during maximal exercise should prompt invasive hemodynamic assessment, and if necessary, with dynamic testing i.e. fluid challenge, exercise cardiac catheter, and or incremental pacing to detect heart related adverse hemodynamic responses [15, 17].

In the 2018 AHA/ACC Guideline for Management of Adults with Congenital Heart Disease following up surveillance recommendations include:

- Annual echocardiogram or cardiac MRI
- CPET every 1–3 years
  - Fontan patients with a peak $VO_2 < 16.6$ mL/kg/min may have a greater risk of morbidity and mortality compared to patients with

more normal VO_2 values [23]. This is however controversial as data is mixed.

- Serial CPET has been shown to have prognostic significance when the following are present:

A decline of percent predicted peak VO_2 >3%/year predictor of 5 year risk of cardiac event [24] and for every 10% decline in peak VO_2, there is a doubling of the hazard for death/transplant [25]

Routine cardiac catheterization during adolescence before transfer to adult care, may help identify occult hemodynamic problems.

Non-invasive Therapeutic Interventions

Exercise cardiopulmonary rehabilitation: A comprehensive cardiopulmonary rehabilitation improves functional capacity in individuals with a Fontan with completion of a 12-week supervised cardiopulmonary rehabilitation program that included 60 min exercise sessions focused on increasing aerobic capacity and muscular strength demonstrated both an improvement in peak VO_2 and oxygen pulse in 10 Fontan patients [26] (Fig. 15.4). Rehabilitation may also improve in submaximal and maximal VO_2 and oxygen pulse in rehabilitation programs ranging in time from 12 weeks to 8 months [27–29].

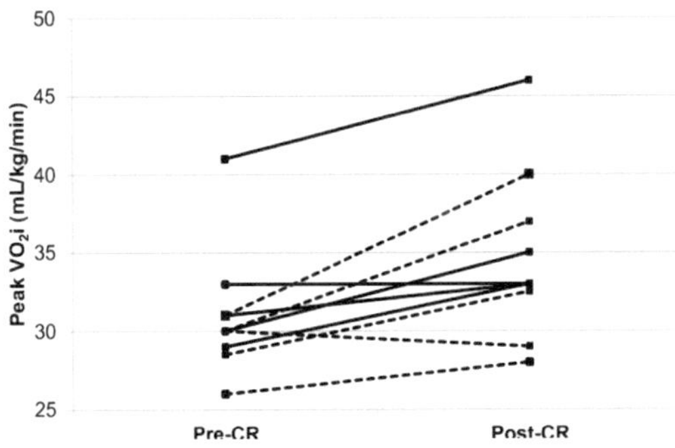

Fig. 15.4 Improved peak indexed oxygen consumption (VO2i) after cardiac rehabilitation (CR). Dashed lines correspond to individual patients with hypoplastic left heart syndrome s/p Fontan, solid lines correspond to those with tricuspid atresia s/p Fontan

Beyond structured cardiopulmonary rehabilitation, increased habitual activity is associated with lower body mass index in Fontan patients [30].

Respiratory muscle strengthening may be of benefit. Twelve weeks of inspiratory muscle training using a threshold inspiratory muscle training device is associated with statistically significant improvement in work rate and trended towards improved peak VO_2 and VE/VCO_2 slope [31]. Six weeks inspiratory muscle training associated with improvement in maximal inspiratory pressure, resting cardiac output and ejection fraction [32]. Twelve weeks of yoga focusing on "breathing training" demonstrates that such exercise program is safe, feasible and have potential to improve muscle strength as well as QoL [33].

Weight loss is important. The Obesity prevalence in paediatric Fontan patients is comparable with United States national data and is highly predictive of obesity in adults patients with a Fontan [34]. Obesity is associated with a significantly shorter transplant free survival [35], symptomatic heart failure and mortality [36]. Based on these observations weight loss therefore has considerable potential prognostic benefits.

Drugs acting on the pulmonary vascular bed: After several placebo-controlled trials, 2 randomized placebo controlled cross-over trials, and at least 7 observational trials in Fontan patients, the specific clinical phenotypes among Fontan patients that might benefit from chronic pulmonary vasodilator therapy in terms of exercise capacity benefit, remains elusive. For summary of trial see Table 15.1.

Acute trials in contrast have demonstrated hemodynamic benefit

- Sildenafil appears to improve ventilatory efficiency by decreasing pulmonary vascular resistance and increasing stroke volume
- Results of the FUEL trial evaluating effect of Udenafil on exercise capacity demonstrated no significant improvement in oxygen consumption at peak exercise but some improvement at ventilatory anaerobic threshold [37]

Table 15.1 Summary of research demonstrating benefit on exercise capacity with both acute and chronic therapy

Study	Intervention	Results
Wittekind et al. 2018 [26]	12 weeks cardiopulmonary rehabilitation	Improvement in peak VO_2 and oxygen pulse
Wu et al. 2018 [31]	12 weeks inspiratory muscle training	Improvement in work rate and VE/VCO_2 slope
Laohachai et al. 2017 [32]	6 weeks inspiratory muscle training	Improvement in max inspiratory pressure, resting cardiac output and ejection fraction
Charla et al. 2019 [33]	12 weeks yoga and breathing exercise	Increased strength and QoL
Goldberg et al. 2019 [37]	Udenafil	Improvement VO_2 at anaerobic threshold but not peak exercise
Rhodes et al. 2013 [38]	Inhaled Iloprost	Improvement in peak VO_2 and oxygen pulse
Giardini et al. 2008 [39]	Sildenafil	Improvement in peak VO_2 after single dose when tested on same day
Goldberg et al. 2011 [40]	Sildenafil	Improved VE/VCO_2 slope but not peak VO_2
Shang et al. 2016 [41]	Bosentan	Improved 6 min walk test distance
Cedars et al. 2016 [42]	Ambrisentan	Improved peak VO_2 in adult patients

- Inhaled Iloprost (prostacyclin analogue) led to increase peak oxygen consumption and oxygen pulse [38]

Drugs Acting on the Ventricular Myocardium

Angiotensin Converting Enzyme Inhibitors and Angiotensin Receptor Antagonists: Despite the potential neurohormonal effects of ACE inhibitors in Fontan patients, no trial to date has demonstrated favourable hemodynamic nor exercise capacity benefits. Six weeks of Enalapril did not improve cardiac index or exercise capacity in stable and well Fontan patients with normal ventricular systolic function [43].

Digoxin: To date there are no published trials demonstrating beneficial effects of digitalis on exercise capacity or hemodynamics in patients with a Fontan.

Tailored drug therapy approach: A combination of ACE inhibition, isosorbide dinitrate and diuretics when uptitrated as an inpatient, was demonstrated in a small trial, to reduce venous pressures [8.9 vs. 14 mmHg] whilst preserving cardiac output relative to control subjects [44]. However, the effects on exercise capacity were not assessed. There have also been other experimental pharmacologic approaches including probenecid and pimobendan.

Devices improving electromechanical coupling: Sinus node dysfunction as intraventricular dyssynchrony is relatively common in patients with a Fontan. Pacing devices that re-establish atrio-ventricular synchrony as well as mechanical synchrony have the potential to improve ventricular preload, and myocardial contractility.

Intermittent External Ventilation: Short-term, external ventilation (Hayek RTX) has been shown to significantly augment pulmonary blood flow and cardiac output safely and effectively in adult Fontan subjects in ambulatory settings. In this study below, two ventilator modes were tested. Among the two modes, biphasic cuirass ventilation (BCV) had greater impact and was well tolerated compared to continuous negative pressure ventilation (CNEP) [45].

Intermittent pneumatic compression devices: Pneumatic compression devices act by uniformly applying circumferential pressure to the lower extremities. The application of pneumatic compression devices for 2–4 h daily over a week resulted in larger exercise time, peak VO_2, and ventilatory threshold on Bruce treadmill testing compared to baseline [46].

Ventricular Assist Devices (VADs): Mechanical circulatory support may be used as a treatment for Fontan failure. Minimal study has been performed on exercise performance in Fontan patients with a VAD, but numerical models with physiologic control algorithms have been proposed to improve hemodynamics during exercise [47].

Total Artificial Heart (TAH): The total artificial heart has been used as a bridge to transplantation in the patient with the failing Fontan [48]. There is minimal research on exercise capacity in this population and whether rehabilitation could result in improved exercise capacity and/or transplant outcomes.

Summary

The Fontan circulation is almost uniformly associated with exercise impairment. Only 20% of asymptomatic Fontan patients appear to have normal exercise capacity. This exercise limitation is characterised by preload limitation to the systemic ventricle. There are multiple potential anatomic and functional reasons for this preload limitation as discussed above.

Interventional strategies that may be helpful include regular systematic surveillance as recommended in the recent AHA Position Statement on the management of Fontan patients. This may assist in earlier recognition and treatment of pathology. Other interventions include exercise rehabilitation, respiratory muscle strengthening, weight loss if obese, pulmonary vasodilatory medication, and a tailored drug therapy approach.

The recent addition of a variety of devices to the treatment options hold great promise but need further trials to better their specific indications and benefits. These devices include intermittent external ventilation, intermittent pneumatic compression, ventricular assist devices and total cardiac replacement therapies (devices or transplantation).

References

1. Kempny A, Dimopoulos K, Uebing A, Moceri P, Swan L, Gatzoulis MA, et al. Reference values for exercise limitations among adults with congenital heart disease. Relation to activities of daily-life—single Centre experience and review of published data. Eur Heart J. 2012;33(11):1386–96.

2. Shafer KM, Garcia JA, Babb TG, Fixler DE, Ayers CR, Levine BD. The importance of the muscle and ventilatory pumps during exercise in patients without a subpulmonary ventricle (Fontan operation). J Am Coll Cardiol. 2012;60:2115–21.

3. Masutani A, Kurishima C, Yana A, Kuwata S, Iwamoto Y, Saiki H, et al. Assessment of central venous physiology of Fontan circulation using peripheral venous pressure. J Thorac. 2017;153(4):912–20.

4. Gewillig M, Brown SC, van de Bruaene A, Rychik J. Providing a framework of principles for conceptualising the Fontan circulation. Acta Paediatr. 2019;109:651–8.

5. Mohanakumar S, Telinius N, Kelly B, Lauridsen H, Boedtkjer D, Pedersen M, et al. Morphology and function of the lymphatic vasculature in patients with a Fontan circulation. Circ Cardiovasc Imaging. 2019;12(4):e008074.

6. Dori Y, Keller MC, Fogel MA, Rome JJ, Whitehead KK, Harris MA, et al. MRI of lymphatic abnormalities after functional single-ventricle palliation surgery. AJR. 2014;203(2):426–31.

7. Averin K, Hirsch R, Seckeler MD, Whiteside W, Beekman RH 3rd, Goldstein BH. Diagnosis of occult diastolic dysfunction late after the Fontan procedure using a rapid volume expansion technique. Heart. 2016;104(14):1109–14.

8. Hays BS, Baker M, Laib A, Tan W, Udholm S, Goldstein BH, et al. Histopathological abnormalities in the central arteries and veins of Fontan patients. Heart. 2018;104(4):324–31.

9. Cordina R, O'Meagher S, Gould H, Rae C, Kemp G, Pasco JA, Celermajer DS, et al. Skeletal muscle abnormalities and exercise capacity in adults with a Fontan circulation. Heart. 2013;99(20):1530–4.

10. Rathod RH, Prakash A, Powell AJ, Geva T. Myocardial fibrosis identified by cardiac magnetic resonance late gadolinium enhancement is associated with adverse ventricular mechanics and ventricular tachycardia late after Fontan operation. J Am Coll Cardiol. 2010;55:1721–8.

11. Ho PK, Lai CT, Wong SJ, Cheung YF. Three-dimensional mechanical dyssynchrony and myocardial deformation of the left ventricle in patients with tricuspid atresia after Fontan procedure. J Am Soc Echocardiogr. 2012;25:393–400.

12. Bolger AP, Sharma R, Li W, Leenarts M, Kalra PR, Kemp M, et al. Neurohormonal activiation and the chronic heart failure syndrome in adults with congenital heart disease. Circulation. 2002;106(1):92–9.

13. Godfrey ME, Rathod RH, Keenan E, Gauvreau K, Powell AJ, Geva T, et al. Inefficient ventriculoarterial coupling in Fontan patients: a cardiac magnetic resonance study. Pediatr Cardiol. 2018;39(4):763–73.

14. Claessen G, La Gerche A, Van De Bruaene A, Claeys M, Willems R, Dymarkowski S, et al. Heart rate reserve in Fontan patients: chronotropic incompe-

tence or hemodynamic limitation? J Am Heart Assoc. 2019;8(9):e012008.

15. Senzaki H, Masutani S, Ishido H, Taketazu M, Kobayashi T, Sasaki N, et al. Cardiac rest and reserve function in patients with Fontan circulation. J Am Coll Cardiol. 2006;47(12):2528–35.

16. Pushparajah K, Wong JK, Bellsham-Revell HR, Hussain T, Valverde I, Bell A, et al. Magnetic resonance imaging catheter stress haemodynamics post-Fontan in hypoplastic left heart syndrome. Eur Heart J Cardiovasc Imaging. 2016;17(6):644–51.

17. Navaratnam D, Fitzsimmons S, Grocott M, Rossiter HB, Emmanuel Y, Diller GP, et al. Exercise-induced systemic venous hypertension in the Fontan circulation. Am J Cardiol. 2016;117(10):1667–71.

18. Alsaied T, Sleeper LA, Masci M, Ghelani SJ, Azcue N, Geva T, et al. Maldistribution of pulmonary blood flow in patients after the Fontan operation is associated with worse exercise capacity. J Cardiovasc Magn Reson. 2018;20(85):1–10. https://doi.org/10.1186/s12968-018-0505-4.

19. Avitabile CM, Leonard MB, Zemel BS, Brodsky JL, Lee D, Dodds K, et al. Lean mass deficits, vitamin D status and exercise capacity in children and young adults after Fontan palliation. Heart. 2014;100(21):1702–7.

20. Sandberg C, Crenshaw AG, Elcadi GH, Christersson C, Hlebowicz J, Thilen U, et al. Slower skeletal muscle oxygenation kinetics in adults with complex congenital heart disease. Can J Cardiol. 2019;35:1815–23.

21. Powell AW, Chin C, Alsaied T, Rossiter HR, Wittekind S, Mays WA, et al. The unique clinical phenotype and exercise adaptation of Fontan patients with normal exercise capacity. Can J Cardiol. 2019;36:1499–507.

22. Rychik J, Atz AM, Celermajer DS, Deal BJ, Gatzoulis MA, Gewillig MH, et al. Evaluation and management of the child and adult with Fontan circulation: a scientific statement from the American Heart Association. Circulation. 2019;140(6):e234–84.

23. Fernandes SM, Alexander ME, Graham DA, Khairy P, Clair M, Rodriguez E, et al. Exercise testing identifies patients at increased risk for morbidity and mortality following Fontan surgery. Congenit Heart Dis. 2011;6:294–303.

24. Egbe AC, Driscoll DJ, Khan AR, Said SS, Akintoye E, Berganza FM, et al. Cardiopulmonary exercise test in adults with prior Fontan operation: the prognostic value of serial testing. Int J Cardiol. 2017;235:6–10.

25. Cunningham JW, Nathan AS, Rhodes J, Shafer K, Landzberg MJ, Opotowsky AR. Decline in peak oxygen consumption over time predicts death or transplantation in adults with a Fontan circulation. Am Heart J. 2017;189:184–92.

26. Wittekind S, Mays W, Gerdes Y, Knecht S, Hambrook J, Border W, et al. A novel mechanism for improved exercise performance in pediatric Fontan patients after cardiac rehabilitation. Pediatr Cardiol. 2018;39(5):1023–30.

27. Rhodes J, Curran TJ, Camil L, Rabideau N, Fulton DR, Gauthier NS, et al. Impact of cardiac rehabilitation on the exercise function of children with serious congenital heart disease. Pediatrics. 2005;116(6):1339–45.

28. Opocher F, Varnier M, Sanders SP, Tosoni A, Zaccaria M, Stellin G, et al. Effects of aerobic exercise training in children after the Fontan operation. Am J Cardiol. 2005;95(1):150–2.

29. Cordina RL, O'Meagher S, Karmali A, Rae CL, Liess C, Kemp GJ, et al. Resistance training improves cardiac output, exercise capacity and tolerance to positive airway pressure in Fontan physiology. Int J Cardiol. 2013;168(2):780–8.

30. O'Bryne ML, McBride MG, Paridon S, Goldmuntz E. Association of habitual activity and body mass index in survivors of congenital heart surgery: a study of children and adolescents with tetralogy of Fallot, transposition of the great arteries, and Fontan palliation. World J Pediatr Congenit Heart Surg. 2018;9(2):177–84.

31. Wu FM, Opotowsky AR, Denhoff ER, Gongwer R, Gervitz MZ, Landzberg MJ, et al. A pilot study of inspiratory muscle training to improve exercise capacity in patients with Fontan physiology. Semin Thorac Cardiovasc Surg. 2018;30(4):462–9.

32. Laohachai K, Winlaw D, Selvadurai H, Gnanappa GK, d'Udekem Y, Celermajer D, et al. Inspiratory muscle training is associated with improve ventilatory muscle strength, resting cardiac output and the ventilatory efficiency of exercise in patients with a Fontan circulation. J Am Heart Assoc. 2017;6(8):e005750.

33. Charla P, Shah A, Oechslin E, Granton J, Wald R. The impact of yoga on cardiopulmonary function and quality of life in the fontan population—a pilot study. Abstract presented. Manuscript in review.

34. Chung ST, Hong B, Patterson L, Petit CJ, Ham JN. High overweight and obesity in Fontan patients: a 20-year history. Pediatr Cardiol. 2016;37(1):192–200.

35. Freud LR, Webster G, Costello JM, Tsao S, Rychlik K, Backer CL, Deal BJ. Growth and obesity among older single ventricle patients presenting for Fontan conversion. World J Pediatr Congenit Heart Surg. 2015;6(4):514–20.

36. Martinez SC, Byku M, Novak EL, Cedars AM, Eghtesady P, Ludbrook PA, et al. Increased body mass index is associated with congestive heart failure and mortality in adult Fontan patients. Congenit Heart Dis. 2016;11(1):71–9.

37. Goldberg DJ, Zak V, Goldstein BH, Schumacher KR, Rhodes J, Penny DJ, et al. Results of the Fontan Udenafil exercise longitudinal (FUEL) trial. Circulation. 2019;140(25):E993–4. [Epub ahead of print]

38. Rhodes J, Ubeda-Tikkanen A, Clair M, Fernandes SM, Graham DA, Milliren CE, et al. Effect of inhaled Iloprost on the exercise function of Fontan patients. Int J Cardiol. 2013;168(3):2435–40.

39. Giardini A, Balducci A, Specchia S, Gargiulo G, Bonvicini M, Picchio FM. Effect of sildenafil on haemodynamic response to exercise and exercise capacity in Fontan patients. Eur Heart J. 2008;29(13):1681–7.

40. Goldberg DJ, French B, McBride MG, Marino BS, Mirarchi N, Hanna BD, et al. Impact of oral sildenafil on exercise performance in children and young adults after the fontan operation: a randomized, double-blind, placebo-controlled, crossover trial. Circulation. 2011;123:1185–93.
41. Shang XK, Lu R, Zhang X, Zhang CD, Xiao SN, Liu M, et al. Efficacy of bosentan in patients after Fontan procedures: a double-blind, randomized controlled trial. J Huazhong Univ Sci Technolog Med Sci. 2016;36:534–40.
42. Cedars AM, Saef J, Peterson LR, Coogan AR, Novak EL, Kemp D, et al. Effect of ambrisentan on exercise capacity in adult patients after the Fontan procedure. Am J Cardiol. 2016;117:1524–32.
43. Kouatli AA, Garcia JA, Zellers TM, Weinstein EM, Mahony L. Enalapril does not enhance exercise capacity in patients after Fontan procedure. Circulation. 1997;96(5):1507–12.
44. Kurishima C, Saiki H, Masutani S, Senzaki H. Tailored therapy for aggressive dilation of systemic veins and arteries may result in improved long-term Fontan circulation. J Thorac Cardiovasc Surg. 2015;150(5):1367–70.
45. Charla P, Karur GR, Yamamura K, Yoo SJ, Granton J, Oechslin E, Shah A, Benson L, Honjo O, Mertens L, Alonso RG, Hanneman K, Wald RM. Augmentation of pulmonary blood flow and cardiac output by external ventilation in adult Fontan patients. Heart. 2021;107(2):142–9.
46. Hernandez J, Chopski SG, Lee S, Moskowitz WB, Throckmorton AL. Externally applied compression therapy for Fontan patients. Transl Pediatr. 2018;7(1):14–22.
47. Granegger M, Schweiger M, Schmid Daners M, Meboldt M, Hübler M. Cavopulmonary mechanical circulatory support in Fontan patients and the need for physiologic control: a computational study with a closed-loop exercise model. Int J Artif Organs. 2018;41(5):261–8.
48. Rossano JW, Goldberg DJ, Fuller S, Ravishankar C, Montenegro LM, Gaynor JW. Successful use of the total artificial heart in the failing Fontan circulation. Ann Thorac Surg. 2014;97(4):1438–40.

Part V

Follow Up in Childhood of Fontan Patients

Neuro-developmental Outcomes of Fontan Patients

Paola Cogo, Massimo A. Padalino, Elisa Cainelli, Giovanni Di Salvo, and Patrizia Bisiacchi

Introduction

Over the last four decades, numerous technical modifications to the original Fontan procedure have been proposed, initially for the management of newborns with tricuspid atresia, including the milestone of the intermediate staging with a bidirectional cavo-pulmonary anastomosis, the development of the concept of total cavo-pulmonary anastomosis, and finally the exclusion of the atrial chamber from the Fontan circuit with the lateral tunnel and extracardiac conduit associated with a fenestration in the Fontan circuit [1].

These modifications led to the fact that currently, a wide variety of congenital cardiac defects other than tricuspid atresia are perfectly suitable for a Fontan circulation.

Long-term survival in such patients with a Fontan circulation has improved significantly over the last two decades, ranging from 85 to 97%, as reported in recent publications [2, 3]. As a result, as it happens for other congenital heart diagnoses, the scientific attention of our medical community is moving beyond survival, but focusing instead on long-term functional results, such as health-related quality of life and neurodevelopmental outcome [4–6].

Nowadays, it is well recognized that the stressful conditions (such as those occurring in children with single ventricle physiology prior to and post-birth) in a developing brain can trigger pro-inflammatory processes followed by a cascade of worsening events that can impair the capability of the immature brain for optimal development. This vulnerability becomes more evident when the environment becomes more demanding and competitive, and complex cognitive abilities, such as learning and social relationships, are required, i.e. transition to school-age. Therefore, the preschool years become a critical developmental period, where the building blocks for later success are laid and where those social, behavioural, and neuropsychological skills necessary for social and academic success are acquired [7].

P. Cogo (✉)
Division of Pediatrics, Department of Medicine, University Hospital S Maria della Misericordia, University of Udine, Udine, Italy
e-mail: paola.cogo@uniud.it

M. A. Padalino
Department of Cardio-Thoracic and Vascular Sciences, and Public Health, University of Padova, Padova, Italy

E. Cainelli
Department of General Psychology, University of Padova, Padova, Italy

G. Di Salvo
Department of Woman and Child Health, University of Padova, Padova, Italy

P. Bisiacchi
Department of General Psychology, University of Padova, Padova, Italy

Padova Neuroscience Centre, PNC, Padova, Italy

"

As mentioned above, the medical community focuses on understanding the impact of both the functional single ventricle condition and its treatment on the neurodevelopmental outcome. Thus, we need to define the underlying pathophysiology of the subtle or overt brain damage and how/when to perform a neurodevelopmental follow up to implement a targeted intervention.

Impaired Neurodevelopment in Fontan Physiology

Recent studies indicate that, overall, Fontan patients have impaired neurodevelopmental outcomes compared to their healthy peers at all stages of the treatment pathway [8–15]. In fact, during growth:

- Fontan patients are exposed to increased risk for cyanosis, acidosis, hypoxic-ischemic injury, or shock for duct closure in the early neonatal period, with secondary effects on cognitive, neuropsychological, educational, and behavioural neurodevelopment.
- Also, most patients with CHD with univentricular physiology undergo multiple surgical procedures with cardiopulmonary bypass (CPB), with or without associated deep hypothermic circulatory arrest (DHCA). It has been demonstrated that children with univentricular heart defects—hypoplastic left heart syndrome—exhibit a CPB-related increase of plasma glial fibrillary acidic protein (GFAP), an early marker of brain injury. This increases only after the Norwood procedure, which occurs in the newborn age. Interestingly, the maximum GFAP increase occurred at the end of rewarming [14].
- In infancy and early childhood, failure to thrive is common and may adversely affect motor skills.
- Before the Fontan operation, all patients have chronic hypoxia, which may later impair cognitive function.
- The potential for embolic events exists both before and after completion of the Fontan circulation.

- All individuals are exposed to the psychological stress of having chronic cardiac disease throughout their life.

Several correlates of poor functioning have been identified [16].

- older age
- the presence of a genetic condition
- prematurity
- CHD with aortic arch obstruction
- lower socioeconomic status
- multiple operations and cardiac catheterizations
- a longer length of hospital stay
- complications such as brain injury, Fontan-associated liver disease, kidney failure.
- Despite the presence of multiple risk factors for adverse neurodevelopmental outcomes among patients undergoing a Fontan procedure, most individuals have scores on standardized tests of cognitive ability and academic achievement within the normal range in cross-sectional follow-up studies [17].
- However, as a group, Fontan patients have significantly lower scores on general intelligence, academic achievement, memory, executive functions, visuospatial skills, attention, and social cognition, when compared to the general population [18–20].
- In particular, scores of adolescents with HLHS or other single right ventricle abnormalities, who have undergone a Norwood procedure, are generally lower than those of adolescents who did not have such an operation in early life. Similarly, they also have significantly lower scores in general intelligence, reading, math achievement, and executive function [17, 21].
- In terms of intelligence, verbal skills appear to be stronger in Fontan patients than perceptual reasoning skills. Processing speed is also reported to be relatively weak [22].
- Concerning academic achievement, reading and mathematics skills and mnemonic function are significantly lower than expected in Fontan patients [17].

- In terms of executive functions, parents and teachers perceive more significant executive dysfunction in adolescent Fontan patients than perceived by the adolescents themselves. Visuospatial skills are also often fragile [17].
- The frequency of parent-reported ADHD-related behaviours ranges between 26 and 37% [23, 24].
- Regarding social cognition, Fontan patients score worse in average than others in their ability to identify the emotions behind facial expressions, and they show more concrete "externally-oriented thinking" [17, 24].

While most studies on neurodevelopmental outcomes in this population are cross-sectional, it would be beneficial to obtain longitudinal follow-up data, since the association between neurocognitive function and clinical parameters may highlight modifiable postnatal factors that could be addressed to optimize neurocognitive outcomes.

Factors that may impact on neurodevelopmental outcome after Fontan operation Currently, patients after Fontan surgery show excellent survival. However, about one half may experience major adverse events in the years after surgery, which can significantly impact on neurological outcomes [2–23].

- Early and late risk factors of impaired neurodevelopmental outcome after the Fontan procedure have been highlighted above.
- Early risk factors after Fontan operation are arrhythmias, thromboembolic events and Fontan failure that can significantly affect the length of hospital stay after surgery.
- Late risk factors are Fontan failure, supraventricular tachycardia, thromboembolism, or complete atrioventricular (AV) heart block, which often requires pacemaker implantation, usually later in life, and can also have an impact on neurodevelopment and quality of life.
- Patients undergoing aortic arch re-interventions and extended hospital stay for prolonged pleural effusions after Fontan surgery have worse late neurodevelopmental outcomes.

Neurodevelopmental Assessment in Fontan Patients

- The long-term outcome of patients undergoing a Fontan procedure is still poorly studied, and the current knowledge is based on limited retrospective or short/mid-term longitudinal data. The uncertainty about neurodevelopmental outcomes is increased by the use of different and poorly comparable measures.
- Neurodevelopmental outcomes are measured using standardized tests according to age and aims of the study. Raw scores are age-corrected and converted into standardized scores using published normative data. A global estimate of the individual neurodevelopmental profile is obtained by calculating intelligence (children and adults) and psychomotor (infants) quotients. For example, a psychomotor quotient may be obtained using the Bayley Scales of Infant Development [25, 26]. As more complex cognitive functions emerge, appropriate intelligence tasks may be administered. The most famous are the Wechsler Intelligence Scales, in versions for preschool children (WPPSI-III), children and adolescents (WISC-IV31), and adults (WAIS-IV32) [27].
- Beyond global quotients, standardized measures of different aspects that characterize human behaviour and functioning are available: neuropsychological tests (memory, language, attention), academic achievement, psychopathological questionnaires, and structured interviews.
- Older studies investigating outcomes after the Fontan procedure focused on global intelligence quotients (IQ) and found only modestly abnormal scores [28–31]. However, global IQ scores are not the best choice for capturing the high complexity of the broad range of symptoms that patients with CHD may exhibit [7], and recent work has shown that patients undergoing a Fontan procedure may develop several neuropsychological impairment, including executive dysfunction, visuomotor integration deficits, memory, attention, and motor skills [11, 17, 32]. Learning disorders, psychopathologies such as deficit hyperactiv-

ity disorder (ADHD), and reduced quality of life have also been reported [17, 24, 33]. In conclusion, more than one-third of the patients undergoing the Fontan procedure has demonstrated some degree of abnormal functioning in various neurocognitive domains, and about 15% exhibit severe impairment [18–21].

- Medical risk factors seem to be implicated in the development of cognitive and psychopathological symptoms, such as prematurity [24] and younger age at Fontan surgery [21]. Furthermore, neurodevelopmental impairment has been associated with smaller global brain volumes and white matter injury [21]. In particular, the widespread abnormalities found in white matter microstructure have been related to cognitive performance [34]. These studies demonstrated that the Fontan procedure might be associated with abnormalities of the brain structure and function, with associations described between neurocognitive function and clinical characteristics.
- The population studied belongs to different age ranges (infancy, childhood, adolescence, and adulthood), though most studies include children >10 years and young adults. The age range selected for the follow-up is essential because cognition and personality take several years to develop; cumulative effects may take time to become evident. Studies on CHD have shown that the full range of neurodevelopmental morbidity can be appreciated in follow-up, extending well into late childhood and adolescence, a crucial period for the emergence of underlying vulnerabilities when patients face complex academic and social challenges [17, 35].
- The broad range of mild, moderate, or severe impairment may impact differently on quality of life. Severe impairment may interfere with independent living, self-care, daily functional skills, and work capabilities; people with mild impairment may appear to function normally but can find challenges in complex situations and exhibit "slowness". It is essential to recognize these, as appropriate interventions may be effective, and targeted assistance may facilitate independent adult functioning.

Brain MRI Studies (Fontan Only)

Acquired Brain Injury

The frequency of any acquired abnormality is reported to be 11-fold greater among Fontan patients compared to healthy age-matched individuals [17, 21, 24, 34–37].

- The majority of abnormalities are focal or multifocal, mostly brain mineralization or iron deposits reported in 94%.
- Strokes are reported to range between 13 and 35%.
- White matter Injury accounts for 81% and is classified as mild, moderate, and severe in 114%, 47%, and 40%, respectively.
- Cerebral cortical, white matter or subcortical grey matter injury accounts for 21%, with an incidence and severity of brain injury similar in adolescent and adult subgroups.
- There are no significant differences between age or time since Fontan surgery and the presence of structural brain injury or white matter injury severity.
- The presence/severity of infarction, subcortical grey matter injury and micro-haemorrhage are not associated with worse neurocognitive outcomes in any neurocognitive domain.
- The presence of white matter injury is associated with lower learning z-scores.

Brain Volumetric Injury

Few studies have focused on neurocognitive outcomes and brain morphology in the adolescent and adult Fontan population [21, 32, 38–40].

In a cohort study of 86 Fontan patients (age 13–49 years) more than 5 years post-Fontan procedure, with no genetic or severe intellectual disability, who were compared to 86 age-and-sex-matched healthy controls, the following findings were outlined [21]:

- All global brain volumetric measures were in average significantly smaller in Fontan patients, even when adjusted for intracranial volume (ICV).

- In a region-based analysis controlled for age and sex, patients with Fontan circulation had significantly smaller volumes and surface area in most cerebral cortical regions.
- The differences in brain volume, cortical thickness, and surface area were more prominent in adult rather than adolescent Fontan patients, compared with controls. However, after adjusting for ICV, most differences in regional brain volumes diminished in both age groups, even though several regions with lower cortical thickness persisted in the adult group.
- Brain volumes were weakly associated with height and body mass index, suggesting that somatic growth and brain development are affected by Fontan physiology.
- There was an association between oxygen saturations and smaller global volumes, suggesting that chronic cyanosis may impact on brain morphology.

Neurocognitive Function and Cortical Morphometric and Region-Based Volumetric Injuries

Brain volume and regional cortical volumes are linked to distinct functional brain networks associated with essential neurocognitive functions, including visual, motor and somatosensory processing, associate learning, working memory, and executive function [17, 21, 32, 41]. More specifically:

- Complex neurocognitive processing, such as visual learning and paired associated learning is associated with smaller global volumes in almost all brain and cerebellum areas.
- Smaller brain volumes have been associated with worse cognitive performance in adolescents and adults with Fontan physiology.
- Adults have a worse neurocognitive impairment and more areas of smaller regional brain

volume, cortical thickness, and surface area than adolescents.

- In Fontan adolescents, a reduced left and right mamillary body volume is associated with altered verbal and memory scores, delayed memory recall subscores and visual special and executive function scores.

Limitations

The majority of studies on the neurodevelopmental outcome of Fontan patients rely on single centre cohorts or National Registries. The recorded clinical data are retrospective and not homogeneous, because they are not routinely recorded in all centres.

Socioeconomic status and place of living (rural vs urban area), parental IQ, and incomes can significantly affect neurodevelopment, but they are not available nor well-defined in most studies. Also, genetic testing is not routinely performed, although it may have important implications for brain development and neurocognitive outcomes. While neuropsychological assessment is a relatively well-validated tool, multisite MRI studies can hide a degree of heterogeneity introduced by variation in the hardware between centres.

Overall, the pathological processes contributing to the widespread brain abnormalities and adverse neurocognitive outcomes in the Fontan population remain largely speculative, and longitudinal studies are required to understand the mechanisms, timing, and trajectory of adverse brain development, reported at various time points across the lifespan.

Conclusions

The incidence of neurodevelopmental morbidities is high in patients with a Fontan circulation, and the impact on quality of life is irrefutable. The high incidence of neurocognitive impairment is associated with smaller brain volume and white matter injury. A smaller global brain volume is associated with chronic cyanosis.

Older age, genetic conditions, prematurity, CHD with aortic arch obstruction, lower socio-economic status, numerous operations or other invasive procedures, a longer length of hospital stay and complications, such as brain injury or Fontan-associated liver disease, are risk factors that affect neurodevelopmental outcomes.

However, routine neurological and neurodevelopmental evaluation is rarely included in clinical care. Studies are helping to understand the trajectory of impairment, and research designed to identify potentially modifiable risk factors are highly warranted. Fostering appropriate care pathways and support networks is crucial to improve social and neurodevelopmental long-term outcomes.

References

1. Stellin G. A tribute to the pioneers of right heart bypass: an historical review. World J Pediatr Congenit Heart Surg. 2020;11(2):198–203.
2. D'Udekem Y, Iyengar AJ, Galati JC, Forsdick V, Weintraub RG, Wheaton GR, Bullock A, Justo RN, Grigg LE, Sholler GF, Hope S, Radford DJ, Gentles TL, Celermajer DS, Winlaw DS. Redefining expectations of long-term survival after the Fontan procedure twenty-five years of follow-up from the entire population of Australia. Circulation. 2014;130(suppl 1):S32–8.
3. Hasaniya NW, Razzouk AJ, Mulla NF, Larsen RL, Bailey LL. In situ pericardial extracardiac lateral tunnel Fontan operation: fifteen-year experience. J Thorac Cardiovasc Surg. 2010;140(5):1076–83.
4. Kim SJ, Kim WH, Lim HG, Lee JY. Outcome of 200 patients after an extracardiac Fontan procedure. J Thorac Cardiovasc Surg. 2008;136(1):108–16.
5. Diller GP, Giardini A, Dimopoulos K, Gargiulo G, Muller J, Derrick G, et al. Predictors of morbidity and mortality in contemporary Fontan patients: results from a multicenter study including cardiopulmonary exercise testing in 321 patients. Eur Heart J. 2010;31(24):3073–83.
6. d'Udekem Y, Iyengar AJ, Cochrane AD, Grigg LE, Ramsay JM, Wheaton GR, et al. The Fontan procedure: contemporary techniques have improved long-term outcomes. Circulation. 2007;116(11 Suppl):I-157–64.
7. Cainelli E, Arrigoni F, Vedovelli L. White matter injury and neurodevelopmental disabilities: a cross-disease (dis)connection. Prog Neurobiol. 2021;193:101845.
8. Sistino JJ, Bonilha HS. Improvements in survival and neurodevelopmental outcomes in surgical treatment of hypoplastic left heart syndrome: a metaanalytic review. J Extra Corpor Technol. 2012;44:216–23.
9. Atallah J, Dinu IA, Joffe AR, Robertson CM, Sauve RS, Dyck JD, Ross DB, Rebeyka IM. Two-year survival and mental and psychomotor outcomes after the Norwood procedure: an analysis of the modified Blalock-Taussig shunt and right ventricle-to-pulmonary artery shunt surgical eras. Circulation. 2008;118:1410–8.
10. McCrindle BW, Williams RV, Mitchell PD, Hsu DT, Paridon SM, Atz AM, Li JS, Newburger JW. Relationship of patient and medical characteristics to health status in children and adolescents after the Fontan procedure. Circulation. 2006;113:1123–9.
11. Longmuir PE, Banks L, McCrindle BW. Cross-sectional study of motor development among children after the Fontan procedure. Cardiol Young. 2012;22:443–50.
12. Idorn L, Jensen AS, Juul K, Overgaard D, Nielsen NP, Sorensen K, Reimers JI, Sondergaard L. Quality of life and cognitive function in Fontan patients, a population-based study. Int J Cardiol. 2013;168:3230–5.
13. Sugimoto A, Ota N, Ibuki K, Miyakoshi C, Murata M, Tosaka Y, Yamazaki T, Sakamoto K. Risk factors for adverse neurocognitive outcomes in school-aged patients after the Fontan operation. Eur J Cardiothorac Surg. 2013;44:454–61.
14. Vedovelli L, Padalino M, Simonato M, D'Aronco S, Bertini D, Stellin G, Ori C, Carnielli VP, Cogo PE. Cardiopulmonary bypass increases plasma glial fibrillary acidic protein only in first stage palliation of hypoplastic left heart syndrome. Can J Cardiol. 2016;32(3):355–61.
15. Newburger JW, Sleeper LA, Bellinger DC, Goldberg CS, Tabbutt S, Lu M, Mussatto KA, Williams IA, Gustafson KE, Mital S, Pike N, Sood E, Mahle WT, Cooper DS, Dunbar-Masterson C, Krawczeski CD, Lewis A, Menon SC, Pemberton VL, Ravishankar C, Atz TW, Ohye RG, Gaynor JW. Early developmental outcome in children with hypoplastic left heart syndrome and related anomalies: the single ventricle reconstruction trial. Circulation. 2012;125:2081–91.
16. The International Cardiac Collaborative on Neurodevelopment (ICCON) Investigators. Impact of operative and postoperative factors on neurodevelopmental outcomes after cardiac operations. Ann Thorac Surg. 2016;102:843–9.
17. Bellinger DC, Watson CG, Rivkin MJ, Robertson RL, Roberts AE, Stopp C, Dunbar-Masterson C, Bernson D, DeMaso DR, Wypij D, Newburger JW. Neuropsychological status and structural brain imaging in adolescents with single ventricle who underwent the Fontan procedure. J Am Heart Assoc. 2015;4:e002302.
18. Gunn JK, Beca J, Hunt RW, Goldsworthy M, Brizard CP, Finucane K, Donath S, Shekerdemian LS. Perioperative risk factors for impaired neurodevelopment after cardiac surgery in early infancy. Arch Dis Child. 2016;101:1010–6.

19. Gaynor JW, Gerdes M, Nord AS, Bernbaum J, Zackai E, Wernovsky G, Clancy RR, Heagerty PJ, Solot CB, McDonald-McGinn D, et al. Is cardiac diagnosis a predictor of neurodevelopmental outcome after cardiac surgery in infancy? J Thorac Cardiovasc Surg. 2010;140:1230–7.

20. Mussatto KA, Hoffmann RG, Hoffman GM, Tweddell JS, Bear L, Cao Y, Brosig C. Risk and prevalence of developmental delay in young children with congenital heart disease. Pediatrics. 2014;133:e570–7.

21. Verrall CE, Yang JYM, Chen J, Schembri A, d'Udekem Y, Zannino D, Kasparian NA, du Plessis K, Grieve SM, Welton DT, Barton B, Gentles TL, Celermajer DS, Attard C, Rice K, Ayer J, Mandelstam S, Winlaw DS, Mackay MT, Cordina R. Neurocognitive dysfunction and smaller brain volumes in adolescents and adults with a Fontan circulation. Circulation. 2021;143:878–91.

22. Cassidy AR, Bernstein JH, Bellinger DC, Newburger JW, DeMaso DR. Visual-spatial processing style is associated with psychopathology in adolescents with critical congenital heart disease. Clin Neuropsychol. 2019;33:760–78.

23. Sasaki J, Dykes JC, Sosa LJ, Salvaggio JL, Tablante MD, Ojito J, Danyal M, Hannan RL, Rossi AF, Burk RP, Wernovsky G. Risk factors for longer hospital stay following the Fontan operation. Pediatr Crit Care Med. 2016;17:411–9.

24. Calderon J, Stopp C, Wypij D, DeMaso DR, Rivkin M, Newburger JW, Bellinger DC. Early-term birth in single-ventricle congenital heart disease after the Fontan procedure: neurodevelopmental and psychiatric outcomes. J Pediatr. 2016;179:96–103.

25. Bayley N. Bayley scales of infant development. 2nd ed. San Antonio: The Psychological Corporation; 1993.

26. Griffiths R. In: Huntley M, editor. The Griffiths mental development scales: from birth to 2 years. Oxford: The Test Agency; 1996.

27. Wechsler D. Wechsler preschool and primary scale of intelligence—third edition: Canadian. Pearson Clinical Assessment Canada; 2002.

28. Uzark K, Lincoln A, Lamberti JJ, Mainwaring RD, Spicer RL, Moore JW. Neurodevelopmental outcomes in children with Fontan repair of functional single ventricle. Pediatrics. 1998;101:630–3.

29. Goldberg CS, Schwartz EM, Brunberg JA, Mosca RS, Bove EL, Schork MA, Stetz SP, Cheatham JP, Kulik TJ. Neurodevelopmental outcome of patients after the Fontan operation: a comparison between children with hypoplastic left heart syndrome and other functional single ventricle lesions. J Pediatr. 2000;137:646–52.

30. Wernovsky G, Stiles KM, Gauvreau K, Gentles TL, duPlessis AJ, Bellinger DC, Walsh AZ, Burnett J, Jonas RA, Mayer JE Jr, Newburger JW. Cognitive development after the Fontan operation. Circulation. 2000;102:883–9.

31. Forbess JM, Visconti KJ, Hancock-Friesen C, Howe RC, Bellinger DC, Jonas RA. Neurodevelopmental outcome after congenital heart surgery: results from an institutional registry. Circulation. 2002;106(12 Suppl 1):I95–102.

32. Cabrera-Mino C, Roy B, Woo MA, Singh S, Moye S, Halnon NJ, Lewis AB, Kumar R, Pike NA. Reduced brain mammillary body volumes and memory deficits in adolescents who have undergone the Fontan procedure. Pediatr Res. 2020;87(1):169–75.

33. Goldberg CS, Mussatto K, Licht D, Wernovsky G. Neurodevelopment and quality of life for children with hypoplastic left heart syndrome: current knowns and unknowns. Cardiol Young. 2011;21(2):88–92.

34. Watson CG, Stopp C, Wypij D, Bellinger DC, Newburger JW, Rivkin MJ. Early-term birth in single-ventricle congenital heart disease after the Fontan procedure: neurodevelopmental and psychiatric outcomes. J Pediatr. 2018;200:140–9.

35. Bellinger DC, Wypij D, Rivkin MJ, DeMaso DR, Robertson RL Jr, Dunbar-Masterson C, Rappaport LA, Wernovsky G, Jonas RA, Newburger JW. Adolescents with d-transposition of the great arteries corrected with the arterial switch procedure: neuropsychological assessment and structural brain imaging. Circulation. 2011;124:1361–9.

36. Pike NA, Roy B, Gupta R, Singh S, Woo MA, Halnon NJ, Lewis AB, Kumar R. Brain abnormalities in cognition, anxiety, and depression regulatory regions in adolescents with single ventricle heart disease. J Neurosci Res. 2018;96:1104–18.

37. Peyvandi S, Kim H, Lau J, Barkovich J, Campbell A, Miller S, Duan X, McQuillen P. The association between cardiac physiology, acquired brain injury, and postnatal brain growth in critical congenital heart disease. J Thorac Cardiovasc Surg. 2018;155:291–300.

38. Cordina R, Grieve S, Barnett M, Lagopoulos J, Malitz N, Celermajer DS. Brain volumetric, regional cortical thickness and radiographic findings in adults with cyanotic congenital heart disease. Neuroimage Clin. 2014;4:319–25. https://doi.org/10.1016/j.nicl.2013.12.011.

39. Singh S, Kumar R, Roy B, Woo MA, Lewis A, Halnon N, Pike N. Regional brain gray matter changes in adolescents with single ventricle heart disease. Neurosci Lett. 2018;665:156–62.

40. Watson CG, Stopp C, Wypij D, Newburger JW, Rivkin MJ. Reduced cortical volume and thickness and their relationship to medical and operative features in post-Fontan children and adolescents. Pediatr Res. 2017;81:881–90.

41. Morton PD, Ishibashi N, Jonas RA. Neurodevelopmental abnormalities and congenital heart disease: insights into altered brain maturation. Circ Res. 2017;120:960–97.

Follow-Up in Childhood of Fontan Patients: Quality of Life

Jo Wray, Rodney Franklin, and Suzie Hutchinson

Introduction

Advances in both medical and surgical care have resulted in dramatic improvements in life expectancy for children born with functionally single ventricle defects who undergo a Fontan procedure. Although their anatomy is not corrected by the Fontan-type operation (total cavopulmonary connection, TCPC), increasing numbers are now reaching adulthood and, in common with other congenital heart diagnoses, attention is moving beyond survival and focusing instead on aspects such as health-related quality of life (HRQoL).

Quality of life (QoL) has been defined by the World Health Organisation as "an individual's perceptions of their position in life in the context of the culture and value systems in which they live, and in relation to their goals, expectations, standards and concerns." [1] Within the context of overall QoL, the specific construct of HRQoL has been developed and is defined as "the influ-ence of a specific illness, medical therapy, or health care policy on an individual's QoL" and incorporates the perception that an individual has of their ability to both function in and derive personal satisfaction from various physical, psychological, and social life contexts." [2].

As the focus has moved to understanding the impact on HRQoL of both the functionally single ventricle condition and its treatment, the need to understand how and when to routinely monitor HRQoL and use the information to target and implement interventions has been highlighted.

Factors that May Impact HRQoL

- Recent studies indicate that, overall, single ventricle physiology patients have lower physical and psychosocial HRQoL than their healthy peers at all stages of the treatment pathway [3–6]. Across the age range patients are at increased risk for:
  - psychiatric/psychological (particularly anxiety, post-traumatic stress and Attention Deficit Hyperactivity Disorder (ADHD)) problems
  - cognitive, neuropsychological, educational and behavioural
  - physical limitations and reduced energy levels and exercise performance, all of which can negatively impact HRQoL (Table 17.1) [7–13].

J. Wray (✉)
Great Ormond Street Hospital for Children NHS Foundation Trust, London, UK
e-mail: jo.wray@gosh.nhs.uk

R. Franklin
Royal Brompton and Harefield NHS Foundation Trust, London, UK
e-mail: r.franklin@rbht.nhs.uk

S. Hutchinson
Little Hearts Matter, Birmingham, UK
e-mail: suzie@lhm.org.uk

P. Clift et al. (eds.), *Univentricular Congenital Heart Defects and the Fontan Circulation*, https://doi.org/10.1007/978-3-031-36208-8_17

Table 17.1 Domains of physical and psychosocial functioning which can impact on overall health-related quality of life

Domain	Examples
Physical development and physical abilities	• Delayed attainment of developmental milestones • Delayed puberty • Short stature • Low lean muscle mass • Abnormal bone structure • Physical limitations/low energy levels
Neurodevelopment and neurocognition	• High levels of neurodevelopmental disabilities • Lower IQ • Impaired visual-spatial skills, working memory and processing speed • Poor levels of executive functioning
Education and schooling	• Increased incidence of learning disabilities/lower levels of academic attainment • Poor attention • Impaired social cognition • Difficulties with peer relationships • Higher levels of bullying, school exclusion and social isolation • Increased absence due to condition and treatment related factors, hospital appointments • Reduced energy levels and fatigue at school
Behaviour and emotional functioning	• Increased incidence of attention deficit hyperactivity disorder • Issues with anger management • More autistic-type behaviours • Higher levels of disruptive behaviour • Increased levels of confusion • Increased incidence of symptoms of acute/chronic stress and post-traumatic stress • Elevated levels of depression and anxiety—related to living with the condition, missing out on social events and resulting social isolation, feeling different, others' lack of understanding of their condition, impact of their condition on others, managing the medical aspects, fear of the future (life expectancy, ability to work, ability to have children, living independently) • Negative illness perceptions • Low self esteem • Poor body image
Family functioning/impact on family life	• Increased parental stress, anxiety and depression, particularly related to fear of their child dying, their child's future and their psychosocial wellbeing • Negative impact on siblings and wider family • Negative impact on family activities—e.g., holidays, social events

- – A number of patient and medical correlates of poorer functioning have been identified [14–17].
  - older age
  - the presence of a genetic condition
  - early-term birth
  - lower socioeconomic status
  - more operations and catheterisations
  - longer length of hospital stay
  - complications such as brain injury, Fontan-associated liver disease

- • However, what is also clear at the individual level is that some patients report an excellent HRQoL, supporting the need for an individualised approach to monitoring and evaluation.

Whilst the majority of studies of HRQoL in this population are cross-sectional, it is also evident that HRQoL changes over time—which may or may not be linked to treatment—and that longitudinal evaluation should be part of routine follow-up of this patient group.

Understanding how the myriad of patient, family, medical and psychosocial factors impact HRQoL and affect the individual child or young person is complex but is a crucial component of the holistic care of patients and their families.

In Box 17.1 a case history illustrates the ways in which outcomes of the condition and its treatment can impact the everyday life and HRQoL of a young person with a single ventricle physiology condition.

Box 17.1 Case History Illustrating the Ways in Which Outcomes of the Condition and Its Treatment Can Impact the Everyday Life and Health-Related Quality of Life of a Young Person with a Single Ventricle Condition

Case History

Daniel is a 16-year-old young man with a combination of cardiac anomalies that have resulted in a diagnosis of Hypoplastic Left Heart. He has had Norwood, superior cavopulmonary connection and then Fontan-type operations in his early years. He has regular medical check-ups and has started the transition from Paediatric to Adult services. He is currently prescribed Aspirin and Lisinopril to aid cardiac function.

Physical Effects

Daniel, like many young people with half a working heart, suffers with night time leg pains and severe migraines. These are physically and mentally very debilitating and require a recovery period that affects Daniel's participation in school. These occur because of the changes in circulation created by the Fontan Circulation.

Energy Levels

All young people with half a working heart have depleted energy levels. Their exercise capacity is reduced in comparison to their peers. Most teenagers run at a 100% energy level at rest and are able to increase that to 500% on activity. Daniel runs on a normal level of between 50 and 75% which can only rise to 200% when active. If he uses up all of his energy stores very rapidly, for example walking to school or completing a full day of education, he has to compromise on further activity.

Education

Although Daniel is very bright, recently achieving 12 GCSEs, and currently studying for science-based A levels, he finds managing his school work a challenge. He has a reduced ability to concentrate, organise his work and to retain information. His lack of energy affects his ability to learn. Balancing school and home working is a major challenge. Daniel also shows signs of being on the Autistic spectrum, a common added diagnosis in children with a complex heart condition. This creates added strains on his ability to learn and how he copes in school and social situations.

His school have put a number of support mechanisms in place, a reduced academic timetable, no PE lessons, and he has an Education, Health and Care (EHC) Plan in place.

Emotional Wellbeing

Daniel has faced a number of fairly common, to young people with a single ventricle heart condition, problems at school. He has been bullied because of the differences in his energy capacity. He lacks the energy to be able to socialise with his peers out of school. This has led to self-imposed isolation and anxiety.

As Daniel has grown up he has developed an increasing awareness of his condition and his risk of mortality.

Why Collecting HRQoL Data Is Important

- Collection of HRQoL data has benefits at an individual, institutional and national/international level [18]. For the individual patient and family, collection of HRQoL data can help to

- improve communication between patients, family members and health professionals
- enable monitoring and evaluation of changes over time following medical, interventional or surgical therapies
- provide a mechanism whereby patient and family views and preferences are included in the discussion about treatments or challenges
- facilitate screening for other physical or psychological problems

- Increasingly, the differences in the perspectives of patients, families and clinicians are being acknowledged [19] and a recent study demonstrated the relatively poor ability of clinicians to predict HRQoL of children with heart disease, emphasising the importance of asking patients themselves (and/or their proxies) [20].
- At a national/international level collection of HRQoL data provides a further point of comparison in addition to the more commonly measured physical and physiological parameters when assessing outcomes of different treatments.
- Potential cultural differences in HRQoL and the impact of different approaches to health care delivery and management can also be explored.
- A further benefit which is currently under-appreciated and under-utilised is the value of information about HRQoL and other health-related outcomes to schools and colleges, employers and other public services such as social services and health care providers outside of the specialist centre.
- Understanding HRQoL and the impact of a functionally single ventricle condition is crucial if children and young people are to fulfil their potential in all areas of their lives.

Measuring HRQoL

There are many challenges associated with measuring HRQoL in children due to the wide age range and changing developmental abilities of children as they progress along the age continuum. A further important consideration is the role of the family and who is the most appropriate informant about a child's HRQoL. The role of parent-proxy reporting and how to deal with cross-informant variance is a frequent source of debate and controversy but it may also be that some children are not able to provide information on their HRQoL themselves.

Although children as young as 5 years of age may be able to provide reliable and valid self-reports, cognitive or psychosocial challenges may make this more unlikely in the younger post-Fontan operation population in particular, resulting in a reliance on parent-proxy reporting. Recognition of the ongoing but changing patterns of stress that families endure during the pathway of life-long treatment and care for their child with a functionally single ventricle condition is also pertinent to the debate about how to monitor HRQoL in this population.

Research undertaken by Little Hearts Matter, a UK based charity specifically for the support of children with single ventricle physiology conditions and their families, identified that stress was experienced by families at every outpatient appointment along the disease trajectory, due to their fear about what they would be told by the clinicians caring for their child. Particular stressors were related to:

- what the future holds
- their child's physical symptoms
- awaiting surgery
- issues related to their child's education and relationships and inclusion.

For the parent of the child who has had their Fontan surgery, this milestone brings with it new fears about the future as there are no further formal treatments in the plan for their child's care until transplantation. Depression is common at this time. In the context of the child's HRQoL, parental functioning can not only have a direct affect on their child's HRQoL but it can also impact how parents report their child's HRQoL.

Although children and their parents may have differing perceptions of the child's HRQoL, both sources of information are important.

Understanding the differences in how children, their parents and health professionals perceive HRQoL may offer important insights and be more informative than perceived agreement.

Selecting appropriate measures for HRQoL evaluation can also be challenging. The gold standard for assessing HRQoL is to use both a disease-specific and a generic measure which cover a wide age range and have both patient and parent-proxy (for paediatric populations) reporting. Whilst a disease-specific measure provides greater sensitivity to change and enables discrimination within a specific patient population, a generic measure allows for comparison with healthy or other disease populations. Increasingly, the importance of assessing 'quality' in health care from the patient's perspective is being recognised, and collection of HRQoL data from patients/their proxies is one method of evaluating the effectiveness and impact of care and treatment. However, if collection of HRQoL outcomes is to become "routine", it is vital that measures are perceived as relevant and appropriate by the informant, can be easily administered and completed in a reasonable time frame and are manageable by the organisation collecting the data in terms of data entry, analysis and utilisation. Examples of measures previously used with functionally single ventricle patients are provided in Table 17.2.

Table 17.2 Health-related quality of life measures used with children/young people with congenital heart disease

Instrument type	Instrument	Respondent type	Age range	Domain(s)/scales	Items	Time to complete (min)
Generic	PedsQL 4.0 General Core Scales [21, 22]	Self-report5	5–7, 8–12 13–18, 19–25	Physical Emotional	23	10
		Proxy report	2–4, 5–7, 8–12, 13–18 years	Social School[a]	23	10
	Infant PedsQL Scales [23]	Proxy report	0–12 months 13–24 months	Physical functioning Physical symptoms Emotional functioning Social functioning Cognitive functioning	36 45	10–15
	KINDL [24]	Self-report	4–6, 7–13, 14–17 years	Physical well-being Emotional well-being Self-esteem	12–24 (+6)	5–15
		Proxy report	3–6, 7–17 years	Family Friends Everyday functioning (school or nursery school/kindergarten) Disease—additional 6-item subscale for completion in cases of prolonged illness or hospitalisation	24–46 (+6)	5–15
	TAPQoL [25]	Proxy-report	9 months–6 years	Physical Social Cognitive Emotional	43	10–15
	TACQoL [26]	Self-report	8–15 years	Physical complaints Motor functioning	56	15–20
		Proxy report	6–15 years	Autonomy Cognitive functioning Social functioning Positive and negative emotional functioning	56	15

(continued)

Table 17.2 (continued)

Instrument type	Instrument	Respondent type	Age range	Domain(s)/scales	Items	Time to complete (min)
Disease-specific (CHD)	CHAT [27]	Self-report	11–18 years	Physical symptoms Physical limitations Limitations of physical education at school Social limitations External pressures Concerns (general, social, educational, physical, total)	53	20–30
	ConQoL [28]	Self-report	8–11, 12–16 years	Symptoms Activities Relationships Coping and control	29 or 35	10
Disease-specific (HD)	PCQLI [29]	Self-report Proxy report	8–12, 13–18 years	Disease impact (physical) Psychosocial impact	24 or 30	10
	PedsQL 3.0 Cardiac Module [30]	Self-report Proxy report	5–7, 8–12, 13–18, 2–4, 5–7, 8–12, 13–18 years	Heart problems (symptoms) Treatment (barriers) Perceived physical appearance Treatment anxiety Cognitive problems Communication	27 27	10 10
	P-PCQLI [31]	Proxy report	3–7 years	Physical capacity and functioning Emotional wellbeing and behaviour Social integration Treatment burden Functional development	52	10

CHAT Congenital Heart Adolescent and Teenage questionnaire, *CHD* Congenital heart disease, *PCQLI* Pediatric Cardiac Quality of Life Inventory, *PedsQL* Pediatric Quality of Life Inventory 4.0 Generic Core Scales, *P-PCQLI* Preschool Pediatric Cardiac Quality of Life Inventory, *TAPQoL* TNO-AZL Preschool Children Quality of Life, *TACQoL* TNO-AZL Children Quality of Life

[a] The Physical domain makes up the Physical Health Summary Score, while the Emotional, Social, and School domains make up the Psychosocial Summary Score

Barriers and Facilitators to Collecting and Using HRQoL Data

A number of barriers and facilitators to incorporating the routine assessment of HRQoL in clinical practice have been identified (Fig. 17.1). Time is a major barrier and those clinicians who are most likely to be involved in data collection (such as specialist nurses, health care assistants) have significant workloads and demands on their time and are unlikely to welcome the introduction of routine HRQoL assessment if it is perceived as an additional task that will add to their workload.

A further consideration is how findings are communicated to the wider team in a timely way so that clinicians are able to respond to the findings. There may also be issues of time related to how long it takes for patients to complete the measures as well as identifying the optimal time for this to occur. Clinicians may not all be aware of the potential value of HRQoL assessments and this may also be a barrier.

Other barriers include the financial and administrative burdens associated with the introduction and coordination of HRQoL evaluation, the challenges associated with how to act on the findings

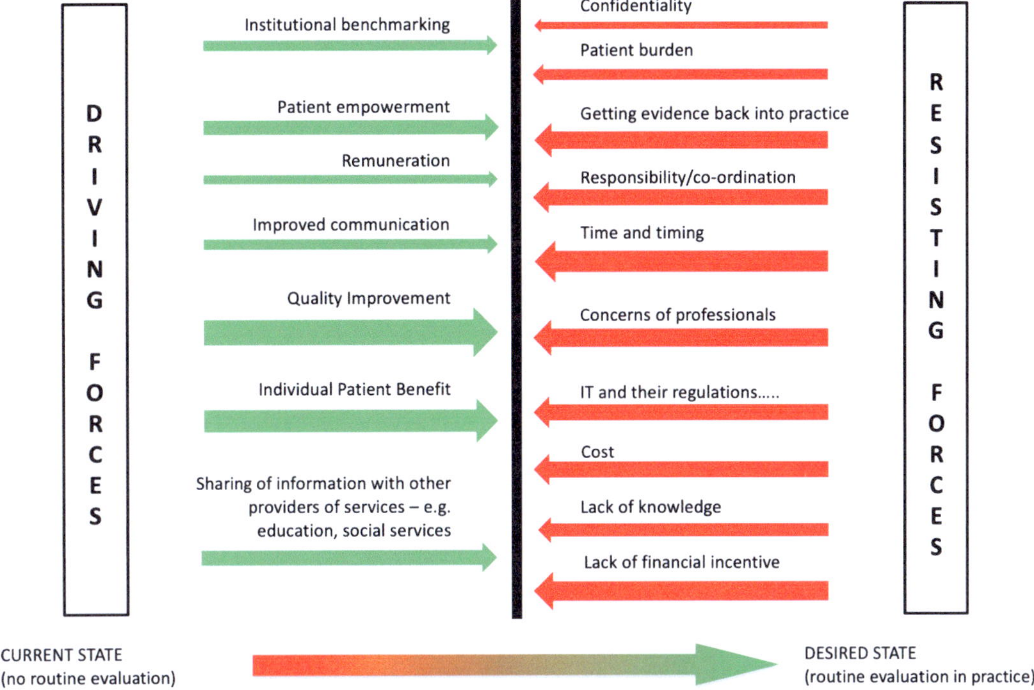

Fig. 17.1 Barriers and facilitators to the implementation of health-related quality of life assessment into routine practice

and get the evidence back into practice at both an individual and an institutional level and concerns about confidentiality, information governance and potential patient burden. Facilitators include the benefit for individual patients and the potential for a positive impact on their care, improved communication between patients and clinicians, patient empowerment through increasing their involvement in their care and quality improvement in the overall service provision through collection of data for the population of functionally single ventricle patients.

Moving the Field on: A Strategy for Routine HRQoL Assessment

If HRQoL evaluation is to be incorporated into the routine follow-up of children with functionally single ventricle conditions it has to be efficient, effective and beneficial for children, families and clinicians. Consideration needs to be given to

- how the data should be collected and analysed (when, where, how and by whom)
- how the data are stored (institutional/registry databases, individual patient notes)
- how the data are disseminated to get the evidence into practice (to inform policy and guideline development, institutional changes in practice and individual patient care).

A key element is implementation of the HRQoL measures and understanding how this should map onto the 'roadmap' [32] of care for children and young people with functionally single ventricle conditions. Such an approach follows the illness and treatment trajectory from the stage of neonatal surgery through to transition to adult care and in the schema shown in Fig. 17.2 suggested time points for collection of HRQoL data are integrated into the clinical course alongside the associated psychosocial and developmental evaluation/support at each stage.

Although there are existing barriers to the collection and use of HRQoL data as outlined above,

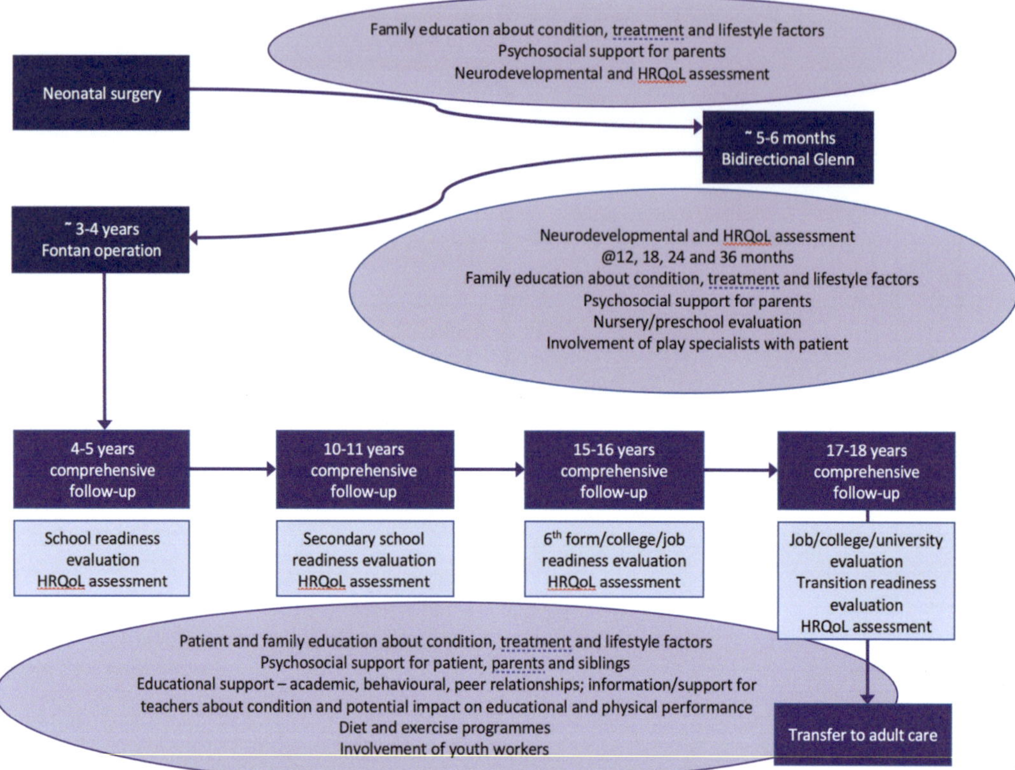

Fig. 17.2 Roadmap for developmental, educational and psychosocial follow-up (adapted from Wernovsky et al. [32])

these can be overcome using a structured approach to follow-up and with the provision of the necessary resources and education of all stakeholder groups (clinicians, managers, commissioners and families) about the benefits of collecting and using HRQoL data and implementing interventions as necessary to improve HRQoL.

ever more pressurised, the case for developing strategies for introducing HRQoL evaluation into routine clinical practice becomes more pressing.

Our aim should be for HRQoL data to sit alongside mortality and physical morbidity data in international databases and for the data to inform and optimise patient care, thereby enabling each individual patient to maximise their potential in all spheres of their life.

Conclusion

The incidence of physical and psychosocial morbidities is high in patients living with single ventricle physiology conditions, wherever they are on the treatment pathway, and the impact on HRQoL is irrefutable. However, routine evaluation of HRQoL is rarely included as part of clinical care. Challenges are numerous but as the demand to improve patient care increases and the need to optimise resource allocation becomes

References

1. WHOQoL Group. Development of the WHOQOL: rationale and current status. Int J Ment Health. 1994;23(3):24–56.
2. Drotar D. Measuring health-related quality of life in children and adolescents: implications for research and practice. London: Psychology Press; 2014.
3. Uzark K, Zak V, Shrader P, McCrindle BW, Radojewski E, Varni JW, et al. Assessment of quality of life in young patients with single ventricle after the Fontan operation. J Pediatr. 2016;170:166–172.e1.

4. Wray J, Franklin R, Brown K, Cassedy A, Marino BS. Testing the pediatric cardiac quality of life inventory in the United Kingdom. Acta Paediatr. 2013;102(2):e68–73.

5. Marino BS, Tomlinson RS, Wernovsky G, Drotar D, Newburger JW, Mahony L, et al. Validation of the pediatric cardiac quality of life inventory. Pediatrics. 2010;126(3):498–508.

6. Idorn L, Jensen AS, Juul K, Overgaard D, Nielsen NP, Sorensen K, et al. Quality of life and cognitive function in Fontan patients, a population-based study. Int J Cardiol. 2013;168(4):3230–5.

7. Rychik J, Atz AM, Celermajer DS, Deal BJ, Gatzoulis MA, Gewillig MH, et al. Evaluation and management of the child and adult with Fontan circulation: a scientific statement from the American Heart Association. Circulation. 2019;140:CIR0000000000000696.

8. DeMaso DR, Calderon J, Taylor GA, Holland JE, Stopp C, White MT, et al. Psychiatric disorders in adolescents with single ventricle congenital heart disease. Pediatrics. 2017;139(3):e20162241.

9. Goldberg CS, Hu C, Brosig C, Gaynor JW, Mahle WT, Miller T, et al. Behavior and quality of life at 6 years for children with hypoplastic left heart syndrome. Pediatrics. 2019;144(5):e20191010.

10. Atz AM, Zak V, Mahony L, Uzark K, D'Agincourt N, Goldberg DJ, et al. Longitudinal outcomes of patients with single ventricle after the Fontan procedure. J Am Coll Cardiol. 2017;69(22):2735–44.

11. Bellinger DC, Watson CG, Rivkin MJ, Robertson RL, Roberts AE, Stopp C, et al. Neuropsychological status and structural brain imaging in adolescents with single ventricle who underwent the Fontan procedure. J Am Heart Assoc. 2015;4(12):e002302.

12. Cassidy AR, Bernstein JH, Bellinger DC, Newburger JW, DeMaso DR. Visual-spatial processing style is associated with psychopathology in adolescents with critical congenital heart disease. Clin Neuropsychol. 2019;33(4):760–78.

13. Holbein CE, Fogleman ND, Hommel K, Apers S, Rassart J, Moons P, et al. A multinational observational investigation of illness perceptions and quality of life among patients with a Fontan circulation. Congenit Heart Dis. 2018;13(3):392–400.

14. Calderon J, Stopp C, Wypij D, DeMaso DR, Rivkin M, Newburger JW, et al. Early-term birth in single-ventricle congenital heart disease after the Fontan procedure: neurodevelopmental and psychiatric outcomes. J Pediatr. 2016;179:96–103.

15. Menon SC, Al-Dulaimi R, McCrindle BW, Goldberg DJ, Sachdeva R, Goldstein BH, et al. Delayed puberty and abnormal anthropometry and its associations with quality of life in young Fontan survivors: a multicenter cross-sectional study. Congenit Heart Dis. 2018;13(3):463–9.

16. Heye KN, Knirsch W, Scheer I, Beck I, Wetterling K, Hahn A, et al. Health-related quality of life in pre-school age children with single-ventricle CHD. Cardiol Young. 2019;29(2):162–8.

17. Daniels CJ, Bradley EA, Landzberg MJ, Aboulhosn J, Beekman RH 3rd, Book W, et al. Fontan-associated liver disease: proceedings from the American College of Cardiology Stakeholders Meeting, October 1 to 2, 2015, Washington DC. J Am Coll Cardiol. 2017;70(25):3173–94.

18. Wray J, Brown K, Marino BS, Franklin R. Medical test results do not tell the whole story: health-related quality of life offers a patient perspective on outcomes. World J Pediatr Congenit Heart Surg. 2011;2(4):566–75.

19. Marino BS, Tomlinson RS, Drotar D, Claybon ES, Aguirre A, Ittenbach R, et al. Quality-of-life concerns differ among patients, parents, and medical providers in children and adolescents with congenital and acquired heart disease. Pediatrics. 2009;123(4):e708–15.

20. Costello JM, Mussatto K, Cassedy A, Wray J, Mahony L, Teele SA, et al. Prediction by clinicians of quality of life for children and adolescents with cardiac disease. J Pediatr. 2015;166(3):679–83.e2.

21. Varni JW, Seid M, Rode CA. The PedsQL: measurement model for the pediatric quality of life inventory. Med Care. 1999;37(2):126–39.

22. Varni JW, Seid M, Kurtin PS. PedsQL 4.0: reliability and validity of the pediatric quality of life inventory version 4.0 generic core scales in healthy and patient populations. Med Care. 2001;39(8):800–12.

23. Varni JW, Limbers CA, Neighbors K, Schulz K, Lieu JE, Heffer RW, et al. The PedsQL™ infant scales: feasibility, internal consistency reliability, and validity in healthy and ill infants. Qual Life Res. 2011;20(1):45–55.

24. Ravens-Sieberer U, Bullinger M. Assessing health-related quality of life in chronically ill children with the German KINDL: first psychometric and content analytical results. Qual Life Res. 1998;7(5):399–407.

25. Fekkes M, Theunissen NC, Brugman E, Veen S, Verrips EG, Koopman HM, et al. Development and psychometric evaluation of the TAPQOL: a health-related quality of life instrument for 1-5-year-old children. Qual Life Res. 2000;9(8):961–72.

26. Vogels T, Verrips GH, Verloove-Vanhorick SP, Fekkes M, Kamphuis RP, Koopman HM, et al. Measuring health-related quality of life in children: the development of the TACQOL parent form. Qual Life Res. 1998;7(5):457–65.

27. Kendall L, Lewin RJ, Parsons JM, Veldtman GR, Quirk J, Hardman GE. Factors associated with self-perceived state of health in adolescents with congenital cardiac disease attending paediatric cardiologic clinics. Cardiol Young. 2001;11(4):431–8.

28. Macran S, Birks Y, Parsons J, Sloper P, Hardman G, Kind P, et al. The development of a new measure of quality of life for children with congenital cardiac disease. Cardiol Young. 2006;16(2):165–72.

29. Marino BS, Shera D, Wernovsky G, Tomlinson RS, Aguirre A, Gallagher M, et al. The development of the pediatric cardiac quality of life inventory: a quality of

life measure for children and adolescents with heart disease. Qual Life Res. 2008;17(4):613–26.

30. Uzark K, Jones K. Parenting stress and children with heart disease. J Pediatr Health Care. 2003;17(4):163–8.

31. Niemitz M, Seitz DC, Oebels M, Schranz D, Hovels-Gurich H, Hofbeck M, et al. The development and validation of a health-related quality of life questionnaire for pre-school children with a chronic heart disease. Qual Life Res. 2013;22(10):2877–88.

32. Wernovsky G, Lihn SL, Olen MM. Creating a lesion-specific "roadmap" for ambulatory care following surgery for complex congenital cardiac disease. Cardiol Young. 2017;27(4):648–62.

Isma Rafiq, Andrew Constantine,
and Konstantinos Dimopoulos

Patients with a Fontan-type circulation are at increased risk of thrombosis and/or embolic events (TE) [1]. Since 1968, the Fontan procedure has undergone a number of modifications to optimize hemodynamics and minimize the rate of complications, including arrhythmias, liver failure, protein-losing enteropathy, and pulmonary and systemic TE [2, 3]. Despite this, all patients with a Fontan-type circulation remain at risk of thromboembolic events and require careful, individualized assessment and management [4].

Epidemiology and Pathophysiology of Thromboembolic Complications

Reported estimates of the prevalence of TE in Fontan patients vary depending on the methodology used. Up to 33% of patients have intracardiac clots on transthoracic or transesophageal echocardiography [5–7], Rosenthal et al. described an incidence of TE of 3.9% per year, 43% of which were asymptomatic [8]. Egbe et al. described the rate of thrombotic and thromboembolic complications in a retrospective cohort of 278 Fontan patients. The event of systemic TE (intracardiac thrombus, ischemic stroke or systemic arterial emboli) was 2.1% per year and that of non-systemic thrombotic or thromboembolic events (Fontan pathway, right atrial or pulmonary thrombi) was 4.4% per year [9]. Multivariable risk factors for thrombotic or thromboembolic events included an AP Fontan and warfarin (but not antiplatelet) therapy.

A recent meta-analysis of 1200 Fontan patients (total follow-up 9620 patient years) reported a total of 122 TE events with a cumulative incidence of 1.3% per year [10]. Incomplete ascertainment of asymptomatic or 'silent' TE means that the true incidence of events likely to be higher than this. These events account for a high proportion of cases in surveillance studies and, though not appearing in reports of clinically manifest TE, contribute to acute or long-term mortality (e.g., through a gradual increase in pulmonary vascular resistance) [10]. Indeed, symptomatic TE is associated with a significant mortality and morbidity in Fontan patients, including stroke or myocardial infarction (from systemic or paradoxical emboli), pulmonary embolism and new or deteriorating heart (Fontan) failure [11–14].

The pathophysiology of TE in patients with a Fontan circulation (Fig. 18.1) is incompletely understood but is widely considered to result from a combination of hematologic, hemodynamic and anatomic/surgical variables (Fig. 18.2).

I. Rafiq · A. Constantine · K. Dimopoulos (✉)
Adult Congenital Heart Centre and Centre for
Pulmonary Hypertension, Royal Brompton Hospital,
London, UK

National Heart and Lung Institute, Imperial College
London, London, UK
e-mail: i.rafiq@rbht.nhs.uk

P. Clift et al. (eds.), *Univentricular Congenital Heart Defects and the Fontan Circulation*,
https://doi.org/10.1007/978-3-031-36208-8_18

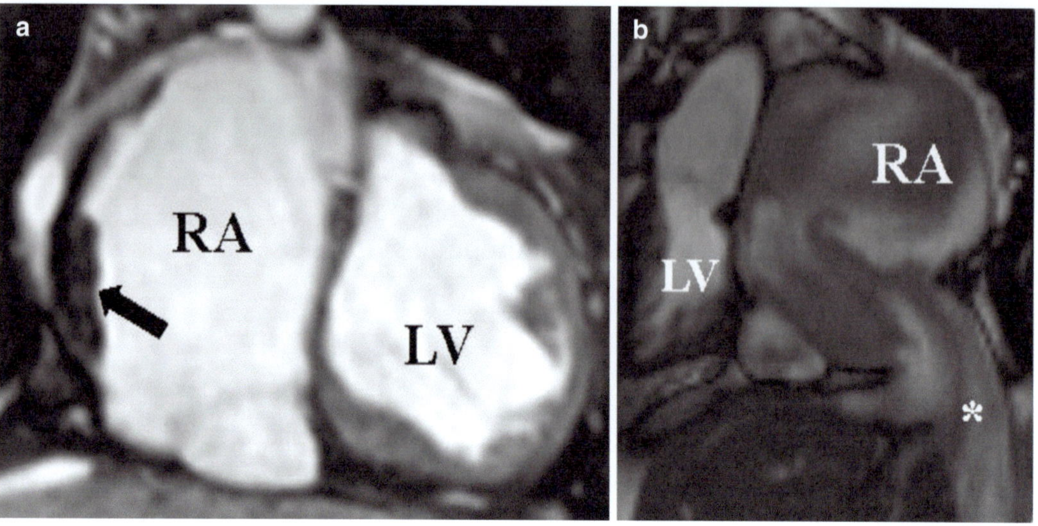

Fig. 18.1 Patient with tricuspid atresia and a single functioning left ventricle (LV) presenting 30 years after atriopulmonary Fontan operation with atrial fibrillation and desaturation. (**a**) Cardiac myocardial resonance imaging revealed a massively dilated right atrium (RA) containing a large crescent-shaped thrombus (arrow). (**b**) Sluggish blood flow from the inferior vena cava (star) giving the appearance of 'smoke' in the RA

Endothelial injury

- Thrombogenic foreign material
- Endothelial dysfunction
- Cardiopulmonary bypass
- Central venous catheters

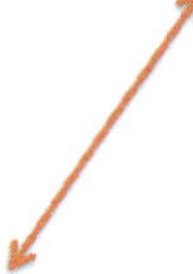

Virchow's Triad in the Fontan circulation

Abnormal blood flow

- Cardiopulmonary bypass
- Abnormal Fontan pathway blood flow
- Non-pulsatile PA blood flow
- Conduit stenosis / valved conduits
- Right-to-left shunting (fenestrations)
- Anatomical dead-ends
- Raised venous pressure
- Ventricular dysfunction
- Atrial or ventricular arrhythmias

Hypercoagulability

- Cardiopulmonary bypass
- Coagulation abnormalities
- Increased platelet activity
- Cyanosis
- Liver dysfunction
- Protein losing enteropathy

Fig. 18.2 Virchow's triad describes the three major variables that determine the formation of venous thrombus: endothelial injury, hypercoagulability and venous stasis. Patients who have undergone Fontan surgery commonly display multiple anatomical, hemodynamic and hematological features which drive venous thrombosis. This can lead to complications in situ, e.g. baffle occlusion, or can result in venous thromboembolism (e.g. pulmonary embolism) or paradoxical arterial thromboembolism (e.g. cerebrovascular accident or myocardial infarction). *PA* pulmonary artery

Hematological abnormalities in both pro- and anticoagulant proteins have been documented in patients who had undergone Fontan surgery, including:

- low concentrations of protein C and plasminogen
- low concentrations of factors II, V, VII and X [15, 16]
- elevated factor VIII levels, documented in a subset of Fontan patients, many of whom had higher systemic venous pressure and a history of TE [15].

Hemodynamic risk factors for TE include:

- severe right atrial dilatation
- sluggish blood flow in the Fontan pathway (low cardiac output and abnormal fluid dynamics)
- arrhythmia [17].

Surgical factors appear to influence the TE risk, including:

- type and extent of surgical material used
- presence of valved versus non-valved conduits.

The specific type of Fontan connection, however, does not appear to impact TE risk: A study of 592 patients failed to show any difference in TE risk between atriopulmonary (AP) Fontan, lateral tunnel and extra cardiac conduits [18].

The interaction between these different factors and their relative importance in individual Fontan patients remains uncertain and is an important target of future research.

Types of Thromboembolism and Predisposing Factors

In the Fontan cohort we come across two types of thrombotic event:

- Venous thrombosis or thromboembolism, including thrombosis in the Fontan pathway which can encompass the right atrium (Fig. 18.1).
- Venous TE may cause pulmonary emboli; systemic TE relating to paradoxical emboli across a fenestration or other right-left shunt, or thrombus formation in the subaortic area, left atrial appendage (especially in the presence of arrhythmia) or pulmonary veins.

Predisposing factors for thrombo-embolic events in Fontan patients include:

- cyanosis, commonly seen in Fontan patients with:
  - a fenestration (allowing flow of blood between the Fontan pathway and the left atrium)
  - arteriovenous collaterals within the lung (with systemic venous blood bypassing the pulmonary capillaries)
  - veno-venous collaterals, with systemic venous blood seeking the path of least resistance, hence bypassing the lungs, and reaching the systemic circulation
  - lateral tunnel leaks (e.g. dehiscence of sutures keeping the patch attached to the right atrial wall to form the lateral tunnel-type total cavopulmonary connection); effectively behaving like a Fontan fenestration.
- atrial arrhythmias, typically atrial tachycardia, or atrial fibrillation
- a failing Fontan circulation, associated with a low cardiac output state, ventricular dysfunction, valve disease, raised central venous pressure, liver disease, protein-losing enteropathy, renal dysfunction, and other complications
- traditional risk factors for venous thromboembolism including a personal history or first-degree relative with a history of venous TE, obesity, use of hormone replacement therapy or estrogen-containing contraceptive therapy, cigarette smoking, pregnancy, major (lower-limb) orthopedic or abdominal surgery and prolonged immobilization.

A retrospective study conducted on 120 patients with Fontan circulation highlighted a number of coagulation abnormalities regardless of having an intra-cardiac thrombus. On the contrary, D-dimer was found to be significantly raised in patients with intracardiac thrombus with a cutoff vale of 1.8 µg/mL with a negative predictive value of 95% [19]. Raised D-dimer levels after stopping anticoagulation in Fontan patients have been correlated to an increased incidence of thrombosis.

Managing the Risk of Thromboembolism in Fontan Patients

A clear consensus on the management of TE risk in Fontan patients is lacking. The benefits of anticoagulation should be weighed against the risk of bleeding and the impact on quality of life in this young population of patients who are likely to remain on anticoagulation for decades (limitations on the types of sport that can be practiced or other activities that carry the risk of injury, need for regular INR measurements and dose adjustments, fear of bleeding etc.). Vitamin K antagonists (VKAs) interact with medication and food, and genetic polymorphisms can affect the response to treatment [20, 21]. The time spent in therapeutic INR range in a single-center Fontan study (median age 19 years) was 84% [22]. Reasons of non-therapeutic INRs included diet change, non-compliance and drug interactions.

Aspirin or dual antiplatelet therapy are also recommended by some experts, especially for patients after total cavopulmonary connection, who are deemed at lower risk of TE than patients with AP Fontan. Antiplatelets may have a lower bleeding risk than warfarin and do not require monitoring, but resistance to antiplatelets is not routinely assessed.

Studies of thromboprophylaxis in Fontan patients have found that either anticoagulation or antiplatelet therapy is beneficial in terms of reducing the risk of TE events, but a consistent clear benefit of anticoagulation over antiplatelet therapy has not been described:

- In a registry of 210 patients (median age 8.5 years), 40% of whom had a lateral tunnel or extracardiac conduit, the lack of treatment with aspirin or warfarin was associated with a higher thromboembolic event rate at 20-year follow-up (48% versus 14% in the treated cohort) [17]. There was no difference, however between aspirin and anticoagulation;

- A trial of 111 children (mean age 5 years) randomized to aspirin versus heparin/warfarin within 2 from Fontan surgery found no difference in thrombotic events at 2 years (24% warfarin versus 14% aspirin, $p = 0.45$) [7] All initial thrombotic events were venous, and the vast majority were detected at routine assessment with only 28% associated with clinical signs and symptoms (e.g., oedema, dyspnea). Twenty of 25 thromboses were in the Fontan circulation and 4 within the pulmonary arteries. In 7 patients, there was recurrent thrombosis;

- Investigators from Australia and New Zealand compared patients with an extracardiac Fontan, treated with warfarin versus aspirin, using propensity score adjustment and matching. In the matched cohort of 328 patients, there was no significant difference in TE events beyond the first year from the Fontan operation [23] TE event rate at 5 years was 6%, and 9% at 12 years. Freedom from TE event or bleeding at 12 years was 54%. Conduit thrombosis (the majority asymptomatic and detected during routine follow-up) and stroke/TIA were the most common events. Almost half (44%) of the patients who suffered a TE on warfarin had an INR < 2 at the time of the event, highlighting issues with compliance and/or the inability to maintain a therapeutic INR. The majority of bleeding events were post-traumatic intracranial hemorrhage or GI bleeding; in one third (36%) of these patients, the INR was >3 at the time of bleeding.

- A retrospective evaluation of 424 Fontan patients with a mean follow-up of 11.2 years reported that warfarin was associated with an increased risk of hemorrhagic events, while no difference was found between patients on antiplatelets or anticoagulation in terms of overall hemostatic (thrombotic or bleeding) events [24].

- A meta-analysis of ten studies (1200 patients, total follow-up time 9620 patient years) showed that treatment with either aspirin or warfarin resulted in a significantly lower rate of TE compared to no TE prophylaxis [10]. No difference in the incidence of TE, however, was detected between aspirin and warfarin therapy early or late after Fontan surgery. This finding persisted when total cavo-pulmonary connection patients were analyzed separately.

The 2018 AHA/ACC adult congenital heart disease (ACHD) guidelines [25] state that:

- anticoagulation with a VKA is recommended for adults with Fontan palliation with known or suspected thrombus, thromboembolic events, or prior atrial arrhythmia, and no contraindications to anticoagulation (class of recommendation I, level of evidence C);
- antiplatelet therapy or anticoagulation with a VKA may be considered in adults after Fontan palliation without known or suspected thrombus, thromboembolic events, or prior arrhythmia (IIb, B).

They also recommend continued surveillance for hemodynamic and anatomic risk factors for thrombosis. Any modifiable risk factor for thrombosis should be treated, e.g., ablation for arrhythmias. Patients may also benefit from anticoagulation if they have a significant residual intracardiac right-to-left shunt or veno-venous collaterals.

The 2020 ESC ACHD guidelines [26] recommend:

- anticoagulation in the presence, or with a history, of atrial thrombus, atrial arrhythmias, or thromboembolic events (I, C).

They also point out the potential for subclinical, recurrent pulmonary embolism (eventually leading to a rise in pulmonary vascular resistance) and systemic embolism that have led to a recommendation, by some, for lifelong anticoagulation in all Fontan patients, but this practice varies between centers as evidence is lacking.

Non-vitamin K Anticoagulants (NOACs)

There are small case studies on the use of NOACs in Fontan patients and ongoing clinical trials however there is currently no robust evidence to recommend their use. NOACs are contraindicated in those with mechanical heart valves or a history of significant mitral or tricuspid (atrioventricular) valve stenosis. Table 18.1 demonstrates the pros and cons of each agent.

A cohort study of 75 Fontan patients on NOACs from the International NOTE (non-vitamin K antagonist oral anticoagulants for thromboembolic prevention in patients with congenital heart disease) registry sheds some light onto the safety and efficacy of these agents in this patient group [27]. The incidence of TE was 2.9% per year and major bleeding was also 2.9% per year, with a minor bleeding incidence of 15.8% per year. NOACs were stopped and reverted to VKAs in 3 patients due to thromboembolic events, in 4 due to bleeding and another 7 for other reasons (e.g., side-effects, pregnancy, patient preference). Less reassuringly, in a subsequent study from the NOTE registry on the overall ACHD population (including 14% Fontan patients), 3 out of 6 patients who had experienced TE and 3 out 7 patients with major bleeding during follow-up were Fontan patients [28].

Georgekutty et al. reported a retrospective cohort of 21 adult Fontan patients (mean age 33 years) in whom NOACs were prescribed mainly for arrhythmia or thrombosis, most commonly because of patient preference or unstable INR levels [29]. Only a single episode of TE was recorded over the total cumulative follow-up period of 316 months, with no major bleeding events.

A systematic review of the available literature suggests that NOACs may be non-inferior to VKAs in preventing thrombosis in Fontan patients [30] even though there are clearly cases of TE events reported in the literature during treatment with a NOAC [28, 31]. Further data are needed to confirm the safety and efficacy of NOACs in Fontan patients.

Table 18.1 Anticoagulants and antiplatelets: Comparison of agents

	Aspirin	Clopidogrel	Warfarin	NOACs
Mechanism of action	Antiplatelet, COX inhibition	Antiplatelet, P2Y12 inhibition	Vitamin K antagonist, Competitive inhibition of VKORC1 Reduces the synthesis of vitamin K-dependent clotting factors	Non-vitamin K antagonist, Thrombin (Dabigatran) or Factor Xa (others) inhibition
Considerations	Drug resistance		Dependent on patient-related factors such as diet, comorbidities and medication	Dose adjustment in renal dysfunction; avoidance in end-stage renal disease
	Gastric issues		Often outside therapeutic range	Higher risk of bleeding in combination with NSAIDs/antiplatelets
Reversibility	Irreversible	Irreversible	Reversible	Reversal agent for some, but not universally available
	Inexpensive	Inexpensive	Inexpensive	Relatively expensive
Anticoagulation monitoring requirements	Not required	Not required	Regular monitoring is required with frequent blood testing Citrate-adjusted bottles for patients with secondary erythrocytosis	Not required
Convenience	Once daily	Once daily	Once daily but variable dose	Once or twice daily depending on agent

Therefore, the AHA/ACC ACHD guidelines stress that NOACs are unstudied and cannot be recommended in Fontan patients. They also voice concerns about liver function vulnerability in Fontan patients, which may theoretically increase the risk of complications with some of these agents [25]. The ESC ACHD guidelines state that robust prospective efficacy data on NOACs in Fontan patients are lacking and these agents cannot be currently recommended as standard therapy [26].

References

1. Rychik J, Atz AM, Celermajer DS, Deal BJ, Gatzoulis MA, Gewillig MH, Hsia TY, Hsu DT, Kovacs AH, McCrindle BW, Newburger JW, Pike NA, Rodefeld M, Rosenthal DN, Schumacher KR, Marino BS, Stout K, Veldtman G, Younoszai AK, D'Udekem Y. Evaluation and management of the child and adult with Fontan circulation: a scientific statement from the American Heart Association. Circulation. 2019;140:E234–84.
2. Cromme-Dijkhuis AH, Hess J, Hählen K, Henkens CM, Bink-Boelkens MT, Eygelaar AA, Bos E. Specific sequelae after Fontan operation at mid- and long-term follow-up. Arrhythmia, liver dysfunction, and coagulation disorders. J Thorac Cardiovasc Surg. 1993;106:1126–32.
3. de Leval MR. The Fontan circulation: what have we learned? What to expect? Pediatr Cardiol. 1998;19:316–20.
4. Monagle P, Cochrane A, McCrindle B, Benson L, Williams W, Andrew M. Editorial: thromboembolic complications after Fontan procedures—the role of prophylactic anticoagulation. J Thorac Cardiovasc Surg. 1998;115:493–8.
5. Fyfe DA, Kline CH, Sade RM, Gillette PC. Transesophageal echocardiography detects thrombus formation not identified by transthoracic echocardiography after the Fontan operation. J Am Coll Cardiol. 1991;18:1733–7.
6. Balling G, Vogt M, Kaemmerer H, Eicken A, Meisner H, Hess J. Intracardiac thrombus formation after the Fontan operation. J Thorac Cardiovasc Surg. 2000;119:745–52.
7. Monagle P, Cochrane A, Roberts R, Manlhiot C, Weintraub R, Szechtman B, Hughes M, Andrew M, McCrindle BW, Fontan Anticoagulation Study Group. A multicenter, randomized trial comparing heparin/warfarin and acetylsalicylic acid as primary thromboprophylaxis for 2 years after the Fontan procedure in children. J Am Coll Cardiol. 2011;58:645–51.
8. Rosenthal DN, Friedman AH, Kleinman CS, Kopf GS, Rosenfeld LE, Hellenbrand WE. Thromboembolic complications after Fontan operations. Circulation. 1995;92:II287–93.
9. Egbe AC, Connolly HM, McLeod CJ, Ammash NM, Niaz T, Yogeswaran V, Poterucha JT, Qureshi MY, Driscoll DJ. Thrombotic and embolic complications associated with atrial arrhythmia after Fontan operation: role of prophylactic therapy. J Am Coll Cardiol. 2016;68:1312–9.
10. Alsaied T, Alsidawi S, Allen CC, Faircloth J, Palumbo JS, Veldtman GR. Strategies for thromboprophylaxis in Fontan circulation: a meta-analysis. Heart. 2015;101:1731–7.

11. Putnam JB, Lemmer JH, Rocchini AP, Bove EL. Embolectomy for acute pulmonary artery occlusion following Fontan procedure. Ann Thorac Surg. 1988;45:335–6.

12. Wilson DG, Wisheart JD, Stuart AG. Systemic thromboembolism leading to myocardial infarction and stroke after fenestrated total cavopulmonary connection. Heart. 1995;73:483–5.

13. Benito Bartolomé F, Prada Martínez F, Bret Zurita M. Pulmonary thromboembolism after Fontan operation. Rev Esp Cardiol. 2002;55:449–51.

14. Chun DS, Schamberger MS, Flaspohler T, Turrentine MW, Brown JW, Farrell AG, Girod DA. Incidence, outcome, and risk factors for stroke after the Fontan procedure. Am J Cardiol. 2004;93:117–9.

15. Cromme-Dijkhuis AH, Henkens CM, Bijleveld CM, Hillege HL, Bom VJ, van der Meer J. Coagulation factor abnormalities as possible thrombotic risk factors after Fontan operations. Lancet. 1990;336:1087–90.

16. Odegard KC, McGowan FX, Zurakowski D, Dinardo JA, Castro RA, del Nido PJ, Laussen PC. Procoagulant and anticoagulant factor abnormalities following the Fontan procedure: increased factor VIII may predispose to thrombosis. J Thorac Cardiovasc Surg. 2003;125:1260–7.

17. Potter BJ, Leong-Sit P, Fernandes SM, Feifer A, Mayer JE, Triedman JK, Walsh EP, Landzberg MJ, Khairy P. Effect of aspirin and warfarin therapy on thromboembolic events in patients with univentricular hearts and Fontan palliation. Int J Cardiol. 2013;168:3940–3.

18. Coon PD, Rychik J, Novello RT, Ro PS, Gaynor JW, Spray TL. Thrombus formation after the Fontan operation. Ann Thorac Surg. 2001;71:1990–4.

19. Takeuchi D, Inai K, Shinohara T, Nakanishi T, Park I-S. Blood coagulation abnormalities and the usefulness of D-dimer level for detecting intracardiac thrombosis in adult Fontan patients. Int J Cardiol. 2016;224:139–44.

20. Linder MW, Looney S, Adams JE, Johnson N, Antonino-Green D, Lacefield N, Bukaveckas BL, Valdes R. Warfarin dose adjustments based on CYP2C9 genetic polymorphisms. J Thromb Thrombolysis. 2002;14:227–32.

21. Holbrook AM, Pereira JA, Labiris R, McDonald H, Douketis JD, Crowther M, Wells PS. Systematic overview of warfarin and its drug and food interactions. Arch Intern Med. 2005;165:1095–106.

22. Faircloth JM, Miner KM, Alsaied T, Nelson N, Ciambarella J, Mizuno T, Palumbo JS, Vinks AA, Veldtman GR. Time in therapeutic range as a marker for thrombotic and bleeding outcomes in Fontan patients. J Thromb Thrombolysis. 2017;44:38–47.

23. Iyengar AJ, Winlaw DS, Galati JC, Wheaton GR, Gentles TL, Grigg LE, Justo RN, Radford DJ, Attard C, Weintraub RG, Bullock A, Sholler GS, Celermajer DS, d'Udekem Y, on behalf of the Australia and New Zealand Fontan Registry. No difference between aspirin and warfarin after extracardiac Fontan in a propensity score analysis of 475 patients. Eur J Cardiothorac Surg. 2016;50:980–7.

24. Ohuchi H, Yasuda K, Miyazaki A, Ono S, Hayama Y, Negishi J, Noritake K, Mizuno M, Yamada O. Prevalence and predictors of haemostatic complications in 412 Fontan patients: their relation to anticoagulation and haemodynamics. Eur J Cardiothorac Surg. 2015;47:511–9.

25. Stout KK, Daniels CJ, Aboulhosn JA, Bozkurt B, Broberg CS, Colman JM, Crumb SR, Dearani JA, Fuller S, Gurvitz M, Khairy P, Landzberg MJ, Saidi A, Valente AM, Van Hare GF. 2018 AHA/ACC guideline for the management of adults with congenital heart disease: a report of the American College of Cardiology/American Heart Association task force on clinical practice guidelines. Circulation. 2019;139:e698–800.

26. Baumgartner H, De Backer J, Babu-Narayan SV, Budts W, Chessa M, Diller G-P, Lung B, Kluin J, Lang IM, Meijboom F, Moons P, Mulder BJM, Oechslin E, Roos-Hesselink JW, Schwerzmann M, Sondergaard L, Zeppenfeld K, ESC Scientific Document Group, Ernst S, Ladouceur M, Aboyans V, Alexander D, Christodorescu R, Corrado D, D'Alto M, de Groot N, Delgado V, Di Salvo G, Dos Subira L, Eicken A, Fitzsimons D, Frogoudaki AA, Gatzoulis M, Heymans S, Hörer J, Houyel L, Jondeau G, Katus HA, Landmesser U, Lewis BS, Lyon A, Mueller CE, Mylotte D, Petersen SE, Sonia Petronio A, Roffi M, Rosenhek R, Shlyakhto E, Simpson IA, Sousa-Uva M, Torp-Pedersen CT, Touyz RM, Van De Bruaene A, Windecker S, Aboyans V, Baigent C, Collet J-P, Dean V, Delgado V, Fitzsimons D, Gale CP, Grobbee DE, Halvorsen S, Hindricks G, Iung B, Jüni P, Katus HA, Landmesser U, Leclercq C, Lettino M, Lewis BS, Merkely B, Mueller C, Petersen SE, Petronio AS, Richter DJ, Roffi M, Shlyakhto E, Simpson IA, Sousa-Uva M, Touyz RM, Hammoudi N, Grigoryan SV, Mair J, Imanov G, Chesnov J, Bondue A, Nabil N, Kaneva A, Brida M, Hadjisavva O, Rubackova-Popelova J, Nielsen DG, El Sayed MH, Ermel R, Sinisalo J, Thambo J-B, Bakhutashvili Z, et al. ESC guidelines for the management of adult congenital heart disease. Eur Heart J. 2020;2020:ehaa554.

27. Yang H, Veldtman GR, Bouma BJ, Budts W, Niwa K, Meijboom F, Scognamiglio G, Egbe AC, Schwerzmann M, Broberg C, Morissens M, Buber J, Tsai S, Polyzois I, Post MC, Greutmann M, Van Dijk A, Mulder BJ, Aboulhosn J. Non-vitamin K antagonist oral anticoagulants in adults with a Fontan circulation: are they safe. Open Heart. 2019;6:e000985.

28. Yang H, Bouma BJ, Dimopoulos K, Khairy P, Ladouceur M, Niwa K, Greutmann M, Schwerzmann M, Egbe A, Scognamiglio G, Budts W, Veldtman G, Opotowsky AR, Broberg CS, Gumbiene L, Meijboom FJ, Rutz T, Post MC, Moe T, Lipczyńska M, Tsai SF, Chakrabarti S, Tobler D, Davidson W, Morissens M, van Dijk A, Buber J, Bouchardy J, Skoglund K, Christersson C, Kronvall T, Konings TC, Alonso-Gonzalez R, Mizuno A, Webb G, Laukyte

M, Sieswerda GTJ, Shafer K, Aboulhosn J, Mulder BJM. Non-vitamin K antagonist oral anticoagulants (NOACs) for thromboembolic prevention, are they safe in congenital heart disease? Results of a worldwide study. Int J Cardiol. 2020;299:123–30.

29. Georgekutty J, Kazerouninia A, Wang Y, Ermis PR, Parekh DR, Franklin WJ, Lam WW. Novel oral anticoagulant use in adult Fontan patients: a single center experience. Congenit Heart Dis. 2018;13:541–7.

30. Stalikas N, Doundoulakis I, Karagiannidis E, Bouras E, Kartas A, Frogoudaki A, Karvounis H, Dimopoulos K, Giannakoulas G. Non-vitamin K oral anticoagulants in adults with congenital heart disease: a systematic review. J Clin Med. 2020;9:9.

31. Pinto C, Samuel BP, Ratnasamy C, Vettukattil JJ. Thrombosis in Fontan patient on apixaban. Int J Cardiol. 2015;182:66–7.

Electrophysiology Considerations After the Fontan Operation

19

Jeremy P. Moore

Introduction

Univentricular heart patients after the Fontan operation are affected by multiple electrical abnormalities, however the problems observed most frequently include:

- Sinus node dysfunction
- Intra-atrial reentrant tachycardia
- Sudden cardiac death
- Ventricular dyssynchrony (Fig. 19.1).

J. P. Moore (✉)
UCLA Medical Center, Ahmanson/UCLA Adult
Congenital Heart Disease Center,
Los Angeles, CA, USA
e-mail: jpmoore@mednet.ucla.edu

© The Author(s), under exclusive license to Springer Nature Switzerland AG 2023
P. Clift et al. (eds.), *Univentricular Congenital Heart Defects and the Fontan Circulation*,
https://doi.org/10.1007/978-3-031-36208-8_19

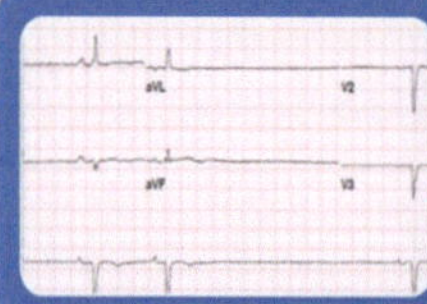

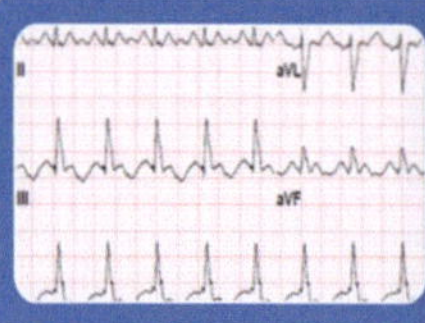

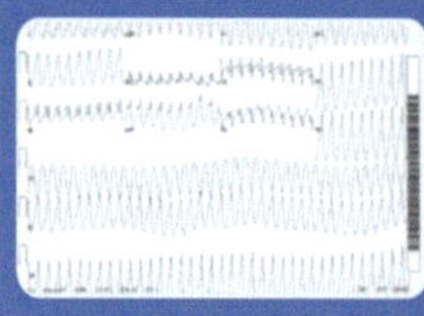

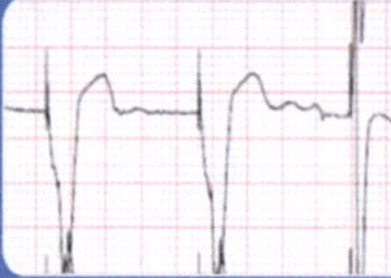

Fig. 19.1 Summary of major electrophysiologic complications after Fontan surgery

Sinus Node Dysfunction (SND)

Fontan Physiology and the Importance of Sinus Rhythm

The cardiac output in Fontan physiology is dependent on downstream pressure in the pulmonary venous atrium as determined by atrial relaxation properties, diastolic and systolic function of the single ventricle, function of the atrioventricular (AV) valve, and presence of AV synchrony.

After Fontan surgery in sinus rhythm, the majority of pulmonary blood flow occurs during ventricular systole, with atrial relaxation and the downward descent of closed AV valve with suction-like effect.

Prolonged junctional rhythm results in loss of forward systolic flow due to simultaneous atrial and ventricular contraction, systolic flow reversal in the pulmonary veins and pulmonary venous pressure that transiently exceeds the Fontan pressure, compromising cardiac output [1, 2].

Junctional rhythm after Fontan operation is poorly tolerated and may result in the development of Fontan failure and protein-losing enteropathy and may be reversible with atrial pacing [3–5].

Scope of the Problem

Potential etiologies of sinus node dysfunction after Fontan surgery (Table 19.1).

Table 19.1 Etiologies of sinus node dysfunction after Fontan surgery

Time course	Etiology
Operative	Manipulation at the cavo-atrial junction
	Surgical autonomic denervation
	Trauma to the sinus node artery
Post-operative	Progressive dilation and fibrosis of the morphologic right atrium

To a degree, mild and asymptomatic sinus bradycardia is expected after the Fontan operation and does not require treatment [6, 7]. Maintenance of sinus rhythm (or even sinus bradycardia) is critical however.

A junctional rhythm is present in 5–6% of Fontan patients at baseline [8] and a clinically significant bradycardia or need for pacemaker placement is observed in ~15% of TCPC patients at 10 years after surgery [9, 10], with no difference between LT and EC Fontan patients that has been demonstrated [10].

Pacemaker Implantation

Pacemaker implantation can be achieved by either the surgical or transvenous route.

Surgical Approach

This is complex often with a densely scarred morphologic right atrium with poor pacing characteristics; pacing of the morphologic left atrium is preferred [11]. A left thoracotomy approach is often utilized to reach viable tissue at the dome of the left atrium.

Recent data suggest higher rates of lead failure and more frequent need for generator replacement for the epicardial as compared to the transvenous route after Fontan operation [12, 13]. Other potential complications include pain, prolonged pleural

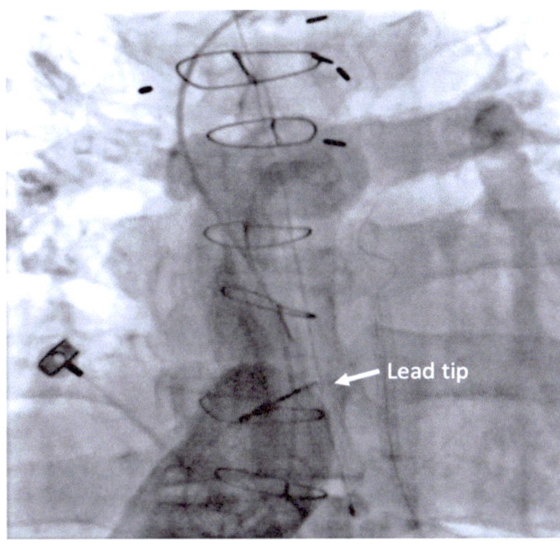

Fig. 19.2 Transvenous pacemaker implantation in a lateral tunnel Fontan. The lead is seen in the lower portion of the Fontan circuit

drainage, pocket infection, and prolonged hospital stay [14].

Transvenous Approach

Transvenous implantation with placement of pacing leads within the Fontan circulation is considered safe and effective after the Fontan operation with similar risk for thromboembolism as compared to the surgical approach [14–16] however chronic anticoagulation is required.

A direct venous route for atrial pacing is also possible for atrio-pulmonary and lateral tunnel Fontan variants, where the SVC still connects to the right atrium (Figs. 19.2 and 19.3).

Modification of this approach, including puncture into the pulmonary venous atrium or fixation of a lead to the epicardial atrial surface is necessary for patients who have undergone extracardiac Fontan operation [18, 19]. Ventricular pacing is possible, but this is usually approached surgically.

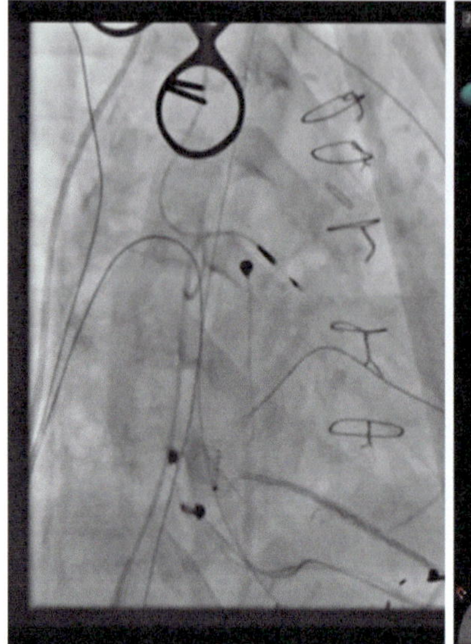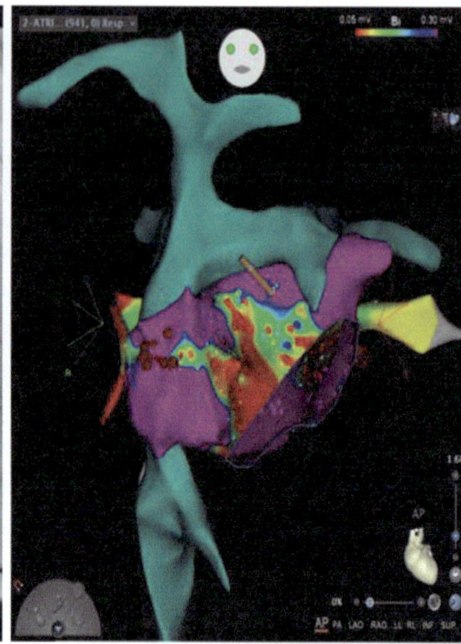

Fig. 19.3 Transpulmonary pacing after extracardiac Fontan surgery. The lead has been placed through the SVC, into the pulmonary artery and screwed into the atrial epicardium [52]

Intra-atrial Reentrant Tachycardia (IART)

Epidemiology

The classical Fontan and subsequent modifications (AP Fontan) is associated with the development of significant atrial arrhythmia in ~50% at 10–15 years [20–23].

Lateral tunnel (LT) Fontan has a lower prevalence of postoperative IART observed in ~25% at 10 years [21], with a significant decrease in atrial arrhythmia burden as compared to modified Fontan. The pathogenesis of atrial arrhythmia for the LT Fontan is understood on the basis of a pre-clinical studies in dogs [24].

The extra-cardiac (EC) Fontan was proposed to further reduce atrial arrhythmia. Initial work did not support a difference in arrhythmia between the two techniques however recently a two- to three-fold reduction in atrial arrhythmia has been shown with longer follow-up and meta-analysis [10, 25].

Management of Atrial Arrhythmia

The development of atrial arrhythmia is associated with increased mortality and adverse events; aggressive management is recommended [26].

Various therapeutic approaches have been described:

- Fontan conversion with arrhythmia surgery: this is generally indicated for drug-refractory atrial arrhythmia and good hemodynamics; patient selection is critical. A modified right atrial Maze should be employed for all patients and a modified Cox III Maze for documented AF.
- In-hospital mortality rates range from 3 to 10% [27–30] with an additional 10% at 1-year in one study [28]. Recurrent arrhythmia occurs in 10–20% at 5 years [27, 28].
- Catheter ablation:
  - (a) In the modified AP Fontan is highly variable, although atriotomy and IVC circuits are common [31, 32]. Ablation has a modest success rate, although improving with

contemporary mapping technologies [32]. Tachycardia recurrence occurs in up to 30% and is often due to novel substrates; [22, 33] therefore multiple procedures may be required

(b) Lateral tunnel ablation: Direct access to the lateral tunnel is possible, with trans-baffle puncture usually required for access to the pulmonary venous atrium. Catheter ablation outcomes are favorable with the cavo-tricuspid isthmus being a frequent target, as well as within the LT chamber [34].

(c) Extra cardiac Fontan ablation: as opposed to other Fontan variants, the extra cardiac conduit poses a significant challenge for access to the pulmonary venous atrium. Approaches include trans-conduit [35], trans-caval [36], and retrograde access (remote magnetic navigation). The CTI also is the most frequent ablation target, with the exception of patients that have undergone Fontan conversion where substrates tend to be highly variable [37]. Long term outcome data are lacking.

- Anti-tachycardia pacing: Some studies support efficacy and safety for CHD, [38] however few Fontan patients are reported in the literature. It is often combined and useful as part of the Fontan conversion strategy [27].

- Drug therapeutic strategies include the use of Class III drugs (sotalol, dofetilide, or amiodarone) and are generally considered poorly effective in the Fontan population [30] (Table 19.2; Figs. 19.4 and 19.5).

Table 19.2 Fontan conversion considerations

Indications
  Atrial arrhythmia
  Fontan pathway obstruction
  Ventricular dysfunction related to arrhythmia
  AV valve insufficiency[a]
  Cyanosis-causing pulmonary AV fistulas
  Residual intracardiac shunts
  Disconnected pulmonary arteries
  Circular venous flow
  Aortic aneurysms/aortic regurgitation
  Anomalous systemic venous drainage
Contraindications
  Severe ventricular dysfunction not related to arrhythmia or pathway obstruction
  Non-compensated protein-losing enteropathy
  Multiple organ dysfunction

[a] Successful AV valve repair considered unlikely

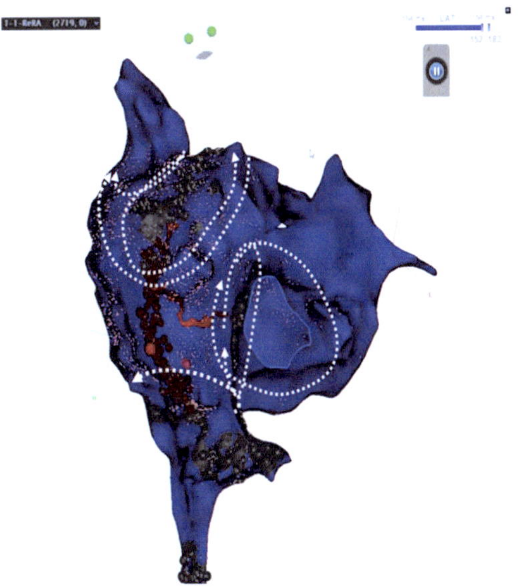

Fig. 19.4 Location of multiple potential atrial reentry circuits after the AP Fontan

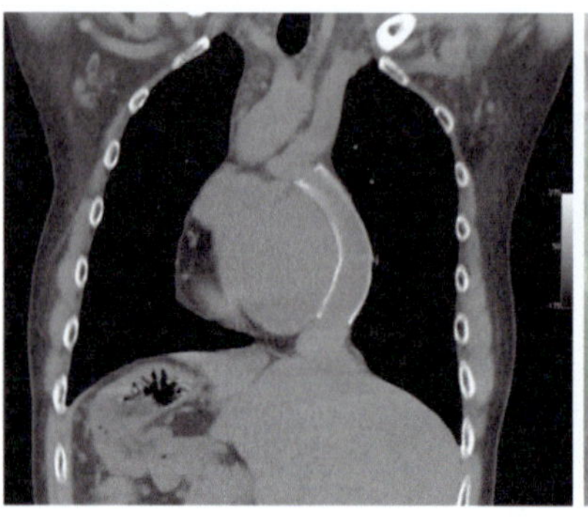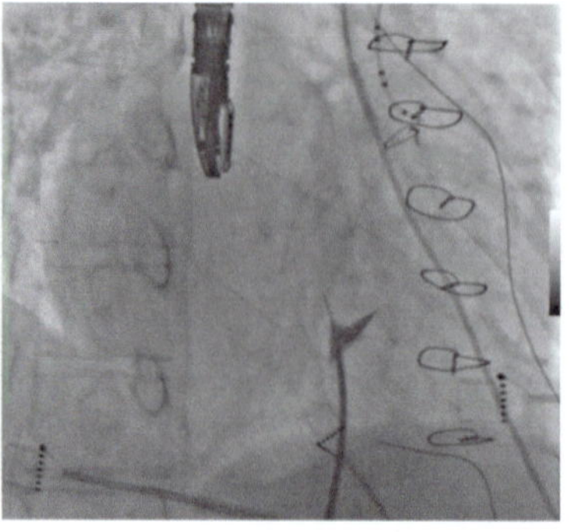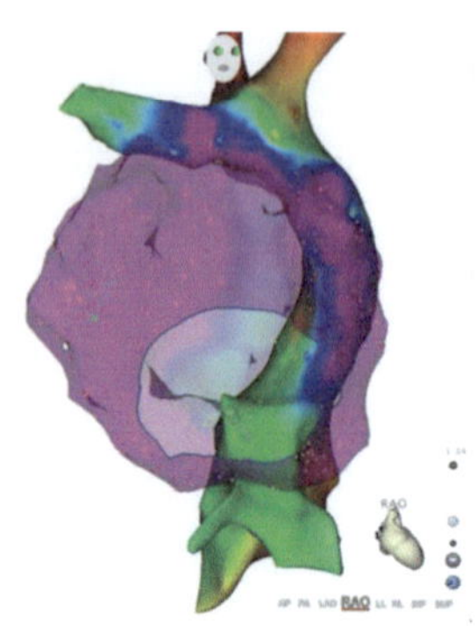

Fig. 19.5 Trans-caval puncture for a patient with heterotaxy syndrome and catheter ablation for twin AV node tachycardia. The preoperative CT scan demonstrated a region of cavo-atrial overlap, facilitating a relatively straightforward access to the pulmonary venous atrium at the procedure

Sudden Cardiac Death

Epidemiology and Risk Factors

Sudden cardiac death is uncommon with an incidence of 3–5% at 10 years follow up. [39, 40]. Modes of death include IART with rapid AV conduction, ventricular tachycardia, AV block, and thromboembolism.

Predictive risk factors have included:

- surgical AV valve repair, [40]
- postoperative Fontan pressure >20 mmHg, [40]
- absence of sinus rhythm [39, 40].

Non-sustained ventricular tachycardia (NSVT) (but not sudden death) can be predicted by MRI late gadolinium enhancement [41]. The ventriculotomy incision as a part of the Sano shunt for hypoplastic left heart syndrome may be proarrhythmic, although this has not yet been demonstrated [42].

Prevention of Sudden Cardiac Death

ICD placement is indicated for Fontan patients with aborted cardiac arrest or sustained ventricular tachycardia. [43] However, primary prevention indications are lacking. The general approach is either surgical or most commonly, the subcutaneous ICD and initial subcutaneous ICD (SICD) experience is favorable [44]. Fontan patients are often reasonable candidates for placement of a subcutaneous ICD [45] and the technology is safe and effective. Caveats are that bradycardia pacing and anti-tachycardia pacing are not available.

Ventricular Dyssynchrony

Scope of the Problem

The negative impact of ventricular pacing was appreciated very early in the Fontan experience [46]. More recently, increased attention has been paid to this phenomenon. Greater than 50% pacing appears to be a strong predictor of negative outcomes [47–49] and is associated with systemic ventricular dysfunction, moderate-to-severe AV valve regurgitation and death/transplantation.

Resynchronization Strategies

Multisite pacing is associated with an improvement in NYHA class and/or systemic EF in two-thirds after Fontan [50]. There is greater freedom from death/transplantation as compared to single site pacing, however of borderline statistical difference at 5-years of follow up. [51]

Apical pacing: is l̲ikely superior to single site pacing, however this is not well studied [49].

Disclosures **None.**

References

1. Rychik J, Fogel MA, Donofrio MT, et al. Comparison of patterns of pulmonary venous blood flow in the functional single ventricle heart after operative aortopulmonary shunt versus superior cavopulmonary shunt. Am J Cardiol. 1997;80:922–6.
2. Hasselman T, Schneider D, Madan N, Jacobs M. Reversal of fenestration flow during ventricular systole in Fontan patients in junctional or ventricular paced rhythm. Pediatr Cardiol. 2005;26:638–41.
3. Cohen MI, Bridges ND, Gaynor JW, et al. Modifications to the cavopulmonary anastomosis do not eliminate early sinus node dysfunction. J Thorac Cardiovasc Surg. 2000;120:891–900.
4. Barber BJ, Burch GH, Tripple D, Balaji S. Resolution of plastic bronchitis with atrial pacing in a patient with Fontan physiology. Pediatr Cardiol. 2004;25:73–6.
5. Dodge-Khatami A, Rahn M, Pretre R, Bauersfeld U. Dual chamber epicardial pacing for the failing atriopulmonary Fontan patient. Ann Thorac Surg. 2005;80:1440–4.
6. Evans WN, Acherman RJ, Restrepo H. Normal sinus rhythm-sinus bradycardia is common in young children post-extracardiac Fontan. Pediatr Cardiol. 2016;37:1377–9.
7. Blaufox AD, Sleeper LA, Bradley DJ, et al. Functional status, heart rate, and rhythm abnormalities in 521 Fontan patients 6 to 18 years of age. J Thorac Cardiovasc Surg. 2008;136:100–107.e1.
8. Anderson PA, Sleeper LA, Mahony L, et al. Contemporary outcomes after the Fontan procedure: a pediatric heart network multicenter study. J Am Coll Cardiol. 2008;52:85–98.
9. Balaji S, Daga A, Bradley DJ, et al. An international multicenter study comparing arrhythmia prevalence between the intracardiac lateral tunnel and the extracardiac conduit type of Fontan operations. J Thorac Cardiovasc Surg. 2014;148:576–81.
10. Ben Ali W, Bouhout I, Khairy P, Bouchard D, Poirier N. Extracardiac versus lateral tunnel Fontan: a meta-analysis of long-term results. Ann Thorac Surg. 2019;107:837–43.
11. Ramesh V, Gaynor JW, Shah MJ, et al. Comparison of left and right atrial epicardial pacing in patients with congenital heart disease. Ann Thorac Surg. 1999;68:2314–9.
12. Huntley GD, Deshmukh AJ, Warnes CA, Kapa S, Egbe AC. Longitudinal outcomes of epicardial and endocardial pacemaker leads in the adult Fontan patient. Pediatr Cardiol. 2018;39:1476–83.
13. Egbe AC, Huntley GD, Connolly HM, et al. Outcomes of cardiac pacing in adult patients after a Fontan operation. Am Heart J. 2017;194:92–8.
14. Hanksy B. Endocardial pacing after Fontan-type procedures. Pacing Clin Electrophysiol. 2005;28:140–8.
15. Takahashi K, Cecchin F, Fortescue E, et al. Permanent atrial pacing lead implant route after Fontan operation. Pacing Clin Electrophysiol. 2009;32:779–85.
16. Segar DE, Maldonado JR, Brown CG, Law IH. Transvenous versus epicardial pacing in Fontan patients. Pediatr Cardiol. 2018;39:1484–8.
17. Hoyt WJ, Moore JP, Shannon KM, Kannankeril PJ, Fish FA. Epicardial atrial pacing after the extra-cardiac Fontan operation: Feasibility of an entirely transvenous approach. J Cardiovasc Electrophysiol. 2022;33(1):128-133. https://doi.org/10.1111/jce.15285. Epub 2021 Nov 24. PMID: 34716972.
18. Moore JP, Shannon KM. Transpulmonary atrial pacing: an approach to transvenous pacemaker implantation after extracardiac conduit Fontan surgery. J Cardiovasc Electrophysiol. 2014;25:1028–31.
19. Arif S, Clift PF, De Giovanni JV. Permanent transvenous pacing in an extra-cardiac Fontan circulation. Europace. 2016;18:304–7.
20. Gelatt M, Hamilton RM, McCrindle BW, et al. Risk factors for atrial tachyarrhythmias after the Fontan operation. J Am Coll Cardiol. 1994;24:1735–41.
21. Cecchin F, Johnsrude CL, Perry JC, Friedman RA. Effect of age and surgical technique on symptomatic arrhythmias after the Fontan procedure. Am J Cardiol. 1995;76:386–91.
22. Weipert J, Noebauer C, Schreiber C, et al. Occurrence and management of atrial arrhythmia after long-term Fontan circulation. J Thorac Cardiovasc Surg. 2004;127:457–64.
23. Quinton E, Nightingale P, Hudsmith L, et al. Prevalence of atrial tachyarrhythmia in adults after Fontan operation. Heart. 2015;101:1672–7.
24. Rodefeld MD, Bromberg BI, Schuessler RB, Boineau JP, Cox JL, Huddleston CB. Atrial flutter after lateral tunnel construction in the modified Fontan operation: a canine model. J Thorac Cardiovasc Surg. 1996;111:514–26.
25. d'Udekem Y, Iyengar AJ, Galati JC, et al. Redefining expectations of long-term survival after the Fontan procedure: twenty-five years of follow-up from the entire population of Australia and New Zealand. Circulation. 2014;130:S32–8.
26. Giannakoulas G, Dimopoulos K, Yuksel S, et al. Atrial tachyarrhythmias late after Fontan operation are related to increase in mortality and hospitalization. Int J Cardiol. 2012;157:221–6.
27. Mavroudis C, Deal BJ, Backer CL, et al. J. Maxwell Chamberlain memorial paper for congenital heart surgery. 111 Fontan conversions with arrhythmia surgery: surgical lessons and outcomes. Ann Thorac Surg. 2007;84:1457–65; discussion 1465–6.
28. Poh CL, Cochrane A, Galati JC, et al. Ten-year outcomes of Fontan conversion in Australia and New Zealand demonstrate the superiority of a strat-

egy of early conversion. Eur J Cardiothorac Surg. 2016;49:530–5; discussion 535.

29. Aboulhosn J, Williams R, Shivkumar K, et al. Arrhythmia recurrence in adult patients with single ventricle physiology following surgical Fontan conversion. Congenit Heart Dis. 2010;5:430–4.

30. Egbe AC, Connolly HM, Khan AR, et al. Outcomes in adult Fontan patients with atrial tachyarrhythmias. Am Heart J. 2017;186:12–20.

31. Mandapati R, Walsh EP, Triedman JK. Pericaval and periannular intra-atrial reentrant tachycardias in patients with congenital heart disease. J Cardiovasc Electrophysiol. 2003;14:119–25.

32. Moore BM, Anderson R, Nisbet AM, et al. Ablation of atrial arrhythmias after the atriopulmonary Fontan procedure: mechanisms of arrhythmia and outcomes. JACC Clin Electrophysiol. 2018;4:1338–46.

33. de Groot NM, Lukac P, Blom NA, et al. Long-term outcome of ablative therapy of postoperative supraventricular tachycardias in patients with univentricular heart: a European multicenter study. Circ Arrhythm Electrophysiol. 2009;2:242–8.

34. Correa R, Sherwin ED, Kovach J, et al. Mechanism and ablation of arrhythmia following total cavopulmonary connection. Circ Arrhythm Electrophysiol. 2015;8:318–25.

35. Dave AS, Aboulhosn J, Child JS, Shivkumar K. Transconduit puncture for catheter ablation of atrial tachycardia in a patient with extracardiac Fontan palliation. Heart Rhythm. 2010;7:413–6.

36. Moore JP, Hendrickson B, Brunengraber DZ, Shannon KM. Transcaval puncture for access to the pulmonary venous atrium after the extracardiac total cavopulmonary connection operation. Circ Arrhythm Electrophysiol. 2015;8:824–8.

37. Moore JP, Shannon KM, Fish FA, et al. Catheter ablation of supraventricular tachyarrhythmia after extracardiac Fontan surgery. Heart Rhythm. 2016;13:1891–7.

38. Kramer CC, Maldonado JR, Olson MD, Gingerich JC, Ochoa LA, Law IH. Safety and efficacy of atrial antitachycardia pacing in congenital heart disease. Heart Rhythm. 2018;15:543–7.

39. Khairy P, Fernandes SM, Mayer JE Jr, et al. Long-term survival, modes of death, and predictors of mortality in patients with Fontan surgery. Circulation. 2008;117:85–92.

40. Pundi KN, Pundi KN, Johnson JN, et al. Sudden cardiac death and late arrhythmias after the Fontan operation. Congenit Heart Dis. 2017;12:17–23.

41. Rathod RH, Prakash A, Powell AJ, Geva T. Myocardial fibrosis identified by cardiac magnetic resonance late gadolinium enhancement is associated with adverse ventricular mechanics and ventricular tachycar-dia late after Fontan operation. J Am Coll Cardiol. 2010;55:1721–8.

42. Wilson WM, Valente AM, Hickey EJ, et al. Outcomes of patients with hypoplastic left heart syndrome reaching adulthood after Fontan palliation: multicenter study. Circulation. 2018;137:978–81.

43. Khairy P, Van Hare GF, Balaji S, et al. PACES/HRS expert consensus statement on the recognition and management of arrhythmias in adult congenital heart disease: executive summary. Heart Rhythm. 2014;11:e81–e101.

44. Moore JP, Mondesert B, Lloyd MS, et al. Clinical experience with the subcutaneous implantable cardioverter-defibrillator in adults with congenital heart disease. Circ Arrhythm Electrophysiol. 2016;9:9.

45. Garside H, Leyva F, Hudsmith L, Marshall H, de Bono J. Eligibility for subcutaneous implantable cardioverter defibrillators in the adult congenital heart disease population. Pacing Clin Electrophysiol. 2019;42:65–70.

46. Paridon SM, Karpawich PP, Pinsky WW. The effects of rate responsive pacing on exercise performance in the postoperative univentricular heart. Pacing Clin Electrophysiol. 1993;16:1256–62.

47. Bulic A, Zimmerman FJ, Ceresnak SR, et al. Ventricular pacing in single ventricles—a bad combination. Heart Rhythm. 2017;14:853–7.

48. Poh CL, Celermajer DS, Grigg LE, et al. Pacemakers are associated with a higher risk of late death and transplantation in the Fontan population. Int J Cardiol. 2019;282:33–7.

49. Kodama Y, Kuraoka A, Ishikawa Y, et al. Outcome of patients with functional single ventricular heart after pacemaker implantation: what makes it poor, and what can we do? Heart Rhythm. 2019;16:1870–4.

50. Cecchin F, Frangini PA, Brown DW, et al. Cardiac resynchronization therapy (and multisite pacing) in pediatrics and congenital heart disease: five years experience in a single institution. J Cardiovasc Electrophysiol. 2009;20:58–65.

51. O'Leary ET, Gauvreau K, Alexander ME, et al. Dual-site ventricular pacing in patients with Fontan physiology and heart block: does it mitigate the detrimental effects of single-site ventricular pacing? JACC Clin Electrophysiol. 2018;4:1289–97.

52. Hoyt WJ, Moore JP, Shannon KM, Kannankeril PJ, Fish FA. Epicardial atrial pacing after the extracardiac Fontan operation: Feasibility of an entirely transvenous approach. J Cardiovasc Electrophysiol. 2022;33(1):128–33. https://doi.org/10.1111/jce.1528510.1111/jce.15285. Epub 2021 Nov 24. PMID: 34716972.

Managing the Pulmonary Circulation

20

Andrew Constantine and Paul Clift

Abbreviations

Ao	Aorta
AP	Atriopulmonary
CMR	Cardiovascular magnetic resonance
eNOS	Endothelial nitric oxide synthetase
PA	Pulmonary artery
PAH	Pulmonary arterial hypertension
PAVM	Pulmonary arterio-venous malformation
PVD	Pulmonary vascular disease
PVR	Pulmonary vascular resistance
TCPC	Total cavo-pulmonary connection
TV	Tricuspid valve

Effective management of pulmonary blood flow in infancy is one of the primary considerations in the patient with a functionally univentricular circulation prior to the creation of a systemic venous-to-pulmonary artery (PA) communication. This may involve measures to augment or maintain pulmonary blood flow, e.g. via prostaglandin E1 infusion to maintain ductal patency, a modified Blalock Taussig shunt, or with medication. Conversely, excessive pulmonary blood flow can be limited by PA banding. The subsequent formation of a Fontan circulation, while greatly improving the outlook for patients with univentricular circulations, places the systemic and pulmonary circulations in series and creates a delicate situation where problems anywhere along the surgical or pulmonary circuit may have a significant adverse impact on the cardiac output. Troubleshooting such problems that may arise early or late following the Fontan operation is the primary focus of this chapter, and are summarised in Table 20.1.

A. Constantine
Adult Congenital Heart Centre and National Centre
for Pulmonary Hypertension, Royal Brompton
Hospital, London, UK

National Heart and Lung Institute, Imperial College,
London, UK

P. Clift (✉)
Department of Cardiology, Queen Elizabeth Hospital,
University Hospitals Birmingham NHS Foundation
Trust, Birmingham, UK
e-mail: paul.clift@uhb.nhs.uk

Table 20.1 Problems with the pulmonary circulation following the Fontan procedure and therapeutic options in selected cases

Problem category	Underlying cause(s)	Therapeutic options
Collateral flow/right-to-left shunt	– Veno-venous collaterals – Aortopulmonary collaterals – Pulmonary arterio-venous malformations – Fenestration/persistent intra-cardiac shunt (with significant cyanosis)	Coil embolisation Fenestration device closure/ASD patch
Inefficient flow dynamics/obstruction to flow	– Older type Fontan repair – Systemic venous pathway obstruction – Pulmonary artery distortion – Pulmonary vein stenosis	Stenting of surgical pathway, branch PAs or pulmonary veins Fontan revision/conversion ± pulmonary artery reconstruction
Rising PVR	– Thrombo-embolism – Endothelial dysfunction – Normal aging	Anti-coagulation PAH therapies Fontan revision (large atrial thrombus)
Pulmonary dysfunction	– Restrictive lung function – Phrenic nerve palsy – Respiratory involvement of a genetic syndrome	Exercise training / yoga Diaphragm plication Involvement of other specialities

ASD atrial septal defect, *PA* pulmonary artery, *PAH* pulmonary arterial hypertension, *PVR* pulmonary vascular resistance

Inefficient Flow Dynamics and Obstruction

Unobstructed flow from the systemic veins to the pulmonary vascular bed is required to maintain transpulmonary flow in the Fontan patient. Problems can occur anywhere on this route (Fig. 20.1), including circuit obstruction, stenosis or distortion of the surgical pathway, hypoplastic or stenotic PAs, and flow mismatch to the 2 lungs. Furthermore, hydrodynamic efficiency is an important concept in a circuit that is reliant on passive flow: the degree of energy dissipation of blood moving through the Fontan circuit increases with turbulence of flow and collision, which is dependent on the design and subsequent distortion of the surgical pathway. The greatest hydrodynamic advantage is gained by the use of an extra-cardiac conduit with offsetting of the conduit and superior vena cava flow streams, but many patients still have older style connections [1]. Obstructed systemic venous flow manifests clinically as worsening systemic venous hypertension, including hepatic congestion, fluid overload (peripheral edema and/or ascites) and cyanosis. Obstruction of the Fontan pathway results from stenosis of the anastomosis of the

superior vena cava to the right PA (Glenn shunt), stenosis of the atriopulmonary connection (suture line), lateral tunnel or extracardiac graft. Features conferring a high risk of systemic venous pathway obstruction include the use of valved conduits in atriopulmonary (AP) or extracardiac repairs, unidirectional ("classical") Glenn shunts with an AP connection to the left PA, or AP connection anterior to the aorta.

Restricted flow at the level of the PAs may result from hypoplasia, distortion or thrombo-embolism. Adequate growth of the PAs depends on the pre-Fontan management of the functionally univentricular patient, and achieving equal or near equal blood flow to both lungs is important to minimise segmental differences in PVR and results in more favourable post-Fontan haemodynamics [2]. While a systemic-to-PA shunt (e.g. Blalock-Taussig shunt) may be necessary to provide adequate pulmonary blood flow to allow growth of the PAs, distortion of the branch PAs post-Fontan repair is a recognised complication of most systemic-to-PA shunts. At the time of cavo-pulmonary connection, these shunts may be occluded, rather than ligated and divided. With subsequent somatic growth, the connection of the PA to a systemic vessel/shunt

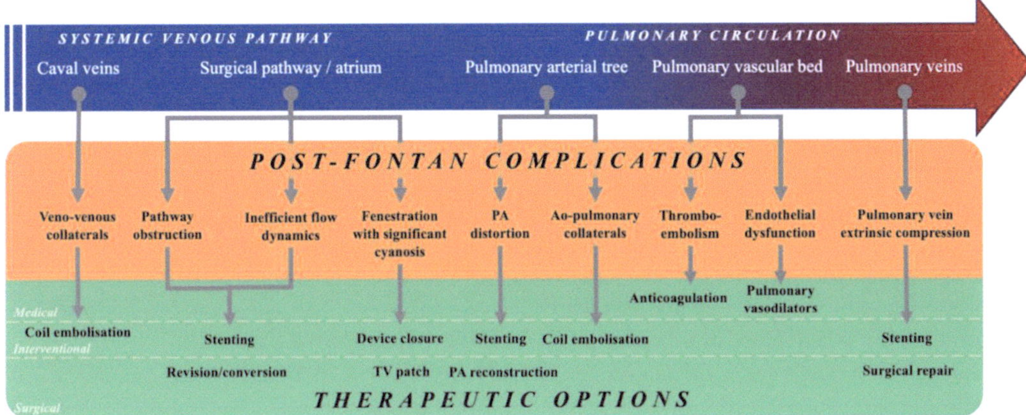

Fig. 20.1 Schematic of the systematic venous pathway and pulmonary circulation following Fontan repair. Problems responsible for attrition of the Fontan circula-tion, along with medical, interventional and surgical ther-apeutic options are shown. *Ao* aorta, *PA* pulmonary artery, *TV* tricuspid valve

can cause distortion. A surgical strategy, which includes ligation of systemic-to-PA shunts, occlusion of collaterals not contributing signifi-cantly to segmental pulmonary blood supply, and resection of all ductal tissue from the cen-tral PAs may minimise the risk of an unbalanced pulmonary vascular bed [3, 4].

Problems with the pulmonary veins usually arise late after Fontan surgery; obstruction of pul-monary venous drainage may be due to severe right atrial dilatation, typically affecting the right-sided pulmonary veins, or coronary sinus dilatation, which affects the left-sided veins.

Trans-thoracic echocardiography, though useful for assessing ventricular function and valve function, rarely provides diagnostic images of the entire Fontan pathway. However, subcos-tal and suprasternal views can detect stenoses at vena cava level, large right atrial thrombi, and the presence and size of fenestrations in the Fontan circuit. Trans-oesophageal echocardiog-raphy is useful for excluding thrombus in the systemic venous pathway, visualising the pulmo-nary veins and assessing atrio-ventricular valve function. Cardiovascular magnetic resonance (CMR) is the modality of choice for assessing the anatomy of the Fontan pathway, branch PAs and pulmonary veins, along with information about the quantity and relative distribution of pulmonary blood flow [5, 6].

At cardiac catheterisation, even small gradi-ents of 1 or 2 mmHg along the Fontan pathway in the context of a low-flow circulation may be hemodynamically significant, i.e. able to increase the impedance of the "Fontan circuit" and may be of clinical importance. In order to reliably detect such small gradients, a 2-catheter technique may be necessary, exchanging catheter positions to assess the gradient with each catheter in the prox-imal or distal position (hence excluding a calibra-tion/zero error). Angiography is also helpful in this setting. Stenting of discrete stenoses is often possible and may postpone the need for surgical intervention. Surgical options include revision of the surgical pathway, conversion from the older AP Fontan to a TCPC, or transplantation.

Pulmonary Vascular Resistance

The importance of a low pulmonary vascular resistance (PVR) to the Fontan circulation is cov-ered fully elsewhere. Even in the setting of a mar-ginally raised PVR, cardiac output declines and the risk of Fontan failure increases [7]. There is increasing evidence of pulmonary vascular dis-ease (PVD) in patients following Fontan opera-tion, although in the setting of a low pulmonary blood flow, the mean PA pressure is rarely ele-vated to the point of fulfilling the guideline definition of pulmonary hypertension (mean PA pressure >20 mmHg) despite a raised PVR [8]. This is magnified in the setting of a "failing Fontan" where a very low pulmonary blood flow (see section) means that a raised PVR can be accompanied by a normal PA pressure, making the calculation of PVR essential to diagnose PVD this group (and more generally in PAH-CHD) [9]. The mechanisms behind the development and progression of PVD in the Fontan population are incompletely understood, but there is growing evidence for endothelial dysfunction due to non-pulsatile pulmonary blood flow [10], as well as a putative role for subclinical microthrombi in the Fontan circulation. This is compounded by the effects of ageing on the pulmonary vasculature, with incrementing PA pressures at rest and on exercise and an increase in mean total pulmonary resistance (mean PA pressure/pulmonary blood flow), leading to a rising PVR [11].

The evidence of progressive pulmonary vasculopathy in this group has formed the rationale for several small trials into the effects of targeted pulmonary arterial hypertension (PAH) therapies in Fontan patients [12–19], with conflicting results. The first trial of oral pulmonary vasodilator therapy was conducted in 27 adult Fontan patients, who received a single dose of the phosphodiesterase-5 inhibitor sildenafil, following which investigators showed a short-term improvement peak VO$_2$, exercise cardiac index and pulmonary blood flow index compared to control subjects [13]. In this and the trials that have followed, effect sizes have been modest at best, with minor improvements in peak exercise capacity or reduced PVR reported. The FUEL trial, a randomised controlled trial of the phosphodiesterase-5 inhibitor udenafil in Fontan patients with a peak VO$_2$ of at least 50% predicted, did not show a significant improvement in peak VO$_2$ compared to placebo after 26 weeks [20]. The recent clinical study assessing the efficacy and safety of macitentan in Fontan-palliated subjects (RUBATO), a double-blind randomized controlled trial in 137 patients, found no significant difference in change in peak VO$_2$ or accelerometer-captured physical activity [21] between treatment and placebo. Several questions remain

with regards to the use of PAH therapies in Fontan patients, including patient selection, use of trial endpoints that better reflect intolerance of submaximal exercise (frequently described by Fontan patients), timing of introduction of therapies, and whether there is a long-term benefit in terms of symptoms and outcome in patients with a failing Fontan.

Thrombosis and Embolic Phenomena in the Fontan Circulation

Thromboembolism is an important cause of mortality in Fontan patients, accounting for 8% of deaths in this patient group [22]. The occurrence of intracardiac thrombi is a greater concern in atrio-pulmonary Fontan patients, in whom sluggish flow in the right atrium predisposes to the formation of, sometimes massive, atrial thrombi [23, 24]. The modern total cavo-pulmonary connection (TCPC) and an increasing use of long-term anticoagulation has reduced the rate of thromboembolism, but imperfect flow dynamics, the presence of foreign surfaces in the venous circulation and intrinsic coagulopathy mean that the risk of thromboembolism persists. The role of anticoagulation or antiplatelet therapy in mitigating this risk and patient selection is the subject of the next chapter.

Collateral Flow

Various types of collateral flow and residual shunting can be encountered in patients with a Fontan circulation and can contribute to the severity of ventricular overload and cyanosis, as well as determine the resistance to pulmonary blood flow, ventilation/perfusion mismatch and efficiency of gas exchange in the lungs. Shunts can be left-to-right (systemic to pulmonary) or right-to-left:

1. Residual or recurrent *left-to-right shunting* may occur due to the presence of aorto-pulmonary collaterals (APCs), failed occlusion of a previous shunt or incomplete ligation of the main pulmonary trunk. Development of

APCs is common in patients with a univentricular circulation, with flow originating from internal mammary arteries, thyrocervical trunks, brachiocephalic vessels, subclavian arteries or, rarely, more distal vessels [25]. They can present pre-Fontan repair in up to 80% of patients [26–28], or can develop in the post-Fontan patient. APCs supply systemic arterial blood to the distal pulmonary vasculature; in the post-Fontan patient APCs may cause "flooding" of segments of the pulmonary vasculature, compete with venous inflow to the lungs, cause energy loss and added volume load to the systemic ventricle [28, 29]. Percutaneous occlusion of APCs can be effective, although selection criteria are multiple and subjective. The following should be taken into consideration: the pulsatility of the branch PAs, ventricular end-diastolic pressures, APC size, the density of pulmonary capillary blush or the opacification of the pulmonary venous return on invasive angiography, step-up in oxygen saturations from the superior *vena cava* to the branch PAs [30].

2. *Right-to-left shunting* in Fontan patients usually occurs via a surgical fenestration in the Fontan pathway, veno-venous collaterals, or pulmonary atrio-venous fistulae.

    (a) A fenestration of the Fontan circuit was routinely created at the time of the Fontan operation in the past, and is currently used in selected high-risk cases. It has been shown to confer short-term benefit, with a reduction in the likelihood of post-operative pleural effusions and a shorter post-operative hospital stay [31–33]. However, as PVR and the filling pressures of the systemic ventricle rise over the long-term, a greater degree of right-to-left shunting may lead to progressive cyanosis and its downstream systemic effects. Device closure may be considered in cases of severe cyanosis although, in a failing Fontan physiology, the fenestration acts as a "relief valve", reduces congestion and helps to maintain cardiac output, and closure should be avoided. In selected cases, fenestration closure has

been shown to improve arterial saturations, and as a result may improve ventilatory efficiency [34], but has not been shown to improve long-term survival [35, 36]. By contrast, in Fontan failure, percutaneous fenestration may be indicated to improve congestive symptoms and avoid cardiac cachexia at the expense of arterial saturations while awaiting cardiac transplantation [37].

    (b) Veno-venous collaterals may occur between the systemic or hepatic veins and the pulmonary veins, left atrium or coronary sinus, or via the Thebesian veins related to the atria [38]. They arise in the setting of chronic systemic venous hypertension, with pressures greater than 18-20 mmHg. In bypassing the pulmonary vascular bed, they decompress the systemic veins, support ventricular preload and can reduce systemic venous pressure, but contribute to cyanosis and volume loading of the systemic ventricle [37]. Occlusion of veno-venous collaterals by transcatheter coiling, other occluder devices, or surgical ligation can improve oxygen saturations and relieve ventricular volume overload, but at the expense of raising the systemic venous pressure and reducing preload. Some investigators have observed that occlusion of veno-venous collaterals appears to be associated with a reduced 5-year survival in Fontan patients [39], hypothesising that the reduction in preload following embolization of veno-venous collaterals may have a negative long-term impact, although data from controlled experiments are lacking.

    (c) Pulmonary arterio-venous malformations (PAVMs), another cause of desaturation following surgery, can be classified as simple or complex, depending on the number of feeding arteries and draining veins [40]. They are much more common in the presence of pulmonary flow that has bypassed the hepatic circulation, as in the case of a Kawashima operation or a (now obsolete) unidirectional Glenn shunt (with PAVMS present in the lung supplied by the Glenn shunt). Unequal distribution of pulmonary flow between the two lungs in a bidirectional Glenn shunt and non-pulsatile flow to the lungs have also been implicated in the pathogenesis of PAVMs, with evidence of aberrant angiogenesis [41, 42]. PAVMs can be diagnosed using contrast echocardiography ("bubble study"), computed tomography (CTPA, adjusting the route and method/rate of contrast administration to the anatomy), magnetic resonance imaging or invasive pulmonary angiography [43–46]. Embolisation may be used to treat isolated PAVMs, but in more diffuse or recurrent disease, surgical redirection of hepatic venous flow to the lungs may be required [47–49].

Respiratory Function

The process of ventilation forms a "thoracic pump", which contributes significantly to pulmonary blood flow and cardiac output, especially in Fontan patients. This interdependence between systems means that optimising respiratory function improves the function of the pulmonary circulation. Fontan patients have smaller lungs than expected for age and sex [50]. Restrictive lung defects are prevalent amongst Fontan patients [51]; in a recent study of 232 Fontan patients with a mean age of 26 years, Callegari et al. reported restrictive lung function in 60% of patients. In a large study of 1188 CHD patients, Alonso-Gonzalez et al. showed that Fontan patients have amongst the lowest FVC values (67 ± 17% predicted) of all types CHD, with at least moderate impairment of lung function in 34.1% [52]. Moderate-to-severe impairment in lung function relates to lower exercise capacity and quality of life, and is an independent predictor of survival in CHD patients [52, 53]. Small programmes of 6–12 weeks of inspiratory muscle or endurance training have been shown to improve respiratory

function in Fontan patients [54–56]. Persistent phrenic nerve palsy is encountered in 5–10% of patients following TCPC and can contribute to restrictive lung function. Patients with clinically significant respiratory or haemodynamic consequences should be assessed for diaphragmatic plication [57].

References

1. Lardo AC, Webber SA, Friehs I, del Nido PJ, Cape EG. Fluid dynamic comparison of intra-atrial and extracardiac total cavopulmonary connections. J Thorac Cardiovasc Surg. 1999;117(4):697–704.
2. Senzaki H, Isoda T, Ishizawa A, Hishi T. Reconsideration of criteria for the Fontan operation. Influence of pulmonary artery size on postoperative hemodynamics of the Fontan operation. Circulation. 1994;89(3):1196–202.
3. Sakamoto K, Ota N, Fujimoto Y, Murata M, Ide Y, Tachi M, et al. Primary central pulmonary artery plasty for single ventricle with ductal-associated pulmonary artery coarctation. Ann Thorac Surg. 2014;98(3):919–26.
4. Elzenga NJ, von Suylen RJ, Frohn-Mulder I, Essed CE, Bos E, Quaegebeur JM. Juxtaductal pulmonary artery coarctation. An underestimated cause of branch pulmonary artery stenosis in patients with pulmonary atresia or stenosis and a ventricular septal defect. J Thorac Cardiovasc Surg. 1990;100(3):416–24.
5. Takawira F, Ayer JG, Onikul E, Hawker RE, Kemp A, Nicholson IA, et al. Evaluation of the extracardiac conduit modification of the Fontan operation for thrombus formation using magnetic resonance imaging. Heart Lung Circ. 2008;17(5):407–10.
6. Fogel MA, Hubbard A, Weinberg PM. A simplified approach for assessment of intracardiac baffles and extracardiac conduits in congenital heart surgery with two- and three-dimensional magnetic resonance imaging. Am Heart J. 2001;142(6):1028–36.
7. Egbe AC, Connolly HM, Miranda WR, Ammash NM, Hagler DJ, Veldtman GR, et al. Hemodynamics of Fontan failure: the role of pulmonary vascular disease. Circ Heart Fail. 2017;10(12):e004515.
8. Dimopoulos K, Wort SJ, Gatzoulis MA. Pulmonary hypertension related to congenital heart disease: a call for action. Eur Heart J. 2014;35(11):691–700.
9. Mitchell MB, Campbell DN, Ivy D, Boucek MM, Sondheimer HM, Pietra B, et al. Evidence of pulmonary vascular disease after heart transplantation for Fontan circulation failure. J Thorac Cardiovasc Surg. 2004;128(5):693–702.
10. Henaine R, Vergnat M, Bacha EA, Baudet B, Lambert V, Belli E, et al. Effects of lack of pulsatility on pulmonary endothelial function in the Fontan circulation. J Thorac Cardiovasc Surg. 2013;146(3):522–9.

11. Kovacs G, Berghold A, Scheidl S, Olschewski H. Pulmonary arterial pressure during rest and exercise in healthy subjects: a systematic review. Eur Respir J. 2009;34(4):888–94.

12. Takahashi K, Mori Y, Yamamura H, Nakanishi T, Nakazawa M. Effect of beraprost sodium on pulmonary vascular resistance in candidates for a Fontan procedure: a preliminary study. Pediatr Int. 2003;45(6):671–5.

13. Giardini A, Balducci A, Specchia S, Gargiulo G, Bonvicini M, Picchio FM. Effect of sildenafil on haemodynamic response to exercise and exercise capacity in Fontan patients. Eur Heart J. 2008;29(13):1681–7.

14. Ovaert C, Thijs D, Dewolf D, Ottenkamp J, Dessy H, Moons P, et al. The effect of bosentan in patients with a failing Fontan circulation. Cardiol Young. 2009;19(4):331–9.

15. Hirono K, Yoshimura N, Taguchi M, Watanabe K, Nakamura T, Ichida F, et al. Bosentan induces clinical and hemodynamic improvement in candidates for right-sided heart bypass surgery. J Thorac Cardiovasc Surg. 2010;140(2):346–51.

16. Goldberg DJ, French B, McBride MG, Marino BS, Mirarchi N, Hanna BD, et al. Impact of oral sildenafil on exercise performance in children and young adults after the Fontan operation: a randomized, double-blind, placebo-controlled, crossover trial. Circulation. 2011;123(11):1185–93.

17. Schuuring MJ, Vis JC, van Dijk APJ, van Melle JP, Vliegen HW, Pieper PG, et al. Impact of bosentan on exercise capacity in adults after the Fontan procedure: a randomized controlled trial. Eur J Heart Fail. 2013;15(6):690–8.

18. Rhodes J, Ubeda-Tikkanen A, Clair M, Fernandes SM, Graham DA, Milliren CE, et al. Effect of inhaled iloprost on the exercise function of Fontan patients: a demonstration of concept. Int J Cardiol. 2013;168(3):2435–40.

19. Hebert A, Mikkelsen UR, Thilen U, Idorn L, Jensen AS, Nagy E, et al. Bosentan improves exercise capacity in adolescents and adults after Fontan operation: the TEMPO (Treatment With Endothelin Receptor Antagonist in Fontan Patients, a Randomized, Placebo-Controlled, Double-Blind Study Measuring Peak Oxygen Consumption) study. Circulation. 2014;130(23):2021–30.

20. Goldberg DJ, Zak V, Goldstein BH, Schumacher KR, Rhodes J, Penny DJ, et al. Results of the Fontan Udenafil Exercise Longitudinal (FUEL) trial. Circulation. 2019;201:1–8.

21. Clift P, Berger F, Sondergaard L, Antonova P, Disney P, Nicolarsen J, Thambo JB et al. The efficacy and safety of macitentan in Fontan-palliated patients: results of the 52-week randomised, placebo-controlled RUBATO trial. European Heart Journal 2022;43(Supp_2):ehac544.1560. https://doi.org/10.1093/eurheartj/ehac544.1560.

22. Khairy P, Fernandes SM, Mayer JE, Triedman JK, Walsh EP, Lock JE, et al. Long-term survival, modes of death, and predictors of mortality in patients with Fontan surgery. Circulation. 2008;117(1):85–92.

23. Dobell ARC, Trusler GA, Smallhorn JF, Williams WG. Atrial thrombi after the Fontan operation. Ann Thorac Surg. 1986;42(6):664–7.

24. Balling G, Vogt M, Kaemmerer H, Eicken A, Meisner H, Hess J. Intracardiac thrombus formation after the Fontan operation. J Thorac Cardiovasc Surg. 2000;119(4):745–52.

25. Triedman JK, Bridges ND, Mayer JE, Lock JE. Prevalence and risk factors for aortopulmonary collateral vessels after Fontan and bidirectional Glenn procedures. J Am Coll Cardiol. 1993;22(1):207–15.

26. Ichikawa H, Yagihara T, Kishimoto H, Isobe F, Yamamoto F, Nishigaki K, et al. Extent of aortopulmonary collateral blood flow as a risk factor for Fontan operations. Ann Thorac Surg. 1995;59(2):433–7.

27. Spicer RL, Uzark KC, Moore JW, Mainwaring RD, Lamberti JJ. Aortopulmonary collateral vessels and prolonged pleural effusions after modified Fontan procedures. Am Heart J. 1996;131(6):1164–8.

28. Kanter KR, Vincent RN, Raviele AA. Importance of acquired systemic-to-pulmonary collaterals in the Fontan operation. Ann Thorac Surg. 1999;68(3):969–74; discussion 974–975.

29. Powell AJ. Aortopulmonary collaterals in single-ventricle congenital heart disease. Circ Cardiovasc Imaging. 2009;2(3):171–3.

30. Stern HJ. Aggressive coiling of aortopulmonary collaterals in single-ventricle patients is warranted. Pediatr Cardiol. 2010;31(4):449–53.

31. Bridges ND, Mayer JE, Lock JE, Jonas RA, Hanley FL, Keane JF, et al. Effect of baffle fenestration on outcome of the modified Fontan operation. Circulation. 1992;86(6):1762–9.

32. Airan B, Sharma R, Choudhary SK, Mohanty SR, Bhan A, Chowdhari UK, et al. Univentricular repair: is routine fenestration justified? Ann Thorac Surg. 2000;69(6):1900–6.

33. Lemler MS, Scott WA, Leonard SR, Stromberg D, Ramaciotti C. Fenestration improves clinical outcome of the Fontan procedure: a prospective, randomized study. Circulation. 2002;105(2):207–12.

34. Meadows J, Lang P, Marx G, Rhodes J. Fontan fenestration closure has no acute effect on exercise capacity but improves ventilatory response to exercise. J Am Coll Cardiol. 2008;52(2):108–13.

35. Hijazi ZM, Fahey JT, Kleinman CS, Kopf GS, Hellenbrand WE. Hemodynamic evaluation before and after closure of fenestrated Fontan. An acute study of changes in oxygen delivery. Circulation. 1992;86(1):196–202.

36. Imielski BR, Woods RK, Mussatto KA, Cao Y, Simpson PM, Tweddell JS. Fontan fenestration closure and event-free survival. J Thorac Cardiovasc Surg. 2013;145(1):183–7.

37. Gewillig M, Brown SC. The Fontan circulation after 45 years: update in physiology. Heart. 2016;102(14):1081–6.

38. Heinemann M, Breuer J, Steger V, Steil E, Sieverding L, Ziemer G. Incidence and impact of systemic venous collateral development after Glenn and Fontan procedures. Thorac Cardiovasc Surg. 2001;49(3):172–8.

39. Poterucha JT, Johnson JN, Taggart NW, Cabalka AK, Hagler DJ, Driscoll DJ, et al. Embolization of venovenous collaterals after the Fontan operation is associated with decreased survival. Congenit Heart Dis. 2015;10(5):E230–6.

40. Kavarana MN, Jones JA, Stroud RE, Bradley SM, Ikonomidis JS, Mukherjee R. Pulmonary arteriovenous malformations after the superior cavopulmonary shunt: mechanisms and clinical implications. Expert Rev Cardiovasc Ther. 2014;12(6):703–13.

41. Kavarana MN, Mukherjee R, Eckhouse SR, Rawls WF, Logdon C, Stroud RE, et al. Pulmonary artery endothelial cell phenotypic alterations in a large animal model of pulmonary arteriovenous malformations after the Glenn shunt. Ann Thorac Surg. 2013;96(4):1442–9.

42. Henaine R, Vergnat M, Mercier O, Serraf A, De Montpreville V, Ninet J, et al. Hemodynamics and arteriovenous malformations in cavopulmonary anastomosis: the case for residual antegrade pulsatile flow. J Thorac Cardiovasc Surg. 2013;146(6):1359–65.

43. Bernstein HS, Brook MM, Silverman NH, Bristow J. Development of pulmonary arteriovenous fistulae in children after cavopulmonary shunt. Circulation. 1995;92(9 Suppl):II309–14.

44. Feinstein JA, Moore P, Rosenthal DN, Puchalski M, Brook MM. Comparison of contrast echocardiography versus cardiac catheterization for detection of pulmonary arteriovenous malformations. Am J Cardiol. 2002;89(3):281–5.

45. Remy J, Remy-Jardin M, Wattinne L, Deffontaines C. Pulmonary arteriovenous malformations: evaluation with CT of the chest before and after treatment. Radiology. 1992;182(3):809–16.

46. Silverman JM, Julien PJ, Herfkens RJ, Pelc NJ. Magnetic resonance imaging evaluation of pulmonary vascular malformations. Chest. 1994;106(5):1333–8.

47. Srivastava D, Preminger T, Lock JE, Mandell V, Keane JF, Mayer JE, et al. Hepatic venous blood and the development of pulmonary arteriovenous malformations in congenital heart disease. Circulation. 1995;92(5):1217–22.

48. Shah MJ, Rychik J, Fogel MA, Murphy JD, Jacobs ML. Pulmonary AV malformations after superior cavopulmonary connection: resolution after inclusion of hepatic veins in the pulmonary circulation. Ann Thorac Surg. 1997;63(4):960–3.

49. McElhinney DB, Kreutzer J, Lang P, Mayer JE, del Nido PJ, Lock JE. Incorporation of the hepatic veins into the cavopulmonary circulation in patients with heterotaxy and pulmonary arteriovenous malformations after a Kawashima procedure. Ann Thorac Surg. 2005;80(5):1597–603.

50. Larsson ES, Eriksson BO, Sixt R. Decreased lung function and exercise capacity in Fontan patients. A long-term follow-up. Scand Cardiovasc J. 2003;37(1):58–63.

51. Opotowsky AR, Landzberg MJ, Earing MG, Wu FM, Triedman JK, Casey A, et al. Abnormal spirometry after the Fontan procedure is common and associated with impaired aerobic capacity. Am J Physiol Heart Circ Physiol. 2014;307(1):H110–7.

52. Alonso-Gonzalez R, Borgia F, Diller G-P, Inuzuka R, Kempny A, Martinez-Naharro A, et al. Abnormal lung function in adults with congenital heart disease: prevalence, relation to cardiac anatomy, and association with survival. Circulation. 2013;127(8):882–90.

53. Callegari A, Neidenbach R, Milanesi O, Castaldi B, Christmann M, Ono M, et al. A restrictive ventilatory pattern is common in patients with univentricular heart after Fontan palliation and associated with a reduced exercise capacity and quality of life. Congenit Heart Dis. 2019;14(2):147–55.

54. Wu FM, Opotowsky AR, Denhoff ER, Gongwer R, Gurvitz MZ, Landzberg MJ, et al. A pilot study of inspiratory muscle training to improve exercise capacity in patients with Fontan physiology. Semin Thorac Cardiovasc Surg. 2018;30(4):462–9.

55. Ait Ali L, Pingitore A, Piaggi P, Brucini F, Passera M, Marotta M, et al. Respiratory training late after Fontan intervention: impact on cardiorespiratory performance. Pediatr Cardiol. 2018;39(4):695–704.

56. Laohachai K, Winlaw D, Selvadurai H, Gnanappa GK, d'Udekem Y, Celermajer D, et al. Inspiratory muscle training is associated with improved inspiratory muscle strength, resting cardiac output, and the ventilatory efficiency of exercise in patients with a Fontan circulation. J Am Heart Assoc. 2017;6(8):e005750.

57. Komori M, Hoashi T, Shimada M, Kitano M, Ohuchi H, Kurosaki K, et al. Impact of phrenic nerve palsy on late Fontan circulation. Ann Thorac Surg. 2019;109:1897–902.

Fontan Failure in Children and Cardiac Transplantation

Milind Chaudhari

Introduction

In 1971 Francis Fontan and Baudet introduced the basic principle of right heart bypass surgery and revolutionized the treatment of functionally single ventricle cardiac anomalies [1]. Over the past five decades, better patient selection [2], modifications of surgical techniques [3–5] and advanced perioperative care has produced excellent results despite the wide-spread application of the procedure to more complex groups of patients, frequently breaching the original ten commandments for eligibility [6–8]. In the long term, however, the elevated central venous pressure and low cardiac output state lead to Fontan failure causing significant morbidity and mortality [9–13]. Both early postoperative and late attrition Fontan failure create unique management challenges and are potentially fatal.

Early Fontan Failure (EFF)

Incidence and Pathophysiology of EFF

Early failure of the Fontan circulation defines a postoperative pathophysiological state characterized by persistent low cardiac output and increased systemic venous pressure [14–16]. This initiates a cascade of events that results in tissue edema, hypoxia, and organ hypoperfusion, culminating in multiorgan failure and death.

These children are in a critical state in the cardiac intensive care unit with an inadequate response to conventional ventilation and inotropic therapy. Significant pleural and pericardial effusions are often accompanied by severe renal and hepatic dysfunction. Arrhythmias are also common and lack of atrioventricular synchrony with junctional ectopic tachycardia further exacerbates Fontan failure.

The incidence of Fontan failure has decreased dramatically in the contemporary era [11–13].

In the Australian and New Zealand Fontan registry [17] the overall incidence of early Fontan failure was 11% in atrio-pulmonary connections (APC), 6% in the lateral tunnel (LT) and 4% in the extracardiac (EC) Fontan procedures respectively. There was progressive reduction in incidence of the early failure from 21 (1975–1990) to 4% (2001–2010).

Evolution of a staged palliative approach, abandoning older APC in favor of more efficient total cavopulmonary connections (TCPC), vastly improved perioperative care and aggressive surgical and catheter interventional strategies dealing with complications are some of the factors responsible for significant decrease in the incidence of early failure after Fontan completion in the current era [11–17].

M. Chaudhari (✉)
Birmingham Children's Hospital, Birmingham, UK
e-mail: milind.chaudhari@nhs.net

© The Author(s), under exclusive license to Springer Nature Switzerland AG 2023
P. Clift et al. (eds.), *Univentricular Congenital Heart Defects and the Fontan Circulation*,
https://doi.org/10.1007/978-3-031-36208-8_21

Prevention of EFF: Patient Selection and Preparation for Fontan

Patient selection is the key to a successful Fontan outcome. Non-cardiac risk factors for poor Fontan outcome (Fig. 21.1) should be recognized and corrected before Fontan completion if feasible.

Alternatively, long term palliation with an aortopulmonary shunt alone or in combination with a superior cavopulmonary shunt or pulmonary artery band should be preferred.

In 1978 Choussat et al. [2] listed ten criteria to select patients and minimize morbidity and mortality with the Fontan procedure. However, in the modern era, only two of the original ten commandments, namely:

- preoperative systemic ventricular function
- preoperative pulmonary artery pressures have been shown to have a significant impact on the early Fontan outcome [6–8].

The emphasis is more on optimum patient preparation which begins in the neonatal period once the diagnosis of functionally single ventricle cardiac anomaly is made.

Preoperative impaired ventricular function (raised ventricular end-diastolic pressure) and elevated pulmonary artery pressures (>15 mmHg) with prolonged cardiopulmonary bypass time (CPB) time are consistently associated with a higher risk of EFF [6–8, 10, 11].

Other associated factors include:

- younger age
- heterotaxy syndrome
- right ventricular morphology
- common atrio-ventricular valve (AVV) [10–12].

In high-risk patients use of fenestration and modified ultrafiltration during CPB is associated with a reduced risk of EFF [4, 7, 11].

Figure 21.2 summarises the critical intervention strategies from the neonatal period through to early childhood en route to successful Fontan completion.

Management of Early Fontan Failure

EFF is a challenging postoperative scenario and demands a meticulous multidisciplinary team approach to management. Prompt cardiac investigations (ECG/Echocardiogram/Cardiac catheterization) are mandatory to ascertain the exact underlying mechanism for failure, exclude correctable anatomical or electrical lesions and guide therapy [13–18].

Lowering PVR will augment pulmonary blood flow and ventricular preload and improve cardiac output. This can be achieved by a ventilation strategy to avoid hypoxia and hypercarbia and maintain functional residual capacity at minimum mean airway pressure [19]. Pleural and peritoneal effusions should be aggressively drained to improve chest compliance. Pulmonary vasodilator therapy with inhaled nitric oxide is beneficial to reduce TPG [19].

Fig. 21.1 Non-cardiac risk factors for poor Fontan outcome

Syndromes:	Airways / Lungs:

Down's syndrome
   Turner's Syndrome
   Williams
   Noonan's
   Alagille
   Heterotaxy
Severe cerebral palsy
Severe Spinal Deformities
Wheelchair dependence
	* CHARGE association
	* Vocal cord palsy
	* Obstructive sleep apnea
	* Tracheal stenosis
	* Diaphragmatic palsy
	* Diaphragmatic hernia
	* Gastro esophageal reflux
	* Restrictive lung function
	* Pulmonary vein stenosis / Sclerosis

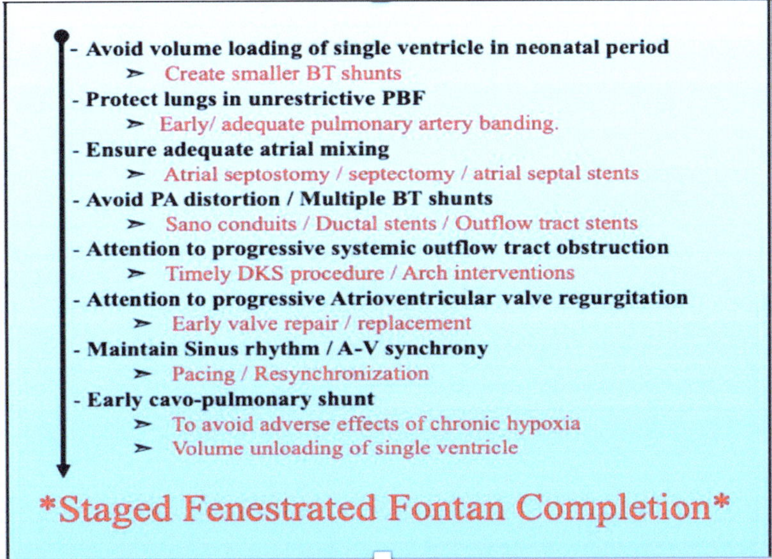

Fig. 21.2 Stepwise approach to Fontan completion

For inotropic support Milrinone: a phosphodiesterase inhibitor with favorable effects on PVR is preferred in combination with catecholamine dobutamine or epinephrine [20].

Multiorgan dysfunction can affect kidneys, liver and gastrointestinal systems and carries a poor prognosis for survival. Renal replacement therapy may be necessary for renal failure.

Coagulation abnormalities with impaired liver function can complicate postoperative bleeding and will need prompt correction.

Early use of parenteral nutrition and selective gut decontamination will prevent gastrointestinal malfunction, maintain nutrition and help reduce chylous fluid losses [21]. Tissue hypoxia, edema, and loss of proteinaceous exudates rich in immunoglobulins and T-Lymphocytes render these patients susceptible to opportunistic infection [19]. Rigorous microbiologic surveillance and treatment with broad-spectrum antimicrobial agents are often required.

Figure 21.3 is an algorithm for the management of EFF based on the predominant mechanism for the failure.

Surgical interventions in the setting of EFF with the added risk of cardiopulmonary bypass are high-risk procedures. However, the efficacy and safety of transcatheter interventions in this scenario is well established [22–24]. Techniques such as balloon dilation/stenting (Fontan conduit/pulmonary artery branches/arch obstruction), device occlusion (aortopulmonary collaterals/anterograde pulmonary flow), creation or closure of Fontan fenestration are well established and safely performed in preference to surgery [22–24].

Maintenance of sinus rhythm is paramount and in addition to medical treatment of arrhythmias pacing for heart block and ablation procedure may be required for persistent tachyarrhythmias.

Surgical intervention is necessary when valve repair/replacement is contemplated, or Fontan takedown is necessary [18]. Fontan takedown can provide an effective bailout option in EFF [14, 15]. However, mortality remains substantially high. In a multicenter European study, Fontan takedown was performed in 38 children with a 30-day mortality of 26.3% and the combined endpoint of mortality or heart transplant was reached in 44.7% patients during follow up [18].

Rescue cardiac transplantation with or without mechanical cardiac support is another option, in particular when EFF is secondary to severe ventricular dysfunction [19].

The recently developed technique of the transcatheter takedown of the Fontan circulation is extremely promising and could become the pro-

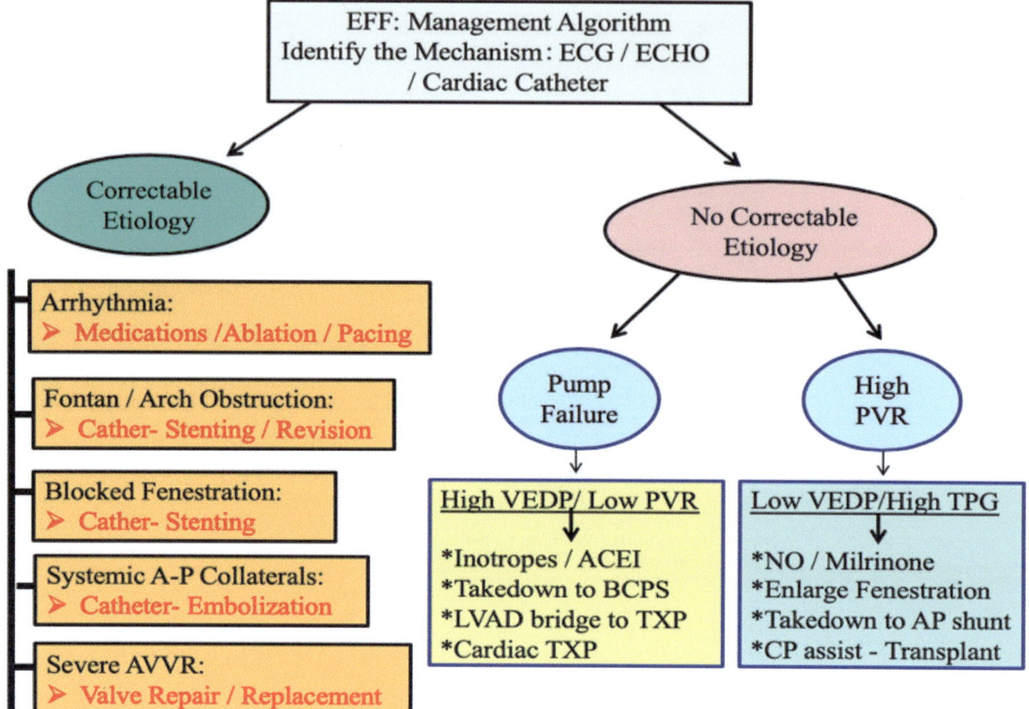

Fig. 21.3 Management of EFF

cedure of choice for initial stabilization in the setting of EFF as a bridge to recovery or cardiac transplantation [25].

Late Fontan Failure (LFF)

The Chronic Burden of Fontan State

With improvements in early survival, the living population with a Fontan circulation is expected to double in the next 20 years [26]. Several longitudinal studies have also shown excellent long-term outcomes in the second, third and fourth decades after Fontan operation [7, 9–13]. These studies, however, are limited by the effect of the era of treatment, the inclusion of old type APC Fontan and a small number of the newer TCPC Fontan procedures.

The pernicious burden of Fontan circulation with its unique anatomical, physiological and electrophysiological components (Fig. 21.4) leads to LFF, a heterogeneous syndrome with multisystem involvement [26–28].

Features of LFF include:

- ventricular dysfunction
- circulatory failure
- cardiac arrhythmias
- protein-losing enteropathy
- plastic bronchitis
- liver fibrosis
- renal dysfunction

These are some of the serious complications seen with increasing frequency as the duration of the follow-up increases after Fontan operation [26–28]. In addition, abnormalities of somatic growth and neurocognitive function are also observed.

Frequent re-interventions are required to prevent gradual attrition in the quality of life and death. Up to 50% of patients will need a catheter-based or/arrhythmia-related intervention by 15 years and 25% will need surgical re-intervention by 20 years post Fontan operation [29, 30]. Patients undergoing re-interventions have worse survival and freedom from failure over the longer term.

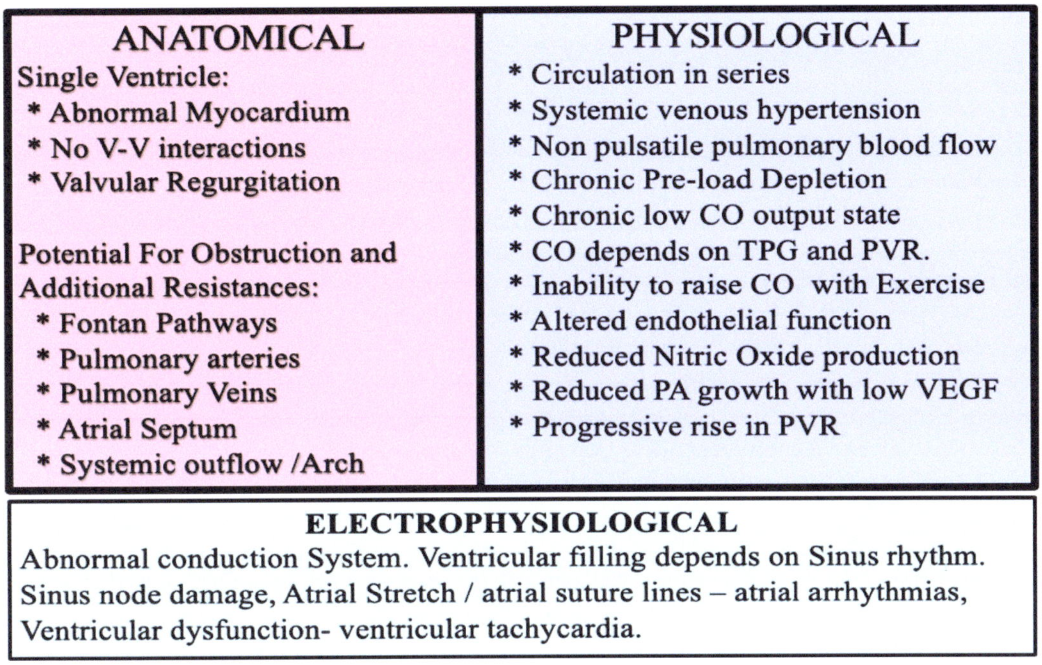

ANATOMICAL	PHYSIOLOGICAL
Single Ventricle: * Abnormal Myocardium * No V-V interactions * Valvular Regurgitation **Potential For Obstruction and Additional Resistances:** * Fontan Pathways * Pulmonary arteries * Pulmonary Veins * Atrial Septum * Systemic outflow /Arch	* Circulation in series * Systemic venous hypertension * Non pulsatile pulmonary blood flow * Chronic Pre-load Depletion * Chronic low CO output state * CO depends on TPG and PVR. * Inability to raise CO with Exercise * Altered endothelial function * Reduced Nitric Oxide production * Reduced PA growth with low VEGF * Progressive rise in PVR

ELECTROPHYSIOLOGICAL

Abnormal conduction System. Ventricular filling depends on Sinus rhythm. Sinus node damage, Atrial Stretch / atrial suture lines – atrial arrhythmias, Ventricular dysfunction- ventricular tachycardia.

Fig. 21.4 The burden of Fontan circulation

Phenotypes of Fontan Failure

Fontan failure has several pathophysiological mechanisms leading to complex multisystem interactions [31, 32]. Brooks et al. [32] have identified four distinct phenotypes as follows:

- Type I with reduced ejection fraction (FFrEF),
- Type II with preserved ejection fraction (FFpEF),
- Type III with normal heart (FFnH) and
- Type IV with abnormal lymphatics (FFaL).

Type I failure is common in children with non-LV morphology Fontan.

- the ventricular ejection fraction is reduced
- end-diastolic pressure is elevated
- systemic vascular resistance is increased due to neurohumoral activation.
- features of pulmonary and systemic congestion are accompanied by cyanosis due to the opening of veno-venous collaterals [32].

- impaired ventricular function predisposes to thromboembolic complications and arrhythmic sudden death.

Type II and Type III Fontan failure phenotypes are mainly seen in adult survivors [31, 32].

Type II failure resembles diastolic heart failure:

- preserved systolic ventricular function
- elevated end-diastolic ventricular pressure.
- presentation mainly with signs of pulmonary venous congestion.

Type III Fontan Failure demonstrates normal cardiac hemodynamic with raised PVR and multi-organ involvement including:

- portal hypertension
- liver fibrosis
- renal dysfunction.

Type IV Fontan Failure relates to abnormalities of the lymphatic system.Systemic venous hypertension impedes normal lymph drainage and causes retrograde flow from thoracic duct into abnormal connections:

- within the lungs (Plastic Bronchitis)
- within the gastrointestinal tract (PLE).

Management of LFF

Aggressive approach to early detection and correction of anatomical and electrical complications of Fontan burden followed by a strategy of phenotype driven management [31, 32] is shown to improve long term Fontan outcome (Fig. 21.5).

Some of the advances in the management of acquired heart failure in adults can be cautiously extrapolated to failing Fontan circulation, provided a meticulous assessment of the cardiac hemodynamics, end-organ function, and metabolic state is performed [32]:

- Fontan failure due to severe ventricular dysfunction can be treated with loop diuretics / spironolactone / ACE inhibitors and cardiospecific beta-blockers.
- ACE inhibitors should be avoided in the presence of advanced liver disease which reduces systemic vascular resistance to avoid hepatorenal syndrome.
- Beta-blockers should be avoided in the presence of sinus node dysfunction and bradyarrhythmia.
- Pulmonary vasodilators are a useful adjunct in the presence of elevated PVR, however, they should be avoided in the presence of diastolic ventricular dysfunction and pulmonary venous congestion [32].

In addition to optimizing Fontan circulation, organ-specific therapy may be directed at the lungs and the gut. Inhaled TPA/vest therapy and steroids/heparin are recommended for plastic bronchitis and PLE respectively.

A diligent search for lymphatic system abnormalities and treatment with interventional (lymphatic embolization) and surgical thoracic duct decompression is beneficial in selected cases of type IV Fontan failure [33, 34].

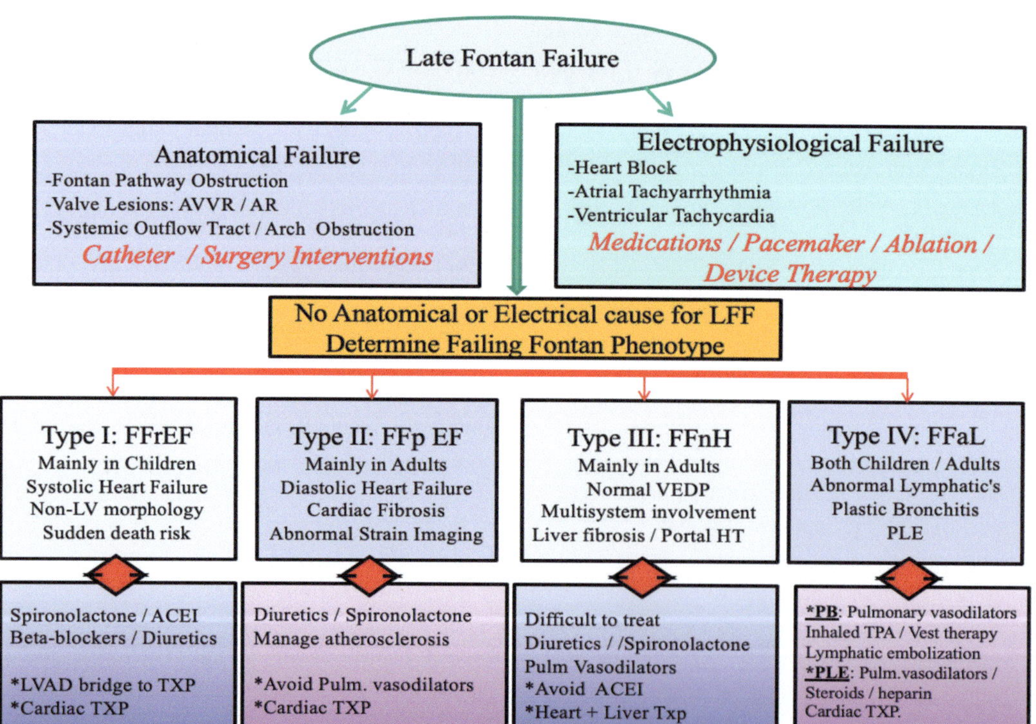

Fig. 21.5 Schematic of causes and treatments of Fontan failure in children

Cardiac transplantation is the final palliation in the Fontan journey and is most successful in patients with severe impairment of ventricular function [35, 36].

Cardiac Transplantation for Failing Fontan Circulation in Children

The evolution of orthotopic heart transplantation (OHT) in children has mirrored the advances in the treatment of single ventricle cardiac anomalies. OHT plays a vital role either as an alternative to high-risk surgery or as a salvage procedure when surgical palliation fails. Significant proportions of pediatric OHT recipients across all age groups have a primary diagnosis of congenital heart disease [37].

Challenges for Transplantation in Failing Fontan

Failing Fontan circulation presents several difficulties during the pre-transplant evaluation, transplant operation, and post-operative management which influence waiting list mortality, operative risk and post-transplant survival (Fig. 21.6) [35–37].

OHT in the setting of a failing Fontan circulation is technically demanding with the longer operative, CPB and ischemic times. Detailed imaging of the cardiac and extra-cardiac anatomy is mandatory to detect anomalies of cardiac position, situs, systemic and pulmonary venous connections.

TheTransplant surgeon needs to request extra donor tissues (veins, aorta and pulmonary arteries) for redirection of systemic venous connections, reconstruction of pulmonary arteries and appropriate siting of an often oversized donor heart [35, 38, 39].Extensive pleural and pericardial adhesions from previous operations increase bleeding risks and difficulties in cannulation.

The presence of multiple arterial and venous collaterals in combination with venous hypertension and coagulopathy further exacerbate the risk of intra-operative bleeding and can potentially compromise flows on CPB and impair vital organ perfusion.

Accurate assessment of PVR and ventricular function is a crucial part of transplant assessment

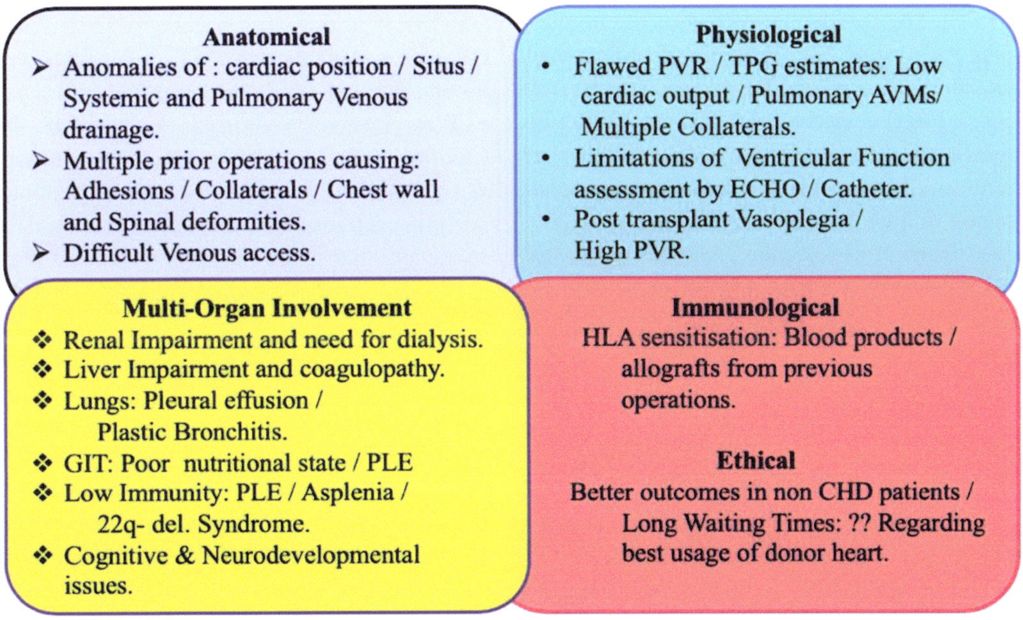

Fig. 21.6 Challenges for transplantation in failing Fontan

and should ideally combine invasive catheter hemodynamic study and magnetic resonance imaging.

Measurement of PVR in the failing Fontan circulation can be inaccurate due to

- low cardiac output state
- poor non-pulsatile distal lung recruitment
- endothelial dysfunction
- presence of collaterals
- pulmonary AVMs and pulmonary micro thromboembolism [19].

Restoration of pulsatile pulmonary blood flow post-transplant is shown to unmask elevated PVR [40] and has implications for right ventricular function during recovery. Oversizing the donor heart, creation of a small atrial septal defect and pulmonary vasodilator therapy are some of the strategies to overcome this problem.

Besides, these patients frequently have poor nutritional state, diminished immunity, renal and hepatic dysfunction, all of which can further complicate post-transplant recovery [26–28].

Immunologically these patients are at risk of sensitization to human leukocyte antigen (HLA) antibodies due to exposure to blood products and homograft tissues during surgical interventions [37, 38]. The degree of sensitization has implications for waiting list times and post-transplant outcomes. A higher degree of sensitization (>50% PRA) is associated with long waiting list times and poor outcomes [37, 38]. Pre-transplant de-sensitization together with post-transplant intense immunological surveillance and aggressive treatment of rejection are some of the factors responsible for recent improvements in the outcome of highly sensitized patients [37, 38, 41].

Mechanical Cardiac Support (MCS) for Failing Fontan Circulation

Currently available MCS devices are not ideal for supporting failing Fontan physiology due to lack of sub-pulmonary ventricle [42]. Various MCS devices are used for bridging failing Fontan to OHT. There is however no consensus on the optimal strategy and both pre and post-transplant outcomes remain poor.

ECMO offers short term cardiorespiratory support which is not reliable as a bridge to transplant [43, 44]. The experience with durable MCS for Fontan failure is limited to short case series or case reports [45–47].

Univentricular ventricular assist devices are reported to support failing single ventricle, leaving the cavopulmonary circulation unassisted. Separation of the systemic and pulmonary circulations and assisting both with two VADs or total artificial heart (TAH) may be required when Fontan physiology failure is associated with preserved ventricular function [42, 46].

Outcome of Cardiac transplantation for Fontan Failure in Children

Notwithstanding all its challenges, OHT is a viable treatment option for children with the failing Fontan circulation. The outcomes have improved remarkably in the modern era and there is no difference in post-transplant mortality as compared to transplants for other CHD patients [37]. Current estimates of survival for OHT in children with failing Fontan operation are 89% at 1 year and 78%% at 5 years respectively [38]. Within this group, patients with LFF or impaired ventricular function tend to do better than those with EFF or preserved ventricular function [48, 49]. Children with hypoplastic left heart syndrome and previous Norwood procedure have high mortality on the transplant waiting list (23%) and fare worse after transplant (53% survival at 10 years) irrespective of the physiological stage of palliation [41].

The success of OHT for failing Fontan circulation is limited by a shortage of donor organs and lack of reliable MCS strategy for bridging to transplantation resulting in high waiting list mortality. Innovations [50] and miniaturisation of VAD technology aided by better patient selection and development of MCS protocols for heterogenous Fontan failure phenotypes is likely to improve overall outcomes.

Conflict of Interests   None.

References

1. Fontan F, Baudet E. Surgical repair of tricuspid atresia. Thorax. 1971;26:240–8.
2. Choussat A, Fontan F, Besse P, Vallot F, Chauve A. Selection criteria for Fontan's procedure. In: Anderson R, Shinebourne E, editors. Pediatric cardiology. Edinburgh: Churchill Livingstone; 1978. p. 559–66.
3. de Leval MR, Kilner P, Gewillig M, Bull C, McGoon DC. Total cavopulmonary connection. A logical alternative to atriopulmonary connection for complex Fontan operation. J Thorac Cardiovasc Surg. 1988;96:682–95.
4. Bridges ND, Lock JE, Castaneda AR. Baffle fenestration with subsequent transcatheter closure. Modification of the Fontan operation for patients at increased risk. Circulation. 1990;82:1681–9.
5. Marcelletti C, Corno A, Giannico S, Marino B. Inferior vena cava–pulmonary artery extracardiac conduit. A new form of right heart bypass. J Thorac Cardiovasc Surg. 1990;100:228–32.
6. Cetta F, Feldt RH, O'Leary PW, Mair DD, Warnes CA, Driscoll DJ, et al. Improved early morbidity and mortality after Fontan operation: the Mayo Clinic experience, 1987 to 1992. J Am Coll Cardiol. 1996;28:480–6.
7. Gentles TL, Mayer JE, Gauvreau K, Newburger JW, Lock JE, Kupferschmid JP, et al. Fontan operation in five hundred consecutive patients: factors influencing early and late outcome. J Thorac Cardiovasc Surg. 1997;114:376–91.
8. Hosein RBM, Clarke AJB, McGuirk SP, Griselli M, Stumper O, De Giovanni JV, et al. Factors influencing early and late outcome following the Fontan procedure in the current era. The 'two commandments'? Eur J Cardiothorac Surg. 2007;31:344–52; discussion 353
9. Khairy P, Fernandes SM, Mayer JE Jr, Triedman JK, Walsh EP, Lock JE, et al. Long-term survival, modes of death, and predictors of mortality in patients with Fontan surgery. Circulation. 2008;117:85–92.
10. Tweddell JS, Nersesian M, Mussatto KA, Nugent M, Simpson P, Mitchell ME, et al. Fontan palliation in the modern era: factors impacting mortality and morbidity. Ann Thorac Surg. 2009;88:1291–9.
11. Rogers LS, Glatz AC, Ravishankar C, Spray TL, Nicolson SC, Rychik J, et al. 18 years of the Fontan operation at a single institution: results from 771 consecutive patients. J Am Coll Cardiol. 2012;60:1018–25.
12. d'Udekem Y, Iyengar AJ, Galati JC, Forsdick V, Weintraub RG, Wheaton GR, et al. Redefining expectations of long-term survival after the Fontan procedure: twenty-five years of follow-up from the entire population of Australia and New Zealand. Circulation. 2014;130(suppl 1):S32–8.
13. Pundi KN, Johnson JN, Dearani JA, Pundi KN, Li Z, Hinck CA, Dahl SH, et al. 40-year follow-up after the Fontan operation: long-term outcomes of 1,052 patients. J Am Coll Cardiol. 2015;66:1700–10.
14. Almond CSD, Mayer JE, Thiagarajan RR, Blume ED, del Nido PJ, McElhinney DB. Outcome after Fontan failure and takedown to an intermediate palliative circulation. Ann Thorac Surg. 2007;84:880–7.
15. Ovroutski S, Sohn C, Barikbin P, Miera O, Alexi-Meskishvili V, Hübler M, et al. Analysis of the risk factors for early failure after extracardiac Fontan operation. Ann Thorac Surg. 2013;95:1409–16.
16. Murphy MO, Glatz AC, Goldberg DJ, Rogers LS, Ravishankar C, Nicolson SC, et al. Management of early Fontan failure: a single-institution experience. Eur J Cardiothorac Surg. 2014;46:458–64.
17. Iyengar AJ, Winlaw DS, Galati JC, Celermajer DS, Wheaton GR, Gentles TL, et al. Trends in Fontan surgery and risk factors for early adverse outcomes after Fontan surgery: the Australia and New Zealand Fontan registry experience. J Thorac Cardiovasc Surg. 2014;148:566–75.
18. van Melle JP, Wolff D, Hörer J, Belli E, Meyns B, Padalino M, et al. Surgical options after Fontan failure. Heart. 2016;102(14):1127–33.
19. Chaudhari M, Sturman J, O'Sullivan J, Smith J, Wrightson N, Parry G, et al. Rescue cardiac transplantation for early failure of the Fontan-type circulation in children. J Thorac Cardiovasc Surg. 2005;129:416–22.
20. Hoffman TM, Wernosky G, Atz AM, Kulik TJ, Nelson DP, Chang AC, et al. Efficacy and safety of milrinone in preventing low cardiac output syndrome in infants and children after corrective surgery for congenital heart disease. Circulation. 2003;107(7):996–1002.
21. Meier Hellmann A, Reinhart K, Bredle DL, Sakka SG. Therapeutic options for management of impaired gut function. Am Soc Nephrol. 2001;12(suppl):S65–9.
22. Stümper O, Gewillig M, Vettukattil J, Budts W, Chessa M, Chaudhari M, et al. Modified technique of stent fenestration of the atrial septum. Heart. 2003;89(10):1227–30.
23. Boshoff DE, Brown SC, De Giovanni J, Stumper O, Wright J, Mertens L, et al. Percutaneous management of a Fontan fenestration: in search for the ideal restriction occlusion device. Catheter Cardiovasc Interv. 2010;75(1):60–5.
24. Bhole V, Wright JG, De Giovanni JV, Dhillon R, Miller PA, Desai T, et al. Transcatheter interventions in the early postoperative period after the Fontan procedure. Catheter Cardiovasc Interv. 2011;77(1):92–8.
25. Hallbergson A, Mascio CE, Rome JJ. Transcatheter Fontan takedown. Catheter Cardiovasc Interv. 2015;86(5):849–54.
26. Rychik J, Atz AM, Celermajer DS, Deal BJ, Gatzoulis MA, Gewillig MH, et al. Evaluation and management of the child and adult with Fontan circulation: a scientific statement from the American Heart Association. Circulation. 2019;140:e234–84.
27. Gewillig M, Brown SC. The Fontan circulation after 45 years: update in physiology. Heart. 2016;102:1081–6.

28. Rychik J. The relentless effects of the Fontan paradox. Semin Thorac Cardiovasc Surg Pediatr Card Surg Annu. 2016;19:37–43.

29. Dennis M, Zannino D, du Plessis K, Bullock A, Disney PJS, Radford DJ, et al. Clinical outcomes in adolescents and adults after the Fontan procedure. J Am Coll Cardiol. 2018;71(9):1009–17.

30. Downing TE, Allen KY, Goldberg DJ, Rogers LS, Ravishankar C, Rychik J, et al. Surgical and catheter-based reinterventions are common in long-term survivors of the Fontan operation. Circ Cardiovasc Interv. 2017;10:e004924.

31. Hebson CL, McCabe NM, Elder RW, Mahle WT, McConnell M, Kogon BE, et al. Hemodynamic phenotype of the failing Fontan in an adult population. Am J Cardiol. 2013;112:1943–7.

32. Book WM, Gerardin J, Saraf A, Marie Valente A, Rodriguez F. Clinical phenotypes of Fontan failure: implications for management. Congenit Heart Dis. 2016;11:296–308.

33. Dori Y, Keller MS, Fogel MA, Rome JJ, Whitehead KK, Harris MA, et al. MRI of lymphatic abnormalities after functional single ventricle palliation surgery. AJR Am J Roentgenol. 2014;203:426–31.

34. Hraška V. Decompression of thoracic duct: new approach for the treatment of failing Fontan. Ann Thorac Surg. 2013;96:709–11.

35. Carey JA, Hamilton JR, Hilton CJ, Dark JH, Forty J, Parry G, et al. Orthotopic cardiac transplantation for the failing Fontan circulation. Eur J Cardiothorac Surg. 1998;14:7–14.

36. Kanter KR, Mahle WT, Vincent RN, Berg AM, Kogon BE, Kirshbom PM. Heart transplantation in children with a Fontan procedure. Ann Thorac Surg. 2011;91:823–30.

37. Dipchand AI, Edwards LB, Kucheryavaya AY, Benden C, Dobbels F, Levvey BJ, et al.; International Society of Heart and Lung Transplantation. The registry of the International Society for Heart and Lung Transplantation: seventeenth official pediatric heart transplantation report–2014; focus theme: retransplantation. J Heart Lung Transplant. 2014;33:985–995.

38. Kovach JR, Naftel DC, Pearce FB, Tresler MA, Edens RE, Shuhaiber JH, et al. Comparison of risk factors and outcomes for pediatric patients listed for heart transplantation after bidirectional Glenn and after Fontan: an analysis from the pediatric heart transplant study. J Heart Lung Transplant. 2012;31:133–9.

39. Iyengar AJ, Sharma VJ, Weintraub RG, Shipp A, Brizard CP, d'Udekem Y, et al. Surgical strategies to facilitate heart transplantation in children after failed univentricular palliations: the role of advanced intraoperative surgical preparation. Eur J Cardiothorac Surg. 2014;46:480–5.

40. Mitchell MB, Campbell DN, Ivy D, Boucek MM, Sondheimer HM, Pietra B, et al. Evidence of pulmonary vascular disease after heart transplantation for Fontan circulation failure. J Thorac Cardiovasc Surg. 2004;128:693–702.

41. Alsoufi B, Mahle WT, Manlhiot C, Deshpande S, Kogon B, McCrindle BW, et al. Outcomes of heart transplantation in children with hypoplastic left heart syndrome previously palliated with the Norwood procedure. J Thorac Cardiovasc Surg. 2016;151:167–74.

42. Miller JR, Lancaster TS, Callahan C, Abarbanell AM, Eghtesady P. An overview of mechanical circulatory support in single-ventricle patients. Transl Pediatr. 2018;7(2):151–61.

43. Rood KL, Teele SA, Barrett CS, Salvin JW, Rycus PT, Fynn-Thompson F, et al. Extracorporeal membrane oxygenation support after the Fontan operation. J Thorac Cardiovasc Surg. 2011;142:504–10.

44. Almond CS, Singh TP, Gauvreau K, Piercey GE, Fynn-Thompson F, Rycus PT, et al. Extracorporeal membrane oxygenation for bridge to heart transplantation among children in the United States. Circulation. 2011;123:2975–84.

45. Nathan M, Baird C, Fynn-Thompson F, Almond C, Thiagarajan R. Successful implantation of a Berlin heart biventricular assist device in a failing single ventricle. J Thorac Cardiovasc Surg. 2006;131:1407–8.

46. Weinstein S, Bello R, Pizarro C, Fynn-Thompson F, Kirklin J, Guleserian K, et al. The use of the Berlin heart EXCOR in patients with functional single ventricle. J Thorac Cardiovasc Surg. 2014;147:697–705.

47. Niebler RA, Ghanayem NS, Shah TK, Bobke AD, Zangwill S, Brosig C. Use of a HeartWare ventricular assist device in a patient with failed Fontan circulation. Ann Thorac Surg. 2014;97:e115–6.

48. Griffiths ER, Kaza AK, Wyler von Ballmoos MC, Loyola H, Valente AM, Blume ED, et al. Evaluating failing Fontans for heart transplantation: predictors of death. Ann Thorac Surg. 2009;88:558–63.

49. Murtuza B, Hermuzi A, Crossland DS, Parry G, Hudson M, Chaudhari MP, et al. Impact of mode of failure and end-organ dysfunction on the survival of adult Fontan patients undergoing cardiac transplantation. Eur J Cardiothorac Surg. 2017;51:135–41.

50. Rodefeld MD, Marsden A, Figliola R, Jonas T, Neary M, Giridharan GA. Cavopulmonary assist: long-term reversal of the Fontan paradox. J Thorac Cardiovasc Surg. 2019;158(6):1627–36.

Part VI

Transition, Education and Lifestyle

Transition to Adult Life

Danielle Massarella, Rachel Wald, Lorna Swan, and Rafael Alonso-Gonzalez

Transitional Care Arrangements

Transition is a process that starts in the pediatric setting and continues into adulthood, while transfer is a single event where the Adult Congenital Cardiologist becomes the primary care provider. Whilst the young person's understanding of their cardiac anatomy and ownership of their condition is important, a comprehensive approach to transition should also address lifestyle, health and career advice. As suggested throughout this chapter, a well-structured multidisciplinary transition program, including doctors, nurses, psychologists and social workers, is required to support patients and families fully throughout the process.

Transition Programs of Patients with Congenital Heart Disease

Even though most experts agree on the importance of a structured transition from pediatric to adult care, there is little evidence or consensus on how a smooth transition should be achieved.

D. Massarella · R. Wald · R. Alonso-Gonzalez (✉)
Division of Cardiology, Department of Medicine, Toronto General Hospital, University Health Network, University of Toronto, Toronto, ON, Canada
e-mail: Rafa.Alonso@uhn.ca

L. Swan
ACHD Unit, Golden Jubilee Hospital, Glasgow, UK

Transition is a process spanning several years and includes the transfer of care, that occurs at a single time point, usually between the age of 16 and 18 years. Transition should start by the age of 12 years and should ideally consist of a series of encounters aimed at providing age-appropriate information and education to patients. The Transition service overlaps pediatric and ACHD services, and is provided by a multidisciplinary team of doctors, nurses and other healthcare workers with knowledge and training in the care of adolescents with chronic heart conditions.

The topics covered during transition clinics should include the following topics (which should be documented in a dedicated care pathway):

- Explanation of the transition and transfer of care
- Diagnosis, previous interventions, comorbidities and disabilities
- Medication and allergies
- Lifestyle issues, including diet, travel, exercise, alcohol, drugs, tattoos and piercings
- Endocarditis
- Reproductive health
- Psychosocial issues
- Education and employment
- Supportive literature and charitable/patient organizations

Psychological Impact of Chronic Disease in Adult Life

Growing up with chronic disease has a pervasive impact on development and on almost every aspect of adult life. Children with congenital heart disease face important social and psychological challenges and are at risk of achieving fewer milestones, or achieving them later than their peers [1]. In addition, psychiatric disorders are prevalent, with up to one-third of patients meeting diagnostic criteria for internalizing disorders, such as depression or anxiety. [2, 3]

Acceptance of their medical condition and interacting with the medical team can be challenging for young people with congenital heart disease. These challenges can be associated with severe detrimental psychologic effects [4]. Fear, loss of control and decreased self-esteem are common and should be addressed during transition. In addition, peer-to-peer interaction during adolescence is one of the most important factors influencing future aspects of wellbeing. While risk-taking behaviors are common during adolescence, patients with a single ventricle do have objective and perceived limitations. This will preclude their participation in certain activities, affecting social acceptance and peer group integration [5].

Table 22.1 Recommendations to address and minimise the psychological impact in CHD

1. Help the adolescent to identify and be involved with adults or older role models
2. Encourage patients to participate in age-appropriate support groups and/or organizations relevant to their healthcare needs
3. Be aware of the risk of comorbid mood disorders and screen/manage these appropriately
4. Involve the adolescent in their medical decisions early in life
5. Encourage self-advocacy skills
6. Routinely take a developmentally appropriate social history
7. Facilitate early access to psychological services
8. Adequate patient preparation for upcoming interventions

While there has been a significant improvement in medical care for this population, less attention has been paid to the psychological morbidity of this population. A successful transition program should include all these aspects, to prepare the young person for adulthood. Addressing psychological issues is difficult, but essential. The recommendations listed in Table 22.1 should be considered.

Lifestyle Advice

Single ventricle physiology confers multifaceted effects on an individuals' lifestyle, affecting routine daily activities, sports, substance use, cosmetic procedures, etc.

Exercise

Patients with Fontan circulation should, in general, be encouraged to lead as active lifestyles as possible. Exercise restrictions that are placed on patients without clear indication can negatively impact on quality of life. Patients and their parents/caregivers have discrepant perceptions of the patient's ability to exercise safely. The vast majority (80%) of parents underestimate their child's exercise tolerance. Patients and their families should be reassured that exercise can be safe, and regular participation in physical activity is to be encouraged.

To avoid confusion among patients and carers regarding activity restrictions (or lack thereof), specific exercise prescriptions should be issued to patients, and recommendations should be revisited at each routine follow up.

Alcohol/Drugs

Certain higher-risk lifestyle choices may tax an already strained cardiovascular system with limited reserve. Specifically, individuals with congenital heart disease may conceivably be at greater risk of adverse reactions to recreational drugs that are known, even in the general population, to predispose to arrhythmia, coronary vasospasm, or cardiomyopathy with either acute or chronic exposure.

Particularly relevant to patients with the Fontan circulation, lung or liver disease related to smoking or alcohol intake may impact on outcome and preclude future cardiac transplantation. The latter may compound or accelerate Fontan associated liver disease.

Piercing, Tattoos and Endocarditis

While the incidence of bacteremia associated with body art such as piercings and tattoos is not known, cases of infective endocarditis have been reported in patients with and without congenital heart disease following such procedures. Nasal and oral piercings place patients at particular risk [6]. In those with congenital heart disease, the endocarditis tends to involve the location of their lesion, and surgical therapy is more likely to be required as an adjunct to intravenous antibiotics [6, 7].

Patients should be counseled regarding the risk of endocarditis as a complication of body art procedures, particularly those performed by amateur artists. They should be strongly advised against tattoos and piercings, urged to follow aftercare instructions meticulously if they do decide to proceed, and contact their cardiologist should any symptoms of systemic illness/sepsis develop within 1–2 weeks of the procedure (Table 22.2).

Table 22.2 Recommendations to address impacts of Fontan physiology on lifestyle

1. Issue an exercise prescription at every visit, detailing frequency, intensity, time and type of activity (FITT principle)
2. Encourage hobbies and leisure activities
3. Inquire about high risk behaviors at every visit, and provide counselling and treatment where appropriate (i.e. smoking cessation support, reduce alcohol intake)
4. Address body art recommendations as part of routine discussions regarding endocarditis risk

Sexual Health, Contraception and Pregnancy Advice in Fontan Patients

The importance of addressing reproductive health in patients with complex congenital heart disease prior to the onset of sexual activity cannot be overstated. Pregnancy poses a significant risk of morbidity in patients with Fontan physiology in particular (see also Sect. 10) [8].

Pediatric cardiologists may be uncomfortable making recommendations regarding engagement in sexual activity or specific contraceptive methods, placing patients at unnecessary and avoidable risk. Congenital heart patients are often poorly supported with respect to reproductive health, as 43% of women with congenital heart disease do not receive contraception counselling, and a similar proportion are uninformed about pregnancy-related risks [9]. Seventy-four percent of sexually active adolescents with congenital heart disease have engaged in one or more types of risky sexual behavior [9]. Unfortunately, some adolescents transition abruptly from the pediatric to adult care setting as a result of an unplanned pregnancy [10]. While Fontan patients do have an increased risk of pregnancy related complication and fertility issues, pregnancy is possible.

A structured transition process is essential for educating patients early, starting age-appropriate discussions from the age or 11–12 years and continuing well after the patient's care has been transferred to an ACHD team (Table 22.3). Unplanned pregnancies should be avoided, by educating young patients on the use of the most effective contraception available. Specific cardiac lesions, including the Fontan physiology, predispose patients to thrombotic phenomena, and in such cases ethinyloestradiol containing contraceptive formulations should be avoided. Providers must be familiar with the types of progesterone -based contraceptive options available for their patients and be prepared to discuss and support their patients' access to them (see Sect. 10). It should also be noted that Fontan patients who choose intrauterine device placement (IUD) should only undergo this procedure in a clinical

Table 22.3 Recommendations to address reproductive health in Fontan patients

1. Discuss relationships, sexuality and personal safety with adolescents
2. Begin to address patient goals and expectations regarding family planning in adolescence
3. Take a sexual history at every routine visit
4. Provide counseling regarding, and facilitate timely access to, safe and reliable contraception at the onset of menarche
5. Fontan patients should use contraceptive formulations containing progestin only
6. Emergency contraceptive formulations can be used in Fontan patients
7. IUD placement in Fontan patients should occur only in an appropriately supervised and supported setting
8. Fontan patients should be offered preconception counselling at a high-risk pregnancy center jointly with ACHD and maternal fetal medicine professionals
9. Pregnant Fontan patients should receive care throughout pregnancy, labour and delivery at a high-risk pregnancy center, in collaboration with experts in ACHD and maternal fetal medicine

Table 22.4 Recommendations to optimize educational and occupational status of individuals with CHD

1. Begin asking about career goals in childhood, when developmentally appropriate
2. Explore possible career options with adolescents
3. If considering post-secondary education, encourage and support adolescents in working with campus services to arrange appropriate accommodation and support, as needed
4. Facilitate, where appropriate, engagement with vocational rehabilitation services professionals or organizations

setting equipped to provide resuscitation in the event of a vasovagal response inciting hemodynamic instability. Finally, Fontan patients should be advised that emergency contraception in the form of progestin only formulations or progestin receptor modulators can be used if needed [8].

Patients with significant Fontan complications, such as cyanosis or ventricular dysfunction, should be advised against pregnancy [8]. In the instance of successful conception, even 'uncomplicated' Fontan patients are at high risk of atrial arrhythmias, a decline in functional class, worsening ventricular function, cyanosis, and peripartum hemorrhage. There is also a high miscarriage rate, and increased risk of fetal prematurity, growth restriction, perinatal mortality and transmission of congenital heart disease. [8]

Educational and Occupational Status

Education and career are two of the most important domains that impact on the quality of life of adults with congenital cardiac disease. Patients with complex cardiac disease exhibit decreased

job participation, but unemployment rates in this population are unaffected by defect complexity [2, 11]. Patients who are employed report better quality of life than those who are not [2]. Employability and occupational status can be optimized by providing early, specific guidance in the pediatric/transition and adult clinical settings. Providers should routinely elicit discussion of a young person's interests, skill set and career and education goals, primarily to dispel possible misconceptions about restrictions, but also to facilitate insightful discussion about long-term goal setting. Certain congenital lesions may impose unique occupational restrictions which, if unanticipated by the patient, stand to derail long-term plans and cause significant stress. For example, a patient with Fontan circulation who plans to join the police forces or military needs to be informed that he, or she, might not be eligible depending on entry criteria.

The transition team should be prepared to discuss the principles and applicable laws related to equal opportunity employment with patients and their employers. Individuals with congenital heart disease have an increased likelihood of being employed if they have received structured career advice, and this highlights the importance of this aspect of transitional ACHD care (Table 22.4) [2].

Dental Health

As patients approach the age of transfer of care, they must be encouraged to secure continued access to dental care into adulthood. Maintaining

Table 22.5 Recommendations to address dental health in Fontan patients

1. Start exploring future dental and healthcare coverage in late adolescence
2. Take a dental health history at every visit
3. Review the indications for endocarditis prophylaxis at every visit
4. Counsel patients on the risks/safety of undergoing dental procedures requiring sedation in an outpatient setting
5. Fontan patients should typically not undergo dental procedures requiring sedation or general anesthesia in an outpatient setting
6. Patients should undergo a comprehensive dental assessment prior to any elective/non-emergency cardiothoracic surgery

Table 22.6 Recommendations for travel with Fontan circulation

1. Assist patients in assembling vital medical information in the form of a health passport, for presentation to health care providers abroad if needed
2. Provide supporting documentation as needed for the patient to establish insurance coverage for travel
3. Be familiar with existing travel directories and advise patients to be aware of the nearest referral center(s) prior to departure
4. Plan anticoagulation checks
5. Ensure adequate medication for the entire trip

oral hygiene with regular dental and hygienist visits, as well as meticulous brushing and flossing is paramount for reducing the risk of endocarditis [12]. Comprehensive dental assessment is an indispensable part of any transition service, and should precede any non-emergent cardiothoracic surgical procedure.

The costs associated with dental care should be discussed with the patient during the transition period, as they might not be covered by the healthcare system.

Recommendations regarding the prophylaxis of spontaneous bacterial endocarditis (SBE) have changed over time and may vary by country. Indications for endocarditis prophylaxis must be reviewed at every visit, as the patient's eligibility might also change over time. Dental procedures requiring sedation or general anaesthesia pose a potential risk to the patient with a univentricular cardiac physiology; such patients should be counselled and referred to a specialist dental service with anaesthetic expertise in congenital heart disease (Table 22.5).

Travel with a Fontan Circulation

In general, there are no absolute contraindications to travel for stable individuals with a Fontan circulation (Table 22.6).

Patients should be counseled regarding contingency planning if they require medical attention while abroad. Namely, they should carry with them their most recent clinic notes and/or health passport, baseline ECG, and any relevant device cards.

Travel insurance, including medical transport and repatriation should certainly be obtained.

The patient should be familiar with the name of the congenital center nearest to their planned destination prior to departure. Patient advocacy groups such as the Adult Congenital Heart Association maintain travel directories for this purpose.

Adequate mobilization and hydration in long-haul flights should minimise the risk of thrombosis. Cyanotic patients usually tolerate flights in commercial airliners well, but some may require supplemental oxygen on the flight. Excessive efforts, and heavyweight lifting should be avoided.

Patients on anticoagulation should ensure INR checks around (and if necessary during) the trip.

Patients should ensure they bring with them enough medication to last the entire trip, together with their prescription in case of checks in the airport.

References

1. Last BF, Stam H, Onland-van Nieuwenhuizen AM, Grootenhuis MA. Positive effects of a psychoeducational group intervention for children with a chronic disease: first results. Patient Educ Couns. 2007;65(1):101–12.
2. Kovacs AH, Verstappen A. The whole adult congenital heart disease patient. Prog Cardiovasc Dis. 2011;53(4):247–53.
3. Stam H, Hartman EE, Deurloo JA, Groothoff J, Grootenhuis MA. Young adult patients with a his-

tory of pediatric disease: impact on course of life and transition into adulthood. J Adolesc Health. 2006;39(1):4–13.

4. Sable C, Foster E, Uzark K, Bjornsen K, Canobbio MM, Connolly HM, et al. Best practices in managing transition to adulthood for adolescents with congenital heart disease: the transition process and medical and psychosocial issues: a scientific statement from the American Heart Association. Circulation. 2011;123(13):1454–85.

5. Shaughnessy L, Alonso-Gonzalez R. Preparing adults with congenital heart disease for surgery or intervention. In: Da Cruz E, Macrae D, Webb GD, editors. Intensive care of the adult with congenital heart disease. Springer; 2019. p. 75–85.

6. Armstrong ML, DeBoer S, Cetta F. Infective endocarditis after body art: a review of the literature and concerns. J Adolesc Health. 2008;43(3):217–25.

7. Cetta F, Graham LC, Lichtenberg RC, Warnes CA. Piercing and tattooing in patients with congenital heart disease: patient and physician perspectives. J Adolesc Health. 1999;24(3):160–2.

8. Regitz-Zagrosek V, Roos-Hesselink JW, Bauersachs J, Blomstrom-Lundqvist C, Cifkova R, De Bonis M, et al. 2018 ESC guidelines for the management of cardiovascular diseases during pregnancy. Eur Heart J. 2018;39(34):3165–241.

9. Moceri P, Goossens E, Hascoet S, Checler C, Bonello B, Ferrari E, et al. From adolescents to adults with congenital heart disease: the role of transition. Eur J Pediatr. 2015;174(7):847–54.

10. Knauth A, Verstappen A, Reiss J, Webb GD. Transition and transfer from pediatric to adult care of the young adult with complex congenital heart disease. Cardiol Clin. 2006;24(4):619–29, vi.

11. Lyon ME, Kuehl K, McCarter R. Transition to adulthood in congenital heart disease: missed adolescent milestones. J Adolesc Health. 2006;39(1):121–4.

12. Baddour LM, Wilson WR, Bayer AS, Fowler VG Jr, Tleyjeh IM, Rybak MJ, et al. Infective endocarditis in adults: diagnosis, antimicrobial therapy, and management of complications: a scientific statement for healthcare professionals from the American Heart Association. Circulation. 2015;132(15):1435–86.

Part VII

Follow Up in Adult Life

Considerations When Developing a Multidisciplinary Adult Fontan Clinic

Adam M. Lubert, Tarek Alsaied, and Alexander R. Opotowsky

Goals of Multidisciplinary Fontan Programs

Over the past decade, multiple congenital heart centers have developed multidisciplinary clinics to provide standardized, subspecialty Fontan care [1]. While the primary goals of these multidisciplinary programs vary for each institution, most programs strive to achieve the goals listed in Table 23.1.

Table 23.1 Goals of multidisciplinary Fontan programs

Early detection and treatment of complications

Prevention of adverse events

Early referral for consideration of heart transplant and advanced heart failure therapies

Improve quality of life

Increase survival

Decrease care variability

Creation of databases for quality improvement and clinical research

Develop a network of diverse medical subspecialists with Fontan expertise

Define quality metrics

Patient education

Benefits of a Multidisciplinary Fontan Clinic

Dedicated multidisciplinary Fontan programs provide several benefits (Fig. 23.1). Fontan patients who require care by multiple subspecialists save time and money with the coordination of these visits and testing. This goes beyond simply avoiding additional travel and time off, since there may be only one clinic registration, one period of time in a waiting room, and one set of vital signs taken. In countries with private-pay insurance, such a visit may incur only a single facility fee and, thereby, decrease cost to the patient and healthcare system. Surveillance testing and evaluation can be decided upon jointly, performed in a single system and made available to all providers. This eliminates the cost of dupli-

A. M. Lubert · T. Alsaied
Department of Pediatrics, Cincinnati Children's Hospital Heart Institute, University of Cincinnati College of Medicine, Cincinnati, OH, USA
e-mail: alsaiedt@upmc.edu

A. R. Opotowsky (✉)
Department of Pediatrics, Cincinnati Children's Hospital Heart Institute, University of Cincinnati College of Medicine, Cincinnati, OH, USA

Department of Cardiology, Boston Children's Hospital, Harvard Medical School, Boston, MA, USA

Department of Medicine, Brigham and Women's Hospital, Harvard Medical School, Boston, MA, USA
e-mail: Sasha.Opotowsky@cchmc.org

P. Clift et al. (eds.), *Univentricular Congenital Heart Defects and the Fontan Circulation*,
https://doi.org/10.1007/978-3-031-36208-8_23

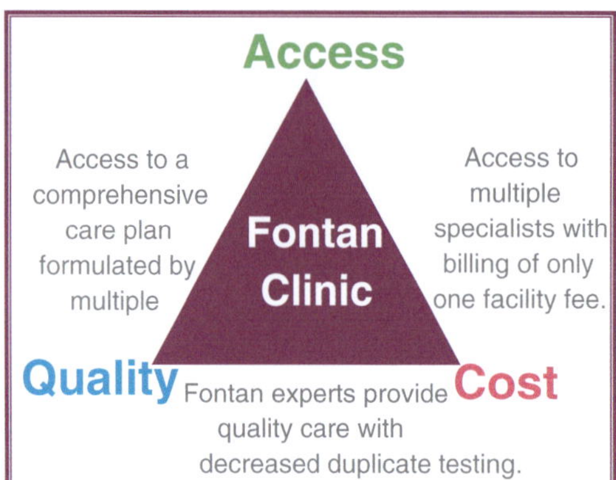

Fig. 23.1 Benefits of a dedicated Fontan programme

cate testing, a common occurrence in a healthcare system where images and results are not always easily accessible. Most importantly, a Fontan-focused clinic provides patients access to quality care from a group that is dedicated to delivering comprehensive, up-to-date, evidence-based Fontan care.

One concern with multidisciplinary Fontan clinics is the potential for over-testing of clinically well patients at low absolute risk for adverse events over the short term. This is a fair concern. Some patients are likely to benefit from multiple subspecialist visits, while others have little use for specialized input. Therefore, a one-size-fits-all model is inappropriate. Firstly, extensive evaluation is likely wasteful in some patients. Secondly an asymptomatic patient who is doing well and attends a multidisciplinary clinic with evaluations by a cardiologist, hepatologist, nephrologist, and pulmonologist may rightfully question the value of this endeavor and be less likely to maintain appropriate care.

Therefore, to the extent possible, testing and evaluation should be tailored to each patient, while maintaining an overarching protocol to enhance reproducibility and the capacity to improve quality of care over time. Decisions on appropriate evaluation for each patient may be achieved via regular (e.g., weekly) care conferences, to allow for review of patients scheduled in an upcoming Fontan clinic. In this setting, the Fontan subspecialty team reviews the patients,

determines which subspecialists would add value to the patient's care for the upcoming visit and discuss frequency of follow-up. Patients who attend our Fontan clinic see a cardiologist on every visit, a hepatologist at baseline and on all visits if they have any liver lesion, and other subspecialists as needed.

Clinic Models

There are different ways to organize a Fontan multidisciplinary clinic, with programs across North America using several different strategies. The choice of which model to adopt depends on the goals of the program and the investment the institution is willing and able to commit to the program. Clinic models are listed below:

- *Consult for all*—All patients with a Fontan circulation are seen in the Fontan clinic at a predetermined frequency but maintain follow-up with a primary cardiologist.
- *Optional consult*—It remains at the discretion of the primary cardiologist when the patient should be seen for a consult in the Fontan clinic. Patients otherwise continue regular follow-up with their primary cardiologist.
- *Transfer of care for all*—All Fontan patients in the center are primarily followed in the Fontan clinic.
- *Optional transfer of care*—The primary cardiologist has the option to transfer their Fontan patients for ongoing care in the Fontan clinic.
- *Primary cardiologist model*—The primary cardiologist sees the patient in the Fontan clinic with the support of the subspecialties and infrastructure available at the institution.
- *Mixed models*—A combination of the above models.

Currently, many Fontan clinics operate on a monthly or bimonthly basis, but this is dependent on volume and resources. Clinics can be designed such that specified subspecialists are physically present for all clinics or are only present as needed. The decision about who is present in clinic will depend on availability, health care system organization, resources and patient needs. Below we will discuss potential members of a Fontan multidisciplinary team.

Fontan Team Members

With increasing recognition of the multiorgan sequelae of the Fontan circulation, it is essential to build a team of multiple disciplines to provide comprehensive care. This team requires a clinical "champion", often a cardiologist, to be the coordinator in assembling and maintaining a cohesive team. Additionally, a dedicated nurse or mid-level provider (typically a nurse practitioner or physician assistant) dedicates time to the Fontan program; this is invaluable and appears to correspond to a much greater likelihood of success. Listed in Table 23.2 are considerations for team members and the services or expertise that each provides for a Fontan patient. Many Fontan clin-

Table 23.2 Potential members of a Fontan Care Team

Nurse coordinator	Scheduling and arranging visits and testing Fielding calls and following up on testing Creating an environment of a cohesive medical home
Cardiology	
Pediatric cardiology	Cardiac and coordinated evaluation of individuals with a Fontan circulation < 18 years old
Adult congenital cardiology	Cardiac and coordinated evaluation of individuals with a Fontan circulation age ≥ 18 years old
Heart failure/transplant cardiologist	Assessing patients with circulatory failure for mechanical support or transplantation
Interventional cardiology	Performing catheterizations including hemodynamics, Fontan or pulmonary artery stenting
Cardiac imaging	Interpreting imaging (e.g. cardiac CT or MRI) Guidance on protocols for Fontan (e.g. pulmonary embolism evaluation)
Electrophysiology	Medical or invasive management of arrhythmias Risk stratification for implantable cardioverter defibrillators
Hepatology/Liver transplant team	Management of Fontan associated liver disease Management of liver lesions/hepatic neoplasms
Pulmonology	Evaluation and management of lung disease, respiratory muscle weakness, hemoptysis, and plastic bronchitis
Endocrinology	Diagnosis and management of growth restriction Management of abnormal bone density
Nephrology	Management of chronic kidney disease
Gynecology	Counseling and management of contraception Management of dysfunctional uterine bleeding
Maternal fetal medicine	Pre-conception counselling Pregnancy management
Pharmacy	Anticoagulation management Dosing of medications (e.g. antiarrhythmics)
Sleep medicine	Evaluation for obstructive sleep apnea Assessment of risks of positive airway pressure
Hematology	Management of coagulopathy
Nutrition therapy	Optimize weight gain/growth in pediatrics Aid in limiting excessive weight gain in older patients
Exercise physiology	Enhance exercise performance and alleviate symptoms of effort intolerance Improvement in sarcopenia
Pathology	Interpreting liver biopsies within context of a Fontan circulation
Psychology/Psychiatry	Management of disease-related anxiety, depression, post-traumatic stress disorder, or other psychological and psychiatric diagnoses
Social work	Aid in navigating the health care system Health insurance guidance
Research coordinator	Development of a data registry Enrolling patients in research studies

ics have some of the subspecialists involved in the clinic and the model evolves based on patient volume, specific needs of the local patient population, and the available resources.

Pre-clinic Meetings

As mentioned above, regular meetings or huddles help streamline, coordinate, and standardize care. At our center, the Fontan nurse manager presents each patient's history including their anatomy, recent health problems, and current symptoms. The cardiologists then present the recent imaging including echocardiograms, cardiac magnetic resonance imaging (MRI), and angiograms. We have found having a radiologist with expertise in Fontan associated liver disease present at these meetings to be extraordinarily beneficial. The radiologists present the most up-to-date liver imaging. This includes discussion of liver lesions, determining which lesions are high-risk and require more frequent follow-up or targeted biopsy. The team then determines what surveillance testing is necessary and which subspecialist will see each patient. We use *The Advanced Cardiac Therapies Improving Outcomes Network* (ACTION) proposed criteria to help identify which patients should referred to be seen by a heart failure/transplant cardiologist (Fig. 23.2) [2].

Considerations for referral by type of clinical Fontan dysfunction
(recognizing overlap exists between categories)

Cardiac/Systemic Ventricular Dysfunction

1) Severe[1] systolic dysfunction by echocardiogram, MRI, or cardiac catheterization.
2) Moderately depressed (by qualitative assessment) systolic function on imaging when accompanied by ≥moderate systemic AV valve regurgitation.
3) Significant growth derangement or failure to thrive including cachexia or linear growth failure
4) Decreasing exercise tolerance by patient report or as measured on sequential formal exercise testing or 6-minute walk
5) Significant electrophysiologic abnormalities, including recurrent arrhythmias despite therapy, implantation of a cardiac pacemaker, or aborted sudden cardiac death event

Fontan Pathway Dysfunction

1) Symptomatic, chronic fluid overload persisting despite new or increasing diuretic therapy
2) Occurrence of chronic pleural effusions or ascites, chylous or nonchylous, refractory to therapy and occurring outside the initial Fontan post-operative period
3) Major hemodynamic disturbance *resulting in symptoms* despite therapy including: low systemic cardiac output, diastolic ventricular failure, significantly elevated Fontan pressure, or symptomatic cyanosis

Lymphatic Dysfunction

1) Protein-losing enteropathy that has failed medical therapy and requires multiple hospital admissions in a 12-month period or PLE requiring repeated albumin infusions to treat symptoms despite standard PLE medical therapy
2) Plastic bronchitis requiring chronic therapy

Extra-cardiac Dysfunction

1) Hemoptysis requiring evaluation that is unrelated to an infection and persists after standard intervention
2) Liver disease with impaired synthetic function/abnormal liver function testing or undergoing evaluation for liver transplantation
3) Chronic kidney disease – Stage 3 or greater[2]

---

[1] Severe systolic dysfunction in a single ventricle can be graded by a qualitative assessment or by using calculated ejection fractions as follows: < 35% by echocardiogram or MR for a single LV; < 30% by MR for a single RV.
[2] Stage 3 CKD is an eGFR between 30 and 60 mL/min per 1.73 m^2

Version 1, Last Updated 5/30/18
Kurt Schumacher, MD, Steve Kindel, MD, &
ACTION Peds/Adult CHD Committee Members

www.actionlearningnetwork.org

Fig. 23.2 Referral types for Fontan Dysfunction

In-clinic flow

Clinic space should be able to accommodate a multidisciplinary team—ideally with a team-room for providers awaiting patient encounters. These multidisciplinary clinics often occur within a defined cardiology clinic space, to facilitate same-day cardiac testing, including electrocardiography and transthoracic echocardiography.

The Fontan nurse or medical assistant should administer an intake questionnaire that is specific to potential Fontan complications. An example of topics to address at intake is shown in Table 23.3.

The multidisciplinary team can then choose to see the patient in tandem or separately. However, for optimal care, the team should discuss the patient prior to the conclusion of the visit, to agree upon a care plan. At the conclusion of each clinic session, patients are reviewed in a brief team huddle to determine what treatment, testing, or consultations require follow-up and who will be responsible for each task.

Table 23.3 Potential topics to address in an intake questionnaire

Cardiovascular	Dyspnea
	Orthopnea
	Paroxysmal nocturnal dyspnea
	Change in exercise tolerance
	Edema
	Palpitations
	Syncope
	Varicose veins
GI	Abdominal pain
	Ascites
	Changes in stool character
	Jaundice
Pulmonary	Cough
	Hemoptysis
	Production of bronchial casts
Hematology	Current thromboprophylaxis
	Family history of blood clots
Neurology	Symptoms of TIA/stroke
Women's Health	Gynecologic concerns
	Contraception use
Sleep	Sleep apnea screening
Psychology	Depression, anxiety, and post-traumatic stress disorder screening
	Quality of life assessment

Frequency of Testing and Subspecialist Care

A recent survey of 11 Fontan care programs revealed marked variability in care and surveillance strategies [1]. In 2019, the American Heart Association (AHA) published the first comprehensive scientific statement on Fontan circulation, which included suggested surveillance practices shown in Table 23.4 [3]. However, the optimal frequency of testing remains unclear in the absence of rigorous research, and the Scientific Statement included the caveat that there is "insufficient evidence base, as strictly defined by the AHA guidelines for developing and grading recommendations, to support recommendations for specific tests or for the frequency/interval of testing". Screening should, therefore, be tailored to the patient's clinical status and also according to the patient's wishes. It is, as yet, unclear at what point more intensive screening starts providing diminishing returns.

One of the most concerning late complications of the Fontan circulation is hepatocellular carcinoma (HCC). The lifetime incidence of HCC in Fontan patients estimated at 1–5% [4, 5]. There is little information about risk factors for HCC within the Fontan population. HCC has been identified in patients as young 12 years old [4] and in patients without advanced liver disease on liver biopsy [6]. It is unclear how quickly these tumors develop, and, therefore, how frequently to screen. Fontan programs have had to develop liver screening guidelines in this environment. We recommend annual imaging for liver lesion screening in adults, usually alternating between ultrasound and MRI. Ultrasound is less sensitive [7], so any patient with an MRI-identified liver lesion should generally be followed with MRI alone. Ultrasound with contrast may be useful in a subset. We also recommend measuring serum alpha-fetoprotein annually, although there is limited sensitivity so a low level should not be overly reassuring as to the absence of a hepatic neoplasm. Further studies to identify risk factors for HCC and optimal screening practices are needed.

Unnecessary screening waste resources and poses a risk to the patient. Imaging studies are associated with a finite probability of incidental find-

Table 23.4 AHA proposed adult organ system surveillance testing toolkit [3]

Organ system	Basic	In-depth	Investigational
	CMP[a]	FibroSure biomarkers[a]	Liver biopsy
	Platelet count[a]	Alpha-fetoprotein[a]	
	GGT[a]	Liver imaging via CT or MRI	
	PT/INR[a]	Liver elastography (ultrasound or MRI)	
	Lipids[a]		
	Abdominal (liver) ultrasound		
Kidney	BUN[a], creatinine[a]	Urinalysis Urine albumin/creatinine ratio	Nuclear scan GFR
	Cystatin C[a]	Renal ultrasound with Doppler	
Lymph	Albumin[a], total protein[a]	IgG[a]	T2-weighted MRI lymphatic imaging
	Lymphocyte count[a]	Fecal alpha-1 antitrypsin level	Lymphatic angiography
Endocrine/metabolic	Calcium[a]	Parathyroid hormone[a]	Insulin-like growth factor[a]
	25-OH vitamin D[a]	Bone densitometry/DXA scan	
	Nutritional evaluation and consultation		
Hematology	CBC[a], Hgb[a], Hct[a]	Iron[a], TIBC[a], ferritin[a]	Coagulation factors[a]
Lungs	Pulmonary function testing	Chest x-ray	
Neurological/Psychological	Psychological evaluation and consultation	Neurodevelopmental/cognitive testing	Brain MRI

BUN blood urea nitrogen, *CBC* complete blood cell count, *CMP* comprehensive metabolic panel, *CT* computed tomography, *DXA* dual energy x-ray absorptiometry, *GFR* glomerular filtration rate, *GGT* γ-glutamyl transferase, *Hct* hematocrit, *Hgb* hemoglobin, *IgG* immunoglobulin G, *INR* international normalized ratio, *MRI* magnetic resonance imaging, *PT* prothrombin time, *TIBC* total iron-binding capacity

[a] Indicates blood test

ings, which can lead to invasive testing. For example, our program recently performed an abdominal MRI for liver lesion screening on a 32-year-old woman. There was a mildly concerning liver lesion that required a six-month follow-up with MRI. While that study concluded that this lesion was a benign focal nodular hyperplasia (FNH) lesion, an incidental breast mass was discovered. Appropriate follow-up was coordinated, including consultation with a surgical oncologist and additional testing—eventually concluding the mass to be benign. The anxiety and fear of possible breast and liver malignancies negatively affected the quality of life for a patient, exacerbating a comorbid anxiety disorder.

Conclusion

There is now a generation of adult adults with a Fontan circulation who have benefited from a revolution of better knowledge, health care, operative and cardiac intensive care unit techniques. These adults are at risk to develop cardiovascular, hepatic, renal, pulmonary and psychosocial morbidities. Multidisciplinary Fontan clinics have been developed with the goal to detect these morbidities early, improve the quality of life and ultimately the survival for this patient population. We discussed our approach to the Fontan clinic, but one size may not fit all, and each institution may develop a slightly different version of this service.

References

1. Di Maria MV, Brown DW, Cetta F, Ginde S, Goldberg D, Menon SC, et al. Surveillance testing and preventive care after Fontan operation: a multi-institutional survey. Pediatr Cardiol. 2019;40(1):110–5. https://doi.org/10.1007/s00246-018-1966-9.
2. Schumacher KR, Kindel SJ, Committee A. Considerations for advanced heart failure consultation in Fontan patients. https://www.actionlearningnetwork.org/clinicians.
3. Rychik J, Atz AM, Celermajer DS, Deal BJ, Gatzoulis MA, Gewillig MH, et al. Evaluation and manage-

ment of the child and adult with Fontan circulation: a scientific statement from the American Heart Association. Circulation. 2019;140:e234–84. https://doi.org/10.1161/cir.0000000000000696.

4. Egbe AC, Poterucha JT, Warnes CA, Connolly HM, Baskar S, Ginde S, et al. Hepatocellular carcinoma after Fontan operation. Circulation. 2018;138(7):746–8. https://doi.org/10.1161/circulationaha.117.032717.

5. Asrani SK, Warnes CA, Kamath PS. Hepatocellular carcinoma after the Fontan procedure. N Engl J Med. 2013;368(18):1756–7. https://doi.org/10.1056/NEJMc1214222.

6. Mazzarelli C, Cannon MD, Hudson M, Heaton N, Sarker D, Kane P, et al. Hepatocellular carcinoma as a complication of vascular disease of the liver after Fontan procedure. Hepatology. 2019;69(2):911–3. https://doi.org/10.1002/hep.30194.

7. Snowberger N, Chinnakotla S, Lepe RM, Peattie J, Goldstein R, Klintmalm GB, et al. Alpha fetoprotein, ultrasound, computerized tomography and magnetic resonance imaging for detection of hepatocellular carcinoma in patients with advanced cirrhosis. Aliment Pharmacol Ther. 2007;26(9):1187–94. https://doi.org/10.1111/j.1365-2036.2007.03498.x.

Echocardiography and the Adult Fontan Patient

Flavia Fusco and Wei Li

Introduction

Patients with univentricular physiology and Fontan palliation are an extremely heterogeneous group in terms of anatomy and physiology. Before starting to scan a patient with Fontan circulation, a full understanding of Fontan physiology and possible late complications is necessary. It is essential to review the patient's diagnosis and past medical history, including the:

- underlying cardiac anatomy
- surgical history
- type of Fontan operation and perioperative complications
- long-term complications
- recent symptomatology

Based on the available information, a protocolised approach to the echocardiographic investigation is followed, tailored to the needs of each patient.

Fontan Echo Protocol

The protocol must include assessment of:

- the basic cardiovascular anatomy, including situs, the position of the heart, atrio-ventricular (AV) and ventriculo-arterial (VA) connections
- the Fontan (atriopulmonary, Glenn or total cavopulmonary) connections
- ventricular function (systolic and diastolic)
- AV valve(s) anatomy and function
- systemic outflow tract and possible obstruction at valve, supravalvar or subvalvar level, including a restrictive ventricular septal defect (VSD) in the presence of VA discordance.
- pulmonary branches, and residual flow through the main pulmonary artery
- intracardiac shunts, e.g. surgical fenestration, residual Blalock-Taussig shunts, major aortopulmonary collaterals etc.
- exclusion of common complications, e.g. thrombosis of the Fontan pathway.

Basic Cardiac Anatomy

Systematic assessment according to the rules of sequential cardiac segmental analysis must be followed to establish:

- the cardiac position: levo, dextro or mesocardia
- the atrial arrangement: situs solitus or usual arrangement, situs inversus, left or right atrial isomerism, often judged on echo based on the

F. Fusco · W. Li (✉)
Royal Brompton Hospital, National Heart Lung Institute, Imperial College, London, UK
e-mail: w.li@rbht.nhs.uk

position of the inferior vena cava (if present) in relation to the descending aorta on subcostal windows.

- the AV connections: concordant, discordant or double inlet ventricle.
- the VA connections: concordant or discordant, with emphasis on the ventricle (main or rudimentary) from which the aorta arises.

Type of Fontan Connection and Its Patency

Type of Fontan connections include: atriopulmonary connection (Fig. 24.1a), total cavopulmonary connection with lateral tunnel conduit (Fig. 24.1b), total cavo-pulmonary connection with extra-cardiac conduit (Fig. 24.1c) and right atrium-to-right ventricular outflow tract connection (Bjork procedure) (Fig. 24.2a and b).

Flow in Fontan pathway is usually low-velocity (<20–30 cm/s) [1], and phasic with respiration. Flow should be assessed by both colour Doppler (adjusting the Nyqist limit) and pulsed wave Doppler and the mean gradient during one cardiac cycle should be measured. In case of obstruction, there is an increase in flow velocity across the pathway and flow becomes continuous throughout the respiration. A peak velocity > 1 m/s or continuous blood flow in the Fontan pathway or Glenn anastomosis should raise the suspicion of Fontan pathway obstruction, to be investigated with other imaging modalities (e.g. magnetic resonance imaging or CT).

Useful echocardiographic views for assessing the Fontan circulation include the:

- subcostal window, which demonstrates flow from the IVC towards the Fontan pathway
- apical window (4-chamber view and 2-chamber view), which provide a short and long axis view of the pathway (Fig. 24.3a–c).
- right suprasternal long axis view, which is best for showing the Glenn connection: with the assistance of colour Doppler, this view shows the flow down the SVC towards the right pulmonary artery (Fig. 24.4a–c). In case of bilateral SVC a left Glenn connection should be also searched.

In adult patients with an atriopulmonary (AP) connection, the right atrium (RA) is part of the Fontan pathway and is often severely dilated, promoting arrhythmias and blood stasis with spontaneous echo-contrast and thrombus formation. Lateral tunnels may also increase in size over time.

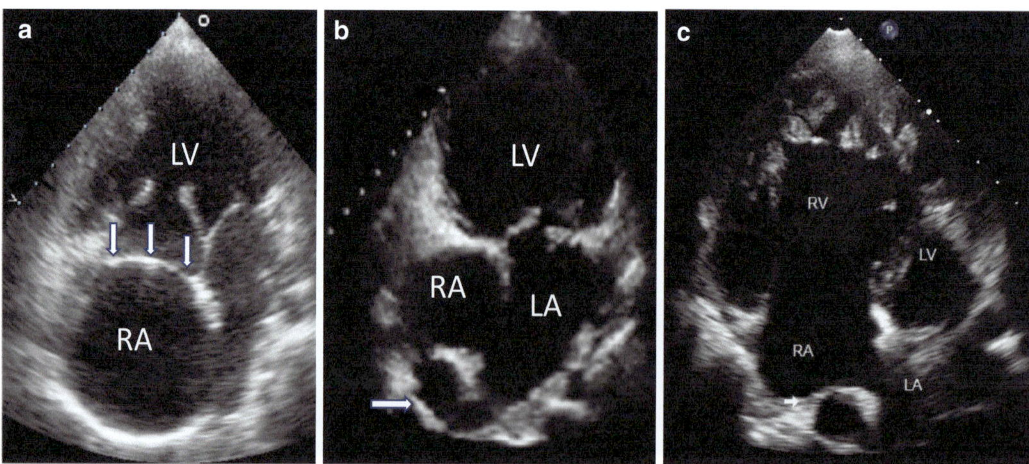

Fig. 24.1 (**a**) Double inlet LV with atrial pulmonary connection, arrow indicate patch above right AV valve, RA dilatation. (**b**) Absent right atrioventricular connection and TCPC with lateral tunnel connection (arrow). (**c**) Hypoplastic left heart and TCPC with an extra cardiac conduit (arrow)

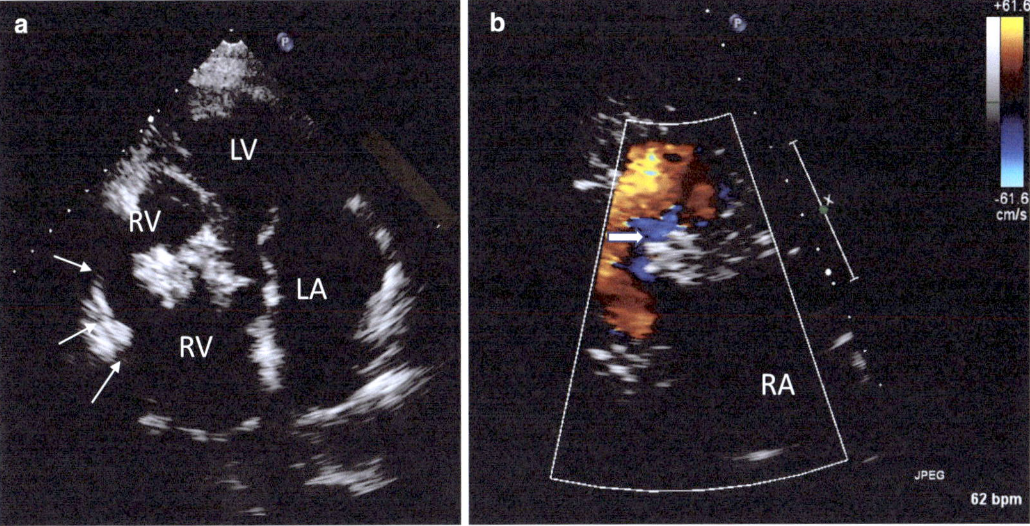

Fig. 24.2 (**a**) Tricuspid atresia, post right atrial to right ventricular outflow tract connection (Bjork procedure, arrow). (**b**) Colour Doppler flow through the RA-RVOT connection

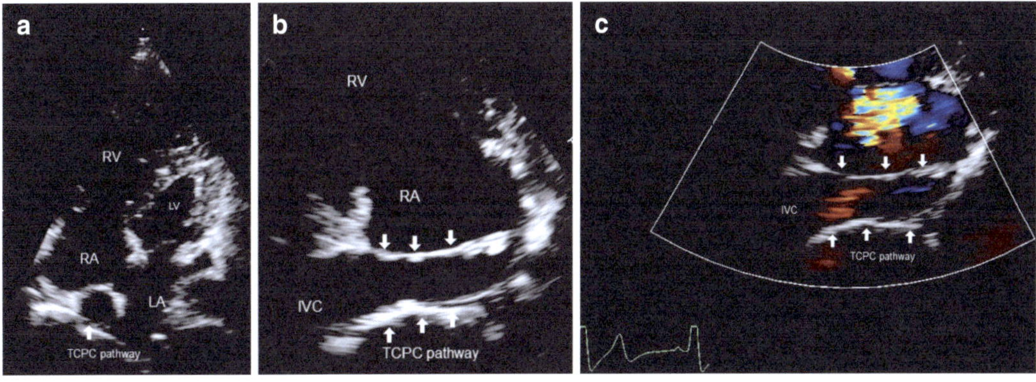

Fig. 24.3 (**a**) Hypoplastic left heart, apical four chamber view shows a short axis view of TCPC pathway (arrow). (**b**) Apical 2 chamber view shows long axis view of the pathway, (**c**) Colour flow from the same image as (**b**) demonstrating lamina flow through the TCPC pathway (arrow)

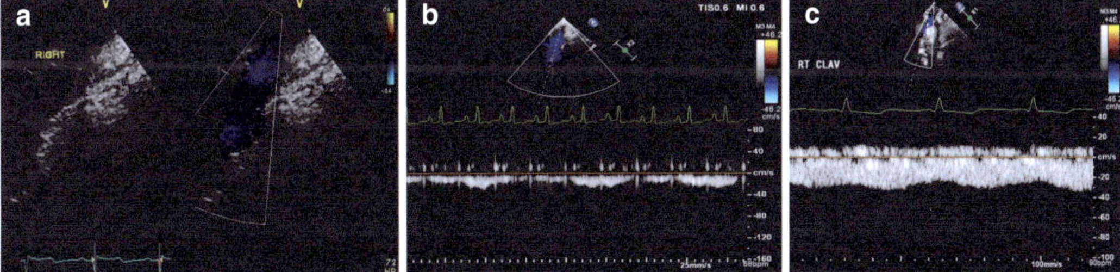

Fig. 24.4 (**a**) Right suprasternal long axis view shows Glenn connection and colour Doppler showed laminal flow in the SVC indicating patent Glenn connection. (**b**) Pulse wave Doppler recording of unobstructed flow in the SVC showing low velocity pulsatile flow increase with inspiration characteristic for patient after TCPC connection. (**c**) Pulse wave Doppler recording of flow in SVC in patient post TCPC, demonstrates low velocity but continuous flow suggestive of obstruction

Ventricular Systolic and Diastolic Function

Ventricular dysfunction, both systolic and diastolic, can impact significantly on the function of the Fontan circulation and cause heart failure and a low cardiac output state. The evaluation of ventricular function may be very challenging in this setting, as standard methods for the assessment of systolic and diastolic function are often not applicable [2] due to underline ventricular morphology, geometry and position, as well as the Fontan pathophysiology (e.g. reduced pulmonary venous return).

A visual estimate of systolic ventricular function (in semiquantitative terms, i.e. normal, or mild-moderate-severe dysfunction) should be provided, but is highly subjective and lacks reproducibility. Quantitative assessment of ventricular function includes:

- Simpson's biplane method: this is most reproducible in patients with a single ventricle of left ventricular (LV) morphology [3], LV volumes and ejection fraction measured by 3-dimensional echocardiography may be more accurate than 2D methods and should be pursued when possible (Fig. 24.5).
- Fractional area change (FAC) is an alternative to Simpson's method, especially for systemic (dominant) right ventricles (RVs) but lacks accuracy (single plane method).
- Advanced echo techniques such as speckle tracking strain (Fig. 24.6) may provide further information on myocardial deformation and asynchrony, but data are lacking on normal reference values for Fontan patients.
- Atrioventricular systolic-to-diastolic duration ratio (S/D ratio, Fig. 24.7): this uses pulse wave or continuous wave Doppler to assess the ratio between the duration of AV valve

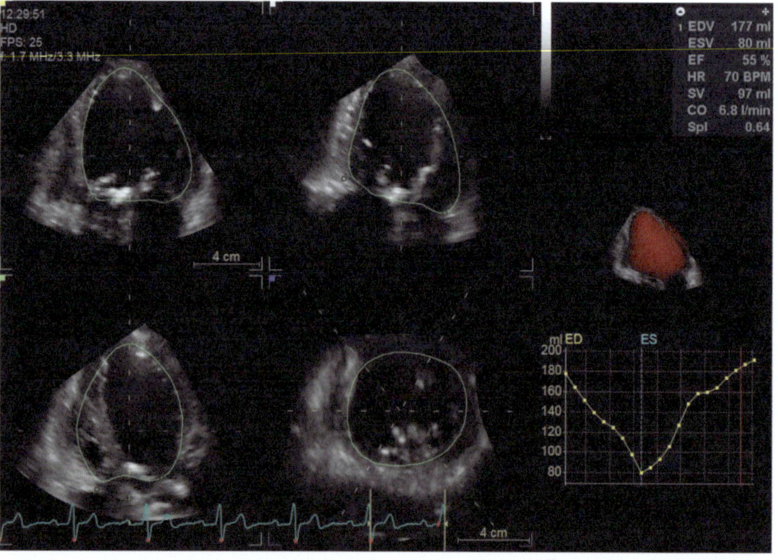

Fig. 24.5 Three-dimensional echocardiography assessment of LV volume and Ejection Fraction in a patient with double inlet left ventricle

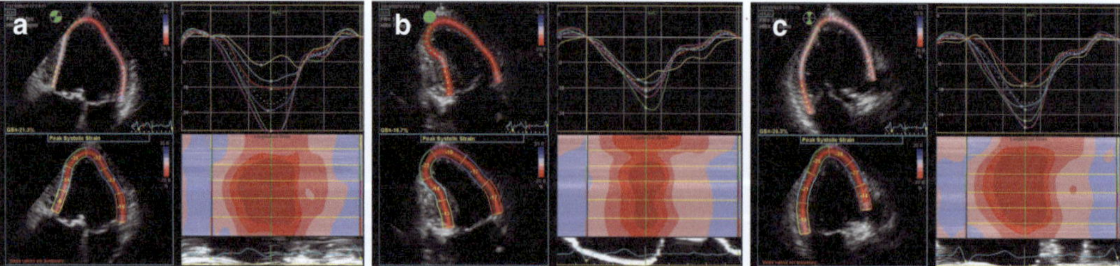

Fig. 24.6 Speckle tracking Echocardiography recording of LV longitudinal strain from (**a**) apical four chamber view (**b**) apical two chamber view and (**c**) apical long axis view from a patient with double inlet left ventricle

Fig. 24.7 Continuous wave Doppler of trans-tricuspid flow. Diastolic duration measured as time during ventricular filling (D) and Systolic duration measured as time duration between the two consecutive filling (S)

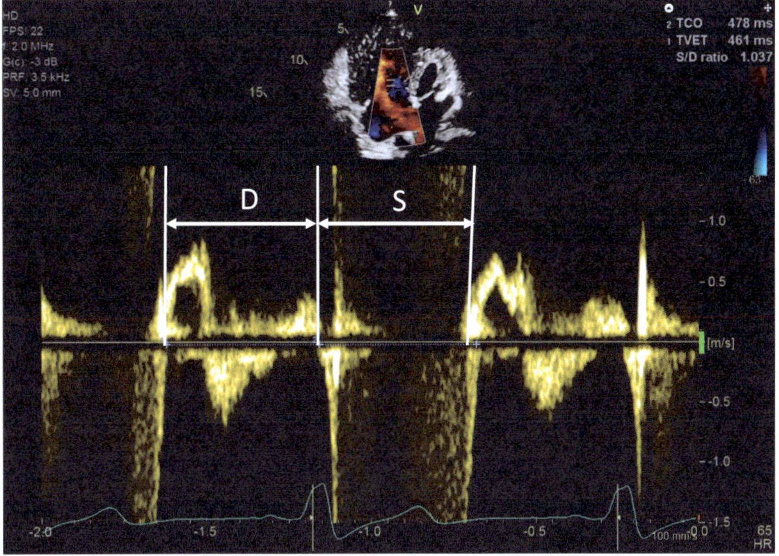

regurgitation (systole) to the duration of ventricular inflow (diastole). Ventricular dysfunction is typically associated with prolongation of the time of AV valve regurgitation. It is a simple parameter that reflects global ventricular systolic and diastolic function and relates to ventricular end-diastolic pressure [3]. An S/D ratio >1.1, together with NYHA functional class >II, were predictors of mortality in adults with Fontan circulation [4].

- Pulmonary vein Doppler: the difference in duration between the pulmonary vein A wave and atrioventricular valve A wave correlates with ventricular filling pressures.
- Pulse wave (PW) Doppler across the AV valve to assess E wave velocity, E/A ratio, and E-wave deceleration time could be used to assess filling pressures in adult Fontan patients. An E velocity of >75 cm/s, deceleration time <135 ms and E/A ratio > 1.7 had good sensitivity and specificity for predicting a PAWP >12 mmHg [5].

Advantages and disadvantages of echocardiographic parameters for assessing ventricular function in Fontan patients are summarised in Table 24.1.

Atrioventricular Valve Function

AV valve regurgitation, even when moderate, can have a significant negative impact on Fontan haemodynamics by reducing effective ventricular output and raising pulmonary venous pressures, increasing total pulmonary resistance and systemic venous pressures.

There are no specific standardised criteria for quantifying AV valve regurgitation in this population. Hence, methods and ranges of normal validated for biventricular hearts are routinely used.

Criteria suggestive of significant regurgitation include:

- vena contracta >6 (PISA method)
- dense spectral Doppler trace
- systolic flow reversal in the pulmonary veins

The PISA method may also be used for serial comparison.

3D and transoesophageal echocardiography (TOE) may be useful in clarifying the mechanism and quantifying the severity of AV valve regurgitation.

Table 24.1 Functional parameters can be included in routine Echo assessment of univentricular heart

Echo parameter	Advantages	Disadvantages
MAPSE TAPSE Tissue Doppler	– Easy to measure – Highly reproducible – Useful for serial assessment during FU	– Reflects only longitudinal shortening – Not reliable in case of AV valve regurgitation – Low sensibility for subtle systolic function changes
FAC	– Radial systolic function – Useful for unusual ventricular geometry	Highly observer-dependent
Simpson's biplane	– More accurate systolic function estimation in morphological left ventricle	Not feasible in case of morphological right ventricle, indeterminant ventricle
S/D duration ratio	– Easily measurable – Reflets global systolic and diastolic function – High positive predictive value for raised end-diastolic pressure – Predictor of mortality	Study was based on small number of patients
E/A	– Easy to measure and interpret – Load dependent	Standard adult population derived criteria for diastolic dysfunction and no proven normal values in Fontan patients
E/E' lateral	– Easy to measure and interpret	
Strain	– High sensitivity for subtle systolic function changes	– No reference values for this population – Difficulties related to unusual ventricular shape
3D volumes	– More accurate volumes and systolic function estimation especially for unusual ventricular shape	– Lack of availability – No reference values for this population

MAPSE mitral annulus plane systolic excursion, *TAPSE* tricuspid annulus plane systolic excursion, *FAC* fractional area change, *S/D* systolic-to-diastolic ratio

Systemic Ventricular Outflow Tract Obstruction and Aortic Regurgitation

Obstruction should be excluded at:

- Subaortic level
- Aortic valve level
- Ascending aorta
- Aortic arch

In patients with double inlet left ventricle or absent right AV connection and VA discordance, the aorta arises from a rudimentary (right) ventricle and the main (left) ventricle is in communication with the rudimentary chamber through a ventricular septal defect (VSD). This VSD may become restrictive, thus hemodynamically acting as subaortic stenosis, which can be very detrimental to cardiac output in patients with a Fontan circulation. This is a particularly challenging diagnosis and an ejection systolic murmur on auscultation should raise the suspicion. The VA relation should be established with certainty on echocardiography and/or other imaging modality. The VSD is assessed on parasternal long-axis view, which demonstrates turbulent colour Doppler flow at the VSD site and the flow velocity can be measured using continuous wave Doppler (Fig. 24.8a–c).

A membranous or fibrous subaortic ring, valvular stenosis, or aortic coarctation may also be present, causing pressure overload to the systemic ventricle and limiting cardiac output. Re-coarctation/stenosis at the site of repair of an interrupted and /or hypoplastic arch should be assessed accordingly. Indirect signs of a significant systemic outflow tract obstruction include a hypertrophied dominant ventricle, with evidence of diastolic dysfunction. Stress echo can be used to delineate a dynamic obstruction and its clinical impact in a patient with exertional symptoms.

Aortic valve regurgitation is not common in this setting but can develop as the result of root/ascending aortic dilatation, or can be iatrogenic,

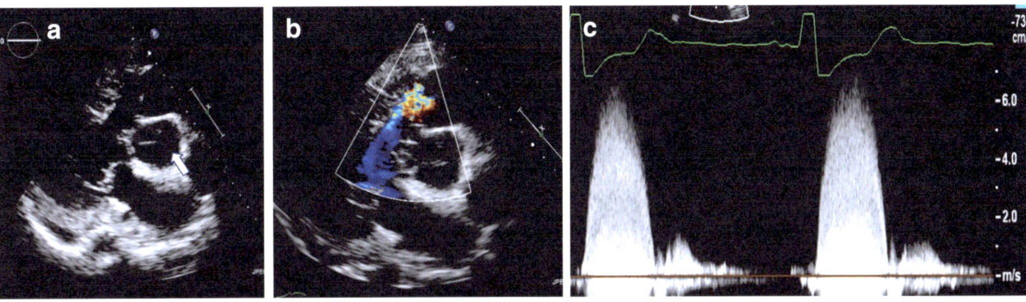

Fig. 24.8 Parasternal long axis view from a patient with absent right atrioventricular connection and ventricular-arterial discordance shows (**a**) a small VSD (arrow) with (**b**) turbulent flow on colour Doppler. (**c**) Continuous wave Doppler recording of flow through the VSD shows high velocity (>6 m/s) suggesting VSD is significantly restrictive

e.g. cusp perforation during emergency retrograde (transaortic) temporary cardiac pacing. Quantification of aortic regurgitation uses the same criteria as for biventricular hearts.

Pulmonary Branches

Visualisation of the pulmonary branches may not be easy in adult Fontan patients. The best view is the suprasternal view, in which the left pulmonary branch is seen below the descending aorta. The right pulmonary branch is best imaged from the right suprasternal view, which is best for showing the Glenn anastomosis (SVC to right pulmonary artery connection). Colour and Pulsed-wave Doppler may be useful to identify pulmonary branch stenoses but, in the presence of passive flow to the lungs, standard criteria do not apply.

Intracardiac and Extra-cardiac Shunts

- Shunt at atrial level: a large non-restrictive communication between the two atria is important after lateral tunnel or extra-cardiac conduit TCPC.
- Shunt at ventricular level: the VSD is usually unrestricted, with low velocity bidirectional flow, depending on VA connection, as explained above. Indeed, in patients with VA discordance and a dominant LV, the blood pumped by the LV must cross the VSD to reach the aorta.
- Fontan fenestration: this is a surgical shunt, which is identified using colour Doppler. The mean gradient across the fenestration can be measured and reflects the pressure difference between systemic venous system (Fontan circulation) and (left) atrial pressure (i.e. the transpulmonary gradient). Agitated saline injection from a femoral or lower limb vein may be used to confirm and quantify the shunt.
- Pulmonary arteriovenous malformations bypass the pulmonary capillaries and can be diagnoses by injecting agitated saline from a peripheral vein on the arm (depending on the anatomy).
- Veno-venous malformations (i.e. systemic venous blood bypassing the lungs, seeking a low resistance route to the systemic ventricle) are difficult to identify but may be suspected when there is reduced blood flow down the SVC and through the Glenn anastomosis (with flow down the azygos vein) or large venous collaterals are seen.

Other Complications (Table 24.2)

Patients with atriopulmonary Fontan connection or a dilated conduit are particularly prone to thrombus formation in the circuit, that could cause obstruction or emboli to the pulmonary circulation, with devastating effect on cardiac out-

Table 24.2 Fontan circuit complications to be ruled out at routine Echocardiography

RA/lateral tunnel dilatation, promoting arrhythmias and thrombus formation
Conduit leak/residual fenestration after percutaneous closure
Fontan connection obstruction (see paragraph on Echo assessment of Fontan pathway)
Thrombus formation (see text)
Pulmonary veins compression (see text)
Single ventricle systolic/diastolic dysfunction (see paragraph)
Significant AV valve/aortic regurgitation (see paragraph)
Outflow tract obstruction

put and systemic venous pressures. Multiple and unconventional views are needed to ensure a complete visualization of the entire Fontan circuit.

Pulmonary vein compression by a giant RA or extra-cardiac conduit is also possible in Fontan patients. Pulsed wave Doppler peak velocity > 1.2 m/s may suggest the pulmonary venous obstruction.

Other complications can be detected or suspected during echocardiography include: stenosis at surgical anastomoses (e.g. if valved conduits were used to construct the Fontan circulation), thrombosis of the Glenn anastomosis (e.g. in a patient with a long venous line or central line), pericardial or pleural effusions, ascites, hepatomegaly and/or splenomegaly and endocarditis.

TOE is often indicated to confirm a suspicion raise by transthoracic echo and to guide interventions (e.g. closure of a fenestration). TOE should also be performed prior to DC cardioversion in patients with atrial tachycardia who are not on effective long-term anticoagulation, to rule out thrombus in the systemic atrium.

References

1. Lai WW, Mertens L, Cohen MS, Geva T. Chapter 28. Echocardiographic assessment of functionally single ventricles after the Fontan operation. In: Echocardiography in pediatric and congenital heart disease. From fetus to adult, 2nd ed. Wiley Blackwell. pp. 541–555.
2. Margossian R, Sleeper LA, Pearson GD, Barker PC, Mertens L, Quartermain MD, Su JT, Shirali G, Chen S, Colan SD, for the Pediatric Heart Network Investigators. Assessment of diastolic function in single ventricle patients following the Fontan procedure. J Am Soc Echocardiogr. 2016;29(11):1066–73.
3. Cordina R, Ministeri M, Babu-Narayan SV, Ladouceur M, Celermajer DS, Gatzoulis MA, et al. Evaluation of the relationship between ventricular end-diastolic pressure and echocardiographic measures of diastolic function in adults with a Fontan circulation. Int J Cardiol. 2018;259(15):71–5.
4. Miranda WR, Warnes CA, Connolly HM, Taggart NW, O'Leary PW, Oh JK, et al. Echo-Doppler assessment of ventricular filling pressures in adult Fontan patients. Int J Cardiol. 2019;284:28–32.
5. Cordina R, von Klemperer K, Kempny A, West C, Senior R, Celermajer DS, et al. Echocardiographic predictors of mortality in adults with a Fontan circulation. JACC Cardiovasc Imaging. 2017;10(2):212–3.

Cardiac MRI Imaging in the Fontan Patient

Paul Clift, Lucy Hudsmith, and Ben Holloway

Abbreviations

2D	Two dimensional
3D	Three dimensional
AP	Atriopulmonary
CMR	Cardiac magnetic resonance imaging
DILV	Double inlet left ventricle
FALD	Fontan associated liver disease
IVC	Inferior vena cava
SVC	Superior vena cava
TCPC	Total cavopulmonary connection
TGA	Transposition of the great arteries

In the early years of the Fontan circulation, there were limited imaging techniques available to monitor the patient's progress. 2D echocardiography allowed serial monitoring of ventricular function and colour flow, continuous wave and pulse waved Doppler allowed for monitoring of flow characteristics and valve function. However, image resolution was at times poor and volumetric assessment was difficult, as the usual geometric assumptions do not apply to a single ventricle. The development of cross-sectional imaging techniques, such as CT and cardiac MRI (CMR) scanning, has significantly improved spatial resolution so routine cardiac catheterisation is no longer necessary. CMR is now considered the imaging modality of choice for complex congenital heart disease, due to its ability to provide both functional and anatomical information, and when necessary, tissue characterisation without ionising radiation.

While CMR is the mainstay for imaging patients with complex congenital disease, it has significant limitations when assessing metal structures, such as stents and occlusion devices, due to susceptibility artefact. However, in controlled conditions, it is rare that metal structures (or a pacemaker) would preclude an MRI scan. Although CMR does provide excellent special resolution, it is below the isotropic resolution (the size of the voxels used in a volume data set) of CT, which may be required for optimal imaging of complications, such as pulmonary arteriovenous malformations, venous collaterals and pulmonary emboli. CT radiation doses have dramatically reduced over the last 15 years, but serial use of CT is not recommended in this young population.

When performing CMR for patients with congenital heart disease it is important to focus on the clinical question that is most pertinent first, as

P. Clift (✉) · L. Hudsmith
Department of Cardiology, Queen Elizabeth Hospital,
Birmingham, UK
e-mail: Paul.clift@uhb.nhs.uk;
Lucy.Hudsmith@uhb.nhs.uk

B. Holloway
Department of Radiology, Queen Elizabeth Hospital,
Birmingham, UK
e-mail: Ben.Holloway@uhb.nhs.uk

P. Clift et al. (eds.), *Univentricular Congenital Heart Defects and the Fontan Circulation*,
https://doi.org/10.1007/978-3-031-36208-8_25

the investigation can be long and some patients may not be able to tolerate lengthy scans (Table 25.1). Assessment is, in general, centred around establishing the anatomy, function and flow of the Fontan circuit and ventricles [2].

Due to specific haemodynamic and anatomical considerations of the Fontan circulation, contrast medium delivery needs special consideration, especially with CT [1]. If delivered from the arm, opacified blood from the SVC will pass to the pulmonary arteries and mix with non-opacified blood from the IVC, which can result in patchy enhancement that can mimic an embolus. This can be overcome with dual leg and arm injection or delaying the phase of image acquisition to improve homogeneity of opacification in the pulmonary arteries. Detailed knowledge of the original anatomy and operations performed is, therefore, essential in planning the scan (such as azygos continuation of the IVC).

Table 25.1 CMR protocol [1]

Target	CMR sequence	Contrast needed
Anatomy	Black blood spin-echo Steady-state free precession (SSFP) in three orthogonal planes Non-enhanced navigator whole heart sequences using b-SSFP	No
Ventricular function	Cine balanced SSFP (b-SSFP) in long and short axis	No
Fontan pathway/ outflow tract/ branch PA	Non-enhanced navigator whole heart sequences using b-SSFP Cine b-SSFP Phase-contrast sequences	No
Flow dynamics and small vessel assessment	Time-resolved MRA	Yes
Myocardial scarring	Delayed enhancement imaging	Yes

CMR for Surveillance and Prognosis

Assessment of Ventricular Function

CMR is the most accurate imaging modality for volume analysis. Modern gated dual source CT scanning allows accurate volume analysis, but comes at the cost of ionising radiation and is, therefore, not suitable for serial monitoring.

Monitoring of single ventricle volumes and function is important. The life of a Fontan patient is characterised by a variable steady state with mild effort intolerance, followed by a later stage of Fontan failure, characterised by rapid decline and multi-organ failure. It is important to identify patients progressing to Fontan failure before they develop advanced liver disease or multi-organ involvement, as this will preclude cardiac transplantation. Early referral for transplantation may improve the chances of a successful outcome. [3] CMR can be useful in the timely referral of Fontan patients for advanced heart failure therapies (Fig. 25.1). Increasing volumes and a cut off of 156 mL/m² predicts transplant-free survival independent of other factors [4], with additional CMR derived parameters, such as ventricular mass, stroke volume and an ejection fraction <40%, also being relevant [5]. Patients with an ICD or pacemaker were not included in the above study, and whilst ICD use is rare in this population, pacemakers (especially epicardial devices) are relatively common [6].

Fontan Pathway Imaging

CMR provides excellent imaging of the Fontan pathway and branch pulmonary arteries (Figs. 25.2 and 25.3) and can identify anatomical narrowing, when present (Fig. 25.4). However, with increasing catheter-based interventions being performed post Fontan surgery [7], implanted devices and stents can often obscure CMR imaging, even when the implanted devices

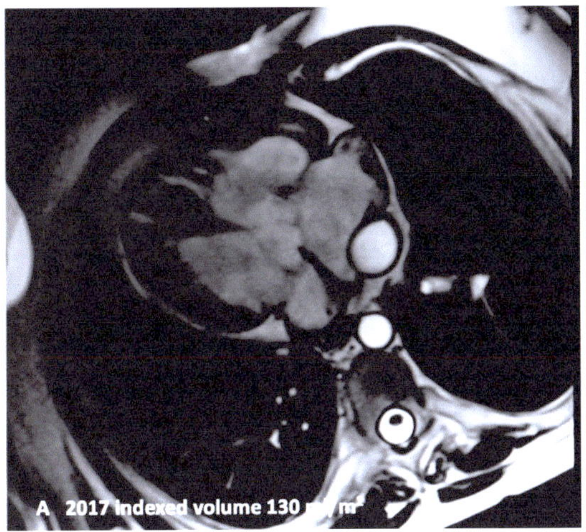

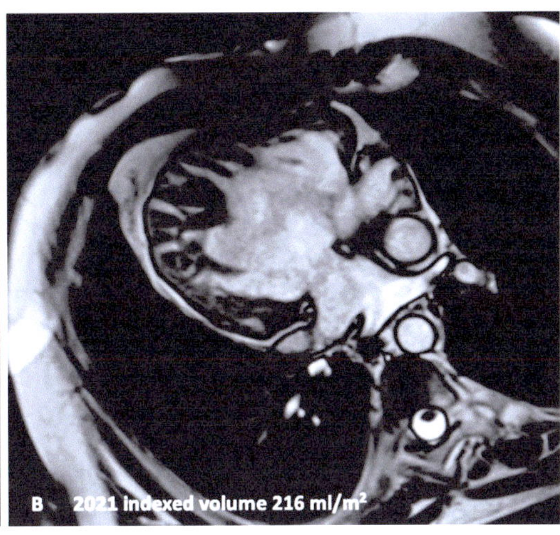

Fig. 25.1 bSSFP cine 4 chamber images of double inlet left ventricle, dextrocardia, situs inversus in an adult with a lateral tunnel TCPC, showing progressive ventricular dilatation associated with symptomatic decline and falling peak VO_2 over a 4-year interval

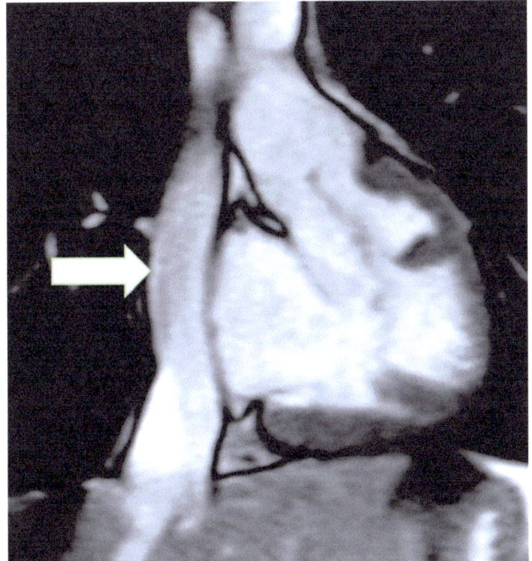

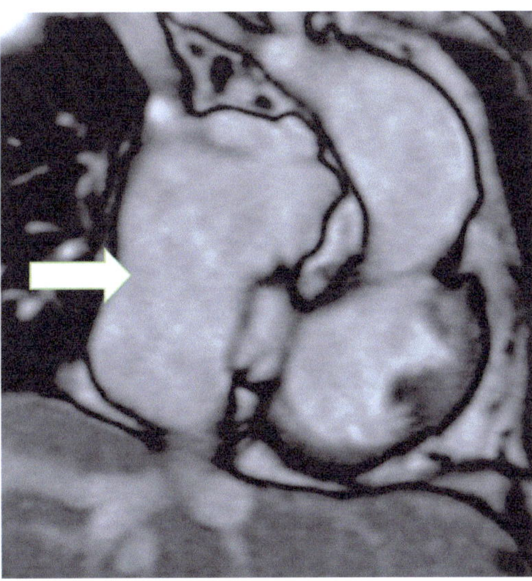

Fig. 25.2 bSSFP coronal image of a 20 mm Goretex extra cardiac conduit TCPC Fontan (white arrow) in a 22-year-old with double inlet left ventricle and transposed great arteries

Fig. 25.3 bSSFP coronal imaging of an atriopulmonary Fontan chamber (white arrow) in a 34-year-old with double inlet left ventricle and transposed great arteries

are MRI compatible (Figs. 25.5 and 25.6). The left pulmonary artery (LPA) is often compressed by the Damus-Kaye-Stansel connection following Norwood surgery for hypoplastic left heart syndrome (HLHS) and stent placement in the LPA is often performed to optimise pulmonary blood flow [8]. Similarly, fenestration of the extra-cardiac conduit is routine in many centres and post Fontan manipulation of the fenestration is frequently performed, either stenting the fenestration open [9] or using a device to close it [10]

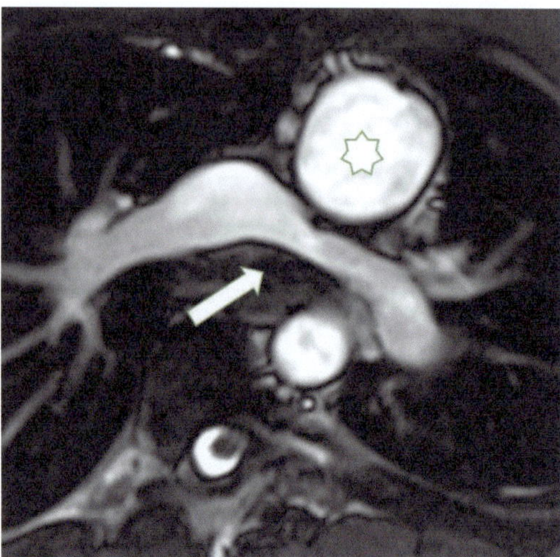

Fig. 25.4 bSSFP cine image of mildly narrowed LPA (white arrow) with no stent behind a Damus-Kaye-Stansel connection (white asterisk) in a 20 years old HLHS post Fontan

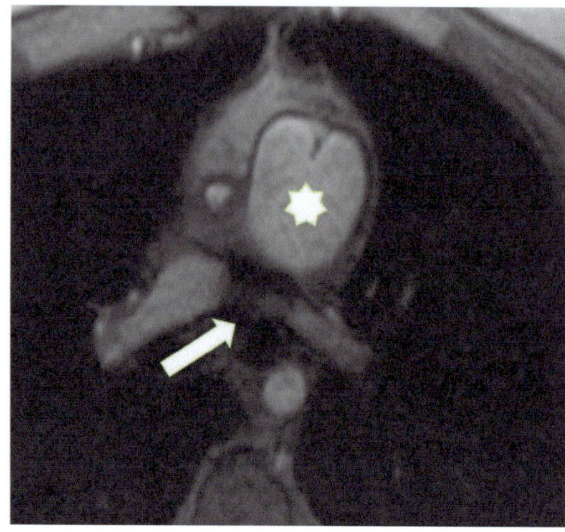

Fig. 25.6 Gradient echo cine of LPA stent (white arrow) behind Damus-Kaye-Stansel connection (white asterisk) in a 21 year old following Norwood palliation for HLHS

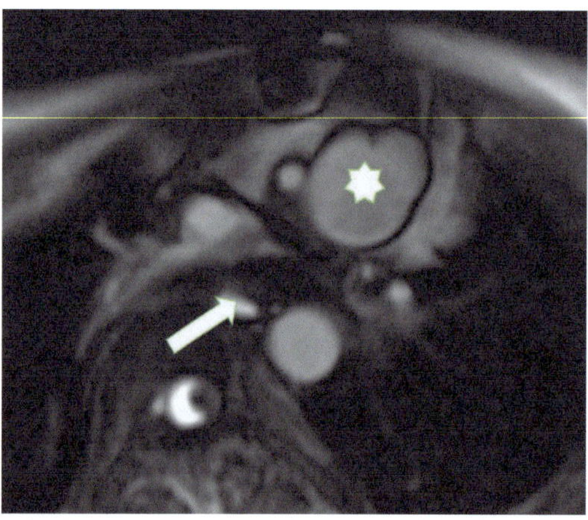

Fig. 25.5 bSSFP showing LPA stent (white arrow) causing signal loss obscuring image behind Damus-Kaye-Stansel connection (white asterisk) in a 19 years old following staged Norwood palliation for HLHS

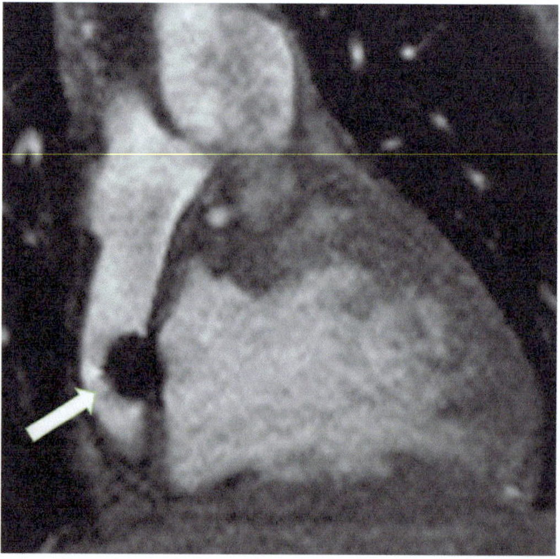

Fig. 25.7 Gradient echo cine of the TCPC. Goretex extra cardiac conduit TCPC with device closure of fenestration (white arrow) in a 20-year-old with HLHS

(Fig. 25.7). In such cases cardiac catheterisation will be required to accurately assess the pressures in the circuit. In addition, following Norwood palliation for HLHS, the Damus-Kaye-Stansel connection can dilate [11] and requires surveillance. There may also be narrowing in the distal aortic arch (Fig. 25.8), which may require balloon dilatation and stenting [12](Fig. 25.9).

Imaging for Fontan Complications

The early modifications of the Fontan operation led to a valveless system, by which the SVC and IVC entered the right atrium, which was baffled to the pulmonary arteries, often via an anastomosis of the right atrial appendage to the pulmonary arteries. Over time, the right atrium dilates sig-

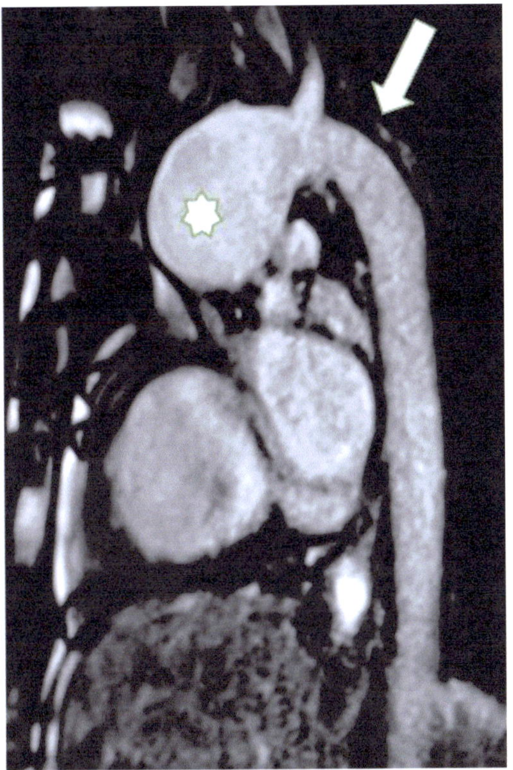

Fig. 25.8 Navigator non-contrast MRA of the aorta showing normal distal arch anastomosis (white arrow) and dilated Damus-Kaye-Stansel (white asterisk) in a young adult post Norwood palliation for HLHS

nificantly, and blood flow within becomes slow and turbulent predisposing to several typical complications, namely arrhythmia (scar-related macro re-entrant atrial tachycardias), thrombus formation and compression of the right sided pulmonary veins. CMR provides excellent imaging of the atrial chamber and can easily detect associated compression of the pulmonary veins (Fig. 25.10). The venous compression, arrhyth-

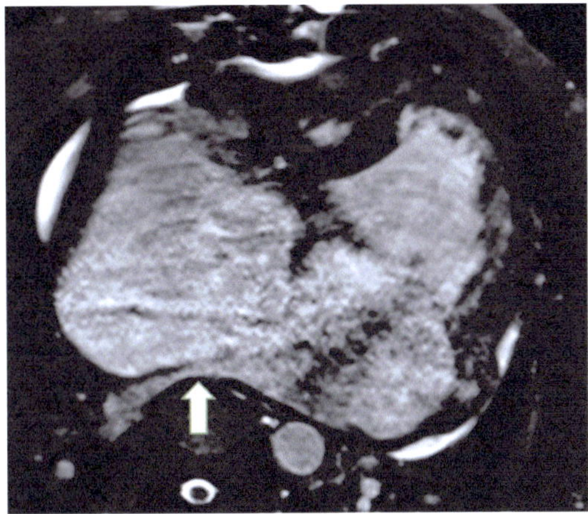

Fig. 25.10 Navigator non-contrast MRA axial showing compression of right lower pulmonary vein by the right atrial chamber in an older adult with tricuspid atresia, classical Glenn and atriopulmonary Fontan

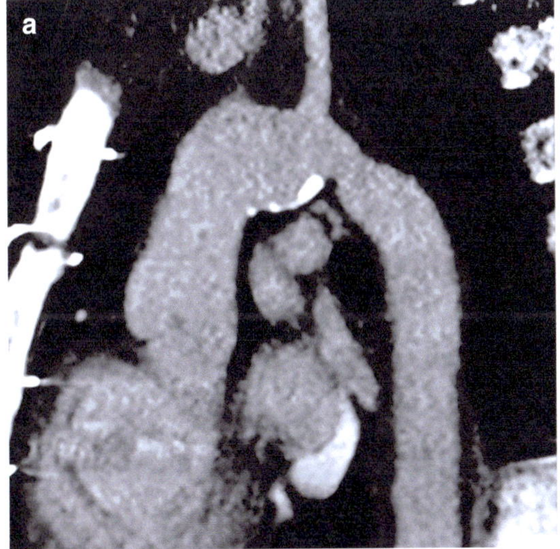

Fig. 25.9 CT angiogram of arch showing narrowing (white arrow, panel **a**) following staged Norwood palliation of congenitally corrected transposition of the great arteries with mitral atresia in a young adult presenting

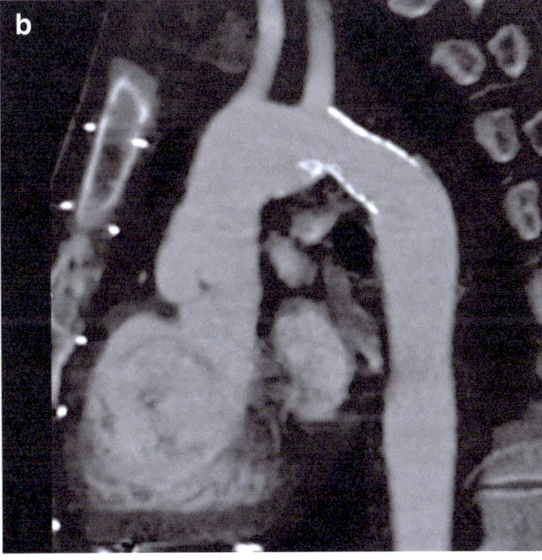

with angina; this was treated by uncovered balloon-expandable stent insertion into the distal arch (white arrow, panel **b**), with resolution of symptoms. CMR was not possible due to epicardial pacing system

mia and energy losses within the dilating chamber are indications for converting an atriopulmonary Fontan to the more energy-efficient total cavopulmonary connection (TCPC) Fontan [13]. Surgery is usually combined with a MAZE operation for addressing the arrhythmia substrate [14]. Pulmonary venous compression is rarely evident in the extra-cardiac TCPC, but could still develop following lateral tunnel TCPC, where atrial tissue persists and can expand.

High systemic venous pressure is required to drive forward flow through the pulmonary circulation, but has an adverse effect on the liver, leading to fibrosis even early after Fontan completion. This is regardless of the type of surgical procedure and is inherent to the Fontan circulation. Fontan associated liver disease (FALD) rarely causes liver dysfunction or clinical features of portal hypertension, however cirrhosis and nodular liver disease are not uncommon and hepatocellular carcinoma is a rare but often fatal outcome of FALD [15] (Fig. 25.11).

The ideal liver surveillance strategy is not yet established but typically includes annual ultrasound surveillance with non-invasive assessments of biomarkers of fibrosis. Many centres use *Fibroscan* assessment for liver fibrosis, although hepatic congestion will in itself lead to abnormal *Fibroscan* readings. Whilst fibrosis is present in most Fontan patients on liver biopsy, it is not predicted by many of the non-invasive tests available [16]. Liver MRI is useful in patients with abnormal ultrasounds scans and for the investigations of liver nodules detected on ultrasound. The clinical utility of magnetic resonance elastography (MRE) [17] and T1 and T2 [17] remain under investigation. MRI diffusion imaging of the liver suggests that the likely aetiology of FALD is abnormal microperfusion within the liver [17, 18].

The slow non-pulsatile flow within the Fontan circulation, predisposes patients to venous thrombo-embolism and occlusive thrombus within the Fontan circuit, especially in patients with an atriopulmonary Fontan circulation (Fig. 25.12). Whether modern Fontan circulations with either lateral tunnel or extra-cardiac conduit have the same risk is uncertain; in theory, the improved laminar flow characteristics in the TCPC should reduce the risk of thrombus formation. In many centres, anti-platelet therapy is often used in TCPC patients, rather than formal anticoagulation with Vitamin K antagonists. The role of direct oral anticoagulants (DOACS) is under investigation. The most sensitive MRI

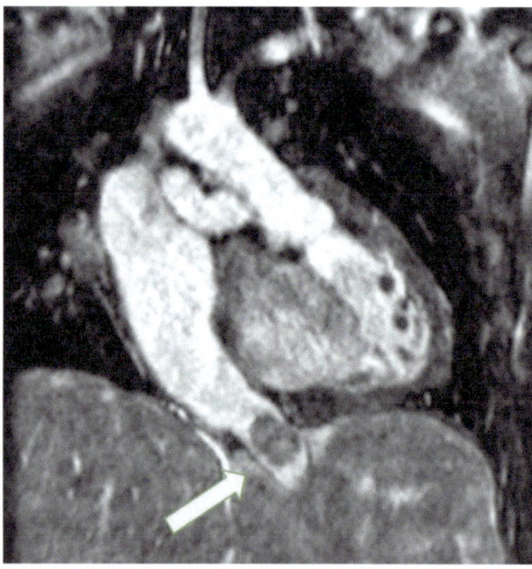

Fig. 25.11 tfi3D nav _3D MRA In a young adult with left atrial isomerism, tricuspid atresia and multiple VSDs with tumour thrombus from a hepatocellular carcinoma arising from left lobe of liver extending into the IVC portion of conduit (white arrow)

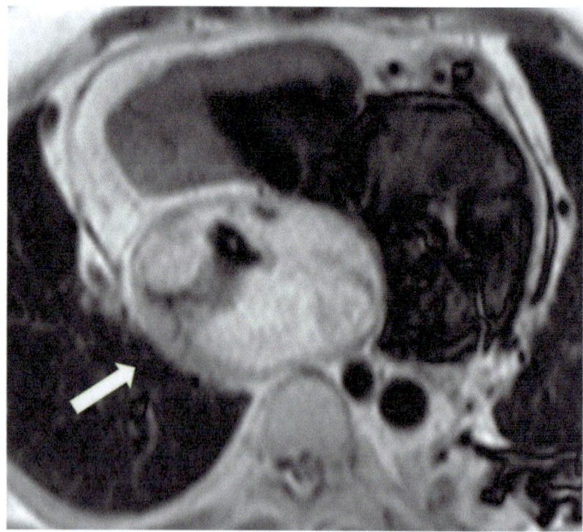

Fig. 25.12 Black blood axial image showing near-occlusion of an atriopulmonary (AP) Fontan chamber in an older adult with tricuspid atresia dextrocardia and a previous classical Glenn and AP Fontan to LPA

sequence to detect thrombus is the early phase inversion recovery scan post Gadolinium contrast although balanced SSFP; black blood and navigator sequences can often detect thrombus as a low-intensity lesion in the Fontan pathway and inversion recovery water-selective fast gradient-echo acquisition may identify hyperintense acute thrombus by nullifying the signals from fat [19].

Identification of venous-venous collaterals and arteriovenous collaterals is best performed with contrast enhanced CT scanning, owing to better spatial resolution. Whilst CMR can assess flow in the collaterals and their impact on ventricular loading, the accuracy of flow assessments by CMR in the Fontan circulation is disputed. In adult practice, collaterals are often not intervened upon unless there is haemoptysis or profound exertional cyanosis.

Other MRI Modalities

Newer CMR techniques require further evaluation in imaging the Fontan patient. Feature tracking allows the assessment of longitudinal and circumferential strain with post acquisition analysis of SSFP cine images, and has been shown to correlate with ejection fraction and ventricular volume, NTproBNP and exercise parameters. However, reproducibility is inconsistent across all ventricular segments. Initial studies suggest it may be a sensitive marker of ventricular dysfunction, but there is currently minimal longitudinal data [20–22].

Myocardial tissue characterisation with T1 and T2 parametric mapping and extracellular volume (ECV) fraction is an evolving area, and analysis can be performed with little additional scanning time [23]. The value of native T1 mapping characteristics is established for several conditions, such as diffuse myocardial fibrosis, oedema, inflammation, infiltrative diseases (e.g. amyloidosis, Fabry disease (FD) and hemosiderosis) [24]. T2 relaxation times relate more to oedema and are, therefore, useful in the detection of acute myocardial infarction, myocarditis, stress cardiomyopathy, sarcoidosis and

cardiac allograft rejection. With the addition of gadolinium enhancement and using T1 mapping techniques, the ECV fraction can be calculated. Expansion of the ECV is typically associated with myocardial fibrosis. Given that diastolic dysfunction is associated with myocardial fibrosis and is thought to be clinically present in patients with a Fontan circulation, T1 mapping and ECV fraction may prove useful in the Fontan population. However, at present, mapping techniques are hampered by inconsistency between scanners (each needing normal range assessment) and this technique is challenging with the complex geometry of the single ventricle.

Phase contrast MRI techniques have been extensively used for modelling of the flow characteristics within the Fontan circulation. Initial *in vitro* modelling of the Fontan circulation by de Leval and colleagues led to the development of the lateral tunnel total cavopulmonary anastomosis. They observed flow in a model of the atriopulmonary Fontan, and calculated power losses and where they occurred. They hypothesised that by removing the atrial pump, directing flow from the IVC to the PA and using a bidirectional Glenn, they could improve the fluid dynamics and reduce energy losses [25]. This pivotal work has led to the modern Fontan operation. Phase contrast MRI techniques have allowed in vivo analysis of flow [26] and continue to direct innovation in Fontan pathway design [27–30], and the creation of personalised Fontan pathways [31]. 4D flow characterisation across the whole of the circulation is being investigated [32–34] and may yet help define the imaging phenotype of the optimal or failing Fontan circulation, albeit at the expense of long scanning times.

CMR has a key role in the surveillance of the patient following Fontan surgery. It provides accurate anatomical and functional data and allows us to better understand the innovations in Fontan surgery through CMR derived flow analysis. Integration of such information with other imaging modalities will further enhance our understanding of what a good or failing Fontan looks like.

References

1. Lewis G, et al. Cross-sectional imaging of the Fontan circuit in adult congenital heart disease. Clin Radiol. 2015;70(6):667–75.
2. Sachdeva R, et al. ACC/AHA/ASE/HRS/ISACHD/SCAI/SCCT/SCMR/SOPE 2020 appropriate use criteria for multimodality imaging during the follow-up care of patients with congenital heart disease: a report of the American College of Cardiology Solution Set Oversight Committee and Appropriate use Criteria Task Force, American Heart Association, American Society of Echocardiography, Heart Rhythm Society, International Society for Adult Congenital Heart Disease, Society for Cardiovascular Angiography and Interventions, Society of Cardiovascular Computed Tomography, Society for Cardiovascular Magnetic Resonance, and Society of Pediatric Echocardiography. J Am Coll Cardiol. 2020;75(6):657–703.
3. McMahon A, McNamara J, Griffin M. A review of heart transplantation for adults with congenital heart disease. J Cardiothorac Vasc Anesth. 2021;35(3):752–62.
4. Meyer SL, et al. Integrated clinical and magnetic resonance imaging assessments late after Fontan operation. J Am Coll Cardiol. 2021;77(20):2480–9.
5. Rathod RH, et al. Cardiac magnetic resonance parameters predict transplantation-free survival in patients with Fontan circulation. Circ Cardiovasc Imaging. 2014;7(3):502–9.
6. Alenius Dahlqvist J, et al. Pacemaker treatment after Fontan surgery—a Swedish national study. Congenit Heart Dis. 2019;14(4):582–9.
7. Bhole V, et al. Transcatheter interventions in the early postoperative period after the Fontan procedure. Catheter Cardiovasc Interv. 2011;77(1):92–8.
8. Noonan P, et al. Stenting of the left pulmonary artery after palliation of hypoplastic left heart syndrome. Catheter Cardiovasc Interv. 2016;88(2):225–32.
9. Anderson B, et al. Novel technique to reduce the size of a Fontan Diabolo stent fenestration. Catheter Cardiovasc Interv. 2010;76(6):860–4.
10. Thatte N, et al. Use of institutional criteria for transcatheter device closure of Fontan fenestration—midterm outcomes. Ann Pediatr Cardiol. 2020;13(4):327–33.
11. Cohen MS, et al. Neo-aortic root dilation and valve regurgitation up to 21 years after staged reconstruction for hypoplastic left heart syndrome. J Am Coll Cardiol. 2003;42(3):533–40.
12. Aldoss O, et al. Acute and mid-term outcomes of stent implantation for recurrent coarctation of the aorta between the Norwood operation and Fontan completion: a multi-center pediatric interventional cardiology early career society investigation. Catheter Cardiovasc Interv. 2017;90(6):972–9.
13. Kreutzer J, et al. Conversion of modified Fontan procedure to lateral atrial tunnel cavopulmonary anastomosis. J Thorac Cardiovasc Surg. 1996;111(6):1169–76.
14. Mavroudis C, et al. Evolving anatomic and electrophysiologic considerations associated with Fontan conversion. Semin Thorac Cardiovasc Surg Pediatr Card Surg Annu. 2007;10:136–45.
15. Egbe AC, et al. Hepatocellular carcinoma after Fontan operation: multicenter case series. Circulation. 2018;138(7):746–8.
16. Munsterman ID, et al. The clinical spectrum of Fontan-associated liver disease: results from a prospective multimodality screening cohort. Eur Heart J. 2019;40(13):1057–68.
17. Silva-Sepulveda JA, et al. Evaluation of Fontan liver disease: correlation of transjugular liver biopsy with magnetic resonance and hemodynamics. Congenit Heart Dis. 2019;14(4):600–8.
18. Dijkstra H, et al. Diminished liver microperfusion in Fontan patients: a biexponential DWI study. PLoS One. 2017;12(3):e0173149.
19. Mendichovszky IA, et al. Combined MR direct thrombus imaging and non-contrast magnetic resonance venography reveal the evolution of deep vein thrombosis: a feasibility study. Eur Radiol. 2017;27(6):2326–32.
20. Callegari A, et al. Myocardial deformation in Fontan patients assessed by cardiac magnetic resonance feature tracking: correlation with function, clinical course, and biomarkers. Pediatr Cardiol. 2021;42(7):1625–34.
21. Meyer SL, et al. Serial cardiovascular magnetic resonance feature tracking indicates early worsening of cardiac function in Fontan patients. Int J Cardiol. 2020;303:23–9.
22. Schmidt R, et al. Value of speckle-tracking echocardiography and MRI-based feature tracking analysis in adult patients after Fontan-type palliation. Congenit Heart Dis. 2014;9(5):397–406.
23. Messroghli DR, et al. Clinical recommendations for cardiovascular magnetic resonance mapping of T1, T2, T2* and extracellular volume: a consensus statement by the Society for Cardiovascular Magnetic Resonance (SCMR) endorsed by the European Association for Cardiovascular Imaging (EACVI). J Cardiovasc Magn Reson. 2017;19(1):75.
24. Kim PK, et al. Myocardial T1 and T2 mapping: techniques and clinical applications. Korean J Radiol. 2017;18(1):113–31.
25. de Leval MR, et al. Total cavopulmonary connection: a logical alternative to atriopulmonary connection for complex Fontan operations. Experimental studies and early clinical experience. J Thorac Cardiovasc Surg. 1988;96(5):682–95.
26. McLennan D, et al. Usefulness of 4D-flow MRI in mapping flow distribution through failing Fontan circulation prior to cardiac intervention. Pediatr Cardiol. 2019;40(5):1093–6.

27. Ensley AE, et al. Fluid mechanic assessment of the total cavopulmonary connection using magnetic resonance phase velocity mapping and digital particle image velocimetry. Ann Biomed Eng. 2000;28(10):1172–83.

28. Frakes DH, et al. New techniques for the reconstruction of complex vascular anatomies from MRI images. J Cardiovasc Magn Reson. 2005;7(2):425–32.

29. Haggerty CM, et al. Comparing pre- and postoperative Fontan hemodynamic simulations: implications for the reliability of surgical planning. Ann Biomed Eng. 2012;40(12):2639–51.

30. Kanter KR, et al. Preliminary clinical experience with a bifurcated Y-graft Fontan procedure—a feasibility study. J Thorac Cardiovasc Surg. 2012;144(2):383–9.

31. Haggerty CM, Yoganathan AP, Fogel MA. Magnetic resonance imaging-guided surgical design: can we optimise the Fontan operation? Cardiol Young. 2013;23(6):818–23.

32. Kamphuis VP, et al. Disproportionate intraventricular viscous energy loss in Fontan patients: analysis by 4D flow MRI. Eur Heart J Cardiovasc Imaging. 2019;20(3):323–33.

33. Kamphuis VP, et al. Hemodynamic interplay of vorticity, viscous energy loss, and kinetic energy from 4D flow MRI and link to cardiac function in healthy subjects and Fontan patients. Am J Physiol Heart Circ Physiol. 2021;320(4):H1687–98.

34. Sjoberg P, et al. Decreased diastolic ventricular kinetic energy in young patients with Fontan circulation demonstrated by four-dimensional cardiac magnetic resonance imaging. Pediatr Cardiol. 2017;38(4):669–80.

CT in Patients with Univentricular Hearts and a Fontan Circulation

26

Tom Semple and Konstantinos Dimopoulos

Introduction

Cardiac computed tomography (CT) has become invaluable in the assessment of many types of congenital heart disease (CHD), especially patients with complex defects. CT provides complementary information to echocardiography and cardiac magnetic resonance on cardiovascular anatomy and physiology and has become the gold standard modality for non-invasive coronary assessment [1–4].

CT provides information on:

- Situs, cardiac position and relative size of cardiac chambers (Fig. 26.1)
- Atrio-ventricular and ventriculo-arterial connections (Fig. 26.2)
- Size and position of the great vessels and outflow tracts (Figs. 26.2 and 26.3)
- Anatomy of the pulmonary vascular bed
- Collateral vessels (e.g. MAPCAs), arteriovenous malformations/collaterals in the lung, or veno-veno collaterals (Fig. 26.4)
- The Fontan pathway and Glenn anastomosis and other surgical shunts (patent or occluded)

- Detailed anatomic information prior to surgical or percutaneous interventions (Fig. 26.5), including providing a roadmap for image integration for EP procedures
- Calcification in prosthetic material and valves (Fig. 26.6)
- Information on the coronary circulation, from anatomic detail (typically "anomalous" origins and courses in patients with a univentricular heart), an to the severity of any atheromatous disease or coronary compression
- Information on the RV-dependent coronary circulation in patients with pulmonary atresia and intact septum
- Cine imaging of metallic and stent valve leaflet function (in more detail than via plain fluoroscopy)
- Intracavitary clots and pulmonary emboli
- Position of fenestrations
- Other complications, including pulmonary venous stenosis, subaortic stenosis
- Associated lesions (e.g. aortic coarctation)
- Assessment of relevant extracardiac disease (lung disease such as bronchiectasis in the context of primary ciliary dyskinesia, liver nodules in cardiac cirrhosis, whole body vascular access prior to transplant etc.)

Particular attention is needed when assessing Fontan patients for pulmonary emboli. The anatomy and resultant potential for contrast mixing artefacts needs to be taken into consideration when

T. Semple
Radiology Department, The Royal Brompton Hospital, London and National Heart and Lung Institute, Imperial College, London, UK

K. Dimopoulos (✉)
Adult Congenital Heart Centre, Royal Brompton and Harefield NHS Foundation Trust, Harefield, UK

P. Clift et al. (eds.), *Univentricular Congenital Heart Defects and the Fontan Circulation*,
https://doi.org/10.1007/978-3-031-36208-8_26

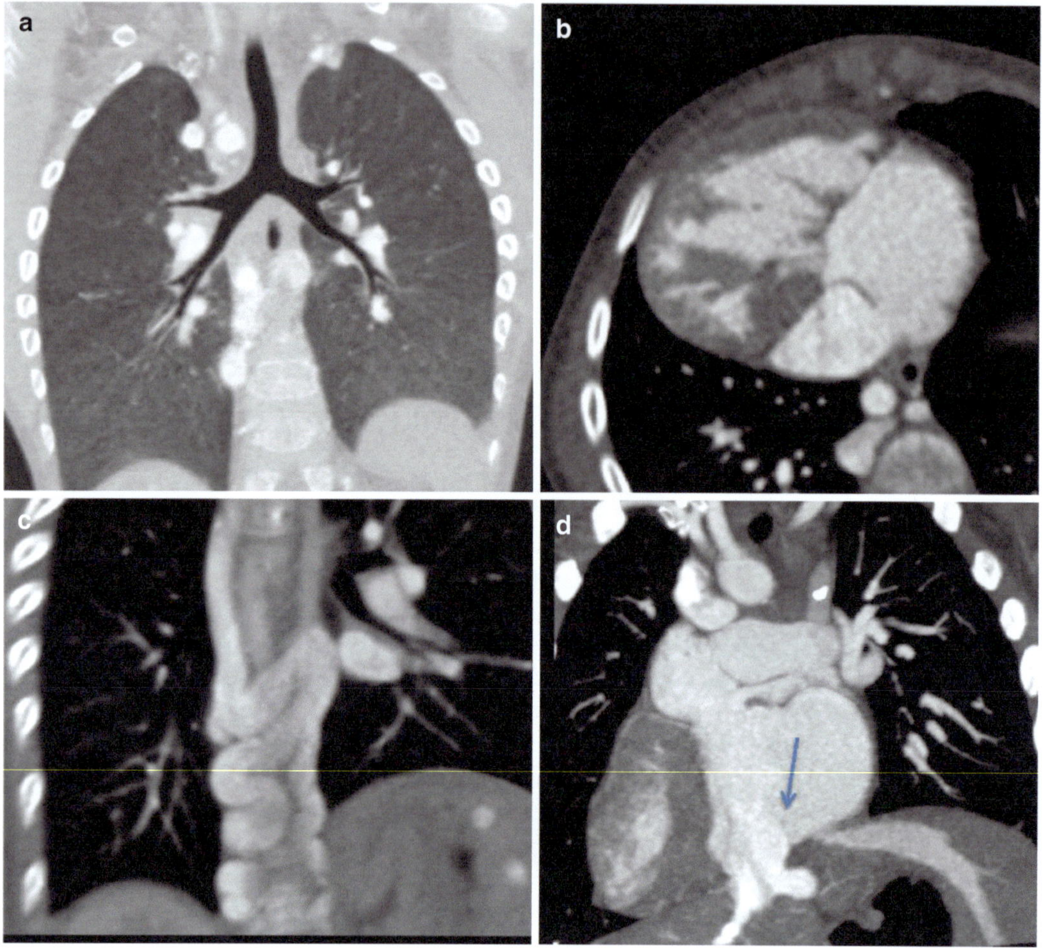

Fig. 26.1 Visceral situs, cardiac position and chamber size in right atrial isomerism. In, (**a**) symmetric bronchial branching with bilateral "right sided" anatomy with epiarterial bronchi. (**b**) Dextrocardia with dilatation of the left atrium and ventricle. (**c**) There is azygous continuation draining the lower body to the SVC via a tortuous, dilated azygous system (also demonstrated in **b**). (**d**) Venous return from the mid-line liver is via two separate hepatic veins draining either side of the atrial septum (arrow)

interpreting filling defects in the pulmonary arteries. Outside of congenital heart disease, much of the mixing of contrast media with blood occurs via right ventricular contraction, resulting in homogeneous enhancement of the pulmonary arterial system. All TCPC patients, and patients with AP Fontan and a Glenn anastomosis, will not achieve this RV dependant mixing of contrast media with unopacified blood, resulting in apparent filling defects that can very convincingly mimic the appearance of pulmonary emboli. Clinical context is key and these "pseudo pulmonary emboli" are generally so extensive that the apparent embolic burden far outweighs the patient's symptoms. There are several contrast administration methods in use that reduce the incidence of pseudo pulmonary emboli in these patients:

1. Paired first and second pass (second pass being 60 s post initial acquisition) imaging
2. Simultaneous injection via cannulae in the upper and lower limbs
3. Dual/multi-phase contrast media injection (for example the modified Bastion Wheel)

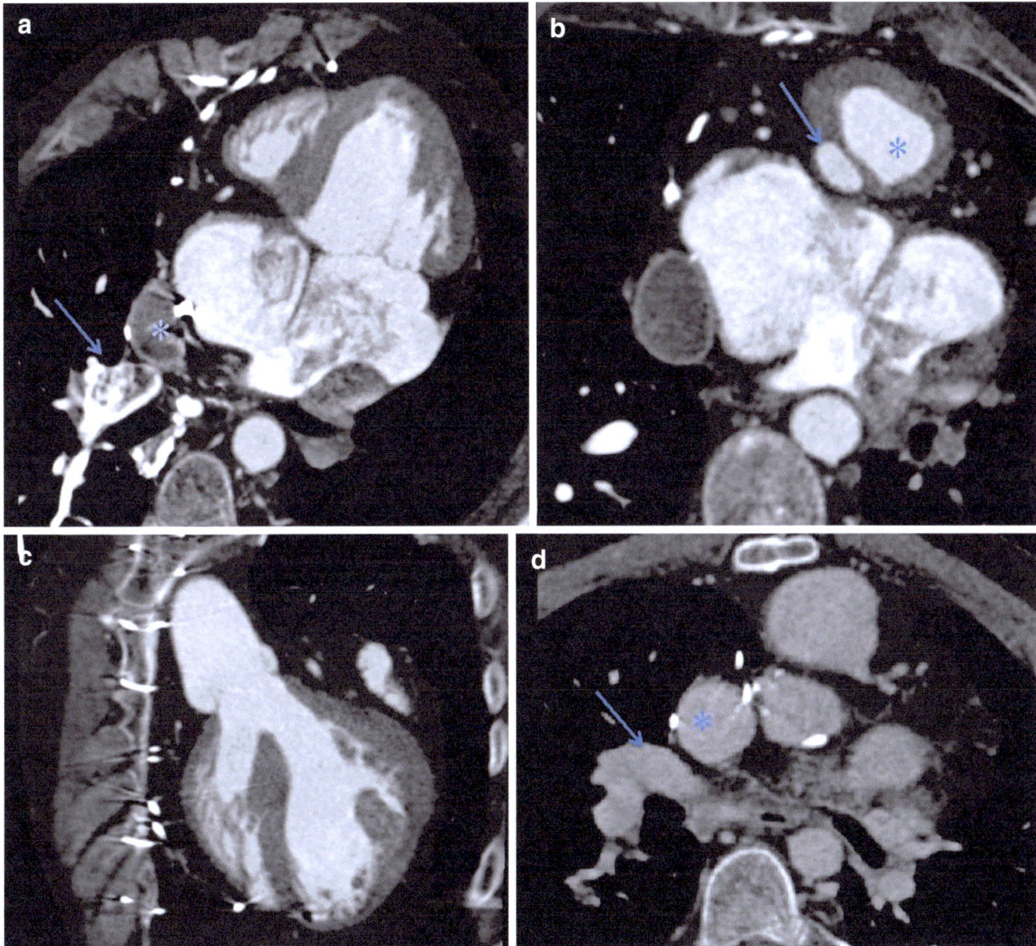

Fig. 26.2 AV and VA connection assessment. In, (**a**) Levocardia with absent right AV connection and a hypoplastic right ventricle. Note that blood returning via the lateral tunnel TCPC (*) is not contrast-opacified, leading to extensive mixing artefact in the pulmonary arteries (arrow) from contrast enhanced blood arriving via a Glenn anastomosis (not shown). (**b**) The aorta (*) is anterior and to the left of the very small pulmonary artery trunk (arrow) and arises from the right ventricle (**c**), superior to a large outlet VSD. (**d**) Delayed acquisition at 120 s post contrast media injection demonstrates homogeneous enhancement of the lateral tunnel TCPC (*) and pulmonary arteries (arrow) now that adequate mixing has been achieved

Paired first and second pass imaging obtains two acquisitions using a conventional injection protocol. The first acquisition can be timed to provide good quality coronary and aortic opacification, but will suffer from the mixing artefacts, whilst the second acquisition confirms there is no true pulmonary arterial thrombus. The advantage of this approach is low contrast volume and good arterial opacification, the disadvantage is that the radiation exposure is doubled. Simultaneous injection via upper and lower limb cannulae will overcome the problem of mixing of upper and lower body blood pools in patients with a TCPC, but mixing artefact is still possible from the short distance from the upper limb cannula to the Glenn anastomosis and the technique requires the placement of a foot cannula—particularly traumatic in children and adults with learning disabilities.

The preferred technique at our institution is a multiphasic injection protocol based on the so-called "Bastion wheel". The original protocol was devised to provide simultaneous arterial and abdominal visceral parenchymal enhancement in

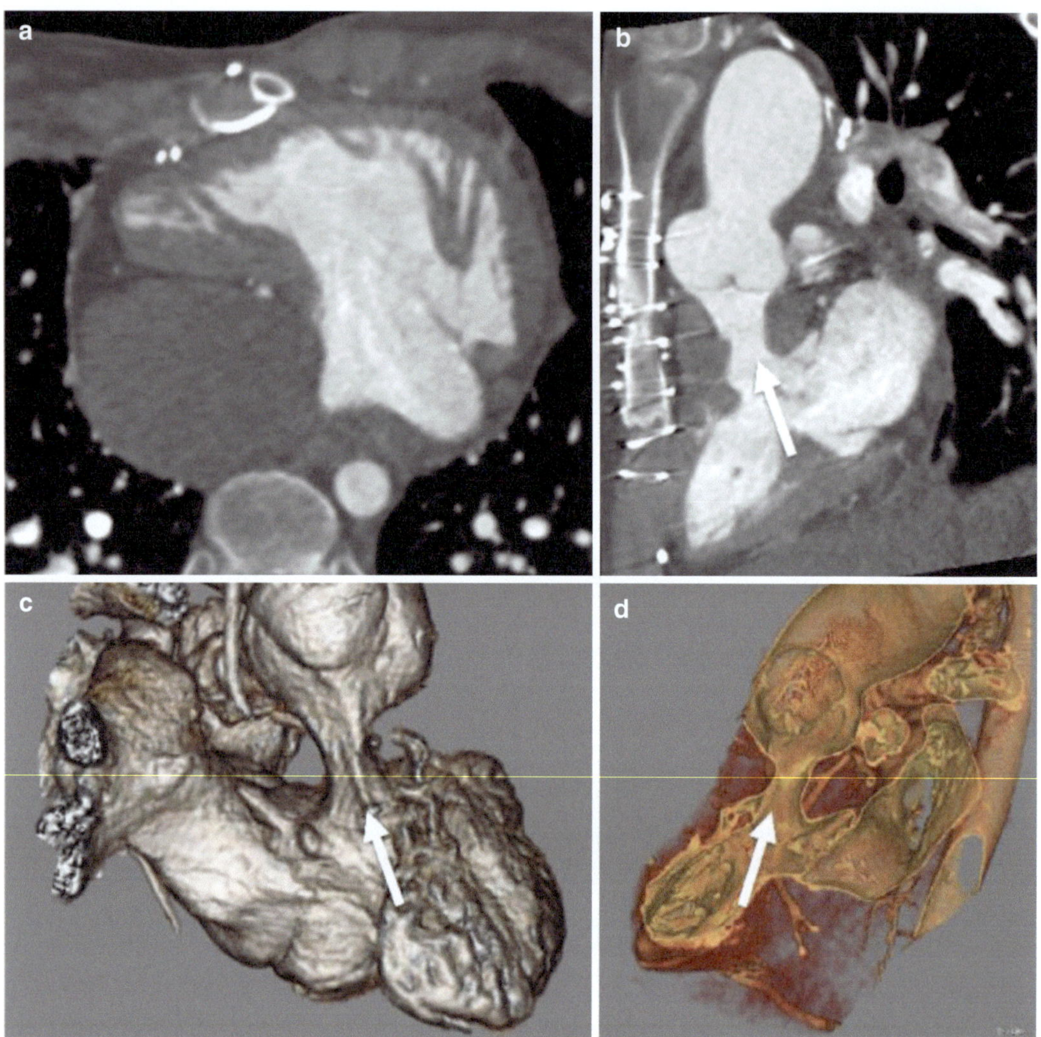

Fig. 26.3 Outflow tract anatomy. In, (**a**) Mesocardia, absent right AV connection, ventricular septal defect (VSD), transposition of the great arteries (not shown) and atriopulmonary Fontan. (**b**) The restrictive VSD forms a long aortic infundibulum (arrow) resulting in sub-aortic stenosis. (**c**) Volume rendered and (**d**) surface rendered reconstructions demonstrate the outflow tract anatomy in 3D

victims of major trauma at Camp Bastion during the war in Afghanistan [5]. A slow injection of contrast is followed by a more rapid injection with single phase imaging a set delay thereafter. At the time of imaging, the first part of the injected contrast media is returning to the thorax in the systemic venous system and the latter part of the injection provides better arterial enhance-ment. Based on personal experience, we have modified the timing of the Bastion Wheel proto-col specifically for Glenn and Fontan imaging, with acquisition at 90 s from the start of injection instead of the 70 s delay used by the original protocol.

Beyond single phase imaging, lack of the need for foot cannulation and the reduction in

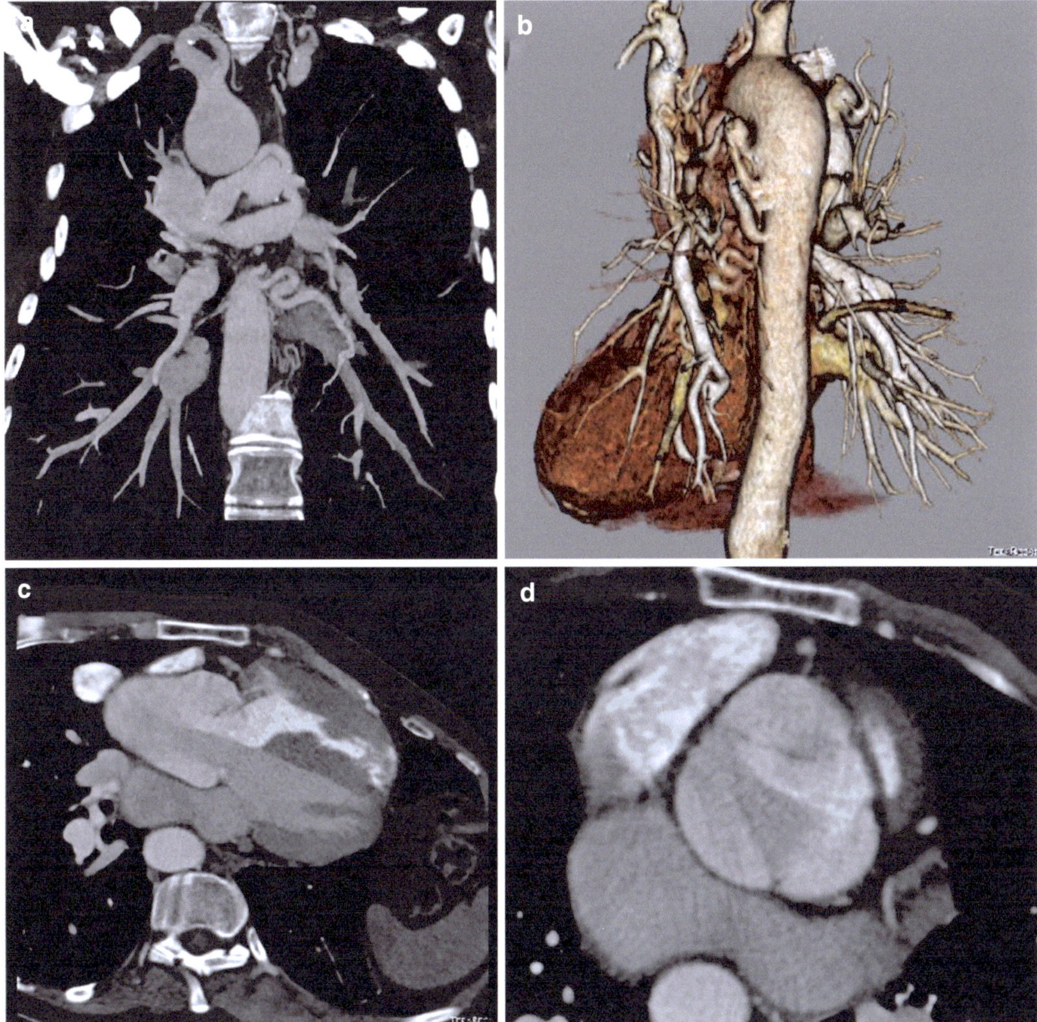

Fig. 26.4 Pulmonary atresia, VSD and MAPCAs. In (**a**) and (**b**), coronal section and 3D reconstruction, respectively, demonstrating the positions of multiple major aorto-pulmonary collateral arteries (MAPCAs). In (**c**) and (**d**) the aorta overrides a large VSD. The contrast timing with differential enhancement of the right and left ventricles demonstrates 50:50 split flow from each ventricle to the dilated aortic root

pseudo pulmonary emboli, the modified Bastion wheel has additional benefits in demonstrating bilateral superior vena cavas and bilateral bidirectional Glenn anastomoses irrespective of the location of the peripheral cannula (conventional acquisitions often result in contrast from the arm preferentially opacifying the ipsilateral lung and in patients with Glenn anastomosis with a high pulmonary vascular resistance, contrast from the arm is likely to preferentially enter the azygos system or other veno-venous collaterals).

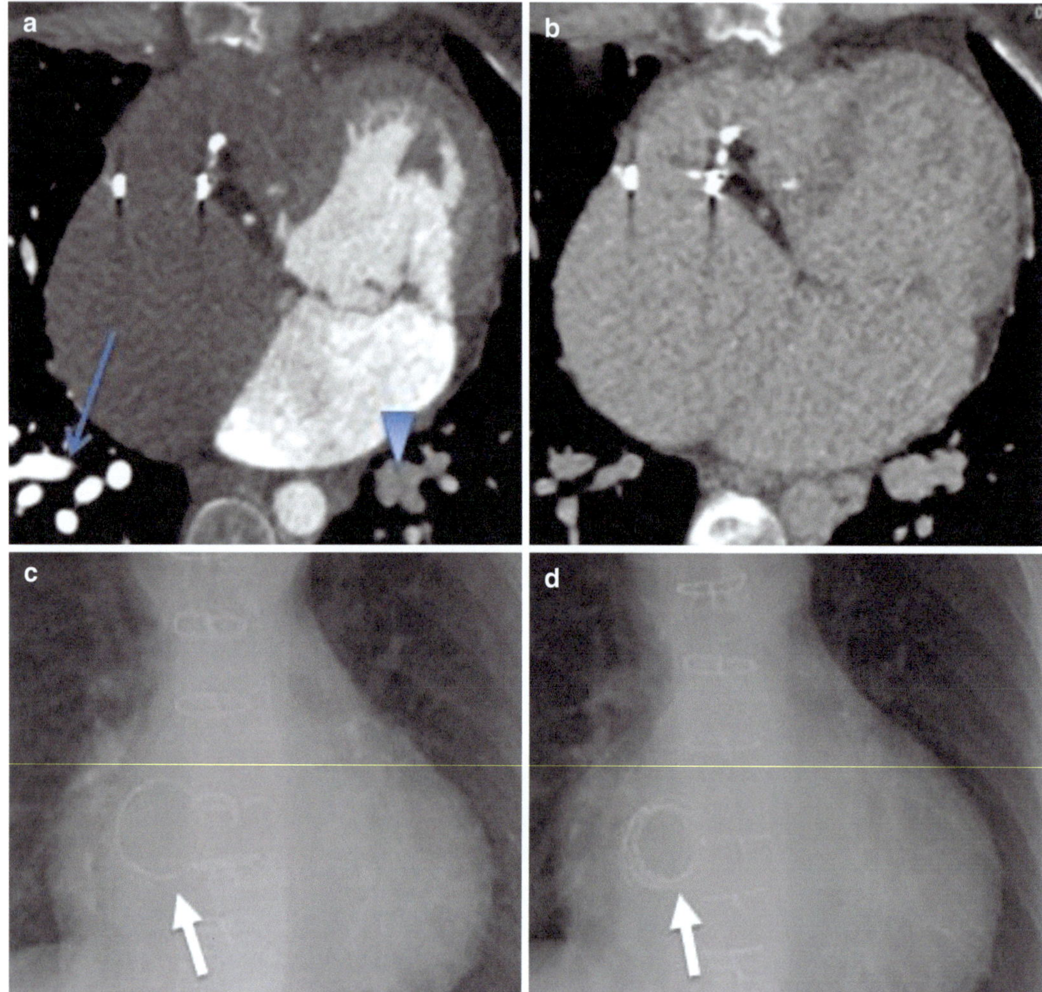

Fig. 26.5 Bjork modification of the Fontan circulation in tricuspid atresia. In, (**a**) first pass imaging (for coronary imaging) contrast fills the right pulmonary vessels (arrow) via a Glenn anastomosis with poor opacification of the left pulmonary vessels (arrow head). Supply to the right atrium, RA-RV conduit (the Bjork modification) is from the lower body venous system and as a result is completely unopacified. (**b**) Second pass imaging demonstrates symmetric opacification of the right and left pulmonary vessels and of the whole heart including the RA-RV conduit and its bioprosthesis. The CT was used to plan valve in valve interventional insertion of a stented percutaneous valve into the RA-RV conduit (see chest radiographs before (**c**) and after (**d**) stent valve insertion

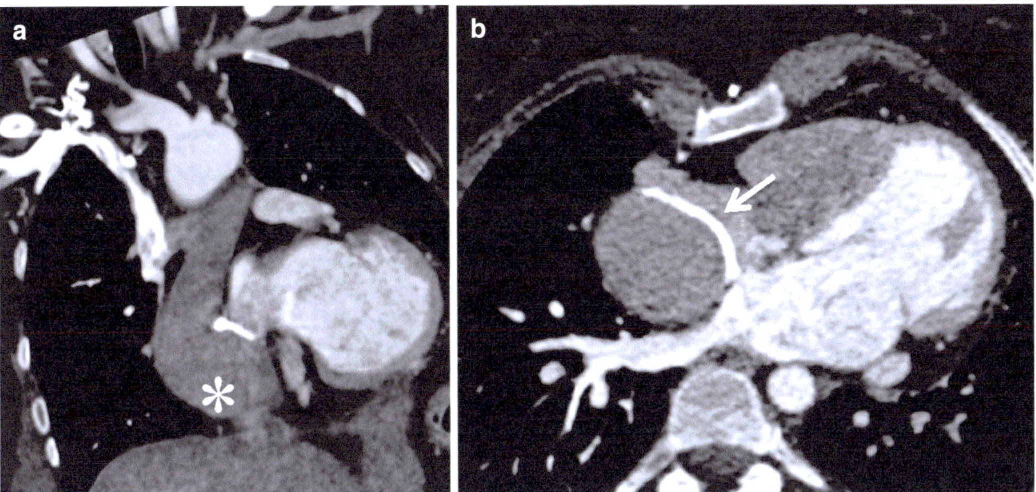

Fig. 26.6 Pulmonary atresia intact ventricular septum post TCPC. In, (**a**) contrast administration via the right arm preferentially fills the right pulmonary arterial system, with unopacified blood via the lateral tunnel TCPC (*) preferentially supplying the left lung. On this first pass acquisition, calcification of the TCPC conduit is clearly demonstrated, also shown in axial section—arrow in (**b**)

References

1. Loughborough WW, Yeong M, Hamilton M, Manghat N. Computed tomography in congenital heart disease: how generic principles can be applied to create bespoke protocols in the Fontan circuit. Quant Imaging Med Surg. 2017;7:79–87.
2. Hauser JA, Taylor AM, Pandya B. How to image the adult patient with Fontan circulation. Circ Cardiovasc Imaging. 2017;10:10.
3. Sandler KL, Markham LW, Mah ML, Byrum EP, Williams JR. Optimizing CT angiography in patients with Fontan physiology: single-center experience of dual-site power injection. Clin Radiol. 2014;69:e562–7.
4. Kelly Han B, et al. Computed tomography imaging in patients with congenital heart disease part I: rationale and utility. An expert consensus document of the Society of Cardiovascular Computed Tomography (SCCT): Endorsed by the Society of Pediatric Radiology (SPR) and the North American Society of Cardiac Imaging (NASCI). SCCT guidelines. J Cardiovasc Comput Tomogr. 2015;9(6):475–92. https://doi.org/10.1016/j.jcct.2015.07.004. Epub 2015 Jul 23.
5. Carter NJ, Kirkwood GW, Mils R, Gay DAT. The inception of the Bastion protocol for trauma CT scanning. J R Nav Med Serv. 2018;104(3):183–6.

Physiological Testing and Basics of Cardiac Catheterisation in Fontan Patients

A. Constantine and Konstantinos Dimopoulos

Abbreviations

6MWT	6-minute walk test
(A)CHD	(Adult) congenital heart disease
BP	Blood pressure
$C(a - \underline{v})O_2$	Arterial-mixed venous O_2 content difference
CMR	Cardiovascular magnetic resonance
CO	Cardiac output
CO_2	Carbon dioxide
CPET	Cardiopulmonary exercise test
HR	Heart rate
HRR	Heart rate reserve
IVC	Inferior vena cava
MVV	Maximal voluntary ventilation
O_2	Oxygen
pVO_2	Peak oxygen uptake
RER	Respiratory exchange ratio
SpO_2	Peripheral oxygen saturation
SV	Stroke volume
SVC	Superior vena cava
TCPC	Total cavo-pulmonary connection
VAT	Ventilatory anaerobic threshold
VE_{max}	Minute ventilation at peak exercise
VE/VCO_2	Ventilatory equivalent for CO_2
VO_2	Oxygen consumption (L/min)
VR	Ventilatory reserve

A. Constantine · K. Dimopoulos (✉)
Adult Congenital Heart Centre and National Centre for Pulmonary Hypertension, Royal Brompton Hospital, London, UK

The National Heart and Lung Institute, Imperial College, London, UK

Most investigations in the physician's toolkit provide a picture of the patient at rest, but many common symptoms occur on effort. This is especially true in patients with a Fontan circulation, who are often well when resting, but in whom exercise limitation is prevalent [1–3]. An inability to exercise and perform ordinary activities reduces quality of life and physical, psychological and social welfare. Hence, physiological stress testing is crucial to fully assess an individual's health.

Cardiopulmonary Exercise Testing

Cardiopulmonary exercise testing (CPET) allows an integrative assessment of the cardiovascular and respiratory response to a tailored exercise protocol, assessing the ability of an individual to sufficiently augment gas exchange between the tissues and the environment to support an increase in muscle respiration. CPET is the gold-standard investigation for assessing exercise intolerance and has become an essential tool in the evaluation of patients with ACHD. It has several purposes in this patient group, in the:

P. Clift et al. (eds.), *Univentricular Congenital Heart Defects and the Fontan Circulation*, https://doi.org/10.1007/978-3-031-36208-8_27

- assessment of the presence and severity of exercise intolerance
- identification of factors that limit exercise performance (cardiac, respiratory, vascular, muscular etc.), guiding further investigations
- risk stratification of patients: CPET parameters are associated with mortality and morbidity in ACHD cohorts, including Fontan patients
- assessment of disease progression and evaluation of the impact of therapeutic interventions on exercise function through serial CPET [4]. In Fontan patients, clinical guidelines advise routine serial testing at intervals of 12–36 months, depending on clinical status [5].
- determine the timing of referral for advanced heart failure therapies and transplantation
- appropriate exercise prescription.

CPET provides a wealth of data, reflecting the response to exercise of the cardiovascular and ventilatory systems, and at a cellular level, as well as providing an assessment of lung function and monitoring for electrocardiographic changes during exercise (a non-exhaustive list is provided in Table 27.1). The respiratory and cardiovascular responses to exercise are important components of the physiology of exercise:

- The *ventilatory response to exercise* depends on an increase in the tidal volume at low and moderate workloads, followed by an increase in respiratory rate at higher workloads (especially above the anaerobic threshold, when ventilation increases to account for the increase in CO_2 produced by anaerobic metabolism). Conditions that limit ventilation, gas diffusion and exchange between the alveoli and the blood are likely to cause of exercise intolerance and a drop in peak VO_2. A rise in the slope of the relation between ventilation (VE) and CO_2 production (VCO_2) is a marker of inefficient ventilation and is common in patients with heart failure, reduced pulmonary perfusion, and right-left shunting/cyanosis. The VE/VCO_2 slope is also a strong predictor of mortality in heart failure and ACHD.

- In healthy subjects, the *cardiovascular response to exercise* is achieved by increasing the cardiac output (CO) and augmenting the oxygen extraction from the blood. At maximal workloads, a three-fold increase in peripheral oxygen extraction is accompanied by a 1.5-fold increase in the stroke volume (SV) and 2.3 times increase in heart rate (HR). The product of these factors determines oxygen consumption (VO_2). Any condition that affects the body's ability to increase oxygen extraction from the blood, or increase CO and the delivery and utilisation of oxygen in the periphery, is likely to cause exercise intolerance and a drop in the highest VO_2 achieved during maximal incremental exercise (peak VO_2). CPET estimates VO_2 by measuring O_2 concentration in the inspired air, and the minute ventilation using a flowmeter. Careful calibration of both sensors is crucial for obtaining accurate and reproducible results.

Exercise intolerance is prevalent in Fontan patients [1–3]: Exercise capacity improves significantly after the Fontan operation compared to the pre-operative state [6], through relief of the cyanosis and ventricular volume overload. Exercise capacity does, however, remain almost universally reduced compared to healthy age and sex matched patients. Almost one half of adult Fontan patients are severely limited in their objective exercise capacity, achieving <50% of predicted peak VO_2 for age, sex and body habitus [34].

Both the cardiovascular and ventilatory responses to exercise are restricted in Fontan patients due to multiple possible mechanisms.

In Terms of the Cardiovascular Response

- the combination of a reduced SV during submaximal [6, 7, 27] and maximal exercise [8], and chronotropic incompetence (inability to sufficiently increase HR on exercise) contribute to the limited ability to augment CO during exercise.

Table 27.1 CPET variables with adult normal ranges and evidence of dysfunction in patients following Fontan repair

Parameter	Definition	Adult normal ranges	Evidence of dysfunction in Fontan circulation
Peak oxygen uptake (pVO$_2$)	The highest rate of oxygen (O$_2$) transport measured during presumed maximal exercise adjusted for weight. Equivalent to VO$_2$ max if measured during maximal effort	>84% predicted for age and sex	Almost universally reduced peak VO$_2$ with wide variability [1–3, 6–26]. In one European study, 50% of patients had a severely impaired peak VO$_2$ (<50% predicted), while 1% had a normal value for age and sex [3]
VO$_2$ max	The highest achievable VO$_2$ evidenced by failure of VO$_2$ to increment despite increasing work rate. VO$_2$ max = HR × SV × C(a − v) O$_2$	–	
Oxygen (O$_2$) pulse	The quantity of O$_2$ consumed from the volume of blood delivered to the tissues per heartbeat. O$_2$ pulse = SV × C(a − v)O$_2$	>80%	Subnormal due to reduced stroke volume during submaximal [6, 7, 27] and maximal exercise [8]
Peak heart rate (HR)	The maximal heart rate attained during exercise	>90% age predicted	Chronotropic incompetence is prevalent with significantly lower peak HR compared to healthy peers [1–3, 6–14, 17, 18, 20, 23, 24] with a larger HRR. This is compounded by the use of rate-limiting drugs e.g. β-adrenergic blockade, lung disease with impaired ventilatory mechanics, or a poor effort
Heart rate reserve (HRR)	Difference between predicted peak HR (220 − age) and measured HR at peak VO$_2$[a]	<15 bpm	
Arterial blood pressure (BP)	Change in cuff BP measured at 1-min intervals prior to, during and following exercise	At rest: 124/79 mmHg At/near maximal exercise: 200/88 mmHg[‡]	Normal BP response to submaximal exercise [2, 24, 26], unless systemic ventricular outflow tract obstruction is present. Limited evidence of blunted response during maximal effort [28]
Ventilatory reserve (VR)	The reserve capacity of the ventilatory system	MVV − VE$_{max}$ > 11 L or VE$_{max}$/MVV × 100 < 85%	VR at peak exercise is variably affected, with abnormal resting spirometry in a subset of patients [29, 30]
Peripheral oxygen saturation (SpO$_2$)	Percentage of oxygen-saturated haemoglobin relative to the total amount of haemoglobin in the blood	94–98%	Variable depending on presence of fenestration or persistent intracardiac right-to-left shunt, pulmonary arteriovenous malformations, systemic venous collateralisation
Minute ventilation/carbon dioxide (CO$_2$) production ratio (VE/VCO$_2$)	The ventilatory equivalent for CO$_2$ (a measure of ventilatory efficiency)	<34	Elevated VE/VCO$_2$ slope at rest and at peak exercise, reflecting ventilation-perfusion mismatch (e.g. from right-to-left shunting in the case of fenestration or residual shunt) or hypoxia with enhanced ventilatory reflex sensitivity [6, 11, 12, 16, 17, 31]. Exaggerated increase in the respiratory rate in early stages of exercise with a lower tidal volume documented in patients with TCPC [6, 26]

(continued)

Table 27.1 (continued)

Parameter	Definition	Adult normal ranges	Evidence of dysfunction in Fontan circulation
Ventilatory anaerobic threshold (VAT)	An index of exercise capacity, measured as the VO_2 at the onset of blood lactate accumulation i.e. the point at which VE increases disproportionately relative to VO_2	>40% pVO_2	Reduced when available [1, 8, 17]
Respiratory exchange ratio (RER)	The ratio of CO_2 output to O_2 uptake. A value of ≥ 1.1 is indicative of a maximal effort	≥ 1.1	Similar to healthy subjects, although found at a significantly lower pVO_2 [2, 11, 12, 14, 15, 17–19, 23, 24]

BP blood pressure, $C(a-\underline{v})O_2$ arterial-mixed venous O_2 content difference, *CO₂* carbon dioxide, *HR* heart rate, *HRR* heart rate reserve, *MVV* maximal voluntary ventilation, *O₂* oxygen, *pVO₂* peak oxygen uptake, *RER* respiratory exchange ratio, *SpO₂* peripheral oxygen saturation, *SV* stroke volume, *TCPC* total cavo-pulmonary connection, *VAT* ventilatory anaerobic threshold, *VE_max* minute ventilation at peak exercise, *VE/VCO₂* ventilatory equivalent for CO_2, *VR* ventilatory reserve

[a] HRR is sometimes reported as the difference between the measured HR at peak VO_2 and the resting HR
[b] Normal values given are for a sedentary, non-hypertensive males ages 34–74 [32, 33]

- Systolic or diastolic dysfunction of the systemic ventricle, a reduced preload due to limited pulmonary blood flow, and persistent haemodynamic lesions (e.g. valve stenosis or regurgitation, or a restrictive VSD in patients with ventriculo-arterial discordance, acting as subaortic stenosis) are likely to impact on the increase in CO on exercise.

- The lack of a subpulmonary ventricle creates a unique physiological situation in the Fontan patient, where the primary driver of transpulmonary blood flow is the negative pressure created by the systemic atrium during ventricular systole along with the atrial volume increase with the apical descent of a competent atrio-ventricular valve. Generation of CO is, therefore, heavily dependent on ventilatory mechanics and the thoracic and lower extremity muscle pumps in Fontan patients. At rest, the "thoracic pump" of the diaphragm and other respiratory muscles contracting during inspiration generates a negative pressure, aiding transpulmonary flow contributing to up to one third of the resting CO [35]. On exercise, the skeletal muscle pump predominates in augmenting the CO with a smaller, secondary contribution of the ventilatory pump [36].

- Unlike acquired heart failure states, the inability on Fontan patients to adequately increase systemic ventricular preload is also a major driver of SV limitation during exercise. A reduction in preload, as when exercise is combined with an expiratory load, causes SV to drop to baseline levels despite ongoing exercise, suggesting that Fontan patients have little haemodynamic reserve to overcome a decrease in venous return [36].

- Peak VO_2 is also limited by chronotropic incompetence, which affects the majority of Fontan patients; in one study, 84% of patients were unable to achieve a HR of at least 80% predicted [9]. Chronotropic incompetence in Fontan patients is likely related to abnormalities of the sinus node and conduction system, which may be intrinsic (relating to the underlying condition) or related to the previous surgery, medication or permanent pacing [9, 37]. The importance of chronotropic incompetence as a mechanism of functional limitation is exhibited by the fact that a greater heart rate reserve (HRR; the difference between the maximum predicted HR and the maximum achieved HR), but not peak VO_2, has been associated with an increased risk of death or transplantation in this cohort.

- The third variable in the equation for VO_2, oxygen extraction from the blood, is increased in Fontan patients during exercise, in an effort to compensate for the limited increase in CO at a given workload [10, 28].

In Terms of Ventilatory Response

- The ventilatory response to exercise is also impaired to a variable degree in Fontan patients. Following the Fontan procedure, almost 50% of patients have abnormal spirometry, with a forced vital capacity below the lower limit of normal. The cause of abnormal pulmonary physiology remains uncertain, but abnormalities in lung development and mechanical limitations have been documented. The abnormal prenatal and early postnatal environment, and particularly the reduced pulmonary blood flow, may impair vascular and parenchymal lung development, limiting lung growth [38]. In addition, chest wall abnormalities, including scoliosis and pectus deformities, and the sequelae of surgical interventions, including diaphragmatic paralysis, contribute to reduced lung volumes.

- Among Fontan patients with a peak VO_2 <80% predicted, almost a quarter of patients demonstrated a pulmonary mechanical contribution to exercise limitation with a breathing reserve <20% [29]. The VE/VCO_2 slope is also steeper than normal in most Fontan patients (see Table 27.1; Fig. 27.1). The likely cause for this is ventilation-perfusion mismatch due reduced pulmonary blood flow because of the lack of a subpulmonary ventricle, reduced pulmonary vasoreactivity and limited recruitment of pulmonary blood vessels during exercise [39]. Moreover, right-to-left shunting and cyanosis contribute to the physiological dead space and chemoreceptor activation driving ventilation [31].

Serial testing using CPET should be part of the routine follow-up of patients with Fontan circulation, as changes in CPET variables over time often indicate a changing clinical status and need for intervention (Fig. 27.2) [40]. Nomograms for Fontan patients, as for other CHD, allow tracking of the VO_2 over time in our aging patients. However, quality control is important to ensure reproducibility and the ability of CPET to reliably detect changes over time.

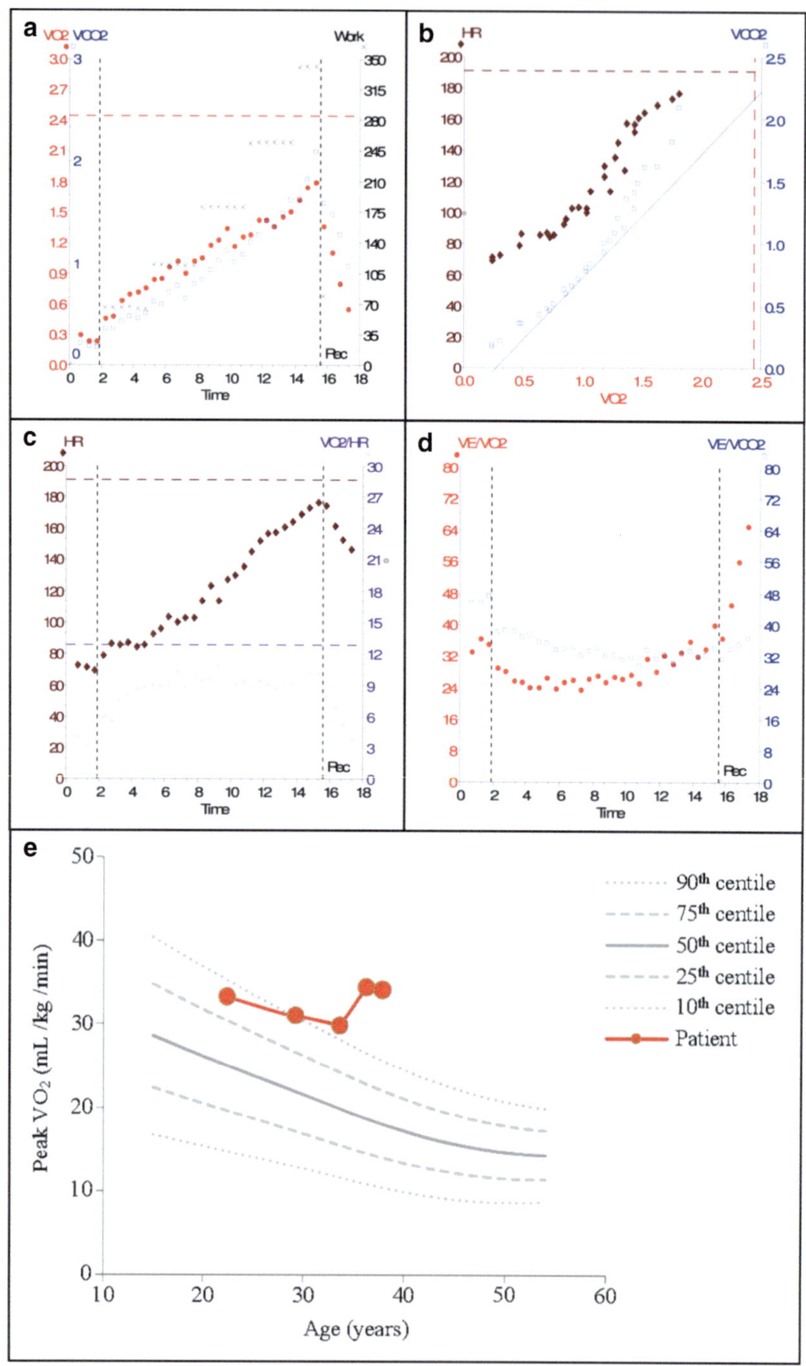

Fig. 27.1 Cardiopulmonary exercise test in a 37-year-old male with tricuspid and pulmonary atresia who underwent bilateral Blalock Taussig shunts followed by a right atrial-pulmonary arterial Fontan aged 7 years. He described no symptoms of exercise limitation (NYHA functional class I). The patient exercised for 13.5 min on a modified Bruce protocol and achieved a peak RER of 1.18, implying adequate effort. The peak VO_2 was 34.1 mL/kg/min (**a**), which is 77% of predicted for age and sex. The anaerobic threshold was also mildly reduced at 24.7 mL/kg/min (**b**). There was a normal heart rate and blood pressure response to exercise, with incrementing O_2 pulse (**c**) and without any desaturation (95% at peak exercise). The VE/VCO_2 slope was within normal limits at 31 (**d**). The trend of peak VO_2 over time provides valuable information and is reassuring, especially when plotted against Fontan reference values (**e**) [34]

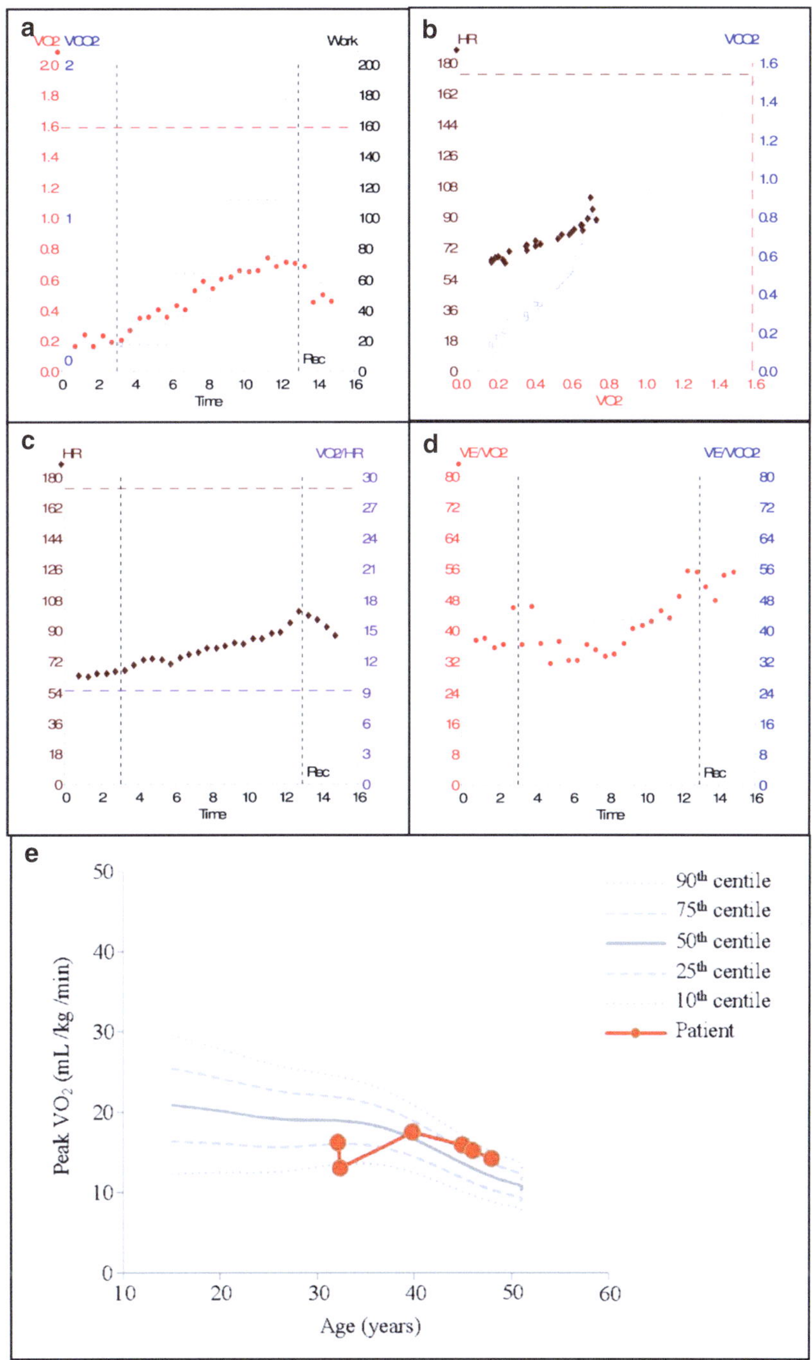

Fig. 27.2 Cardiopulmonary exercise test in a 49-year-old female with left atrial isomerism, a common atrioventricular valve, and double outlet right ventricle with a Glenn connection in childhood followed by a late completion to a lateral tunnel total cavo-pulmonary connection aged 25 years. The patient exercised for 10 min, achieving a peak VO_2 of 14.2 mL/kg/min (48% predicted) at an RER of 1.15 (**a**). The anaerobic threshold was significantly reduced at 11.9 mL/kg/min (**b**). There was a blunted heart rate response to exercise, the heart rate rising to 106 bpm (**c**), with desaturation from 85 to 75%. The VE/VCO_2 slope is steep in keeping with cyanosis and altered ventilatory efficiency with likely V/Q mismatching (**d**). Exercise capacity fell at 33 years of age following recurrent atrial tachycardia but recovered to levels expected for a Fontan patient of her age following ablation of a macro-re-entrant tachycardia around the baffle scar (**e**)

Six-Min Walk Test

The six-min walk test (6MWT) is a simple and reproducible means of assessing exercise capacity in patients with significant exercise limitation. It consists of the patient walking up and down a 15–30 m corridor at their fastest walking speed, without running, for 6 min. The total distance covered, and oxygen saturations, blood pressure and the modified BORG dyspnoea score are recorded at baseline and at the end of the 6 min [41].

Like CPET, it is an approved endpoint for use in randomised controlled trials of pulmonary arterial hypertension therapies [42–44]. In Eisenmenger syndrome, including patients with unrepaired univentricular circulation, 6-min walk distance was a strong predictor of outcome [45]. It is also more likely to detect changes in exercise capacity over time or after medical or other intervention than CPET.

Unlike CPET, however, the 6MWT provides little information on the mechanisms of exercise tolerance. Most importantly, the 6MWT has a "ceiling effect", with a maximum achievable distance of about 600 m, and hence cannot be used in patients with mild or even moderate limitation in exercise capacity.

Cardiac Catheterization

Cardiac catheterization in complex CHD patients, including those with a Fontan circulation, should be undertaken by an experienced operator in a specialist centre. It remains the gold standard investigation for determining pressures in the Fontan circulation and pulmonary arteries, detecting shunts and calculating pulmonary vascular resistance (PVR). Invasive data from the cardiac catheter should be combined with the results of non-invasive tests and clinical assessment when deciding on the management of Fontan patients with symptoms or other complications.

Indications

Indications for catheterization in Fontan patients are driven by symptoms or signs of disease progression, including signs of a "failing Fontan" circulation, as well as the need to evaluate haemodynamics prior to cardiac surgery or catheter-driven interventions [5]. The role for routine invasive haemodynamic monitoring in asymptomatic patients is less clear [40].

Preparation and Access

Prior to undertaking cardiac catheterization in a patient with univentricular physiology, a detailed review of the anatomy and the pathways of blood flow to and from the heart must be undertaken, with a review of clinical documentation, operation notes, prior imaging, and previous catheterization procedures. This will inform the operator about the best point of access, catheter selection, navigational difficulties and persistent shunts, and will reduce the length of the procedure, together with the contrast and radiation dose.

The procedure itself involves obtaining pressures and oxygen saturation measurements at the following points: superior *vena cava* (SVC; high and low), inferior *vena cava* (IVC), right atrium or the Fontan pathway, the subpulmonary ventricle (in the Björk modification of the Fontan operation), pulmonary arteries, and the pulmonary artery wedge position [46]. Systemic pressures and saturations, by invasive or non-invasive measurement, are also required for calculations. Left-sided pressures can be obtained by crossing a fenestration or through a retrograde approach from the aorta (arterial access).

Planning access is important in Fontan patients. Ultrasound guidance is recommended for all cases to ensure vessel patency, position and size. Femoral venous access allows the operator to collect data on the Fontan circulation and pulmonary arteries in patients with atriopulmonary Fontan. In the presence of a bidirectional Glenn anastomosis, access via the arm (basilica or cephalic vein) or neck (internal jugular vein) is required to allow the operator to collect data from the SVC and pulmonary arteries. In patients with a total cavopulmonary connection (TCPC), a femoral approach may be sufficient to collect data in the Fontan circulation and pulmonary arteries, even though manipulation of catheters to the SVC may be difficult depending on the surgical anatomy. In the presence of left atrial isomerism and azygos continuation to the SVC, a femoral approach may allow assessment of pulmonary artery pressure, depending on the size of the patient and the length of the catheter used (which will need to enter the azygos vein from the IVC, at a level above the renal veins and below the absent hepatic segment, following its course cephalad to the SVC before reaching the pulmonary arteries). Alternatively, an arm or neck approach may be preferable, also when bilateral bidirectional Glenn shunts are present (right and persistent left SVC connected to the right and left PA, respectively). In such cases, it is useful to know whether a bridging innominate vein is present.

Catheters

Catheter selection depends on operator preference and the planned investigation.

A Swan-Ganz catheter is a soft, balloon-tipped, end-hole catheter that allows the operator to obtain wedge pressure measurements (e.g. in the pulmonary arteries and hepatic veins). The hole in the tip also allows the use of a guidewire and exchange with other end-hole catheters for angiography or other issues (e.g. inability to access structures). Thermodilution may also be performed to measure pulmonary blood flow but should be avoided when shunts are present. A

Swan-Ganz catheter should not be used for angiography.

The Berman catheter is also a balloon-tipped catheter with no end-hole. It can be used for angiography but cannot be used with a guidewire or exchanged for other catheters.

A 5F pigtail catheter can also be used with a hydrophilic or other guidewire to obtain access to the Fontan circulation and pulmonary arteries and perform angiography. It cannot, however, provide wedge pressure measurements.

Angiography

With modern imaging, the indications for invasive angiography are nowadays limited to answering specific questions, such as:

- Identify stenoses in the Fontan pathway and visualise flow towards the pulmonary arteries
- Assess the size of the pulmonary arteries and presence of peripheral pulmonary artery stenoses
- Identify arteriovenous malformations
- Identify veno-venous collaterals and flow from the SVC
- Visualise fenestrations or patch leaks
- Assess pulmonary venous return

In Fontan patients, angiograms may be obtained at the:

- SVC and Glenn anastomosis
- Pulmonary arteries (central and selective) to assess size and collateral circulation and/or pulmonary venous return, presence of arteriovenous malformations
- Low IVC to assess anatomy and right atrial junction
- Right atrium to assess the anastomosis to the pulmonary arteries, presence of clots, fenes-

trations, patch leaks (e.g. right atrioventricular patch) and patterns of flow within the atrium;

- Systemic ventricle, to assess ventricular and atrioventricular valve function
- Aorta, to assess its size, shape and presence of collateral arteries to the lungs
- Coronary arteries, in older patients with suspected atherosclerotic disease, on to assess possible coronary anomalies/fistulae.

Calculations and Reporting

The cardiac catheter report should include all information collected, calculations and expert interpretation of the results in light also of the results on non-invasive investigations. An essential component of the report are the pressures in the Fontan circuit and pulmonary arteries, filling pressures of the systemic ventricle and a PVR estimate. Indeed, it important to detect an increase in PVR that can occur without a significant increase in PA pressure, because of the drop in pulmonary blood flow/cardiac output.

Unfortunately, the calculation of pulmonary blood flow and PVR may not be straightforward in Fontan patients, especially when there are multiple sources of pulmonary blood flow. This is the case for patients with:

- TCPC, who receive pulmonary blood flow separately from the SVC and IVC
- persistent systemic-to-pulmonary collaterals or surgical shunts
- persistent antegrade flow through the main pulmonary artery
- a unidirectional Glenn shunt with separate right and left lung circulation (classical Glenn anastomosis), in whom one lung typically receives antegrade flow from the ventricle and main pulmonary artery
- bilateral bidirectional Glenn anastomoses (who have bilateral SVCs).

The use of thermodilution to calculate pulmonary blood flow is unlikely to be accurate in the presence of shunts and multiple source flow to the lungs.

The Fick principle is routinely used in congenital heart disease, but also carries significant limitations. The Fick principle relies on the concept that blood flow through an organ (in this case the lung, i.e. pulmonary blood flow, Qp) can be calculated if one knows:

1. the amount of the marker substance (O_2) absorbed by the organ per unit of time (VO_2).
2. the concentration of marker in the arterial blood supplying the organ (pulmonary artery blood).
3. the concentration of marker (O_2) in the venous blood leaving the organ (pulmonary venous blood).

The direct Fick method that requires measurement of VO_2 in the catheter lab is far more accurate that the indirect Fick method that utilizes VO_2 nomograms.

The concentration of O_2 in an artery (CaO_2) or vein (CvO_2), i.e. in the pulmonary venous and artery blood, can be calculated based on arterial oxygen saturation (SaO_2), partial pressure of oxygen (PaO_2) if administering oxygen at a $FiO_2 > 0.30$, and haemoglobin concentration (Hb).

$$CaO_2 = 1.34 \left(\frac{mLO_2}{g} \right) \times Hb \left(\frac{g}{dL} \right) \times SaO_2 \left(decimal \right)$$
$$+ 0.0031 \left(\frac{\frac{mLO_2}{dL\,blood}}{mmHg} \right) \times PaO_2 \left(mmHg \right)$$

Therefore, pulmonary blood flow can be calculated:

$$Qp \left(\frac{L}{min} \right) = \frac{VO_2 \left(\frac{mL}{min} \right)}{CaO_2 \left(\frac{mLO_2}{dL_{blood}} \right) - CvO_2 \left(\frac{mLO_2}{dL_{blood}} \right)} \times 0.1$$

The operator, thus, needs to decide where to sample blood for saturations, to obtain arterial and venous reading that represent the entire lung. In the presence of a single source of pulmonary blood flow to the main PA, sampling within the main PA is sufficient. However, when pulmonary blood flow originates from more than one source e.g. from the Glenn anastomosis and an extracardiac TCPC, it is less clear where sampling should occur (e.g. in both lungs? how distal? is it correct to average the readings from both lungs?) and similarly for other situations listed above.

In recent years, hybrid cardiovascular magnetic resonance (CMR) and fluoroscopic guided cardiac catheterization techniques have been employed increasingly in clinical practice, allowing simultaneous measurement of invasive pressures and CMR quantification of flow. This approach has been validated in congenital cohorts as a more accurate method for PVR assessment than the Fick method [47–49], and has been used to guide management decisions in unpalliated univentricular and Fontan patients [50].

In patients with arteriovenous malformation in one or both lungs, desaturated PA blood bypasses the lung capillaries, effectively shunting right-to-left and causing cyanosis. Calculating shunt fraction for this type of shunt can be challenging. Moreover, estimates of PVR will reflect the resistance across the entire PA tree (that includes both the native vessels and arteriovenous malformations) and should be interpreted with caution when attempting to identify pulmonary vascular disease in the native pulmonary circulation.

References

1. Weipert J, Koch W, Haehnel JC, Meisner H. Exercise capacity and mid-term survival in patients with tricuspid atresia and complex congenital cardiac malformations after modified Fontan-operation. Eur J Cardiothorac Surg. 1997;12(4):574–80.
2. Fredriksen PM, Veldtman G, Hechter S, Therrien J, Chen A, Warsi MA, et al. Aerobic capacity in adults with various congenital heart diseases. Am J Cardiol. 2001;87(3):310–4.
3. Diller G-P, Giardini A, Dimopoulos K, Gargiulo G, Müller J, Derrick G, et al. Predictors of morbidity and mortality in contemporary Fontan patients: results from a multicenter study including cardiopulmonary exercise testing in 321 patients. Eur Heart J. 2010;31(24):3073–83.
4. Fletcher GF, Ades PA, Kligfield P, Arena R, Balady GJ, Bittner VA, et al. Exercise standards for testing and training: a scientific statement from the American Heart Association. Circulation. 2013;128(8):873–934.
5. Stout KK, Daniels CJ, Aboulhosn JA, Bozkurt B, Broberg CS, Colman JM, et al. 2018 AHA/ACC guideline for the management of adults with congenital heart disease: a report of the American College of Cardiology/American Heart Association task force on clinical practice guidelines. J Am Coll Cardiol. 2019;73(12):1494–563.
6. Driscoll DJ, Danielson GK, Puga FJ, Schaff HV, Heise CT, Staats BA. Exercise tolerance and cardiorespiratory response to exercise after the Fontan operation for tricuspid atresia or functional single ventricle. J Am Coll Cardiol. 1986;7(5):1087–94.
7. Cortes RGS, Satomi G, Yoshigi M, Momma K. Maximal hemodynamic response after the Fontan procedure: Doppler evaluation during the treadmill test. Pediatr Cardiol. 1994;15(4):170–7.
8. Harrison DA, Liu P, Walters JE, Goodman JM, Siu SC, Webb GD, et al. Cardiopulmonary function in adult patients late after Fontan repair. J Am Coll Cardiol. 1995;26(4):1016–21.
9. Diller G-P, Dimopoulos K, Okonko D, Uebing A, Broberg CS, Babu-Narayan S, et al. Heart rate response during exercise predicts survival in adults with congenital heart disease. J Am Coll Cardiol. 2006;48(6):1250–6.
10. Larsson ES, Eriksson BO. Haemodynamic adaptation during exercise in Fontan patients at a long-term follow-up. Scand Cardiovasc J. 2003;37(2):107–12.
11. Brassard P, Poirier P, Martin J, Noël M, Nadreau E, Houde C, et al. Impact of exercise training on muscle function and ergoreflex in Fontan patients: a pilot study. Int J Cardiol. 2006;107(1):85–94.
12. Chua TP, Iserin L, Somerville J, Coats AJS. Effects of chronic hypoxemia on chemosensitivity in patients with univentricular heart. J Am Coll Cardiol. 1997;30(7):1827–34.
13. Driscoll DJ, Feldt RH, Mottram CD, Puga FJ, Schaff HV, Danielson GK. Cardiorespiratory response to exercise after definitive repair of univentricular atrioventricular connection. Int J Cardiol. 1987;17(1):73–81.
14. Durongpisitkul K, Driscoll DJ, Mahoney DW, Wollan PC, Mottram CD, Puga FJ, et al. Cardiorespiratory response to exercise after modified Fontan operation: determinants of performance. J Am Coll Cardiol. 1997;29(4):785–90.
15. Garcia JA, McMinn SB, Zuckerman JH, Fixler DE, Levine BD. The role of the right ventricle during hypobaric hypoxic exercise: insights from patients after the Fontan operation. Med Sci Sports Exerc. 1999;31(2):269–76.
16. Grant GP, Mansell AL, Garofano RP, Hayes CJ, Bowman FO, Gersony WM. Cardiorespiratory response to exercise after the Fontan procedure for tricuspid atresia. Pediatr Res. 1988;24(1):1–5.

17. Inai K, Saita Y, Takeda S, Nakazawa M, Kimura H. Skeletal muscle hemodynamics and endothelial function in patients after Fontan operation. Am J Cardiol. 2004;93(6):792–7.

18. Iserin L, Chua TP, Chambers J, Coats AJS, Somerville J. Dyspnoea and exercise intolerance during cardiopulmonary exercise testing in patients with univentricular heart. The effects of chronic hypoxaemia and Fontan procedure. Eur Heart J. 1997;18(8):1350–6.

19. Minamisawa S, Nakazawa M, Momma K, Imai Y, Satomi G. Effect of aerobic training on exercise performance in patients after the Fontan operation. Am J Cardiol. 2001;88(6):695–8.

20. Nir A, Driscoll DJ, Mottram CD, Offord KP, Puga FJ, Schaff HV, et al. Cardiorespiratory response to exercise after the Fontan operation: a serial study. J Am Coll Cardiol. 1993;22(1):216–20.

21. Ohuchi H, Arakaki Y, Hiraumi Y, Tasato H, Kamiya T. Cardiorespiratory response during exercise in patients with cyanotic congenital heart disease with and without a Fontan operation and in patients with congestive heart failure. Int J Cardiol. 1998;66(3):241–51.

22. Rhodes J. Concerning the Fontan patient's excessive minute ventilation during exercise. J Am Coll Cardiol. 1998;32(4):1132.

23. Larsson ES, Eriksson BO, Sixt R. Decreased lung function and exercise capacity in Fontan patients. A long-term follow-up. Scand Cardiovasc J. 2003;37(1):58–63.

24. Strömvall-Larsson E, Eriksson BO, Holmgren D, Sixt R. Pulmonary gas exchange during exercise in Fontan patients at a long-term follow-up. Clin Physiol Funct Imaging. 2004;24(6):327–34.

25. Diller G-P, Dimopoulos K, Okonko D, Li W, Babu-Narayan SV, Broberg CS, et al. Exercise intolerance in adult congenital heart disease: comparative severity, correlates, and prognostic implication. Circulation. 2005;112(6):828–35.

26. Zellers TM, Driscoll DJ, Mottram CD, Puga FJ, Schaff HV, Danielson GK. Exercise tolerance and cardiorespiratory response to exercise before and after the Fontan operation. Mayo Clin Proc. 1989;64(12):1489–97.

27. Gewillig MH, Lundström UR, Bull C, Wyse RKH, Deanfield JE. Exercise responses in patients with congenital heart disease after Fontan repair: patterns and determinants of performance. J Am Coll Cardiol. 1990;15(6):1424–32.

28. Ohuchi H. Cardiopulmonary response to exercise in patients with the Fontan circulation. Cardiol Young. 2005;15(S3):39–44.

29. Opotowsky AR, Landzberg MJ, Earing MG, Wu FM, Triedman JK, Casey A, et al. Abnormal spirometry after the Fontan procedure is common and associated with impaired aerobic capacity. Am J Physiol Heart Circ Physiol. 2014;307(1):H110–7.

30. Takken T, Tacken MHP, Blank AC, Hulzebos EH, Strengers JLM, Helders PJM. Exercise limita-tion in patients with Fontan circulation: a review. J Cardiovasc Med (Hagerstown). 2007;8(10):775–81.

31. Dimopoulos K, Okonko DO, Diller G-P, Broberg CS, Salukhe TV, Babu-Narayan SV, et al. Abnormal ventilatory response to exercise in adults with congenital heart disease relates to cyanosis and predicts survival. Circulation. 2006;113(24):2796–802.

32. Hansen JE, Sue DY, Wasserman K. Predicted values for clinical exercise testing. Am Rev Respir Dis. 1984;129(2P2):S49–55.

33. Robinson TE, Sue DY, Huszczuk A, Weiler-Ravell D, Hansen JE. Intra-arterial and cuff blood pressure responses during incremental cycle ergometry. Med Sci Sports Exerc. 1988;20(2):142–9.

34. Kempny A, Dimopoulos K, Uebing A, Moceri P, Swan L, Gatzoulis MA, et al. Reference values for exercise limitations among adults with congenital heart disease. Relation to activities of daily life—single centre experience and review of published data. Eur Heart J. 2012;33(11):1386–96.

35. Hsia TY, Khambadkone S, Redington AN, Migliavacca F, Deanfield JE, de Leval MR. Effects of respiration and gravity on infradiaphragmatic venous flow in normal and Fontan patients. Circulation. 2000;102(19 Suppl 3):III-148–53.

36. Shafer KM, Garcia JA, Babb TG, Fixler DE, Ayers CR, Levine BD. The importance of the muscle and ventilatory blood pumps during exercise in patients without a subpulmonary ventricle (Fontan operation). J Am Coll Cardiol. 2012;60(20):2115–21.

37. Stout KK, Broberg CS, Book WM, Cecchin F, Chen JM, Dimopoulos K, et al. Chronic heart failure in congenital heart disease a scientific statement from the American Heart Association. Circulation. 2016;133(8):770–801.

38. Balinotti JE, Tiller CJ, Llapur CJ, Jones MH, Kimmel RN, Coates CE, et al. Growth of the lung parenchyma early in life. Am J Respir Crit Care Med. 2009;179(2):134–7.

39. Gewillig M, Brown SC. The Fontan circulation after 45 years: update in physiology. Heart. 2016;102(14):1081–6.

40. Rychik J, Atz AM, Celermajer DS, Deal BJ, Gatzoulis MA, Gewillig MH, et al. Evaluation and management of the child and adult with Fontan circulation: a scientific statement from the American Heart Association. Circulation [Internet]. 2019 [cited 2020 Jul 29];140(6). https://www.ahajournals.org/doi/10.1161/CIR.0000000000000696.

41. ATS Committee on Proficiency Standards for Clinical Pulmonary Function Laboratories. ATS statement: guidelines for the six-minute walk test. Am J Respir Crit Care Med. 2002;166(1):111–7.

42. Galiè N, Beghetti M, Gatzoulis MA, Granton J, Berger RMF, Lauer A, et al. Bosentan therapy in patients with Eisenmenger syndrome: a multicenter, double-blind, randomized, placebo-controlled study. Circulation. 2006;114(1):48–54.

43. Gatzoulis MA, Landzberg M, Beghetti M, Berger RM, Efficace M, Gesang S, et al. Evaluation of Macitentan

in patients with Eisenmenger syndrome. Circulation. 2019;139(1):51–63.

44. Diller G-P, Alonso-Gonzalez R, Dimopoulos K, Alvarez-Barredo M, Koo C, Kempny A, et al. Disease targeting therapies in patients with Eisenmenger syndrome: response to treatment and long-term efficiency. Int J Cardiol. 2013;167(3):840–7.

45. Kempny A, Dimopoulos K, Alonso-Gonzalez R, Alvarez-Barredo M, Tutarel O, Uebing A, et al. Six-minute walk test distance and resting oxygen saturations but not functional class predict outcome in adult patients with Eisenmenger syndrome. Int J Cardiol. 2013;168(5):4784–9.

46. D'Alto M, Dimopoulos K, Budts W, Diller G-P, Di Salvo G, Dellegrottaglie S, et al. Multimodality imaging in congenital heart disease-related pulmonary arterial hypertension. Heart. 2016;102(12):910–8.

47. Razavi R, Hill DLG, Keevil SF, Miquel ME, Muthurangu V, Hegde S, et al. Cardiac catheterisation guided by MRI in children and adults with congenital heart disease. Lancet. 2003;362(9399):1877–82.

48. Muthurangu V, Taylor A, Andriantsimiavona R, Hegde S, Miquel ME, Tulloh R, et al. Novel method of quantifying pulmonary vascular resistance by use of simultaneous invasive pressure monitoring and phase-contrast magnetic resonance flow. Circulation. 2004;110(7):826–34.

49. Kuehne T, Yilmaz S, Schulze-Neick I, Wellnhofer E, Ewert P, Nagel E, et al. Magnetic resonance imaging guided catheterisation for assessment of pulmonary vascular resistance: in vivo validation and clinical application in patients with pulmonary hypertension. Heart. 2005;91(8):1064–9.

50. Pushparajah K, Tzifa A, Bell A, Wong JK, Hussain T, Valverde I, et al. Cardiovascular magnetic resonance catheterization derived pulmonary vascular resistance and medium-term outcomes in congenital heart disease. J Cardiovasc Magn Reson [Internet]. 2015 [cited 2019 Oct 6];17(1). https://www.ncbi.nlm.nih.gov/pmc/articles/PMC4395971/.

Fontan Patients: Psychological Support in Adult Life

28

Lidija McGrath, Andra Eldridge, Abigail Khan, and Craig Broberg

Introduction

Adult congenital heart disease (ACHD) providers are often called upon to screen for psychological distress and coordinate psychological care for their patients. Patients with a Fontan palliation are undoubtedly among the most affected congenital groups in this regard and warrant clinical attention to psychosocial factors affecting their health and wellbeing. Psychological health is coupled to physiologic health. Efforts to understand the underpinnings of any psychological difficulties and their interplay with the cardiovascular status of the individual can lead to an overall health improvement. This chapter summarizes the prevalence of psychologic issues encountered by ACHD patients and reviews treatment options.

Prevalence and Significance of Psychological Distress

Many studies have shown a high prevalence of symptoms of anxiety and depression in ACHD. Notable findings include the following:

- In a study of 150 ACHD patients, 31% met criteria for a mood disorder and 28% met criteria for an anxiety disorder [1].
- In a study of 130 ACHD patients, 42% had elevated anxiety symptoms and 12% had elevated depressive symptoms. Most patients with elevated depressive symptoms (94%) had elevated anxiety symptoms, suggesting that the two conditions often overlap [2].
- It is expected that these findings are even more prevalent in patients with more severe or complex conditions, including Fontan palliation for single ventricle defects.
- Manifestations of anxiety and depression may begin as early as childhood [3]. In a study of 156 adolescents, Fontan patients were five times more likely to have either anxiety, separation anxiety, or social phobia/avoidant behavior than their healthy peers (35% versus 7%, respectively) [4].

Other psychiatric conditions commonly coexist with anxiety and depression, including:

- Post-traumatic stress disorder (PTSD), present in 20% of ACHD patients [5].
- Attention deficit hyperactivity disorder (ADHD), which is five times more common in Fontan teens as compared to their healthy peers [4].
- Neurocognitive challenges, such as poor executive functioning [6]; this and ADHD are

L. McGrath · A. Eldridge · A. Khan · C. Broberg (✉)
Adult Congenital Heart Program, Knight
Cardiovascular Institute, Oregon Health and Science
University, Portland, OR, USA
e-mail: mcgrathl@ohsu.edu; eldriga@ohsu.edu;
khaab@ohsu.edu; brobergc@ohsu.edu

P. Clift et al. (eds.), *Univentricular Congenital Heart Defects and the Fontan Circulation*,
https://doi.org/10.1007/978-3-031-36208-8_28

collectively found in about one third of subjects studied [4].

- Impaired social cognition and other autism-like behaviors [7].

Importantly, the presence of psychological distress also impacts other aspects of an ACHD patient's life. It has been shown that, compared to ACHD patients with no psychological distress, those with both elevated anxiety and depressive symptoms were about half as likely to be in a school or work activity (47% versus 81%, respectively) [2]. Though data are more limited for Fontan patients, they are expected to be similarly affected, if not more so.

Psychological Distress and Quality of Life

Anxiety and depression have been linked with lower quality of life (QOL) [2]. Adolescents with Fontan palliation have a lower QOL than healthy teens based on the PedsQL score, which is specific for physical, emotional, social, and school/work-related QOL [8]. Of these, the scores for emotional functioning are slightly better than for social functioning and school/work functioning. In this same study, the QOL scores of young adults with Fontan palliation were also lower than controls.

Depression and QOL have not been linked in all Fontan studies [9]. Possible explanations that have been cited include the disability paradox, a sense of coherence, and response shift, which are well described elsewhere [9]. Another explanation may be the lack of a "normal" reference, since QOL is largely subjective and congenital heart disease is a lifelong condition [9].

Identification of Psychological Impairment

Symptoms suggestive of significant psychological distress can and should be identified by clinicians during routine outpatient visits.

- At a minimum, clinicians should ask about mental health challenges and explore their impact, when relevant.

- Several formal screening tools are available, each with their strengths and weaknesses.
- When psychological distress is identified, there needs to be a process in place to respond and provide resources to address the problem.
- Established referral pathways greatly facilitate achieving proper mental health care and should be in place to help patients navigate the complex healthcare system, and identify an appropriate mental health provider.

Intervention

Universal screening for psychiatric disorders provides a mechanism that allows to identify psychologic distress early and facilitate treatment [10], which may include psychotherapy and/or pharmacologic treatment [4]. However, questions remain on when or in what context these interventions are most effective. As such, there is need for further studies on the use of these interventions in adults with congenital heart disease [2, 10].

In a recent scientific statement on the management of patients with a Fontan circulation, the sole recommendation about psychosocial intervention was as follows: "Congenital cardiology teams are encouraged to be proactive in their approach to the growing cohort of patients with Fontan circulation, by developing efficient ways to identify psychosocial maladjustment, collaborating with mental health professionals, and developing pediatric based preventive approaches to encourage positive psychosocial adaptation" [6]. Additional recommendations to guide clinical care are urgently needed. Published data in Fontan patients are limited and extrapolation from other groups is necessary, but should be done with caution. Different treatment avenues are discussed below.

Pharmacotherapy

Most patients affected by psychological distress do not receive pharmacotherapy, and the effectiveness of pharmacologic intervention in ACHD is unknown [2]. In acquired heart disease, such as coronary artery disease (CAD) and congestive heart failure

(CHF), the data supporting the use of selective serotonin reuptake inhibitors (SSRIs) is relatively weak [11]. These drugs are, however, well-tolerated in the general population and there is no known adverse effect or contraindication specifically for Fontan patients to warrant hesitancy in their use, when indicated. Sedatives, such as benzodiazepines, are unfavorable long-term treatments given their habit-forming potential [12]. There is no data on the use or effectiveness of antipsychotic medications in Fontan patients. Not surprisingly, only 3% of ACHD patients under active follow-up at a single center over a span of 11 years were treated with antidepressants [13], far less than the expected number with depression in this patient population.

Psychotherapy

Psychotherapy is a non-pharmacologic intervention that avoids the unwanted chemical side-effect of medication and should play a prominent role in the treatment of significant mental health disorders in Fontan patients. Despite the lack of Fontan-specific experience to date, the following points can be applied:

- Psychotherapy is effective in acquired heart disease [14], perhaps more so for depression than anxiety [15].
- For specific anxieties, "exposure-based treatment" has been successful. This involves small, controlled amounts of exposure to the anxiety triggers that allow one to control their reaction [16].
- A pilot clinical trial randomized subjects to cognitive-behavioral therapy for anxiety/depression, including education on living with CHD and cognitive restructuring, with favorable outcomes [17, 18].
- In a study of 75 ACHD patients who underwent psychological treatment consisting of cognitive behavioral therapy, relaxation and communication skills training, 88% of participants reported reduced or absent psychological distress after treatment [19].

Close communication between mental health professionals and other members of the healthcare team is necessary to offer effective treatment. For example, upcoming surgery may be a trigger for anxiety, and may be an important focus of psychotherapy. When a patient's anxiety or depression becomes a major impediment to healthy lifestyle choices, psychological treatment may be necessary for medical treatment to become successful.

Employment and Physical Activity

Fontan patients often face challenges in acquiring a meaningful occupation due to inherent physical, neurocognitive, psychosocial, and educational limitations. ACHD patients with anxiety/depression are half as likely to be in a school or work activity (47% versus 81% in ACHD patients without anxiety or depression) [2], and employment is linked to QOL [20]. Thus, it is likely that establishing a favorable vocational situation, with adaptations as needed, may temper at least some of these symptoms [2]. In a narrative analysis study of patients with complex CHD, several described altering their career choices because of their condition, and 6 out of 10 entered care professions (working with children, vulnerable adults, or healthcare), crediting their childhood experiences with making them more empathic adults [21].

However, employment can also be a source of stress, therefore matching the individual with an occupation suitable to their abilities is key to the success of this strategy.

Physical activity is also a means of improving patients' sense of well-being, including their physical and emotional health. Higher perceived general health and greater QOL have been shown to relate with physical activity [22]. Individualized exercise prescriptions should be given to all Fontan patients, ensuring they remain physically fit throughout their lives and within their abilities, in a safe and effective manner.

Conclusions

Several issues are important when providing psychosocial support for patients with a Fontan palliation. Firstly, a process for identifying psychosocial distress should be incorporated into the routine clinical encounter. Secondly, referral mechanisms to appropriate mental health providers must be readily available. Thirdly, treatment options should be individualized, and include cognitive behavior therapy and/or pharmacologic treatments.

References

1. Westhoff-Bleck M, Briest J, Fraccarollo D, Hilfiker-Kleiner D, Winter L, Maske U, Busch MA, Bleich S, Bauersachs J, Kahl KG. Mental disorders in adults with congenital heart disease: unmet needs and impact on quality of life. J Affect Disord. 2016;204:180–6.
2. Gleason LP, Deng LX, Khan AM, Drajpuch D, Fuller S, Ludmir J, Mascio CE, Partington SL, Tobin L, Kim YY, Kovacs AH. Psychological distress in adults with congenital heart disease: focus beyond depression. Cardiol Young. 2019;29:185–9.
3. Abda A, Bolduc ME, Tsimicalis A, Rennick J, Vatcher D, Brossard-Racine M. Psychosocial outcomes of children and adolescents with severe congenital heart defect: a systematic review and meta-analysis. J Pediatr Psychol. 2019;44:463–77.
4. DeMaso DR, Calderon J, Taylor GA, Holland JE, Stopp C, White MT, Bellinger DC, Rivkin MJ, Wypij D, Newburger JW. Psychiatric disorders in adolescents with single ventricle congenital heart disease. Pediatrics. 2017;139:e20162241.
5. Deng LX, Khan AM, Drajpuch D, Fuller S, Ludmir J, Mascio CE, Partington SL, Qadeer A, Tobin L, Kovacs AH, Kim YY. Prevalence and correlates of post-traumatic stress disorder in adults with congenital heart disease. Am J Cardiol. 2016;117:853–7.
6. Rychik J, Atz AM, Celermajer DS, Deal BJ, Gatzoulis MA, Gewillig MH, Hsia TY, Hsu DT, Kovacs AH, McCrindle BW, Newburger JW, Pike NA, Rodefeld M, Rosenthal DN, Schumacher KR, Marino BS, Stout K, Veldtman G, Younoszai AK, d'Udekem Y. Evaluation and management of the child and adult with Fontan circulation: a scientific statement from the American Heart Association. Circulation. 2019;140:e234–84.
7. Bellinger DC, Watson CG, Rivkin MJ, Robertson RL, Roberts AE, Stopp C, Dunbar-Masterson C, Bernson D, DeMaso DR, Wypij D, Newburger JW. Neuropsychological status and structural brain imaging in adolescents with single ventricle who underwent the Fontan procedure. J Am Heart Assoc. 2015;4:e002302.
8. Uzark K, Zak V, Shrader P, McCrindle BW, Radojewski E, Varni JW, Daniels K, Handisides J, Hill KD, Lambert LM, Margossian R, Pemberton VL, Lai WW, Atz AM. Assessment of quality of life in young patients with single ventricle after the Fontan operation. J Pediatr. 2016;170:166–72.e1.
9. Pike NA, Evangelista LS, Doering LV, Eastwood JA, Lewis AB, Child JS. Quality of life, health status, and depression: comparison between adolescents and adults after the Fontan procedure with healthy counterparts. J Cardiovasc Nurs. 2012;27:539–46.
10. Riley JP, Habibi H, Banya W, Gatzoulis MA, Lau-Walker M, Cowie MR. Education and support needs of the older adult with congenital heart disease. J Adv Nurs. 2012;68:1050–60.
11. Andrade C, Kumar CB, Surya S. Cardiovascular mechanisms of SSRI drugs and their benefits and risks in ischemic heart disease and heart failure. Int Clin Psychopharmacol. 2013;28:145–55.
12. Jackson JL, Leslie CE, Hondorp SN. Depressive and anxiety symptoms in adult congenital heart disease: prevalence, health impact and treatment. Prog Cardiovasc Dis. 2018;61:294–9.
13. Diller GP, Brautigam A, Kempny A, Uebing A, Alonso-Gonzalez R, Swan L, Babu-Narayan SV, Baumgartner H, Dimopoulos K, Gatzoulis MA. Depression requiring anti-depressant drug therapy in adult congenital heart disease: prevalence, risk factors, and prognostic value. Eur Heart J. 2016;37:771–82.
14. Richards SH, Anderson L, Jenkinson CE, Whalley B, Rees K, Davies P, Bennett P, Liu Z, West R, Thompson DR and Taylor RS. Psychological interventions for coronary heart disease. Cochrane Database Syst Rev. 2017;4:CD002902.
15. Ski CF, Jelinek M, Jackson AC, Murphy BM, Thompson DR. Psychosocial interventions for patients with coronary heart disease and depression: a systematic review and meta-analysis. Eur J Cardiovasc Nurs. 2016;15:305–16.
16. Hofmann SG, Asnaani A, Vonk IJ, Sawyer AT, Fang A. The efficacy of cognitive behavioral therapy: a review of meta-analyses. Cognit Ther Res. 2012;36:427–40.
17. Kovacs AH, Bandyopadhyay M, Grace SL, Kentner AC, Nolan RP, Silversides CK, Irvine MJ. Adult Congenital Heart Disease-Coping And REsilience (ACHD-CARE): rationale and methodology of a pilot randomized controlled trial. Contemp Clin Trials. 2015;45:385–93.
18. Kovacs AH, Grace SL, Kentner AC, Nolan RP, Silversides CK, Irvine MJ. Feasibility and outcomes in a pilot randomized controlled trial of a psychosocial intervention for adults with congenital heart disease. Can J Cardiol. 2018;34:766–73.
19. Ferguson M, Kovacs AH. An integrated adult congenital heart disease psychology service. Congenit Heart Dis. 2016;11:444–51.
20. Apers S, Kovacs AH, Luyckx K, Thomet C, Budts W, Enomoto J, Sluman MA, Wang JK, Jackson JL, Khairy P, Cook SC, Chidambarathanu S, Alday L, Eriksen K, Dellborg M, Berghammer M, Mattsson E, Mackie AS, Menahem S, Caruana M, Veldtman G, Soufi A, Romfh AW, White K, Callus E, Kutty S, Fieuws S, Moons P. Quality of life of adults with congenital heart disease in 15 countries: evaluating

country-specific characteristics. J Am Coll Cardiol. 2016;67:2237–45.

21. Keir M, Bailey B, Lee A, Kovacs AH, Lucy RS. Narrative analysis of adults with complex congenital heart disease: childhood experiences and their lifelong reverberations. Congenit Heart Dis. 2018;13:740–7.

22. Holbein CE, Veldtman GR, Moons P, Kovacs AH, Luyckx K, Apers S, Chidambarathanu S, Soufi A, Eriksen K, Jackson JL, Enomoto J, Fernandes SM, Johansson B, Alday L, Dellborg M, Berghammer M, Menahem S, Caruana M, Kutty S, Mackie AS, Thomet C, Budts W, White K, Sluman MA, Callus E, Cook SC, Khairy P, Cedars A. Perceived health mediates effects of physical activity on quality of life in patients with a Fontan circulation. Am J Cardiol. 2019;124:144–50.

Dominica Zentner and Sara Thorne

Introduction

Although this chapter concentrates on pregnancy in women with a Fontan circulation and the surrounding risks and challenges of childbearing, it is important to recognise that childbearing motivates only a small part of sexual activity for most adults. Little work has been done on the sexual well-being of individuals with a Fontan circulation. A recent paper describes a link between sexual problems and physical limitations, particularly for male Fontan patients and between sexual problems and psychosocial well-being, particularly in female Fontan patients [1]. Education regarding contraception, sexually transmitted infections (STI's) and pregnancy should be part of routine care, both during adolescence and the transition period (from paediatric to adult services) [2], and throughout their life. Sexual identity and activity is often very enmeshed with an individual's sense of self, and the capacity for chronic illness to interfere with this should be recognised [3].

Contraception and Fertility Treatment in the Woman with a Fontan Circulation

Contraceptive methods have different efficacy rates, and many have higher than expected unplanned pregnancy rates due to the reliance on perfect user adherence. It is important to recognise this when discussing the benefits and risks of different contraceptive methods with patients (Table 29.1). Also, only condoms convey protection from STI's. Therefore, a 'contraceptive *plus* condom' approach as provision of both contraceptive and sexual health protection should be discussed.

Combined Oral Contraceptive Pill (COCP)

The COCP, like other estrogen-containing preparations such as the contraceptive sponge, has the highest risk of thrombosis, due to its ethinyl oestradiol component. Lower dose ethinyl oestradiol conveys a lesser risk, with data showing reduced

D. Zentner (✉)
Department of Cardiology, Royal Melbourne Hospital, Melbourne, VIC, Australia

Department of Genomic Medicine, Royal Melbourne Hospital, Melbourne, VIC, Australia

Department of Medicine, University of Melbourne, Melbourne, VIC, Australia
e-mail: Dominica.Zentner@mh.org.au

S. Thorne
Peter Munk Cardiac Centre, Toronto General Hospital, University Health Network, Toronto, ON, Canada

University of Toronto, Toronto, ON, Canada
e-mail: sara.thorne@uhn.ca

© The Author(s), under exclusive license to Springer Nature Switzerland AG 2023
P. Clift et al. (eds.), *Univentricular Congenital Heart Defects and the Fontan Circulation*,
https://doi.org/10.1007/978-3-031-36208-8_29

Table 29.1 Efficacy and unplanned pregnancy rates with different contraceptive methods [4, 5]

Contraceptive method	Reported efficacy[a]	Reported unplanned pregnancy rate	Concerns for the woman with a Fontan circulation
Levonorgestrel releasing intrauterine device	99.8%	<1/100 women in 1 year	Needs to be inserted with analgesic cover and cardiac monitoring in hospital, as may induce a vagal response [6]
Etonogestrel implant	99.95%	<1/100 women in 1 year	Bleeding (likely minor only) at insertion site if anticoagulated
Depot medroxyprogesterone acetate	99.8%	6–9/100 women in 1 year	*May* have an increased risk of VTE compared with other progesterone-only contraceptives [7]. Generally considered safe [6]
Combined oral contraceptive pill (COCP)	99.7% (12-h administration window)	6–9/100 women in 1 year	Contraindicated in some guidelines [6] (see below)
Progesterone only mini pill[b]	99.7% (small window of administration (3 h) reduces efficacy)	6–9/100 women in 1 year	None
Desogestrel progesterone only pill[c]	>99% (12-h administration window)	<8/100 women in 1 year	Nil known
Diaphragm	94%	18+/100 women in 1 year	None
Condom	98%	18+/100 women in 1 year	None *ONLY* Contraception with STI protection

VTE venous thromboembolism

[a] Efficacy if adherence of 100%

[b] Often referred to as the mini pill

[c] Not available throughout the world, efficacy closer to that of the COCP than the mini pill, as it also induces anovulation. Safe for women with cardiac disease [8, 9]

risk by lowering the dose to 35 μg [10]. Concern about the sequelae of VTE in the Fontan circulation has led to the use of the COCP being contraindicated in guidelines [6]. However, many follow a pragmatic approach that:

- recognises the far higher risk of VTE associated with pregnancy, and the post-partum period, [10] and
- allows COCP use with:
  - concomitant anticoagulation [11] and
  - absence of a right to left shunt [2, 12].

This explains patient experience patterns reported in Australia and New Zealand, where almost half the women with Fontan surveyed had utilised the COCP [13]. It is important to recognise that there are some general patient factors that preclude prescription of the COCP as they add to the VTE risk, particularly hypertension, smoking, migraine with aura and stroke [14] (please consult reference for a full list).

An additional concern in this population, who have an increased risk of Fontan associated liver disease, is the observation that the COCP can cause hepatocellular adenomas [15]. Prescription of the COCP, requires a frank discussion with patients, and shared decision-making that recognises the known and potential risks and benefits.

Fertility Treatment

Infertility describes a spectrum, from complete sterility to reduced fertility, and is common in the general population, affecting 1 in 6 couples when defined as failure to conceive after 12 months of regular unprotected intercourse [16]. Publications have suggested increased rates of infertility in patients with certain chronic diseases. It is likely that the physiological sequelae of the Fontan circulation, particularly cyanosis, venous hypertension and clotting abnormalities, are significant contributors to reduced fertility in this cohort [17]. Additionally, menarche is delayed [14] and menstrual cycle abnormalities are more common in patients with a Fontan circulation [18].

Failure of conception often leads couples to seek further advice. It is important to sensitively explore whether there are health concerns that suggest that pregnancies may be miscarried, even if the inability to conceive is overcome. Though the data is limited, there are no published reports of pregnancy leading to a livebirth in a woman with a Fontan circulation and resting oxygen saturations <85% [19, 20]. In other congenital heart disease (CHD), the success of livebirth with this degree of maternal cyanosis is quoted at 12% [21].

Fertility treatments (FT) consist of a spectrum of increasing medical intervention, ranging from promotion of ovulation via medical therapy, to in-vitro fertilisation (IVF), where fertilisation occurs outside the body. It is important to also consider surrogacy and adoption as options in the treatment of infertility, particularly if there is concern regarding maternal well-being during pregnancy.

Both investigation and treatment of infertility may adversely affect the Fontan circulation (Table 29.2). We were only able to identify unsuccessful outcomes of IVF in women with a Fontan circulation in the literature (n = 2) [28], though ovulation induction has been described as leading to livebirths [14]. Some have proposed that FT should not be undertaken in women in

Table 29.2 Adverse physiological sequelae from investigation and treatment of infertility

Intervention	Potential adverse effects	Concerns for the woman with a Fontan circulation
Tubal patency investigation		
• Hysterosalpingogram (HSG) • Laparoscopy and dye test	• HSG: cervical manipulation may elicit vagal response. Undertake with analgesia and cardiac monitoring • Laparoscopy: requires abdominal insufflation to achieve a pneumoperitoneum	• Vagal reaction may precipitate severe hypotension and cardiovascular collapse • Increased abdominal pressure may compromise systemic venous return and cause an elevation in systemic vascular resistance, both contributing to reduced CO. Additionally, it may increase pulmonary vascular resistance, further worsening systemic venous return/pressures and CO
Treatment of anovulation—ovulation induction		
• Clomiphene citrate (CC)[a] • Gonadotrophins (GnT)	• Both CC and GnT can cause ovarian hyperstimulation syndrome (OHSS) • OHSS is associated with an increased risk for both VTE and arterial TE events • Pregnancies complicated by OHSS have an increased risk of PET and preterm delivery • Treatment of anovulation increases the risk for multiple pregnancy	• OHSS varies in severity from mild to severe [22]. OHSS is characterised by significant fluid shifts that can cause ascites (with subsequent potential for haemodynamic compromise, see above) and hypovolemia. This is potentially life threatening, especially in women with a Fontan circulation • VTE is more likely in the Fontan circulation and has a higher adverse effect profile. The risk of arterial TE may be raised further by the presence of cyanosis, clotting abnormalities and right-left shunts • Pregnancies in the Fontan circulation are at increased risk for preterm delivery • Concern regarding the additional haemodynamic load of multiple (twin) pregnancy [23] strongly suggests that singleton conception should be the aim in this population. This is also relevant when considering the increased likelihood of preterm delivery and IUGR, and the relationship with fetal outcomes
In-vitro fertilisation		

Table 29.2 (continued)

Intervention	Potential adverse effects	Concerns for the woman with a Fontan circulation

• Includes treatment to induce ovulation (see above)
  –Egg harvesting
  –Embryo transfer
• Increased risk of pregnancy adverse events [24]
  –PIH
  –GDM
  –VTE [25]
  –Placenta praevia
  –Placental abruption
  –APH
  –PPH
  –Preterm and very preterm birth
  –Low and very low birth weight
  –Perinatal mortality
  –Congenital abnormalities
	• See above
	• Requires sedation
	• Variable practice with respect to sedation and cervical dilatation [26]
	• As in column 1
		• See above
		• May occur in a non-hospital setting. Women with a Fontan circulation should have this procedure performed in hospital and with an anaesthetist who is comfortable with the maternal physiology. If the woman is anticoagulated, this needs individualised planning
		• Concerns as above
		• Women with a Fontan circulation are more likely to have adverse haemodynamic consequences from many of the described maternal obstetric complications. Their fetuses are already at increased risk from the described fetal complications of ART
		• An increase in cyanotic CHD has been identified in livebirths from any form of FT as compared with natural conception [27]. As these women represent a cohort with an already increased risk of fetal CHD, they should be educated as to the further increased risk

CO cardiac output, *PET* pre-eclampsia, *IUGR* intra-uterine growth restriction, *ART* assisted reproductive technology, *PIH* pregnancy induced hypertension, *GDM* gestational diabetes mellitus, *VTE* venous thromboembolic disease, *APH* antepartum haemorrhage, *PPH* postpartum haemorrhage, *CHD* congenital heart disease

WHO class III or IV pregnancy risk [25]. This would preclude all women with a Fontan circulation from pursuing assistance with conception; we believe this is too restrictive, given the wide spectrum of functional status that can be observed in these individuals. However, any FT should be done in open consultation with both the woman and her cardiologist, and strong preference should be expressed for the lowest dose hormonal treatment in the setting of ovulation induction, single-embryo transfer and 'natural cycle' or minimal stimulation IVF, to avoid or reduce the risk of ovarian hyperstimulation syndrome (OHSS) [6, 29].

The Cardiac Obstetric Team

All women with a Fontan circulation are deemed high-risk in pregnancy, and should all be managed in a specialised centre by a multidisciplinary team (Class IA recommendation) [6]. The pregnancy heart team consists of a cardiologist, obstetrician and anaesthetist, with additional expertise required throughout the pregnancy and at the time of delivery. For women with a Fontan circulation, the cardiologist should have expertise in congenital heart disease, and the obstetrician should have expertise in high-risk pregnancies (maternal fetal medicine specialists). The team should be flexible and expand to include a haematologist (for women who are anticoagulated), cardiac anaesthetist, midwives, cardiac nurses and a neonatologist as/ when required. An understanding of the likely pregnancy course and possible concerns, that includes anticipatory preparation for the likely earlier delivery of a smaller baby is important.

Although very little research exists into the experience of pregnancy for women with Fontan palliation [30], involving patients in discussions and decision-making is an important means of achieving a flexible maternal approach to pregnancy care and delivery. This is highly desirable in terms of coping with the potential complications of a high risk pregnancy.

Management Plan in the Pregnant Fontan Patient

Pre-conception Assessment

The management of pregnancy in women with a Fontan circulation starts in late childhood/ adolescence, well before conception, with the first conversations on sex, contraception and sexual health. The importance of planned conception, preceded by careful pre-conception assessment of maternal cardiovascular status and well-being, needs to discussed in every clinical encounter in the adult service, without presumption of prior knowledge. Differences have been reported around the world as to the frequency of preconception education. In a Canadian study of women with a range of CHD diagnoses, one third of those at intermediate-to-high risk for pregnancy-related complications did not recall ever being informed of this risk [31]. In contrast, in a more recent study on Fontan women from Australia and New Zealand, 93% of participants recalled being counselled about pregnancy-related risk, with the majority (81%) being aware they were at increased risk and, for some, that pregnancy had been advised against [14].

Preconception assessment should encompass an assessment of maternal cardiac status (medical history review, examination, electrocardiogram (ECG), echocardiogram and blood tests). A cardiac MRI is reasonable (particularly if there isn't a prior assessment with intervening clinical stability) and functional capacity should be objectively documented (exercise test with ECG and oximetry monitoring or cardiopulmonary exercise testing). Experts feel that women with CHD that achieve 9-min with a Bruce protocol treadmill test, or a peak oxygen uptake (pVO$_2$) of >60% predicted during a cardiopulmonary exercise test may be capable of tolerating the haemodynamic challenges of pregnancy. However, the above exercise parameters should be combined with other anatomical clinical information to provide an individualised estimated risk. This includes ongoing medical therapies, as described in Table 29.3).

Maternal and Fetal Risk Models

As part of the preconception assessment and counselling, women need to be educated as to the likely maternal and fetal course in pregnancy, with explanation of risks and outcomes and the observed incidence.

No Fontan-specific prospectively validated pregnancy risk model exists. The WHO pregnancy risk classification predicts maternal outcomes in CHD patients better than either the CARPREG or ZAHARA models [37]. The CARPREG II model was recently published [38], however, it is not possible to tell whether any patients included in the derivation population had a Fontan circulation. To date, no model has been demonstrated to accurately predict fetal risk in a Fontan pregnancy.

A retrospectively-derived risk-scoring system appeared able to identify women with a Fontan circulation who were at particularly high risk of a negative pregnancy outcome: 6.7% livebirths in the highest risk group (small subgroup of 4 women) versus 37.5% livebirths in the lower risk group [39]. Physician experience is, therefore, important when estimating pregnancy-related risk in Fontan women. Indeed, in one study, physician risk assessment in women with WHO III–IV cardiac disease outperformed risk model assessment [40].

Table 29.3 Active preconception medical management in women with a Fontan circulation

Medical concern	Specific/additional assessment[a]	Intervention
Pre pregnancy assessment	As per general population	• Rubella status, immunise if required • Smoking cessation • Ideal weight attainment[b] • Alcohol cessation • Regular exercise • Folic acid supplementation (500 mcg daily, at least 4 weeks pre and 12 weeks post conception. Many formulations come with iron supplementation) • Psychosocial issues – refer if appropriate • Up to date cervical cancer screening • Up-to-date immunisations • Review diet (need adequate iodine, vitamin D, iron, B12 and calcium) • Advice regarding food and supplements to avoid in pregnancy
Arrhythmias	Holter	Consider: • Medical therapy • Radiofrequency ablation • Fontan conversion
Reduced exercise capacity	Exercise stress test/ cardiopulmonary stress test	Consider: • Weight loss if overweight • Regular exercise (may benefit from referral to cardiac rehabilitation program) • Iron status—ensure replete • Re assess after a 6-month period of active intervention
Cyanosis	Oxygen saturation at rest and exercise Cardiac MRI/CT/ angiography[a]	Consider • Shunt closure (for e.g. of fenestration or significant veno-venous collaterals) if clinically significant desaturation present; it is important to appreciate that improvement is often not obtained or sustained longer-term; moreover, such procedures may lead to preload reduction. Test occlusion should be performed to confirm that Fontan pressures do not rise

Medication	Medical history review[a]	Consider
		• Amiodarone is generally contraindicated on fetal grounds in pregnancy[c]
		• ACE inhibitors and ARB's are contraindicated on fetal grounds. Cease. Transition to a beta blocker, if indicated
		• Spironolactone is contraindicated on fetal grounds. Transition to a loop diuretic, if required
		• Anticoagulation: review indication. If indication confirmed, then discuss with woman on the known teratogenic risk with warfarin in the first trimester and advise to immediately transition to LMWH at conception with option to
		  – remain on LMWH throughout gestation or
		  – return to warfarin in the second trimester
		Refer women who are anticoagulated for haematology review before conception
		  – Proactive formulation of anticoagulation plan, including prescription of LMWH, education re LMWH administration and plan for anti-factor Xa monitoring
		  – Regular pregnancy tests to identify pregnancy very soon after conception

Table 29.3 (continued)

Medical concern	Specific/additional assessment[a]	Intervention
Fontan failure PLE ≥ moderate ventricular dysfunction ≥ moderate AVV regurgitation Oxygen saturation < 85%	Review medical file, history, examination and investigation findings[a]	• If no reversible factors are identified, then pregnancy should be advised against • If reversible factors identified, treat and reassess • Consider surgery, Fontan conversion or assessment for heart transplantation as appropriate

ACEI angiotensin converting enzyme inhibitor, *ARB* angiotensin receptor blocker, *LMWH* low molecular weight heparin, *AVV* atrioventricular valve

[a] Note: all Fontan women should receive preconception assessment, as detailed in the table and text

[b] An elevated BMI carries an increased risk of medical complications in pregnancy, as well as increasing the risks of adverse fetal outcomes and Caesarean section. Treatment of obesity pre-conception is currently recommended by both the American [32] and British Obstetrics and Gynaecology [33] societies. However, a small body of animal work suggests that conception during maternal caloric restriction adversely affects the endocrine development in the offspring [34, 35]. Work is planned in humans which will ascertain short term safety of significant pre-conception weight loss [36]. It may be safest to attain an ideal BMI that is then sustainably maintained for some months prior to conception

[c] Consider a preconception trial of beta-blocker to replace amiodarone. If arrhythmias remain suppressed, remain off amiodarone. If arrhythmias cannot be controlled by a beta-blocker or ablation, the fetal risk of continuing amiodarone needs to be balanced against the maternal (and fetal) risk of uncontrolled arrhythmia

Pregnancy Management

These women require frequent monitoring throughout pregnancy (Table 29.4). As this is quite different to the usual societal expectations of pregnancy, this needs to be highlighted in pre-conception counselling.

Delivery Management

Pregnancy management should aim at achieving a vaginal delivery in Fontan patients. This has increasingly been recognised as appropriate for the majority of women with heart disease [6]. However, the reality of maternal cardiac complications, fetal growth restriction and the increased risk of preterm onset of labour and premature rupture of membranes reduce the likelihood of success. If the mother is therapeutically anticoagulated, a clear plan needs to be formulated with haematology and obstetric input ahead of delivery.

Additionally, as women may deteriorate peri-delivery, it is reasonable to consider induction of labour (IOL), aiming to deliver during business hours on a weekday, when the entire team are onsite. IOL can be undertaken with local prostaglandin, artificial rupture of membranes and oxytocin. If a vaginal delivery can be attained, then regional anaesthesia with slow titration of agents, that minimises exertive effort, is appropriate due to the potentially detrimental haemodynamic effect of a maternal Valsalva manoeuvre (pushing with closed glottis) [41].

It is reasonable to monitor the mother with telemetry, oximetry and frequent or continuous blood pressure monitoring. Women with a Fontan circulation tolerate blood loss particularly poorly, so a group and screen of blood type and antibody status is appropriate, and the third stage of labour should be actively managed. It is generally accepted that women with heart disease have higher blood loss at delivery than women with normal hearts. There are several factors that may contribute, including maternal anticoagulation, limitation of active second stage and caution in the use of uterotonics in the third stage of labour [42].

There is a paucity of data regarding the optimal management of the third stage of labour in these women. Ergot alkaloids and prostaglandins

Table 29.4 Pregnancy care

Pregnancy	Routine	Additional tests/ care as clinically indicated
On recognition of conception	Contact pregnancy heart team service who ensure: • the woman knows who to contact with health concerns • a referral for obstetric care (if not at site of Pregnancy Heart team review) • a dating scan organised	• Transition to LMWH for women on warfarin. Contact haematologist regarding dose, follow anti factor Xa levels
First clinic review (*ideally multidisciplinary review with obstetrician and cardiologist*)	• Approximately 10–14 weeks gestation, in recognition of the high likelihood of early pregnancy loss • ECG, echocardiogram, oximetry	• 6-min walk test with oximetry if any concerns about symptoms, well-being (or no prior or preconcetion stress test) • Holter monitor if any concerns regarding arrhythmias • Haematology review if anticoagulated. Anticoagulation should be individualised, and a preconception plan should be in place (see Table 29.3)
Second clinic review (*ideally multidisciplinary review with obstetrician and cardiologist*)	• Approximately 16–20 weeks • ECG, echocardiogram, oximetry • Organise fetal echocardiogram scan (approximately 20 weeks' gestation) • Organise fetal growth scan monitoring	• 6-min walk test with oximetry if any concerns about symptoms, well-being (or no prior or preconcetion stress test) • Holter monitor if any concerns regarding arrhythmias
Third clinic review (*ideally multidisciplinary review with obstetrician and cardiologist*)	• Approximately 24–26 weeks • ECG, echocardiogram, oximetry • Organise obstetric anaesthetic review • Organise fetal growth scan monitoring	• 6-min walk test with oximetry if any concerns about symptoms, well-being or no preconception stress test • Holter monitor if any concerns regarding arrhythmias
Fourth and every subsequent clinic review (*ideally multidisciplinary review with obstetrician and cardiologist*)	• Approximately 28–30 weeks • ECG, echocardiogram, oximetry • Plan for review at least 4-weekly from now until delivery • Support cessation of work and commencement of maternity leave as dictated by maternal well- being • Organise fetal growth scan monitoring	• Consider repeat 6-min walk test with oximetry • Holter monitor if any concerns regarding arrhythmias
Multidisciplinary delivery planning	• Service-specific, but in many centres will consist of a face to face meeting of all members of the medical and nursing team	

should be avoided, due to risks of hypertension and pulmonary hypertension, respectively. A slow intravenous titration of oxytocin is widely used. A recent publication has demonstrated that an additional 2 U given as a slow bolus to a group of CHD patients resulted in a significant reduction in bleeding, with no adverse maternal cardiac events. However, only 1 Fontan patient was included, and only received slow iv administration. The regime used in this study was still associated with higher rates of PPH than seen in the general population [43].

In contrast, a recent retrospective study reported that the regimen used in women without CHD (10 IU IM after a vaginal delivery and 5 IU slow IV after an operative delivery) was safe in women with either CHD or acquired heart disease; blood loss was also comparable. Again, the number of women with a Fontan circulation in this study was limited (n = 2) [42].

Post-partum Management

Although delivery of a baby results in a huge sense of relief for both the parents and the team, the increased risk of PPH and the possibility of haemodynamic deterioration from postpartum fluid shifts require careful ongoing vigilance and monitoring.

Women should be monitored in a higher acuity setting for 48–72 h. Depending on local service capacity, this may be in a telemetry cardiology bed, high dependency or intensive care setting. Unfortunately, and particularly if the delivery has been preterm, this often results in separation of the mother and baby. This possibility should be actively communicated to the woman and her family throughout the pregnancy management.

Prophylactic LMWH to reduce the risk of DVT is mandatory post caesarean section and should be strongly considered in Fontan women even after a vaginal delivery. As the risk of DVT is significantly elevated for several weeks postpartum, it is reasonable to discuss prolonged DVT prophylaxis in women without long-term anticoagulation indication.

Breastfeeding should be encouraged. Realistically, given the high likelihood of maternal and baby separation, initiation will rely on midwifery input and education regarding breast stimulation. The colostrum should be collected and transferred to the baby given its significant antibody profile and associated neonatal benefit.

Routine neonatology review of the baby is important. Parental concern regarding CHD should be allayed as soon as possible.

Maternal anticoagulation, if indicated, should be reinstituted at a time decided collectively by the team, dependent on risk profile and post-delivery bleeding potential. Women should be discharged home with contraceptive advice and planned review with repeat echocardiography at approximately 6 weeks post-partum. Women and their families should know how to access help in case of cardiovascular deterioration or other complication in the intervening time.

Maternal and Fetal Outcomes

The available data on pregnancy complications and outcomes for the mother and baby appear consistent. Unfortunately, the data comes from retrospective publications, and it is unknown whether adverse outcomes have been underreported (e.g. maternal mortality). Additionally, causal inferences between management strategies and outcome data is challenging.

A recent systematic review summarised 6 publications encapsulating the reported outcomes of 133 women and 255 pregnancies [44]. The most sobering outcomes were for the fetus with 115 (45%) miscarriages, 2 (1%) stillbirths and 6 (5%) neonatal deaths. Moreover, there was a significant number of terminations (19, 7%). These should serve as a reminder of the importance of maternal education on contraception, preconception assessment and counselling for all.

Maternal cardiac adverse events were most often supraventricular arrhythmias and heart failure (affecting 8.4% and 3.9% of pregnancies, respectively). Smaller numbers of other events were also reported: pulmonary emboli, bradycardia requiring pacemaker insertion, transient ischaemic attacks, reduced exercise capacity and intracardiac thrombosis.

Obstetric events were characterised by bleeding, as both antepartum and postpartum events. Most births (68%) were premature, and most women (57%) delivered by caesarean section. The livebirth rate was 45% of all pregnancies.

Late Effects Following Pregnancy in Fontan Patients

An important unanswered concern in this population is the potential for pregnancy to impact on long-term maternal survival, health and well-being. This concern is founded on demonstration that pregnancy in normal hearts is

Table 29.5 Published deaths post pregnancy in women with a Fontan circulation

Author and publication details	Post pregnancy cohort descriptor	Follow up (n) and time	Control population	Deaths (and causes if described)
Canobbio [51]	45 women[a] 71 pregnancies (51 livebirths)[b]	• 29 (67%) • Mean 7.74 years (range 1–23 years)	Nil	• 5 late deaths – TE (n = 2) – Heart failure (n = 2) – Unknown (n = 1)
Gouton [52]	37 women 59 pregnancies (36 livebirths[b])	• N = unclear (? All) • Median 2 years (95% CI 8–31 months)	Nil	• No deaths
Pundi [53]	19 women (29 livebirths[b])	• Difficult to ascertain, but paper states "complete follow-up for nearly 50%" • Mean 13.3 ± 4.7 years	Nil	• 1 late death – Cause unknown (11 years pp)
Arif [39]	21 women 55 pregnancies (13 livebirths[b])	• 9 of the 10 women with livebirths • Median 4.8 years (3.3–10)	Nil	• No deaths
Cauldwell [20]	50 women 124 pregnancies (53 livebirths[b])	• 33 women • Median 6 years (range 4 months – 10.4 years)	Nil	• No deaths
Moroney [19][c]	30 women 69 pregnancies (43 livebirths, includes 1 set twins[b])	• 26 • Median 3.6 (1.2–7.5) years	233 women 280 men	• 1 death (2.6 years pp) – TE

TE thromboembolic event, *pp.* post-partum

[a] Please note that this abstract also reports 1 woman who was resuscitated from a cardiac arrest during delivery

[b] Livebirths does not take into account subsequent neonatal deaths in some series

[c] In this publication, the women who had had a pregnancy were a healthier subgroup. Total deaths over follow up from date of Fontan to data ascertainment were: 1/30 pregnancy group; 17/233 non pregnant females and 32/280 males (unpublished data)

accompanied by measurable—though asymptomatic—deterioration in function [45, 46]. Moreover, a decline in ventricular function, and other delayed adverse events, have also been reported in several types of CHD [47–49].Controlled data are lacking, and the tendency for a slow but gradual deterioration in the well-being of patients with a Fontan circulation [50] makes ascertaining the effect of pregnancy on long-term outcome difficult (Table 29.5). Indeed, none of the recent large systematic reviews/meta-analyses on the outcome of Fontan patients appear to have considered pregnancy as a potentially modulating factor [54–56]. Mortality, as an absolute endpoint is also easier to capture than indexes of health-related well-being, which may be affected by pregnancy-related morbidity, or complications of the Fontan operation that are exacerbated by pregnancy. The potential effects of pregnancy include deterioration in ventricular function and an increase in TE events, both related to the volume expansion of pregnancy and mediated by a (postulated) increase in venous pooling in the latter. Individuals with a Fontan circulation are at increased risk for varicose veins [57], and this is likely further exacerbated by the hormonal and weight gain effects of pregnancy.

We have recently published a study looking at post-partum outcomes in women with a Fontan circulation, compared to both women without prior pregnancy and men [19]. Although the post-partum women were significantly older than both comparator groups, they were healthier, with significantly fewer cardiac events. Post-partum, this "healthier status" was lost, with an increased likelihood for VTE (HR 4.84, p = 0.04), but no difference in outcomes after propensity score analysis (possibly due to a significant reduction in sample size). The potential signal for increased VTE informs the earlier comment that prophylactic LMWH may be appropriate in the puerperium, though all the VTE events captured were delayed beyond this time frame.

Unrepaired Univentricular Hearts

A recent paper has summarised the outcomes of 17 women with 21 pregnancies that proceeded to delivery with maternal unrepaired UVH in the literature [58]. There was 1 post-partum maternal death and 1 post-partum embolic event and 2 perinatal deaths. Importantly, this publication only captures women who survived to delivery, and it would be anticipated that the real risks to both mother and baby are significantly underrepresented.

Conclusions

Pregnancy remains, at best, a high-risk undertaking for women with a Fontan circulation. Nonetheless, expert clinical assessment can identify those who may proceed with pregnancy without a significant pregnancy-related mortality. However, the risks of cardiac and obstetric complications are significantly increased for the mother, while the fetus faces a very high risk, with a low livebirth rate. It is still unclear how to best risk assess Fontan women who wish to become pregnant, but outcome relates to baseline functional and cardiovascular status, exercise capacity and oxygen saturations.

There are no data on the role for pre-conception exercise training, but it appears logical that exercise should be encouraged to improve the peripheral pump and respiratory muscle function, and counter some of the physiological challenges imposed by pregnancy in this population. Anticoagulation management remains contentious in this population as a whole. Therapeutic anticoagulation should be continued in all women with a pre-existing indication, including a patent fenestration and those with an atriopulmonary Fontan, given the significantly increased thrombotic risk encountered.

A planned international registry that will collate post-partum outcome data of women matched to never pregnant controls is being developed, to answer questions on long-term outcome.

References

1. Wolff D, van de Wiel HBM, de Muinck Keizer ME, van Melle JP, Pieper PG, Berger RMF, et al. Quality of life and sexual well-being in patients with a Fontan circulation: an explorative pilot study with a mixed method design. Congenit Heart Dis. 2018;13(2):319–26.
2. Zentner D, Celermajer DS, Gentles T, d'Udekem Y, Ayer J, Blue GM, et al. Management of people with a Fontan circulation: a Cardiac Society of Australia and New Zealand position statement. Heart Lung Circ. 2020;29(1):5–39.
3. Helgeson VS, Zajdel M. Adjusting to chronic health conditions. Annu Rev Psychol. 2017;68:545–71.
4. NHS. The progestogen-only pill, your contraception guide. 2018. https://www.nhs.uk/conditions/contraception/the-pill-progestogen-only/.
5. The Royal Women's Hospital and Family Planning Victoria. Contraception—your choices. 2018. https://thewomens.r.worldssl.net/images/uploads/fact-sheets/Contraception-Choices-2018.pdf.
6. Regitz-Zagrosek V, Roos-Hesselink JW, Bauersachs J, Blomstrom-Lundqvist C, Cifkova R, De Bonis M, et al. 2018 ESC guidelines for the management of cardiovascular diseases during pregnancy. Eur Heart J. 2018;39(34):3165–241.
7. Tepper NK, Whiteman MK, Marchbanks PA, James AH, Curtis KM. Progestin-only contraception and thromboembolism: a systematic review. Contraception. 2016;94(6):678–700.
8. Thorne S, MacGregor A, Nelson-Piercy C. Risks of contraception and pregnancy in heart disease. Heart. 2006;92(10):1520–5.
9. Roos-Hesselink JW, Cornette J, Sliwa K, Pieper PG, Veldtman GR, Johnson MR. Contraception and cardiovascular disease. Eur Heart J. 2015;36(27):1728–34, 34a-34b.
10. Practice Committee of the American Society for Reproductive Medicine. Combined hormonal contraception and the risk of venous thromboembolism: a guideline. Fertil Steril. 2017;107(1):43–51.
11. Klok FA, Schreiber K, Stach K, Ageno W, Middeldorp S, Eichinger S, et al. Oral contraception and menstrual bleeding during treatment of venous thromboembolism: expert opinion versus current practice: combined results of a systematic review, expert panel opinion and an international survey. Thromb Res. 2017;153:101–7.
12. Canobbio MM, Warnes CA, Aboulhosn J, Connolly HM, Khanna A, Koos BJ, et al. Management of

pregnancy in patients with complex congenital heart disease: a scientific statement for healthcare professionals from the American Heart Association. Circulation. 2017;135(8):e50–87.

13. Zentner D, Kotevski A, King I, Grigg L, d'Udekem Y. Fertility and pregnancy in the Fontan population. Int J Cardiol. 2016;208:97–101.

14. Black A, Guilbert E, Costescu D, Dunn S, Fisher W, Kives S, et al. No. 329-Canadian contraception consensus part 4 of 4 chapter 9: combined hormonal contraception. J Obstet Gynaecol Can. 2017;39(4):229–68. e5

15. Ponnatapura J, Kielar A, Burke LMB, Lockhart ME, Abualruz AR, Tappouni R, et al. Hepatic complications of oral contraceptive pills and estrogen on MRI: controversies and update—adenoma and beyond. Magn Reson Imaging. 2019;60:110–21.

16. Palomba S, Santagni S, Gibbins K, La Sala GB, Silver RM. Pregnancy complications in spontaneous and assisted conceptions of women with infertility and subfertility factors. A comprehensive review. Reprod Biomed Online. 2016;33(5):612–28.

17. Moroney E, Posma E, Dennis A, d'Udekem Y, Cordina R, Zentner D. Pregnancy in a woman with a Fontan circulation: a review. Obstet Med. 2018;11(1):6–11.

18. Drenthen W, Hoendermis ES, Moons P, Heida KY, Roos-Hesselink JW, Mulder BJ, et al. Menstrual cycle and its disorders in women with congenital heart disease. Congenit Heart Dis. 2008;3(4):277–83.

19. Moroney E, Zannino D, Cordina R, Gentles T, d'Udekem Y, Zentner D. Does pregnancy impact subsequent health outcomes in the maternal Fontan circulation? Int J Cardiol. 2019;301:67–73.

20. Cauldwell M, Steer PJ, Bonner S, Asghar O, Swan L, Hodson K, et al. Retrospective UK multicentre study of the pregnancy outcomes of women with a Fontan repair. Heart. 2018;104(5):401–6.

21. European Society of Gynecology (ESG); Association for European Paediatric Cardiology (AEPC); German Society for Gender Medicine (DGesGM), Regitz-Zagrosek V, Blomstrom Lundqvist C, Borghi C, et al. ESC guidelines on the management of cardiovascular diseases during pregnancy: the task force on the management of cardiovascular diseases during pregnancy of the European Society of Cardiology (ESC). Eur Heart J. 2011;32(24):3147–97.

22. Mathur RS, Drakeley AJ, Raine-Fenning NJ, Evbuomwan IO, Hamoda H. The management of ovarian hyperstimulation syndrome. RCOG; 2016.

23. Kuleva M, Youssef A, Maroni E, Contro E, Pilu G, Rizzo N, et al. Maternal cardiac function in normal twin pregnancy: a longitudinal study. Ultrasound Obstet Gynecol. 2011;38(5):575–80.

24. Qin J, Liu X, Sheng X, Wang H, Gao S. Assisted reproductive technology and the risk of pregnancy-related complications and adverse pregnancy outcomes in singleton pregnancies: a meta-analysis of cohort studies. Fertil Steril. 2016;105(1):73–85. e1–6.

25. Rossberg N, Stangl K, Stangl V. Pregnancy and cardiovascular risk: a review focused on women with

heart disease undergoing fertility treatment. Eur J Prev Cardiol. 2016;23(18):1953–61.

26. Arora P, Mishra V. Difficult embryo transfer: a systematic review. J Hum Reprod Sci. 2018;11(3):229–35.

27. Shamshirsaz AA, Bateni ZH, Sangi-Haghpeykar H, Arian SE, Erfani H, Shamshirsaz AA, et al. Cyanotic congenital heart disease following fertility treatments in the United States from 2011 to 2014. Heart. 2018;104(11):945–8.

28. Cauldwell M, Von Klemperer K, Uebing A, Swan L, Steer PJ, Babu-Narayan SV, et al. A cohort study of women with a Fontan circulation undergoing preconception counselling. Heart. 2016;102(7):534–40.

29. von Wolff M. The role of natural cycle IVF in assisted reproduction. Best Pract Res Clin Endocrinol Metab. 2019;33(1):35–45.

30. Dawson AJ, Krastev Y, Parsonage WA, Peek M, Lust K, Sullivan EA. Experiences of women with cardiac disease in pregnancy: a systematic review and meta-synthesis. BMJ Open. 2018;8(9):e022755.

31. Kovacs AH, Harrison JL, Colman JM, Sermer M, Siu SC, Silversides CK. Pregnancy and contraception in congenital heart disease: what women are not told. J Am Coll Cardiol. 2008;52(7):577–8.

32. The American College of Obstetricians and Gynecologists. ACOG obesity toolkit: obesity screening and assessment of patient readiness for weight loss. 2019. https://www.acog.org/About-ACOG/ACOG-Departments/Toolkits-for-Health-Care-Providers/Obesity-Toolkit.

33. Denison FC, Aedla NR, Keag O, Hor K, Reynolds RM, Milne A, et al. Care of women with obesity in pregnancy: green-top guideline no. 72. BJOG. 2019;126(3):e62–e106.

34. Zhang S, Rattanatray L, MacLaughlin SM, Cropley JE, Suter CM, Molloy L, et al. Periconceptional undernutrition in normal and overweight ewes leads to increased adrenal growth and epigenetic changes in adrenal IGF2/H19 gene in offspring. FASEB J. 2010;24(8):2772–82.

35. Zhang S, Morrison JL, Gill A, Rattanatray L, MacLaughlin SM, Kleemann D, et al. Maternal dietary restriction during the periconceptional period in normal-weight or obese ewes results in adrenocortical hypertrophy, an up-regulation of the JAK/STAT and down-regulation of the IGF1R signaling pathways in the adrenal of the postnatal lamb. Endocrinology. 2013;154(12):4650–62.

36. Price S, Nankervis A, Permezel M, Prendergast L, Sumithran P, Proietto J. Health consequences for mother and baby of substantial pre-conception weight loss in obese women: study protocol for a randomized controlled trial. Trials. 2018;19(1):248.

37. Balci A, Sollie-Szarynska KM, van der Bijl AG, Ruys TP, Mulder BJ, Roos-Hesselink JW, et al. Prospective validation and assessment of cardiovascular and offspring risk models for pregnant women with congenital heart disease. Heart. 2014;100(17):1373–81.

38. Silversides CK, Grewal J, Mason J, Sermer M, Kiess M, Rychel V, et al. Pregnancy outcomes in women with heart disease: the CARPREG II study. J Am Coll Cardiol. 2018;71(21):2419–30.
39. Arif S, Chaudhary A, Clift PF, Morris RK, Selman TJ, Bowater SE, et al. Pregnancy outcomes in patients with a Fontan circulation and proposal for a risk scoring system: single centre experience. J Congenit Cardiol. 2017;1:10.
40. Cauldwell M, Ghonim S, Uebing A, Swan L, Steer PJ, Gatzoulis M, et al. Preconception counseling, predicting risk and outcomes in women with mWHO 3 and 4 heart disease. Int J Cardiol. 2017;234:76–80.
41. Shum KK, Gupta T, Canobbio MM, Durst J, Shah SB. Family planning and pregnancy management in adults with congenital heart disease. Prog Cardiovasc Dis. 2018;61(3–4):336–46.
42. Chong HP, Hodson J, Selman TJ, Hudsmith LE, Thompson PJ, Morris RK, et al. Estimated blood loss in pregnant women with cardiac disease compared with low risk women: a retrospective cohort study. BMC Pregnancy Childbirth. 2019;19(1):325.
43. Cauldwell M, Steer PJ, Swan L, Uebing A, Gatzoulis MA, Johnson MR. The management of the third stage of labour in women with heart disease. Heart. 2017;103(12):945–51.
44. Garcia Ropero A, Baskar S, Roos Hesselink JW, Girnius A, Zentner D, Swan L, et al. Pregnancy in women with a Fontan circulation: a systematic review of the literature. Circ Cardiovasc Qual Outcomes. 2018;11(5):e004575.
45. Zentner D, du Plessis M, Brennecke S, Wong J, Grigg L, Harrap SB. Deterioration in cardiac systolic and diastolic function late in normal human pregnancy. Clin Sci (Lond). 2009;116(7):599–606.
46. Zentner D, du Plessis M, Brennecke S, Wong J, Grigg L, Harrap S. Cardiac function at term in human pregnancy. Pregnancy Hypertens. 2012;2(2):132–8.
47. Zentner D, Wheeler M, Grigg L. Does pregnancy contribute to systemic right ventricular dysfunction in adults with an atrial switch operation? Heart Lung Circ. 2012;21(8):433–8.
48. Tzemos N, Silversides CK, Colman JM, Therrien J, Webb GD, Mason J, et al. Late cardiac outcomes after pregnancy in women with congenital aortic stenosis. Am Heart J. 2009;157(3):474–80.
49. Grewal J, Siu SC, Ross HJ, Mason J, Balint OH, Sermer M, et al. Pregnancy outcomes in women with dilated cardiomyopathy. J Am Coll Cardiol. 2009;55(1):45–52.
50. d'Udekem Y, Iyengar AJ, Galati JC, Forsdick V, Weintraub RG, Wheaton GR, et al. Redefining expectations of long-term survival after the Fontan procedure: twenty-five years of follow-up from the entire population of Australia and New Zealand. Circulation. 2014;130(11 Suppl 1):S32–8.
51. Canobbio MM, Silversides C, Warnes CA, Aboulhosn J, Colman JM. Pregnancy after Fontan operation: early and late outcomes. JACC. 2013;61(10_Suppl):E427.
52. Gouton M, Nizard J, Patel M, Sassolas F, Jimenez M, Radojevic J, et al. Maternal and fetal outcomes of pregnancy with Fontan circulation: a multicentric observational study. Int J Cardiol. 2015;187:84–9.
53. Pundi KN, Pundi K, Johnson JN, Dearani JA, Bonnichsen CR, Phillips SD, et al. Contraception practices and pregnancy outcome in patients after Fontan operation. Congenit Heart Dis. 2016;11(1):63–70.
54. Alsaied T, Bokma JP, Engel ME, Kuijpers JM, Hanke SP, Zuhlke L, et al. Factors associated with long-term mortality after Fontan procedures: a systematic review. Heart. 2017;103(2):104–10.
55. Kverneland LS, Kramer P, Ovroutski S. Five decades of the Fontan operation: a systematic review of international reports on outcomes after univentricular palliation. Congenit Heart Dis. 2018;13(2):181–93.
56. Poh CL, d'Udekem Y. Life after surviving Fontan surgery: a meta-analysis of the incidence and predictors of late death. Heart Lung Circ. 2018;27(5):552–9.
57. Valente AM, Bhatt AB, Cook S, Earing MG, Gersony DR, Aboulhosn J, et al. The CALF (congenital heart disease in adults lower extremity systemic venous health in Fontan patients) study. J Am Coll Cardiol. 2010;56(2):144–50.
58. Wang K, Luo H, Xin Y, Yu H. Successful pregnancy and delivery in patients with uncorrected single ventricle: three new cases and literature review. Int J Cardiol. 2015;184:135–9.

Factors Impacting on the Late Outcome of the Fontan Circulation

30

Paul Clift

Abbreviations

AP	Atriopulmonary Fontan
AVSD	Atrioventricular septal defect
AVV	Atrioventricular valve
BDG	Bidirectional Glenn cavopulmonary anastomosis
DILV	Double inlet left ventricle
DS	Down syndrome
EC-TCPC	Extra-cardiac TCPC Fontan
HLHS	Hypoplastic left heart syndrome
LT-TCPC	Lateral tunnel TCPC Fontan
TCPC	Total cavopulmonary connection Fontan
uAVSD	Unbalanced atrioventricular septal defect

Introduction

Prior to the initial reports of Fontan and Kreutzer, surgical intervention for tricuspid atresia with restricted pulmonary blood flow was primarily with a shunt procedure, often an aortopulmonary shunt in very early life (Potts or Waterston shunt), with Blalock-Taussig shunts more common in infants >6 months of age. The Glenn procedure was favoured in older children or as a second or third procedure later in childhood [1, 2]. Early mortality was high, especially in the very young [1], and late survival was reasonable with >70% surviving >10 years, however shunt adequacy was poor with less than half of survivors showing adequate oxygenation after 10 years [1]. Unoperated survival beyond childhood was rarely reported.

Physiologically, shunt procedures do not alleviate cyanosis but increase volume-loading of the single ventricle, which can have deleterious effects [3]. Fontan surgery alleviates cyanosis and volume loading of the single ventricle and should, therefore, improve long-term survival over shunt surgery alone.

While survival in the current era is generally excellent, data are lacking on the adult outcomes of the Fontan surgery, and we are still unable to accurately predict life expectancy. When considering the outcomes of Fontan surgery in terms of morbidity and mortality, but also quality of life, several factors need to be considered, including the underlying anatomy, comorbidity, era of surgical intervention and type of Fontan procedure performed.

P. Clift (✉)
Department of Cardiology, Queen Elizabeth Hospital, Birmingham, UK
e-mail: pclift@nhs.net

P. Clift et al. (eds.), *Univentricular Congenital Heart Defects and the Fontan Circulation*,
https://doi.org/10.1007/978-3-031-36208-8_30

Era of Surgical Intervention

The teams in Bordeaux and Leiden published the results of the first 100 Fontan procedures performed for tricuspid atresia in 1983. In this paper, they acknowledged the steep learning curve and rapid improvements made in preoperative evaluation, case selection, operative techniques, perioperative management strategy and improved understanding of anatomy required to reduce mortality from this surgery to acceptable levels [4]. The concept of a learning curve for this challenging surgery is widely acknowledged and is reflected in the published case series [5–8]. Given the nature of innovation, initial case series were only published by a small number of centres and operative mortality (15–17%) [7, 9] would be considered high by modern standards. However, all centres report rapid improvement in early outcomes followed by a period of stability [7, 9–11]. By 1990 many centres were running successful Fontan programmes, yet there remained a learning curve and a difference in survival based on era during which the surgery was performed [12, 13].

Modern series have not shown further improvements in survival likely due to the increasing complexity of cases undergoing single ventricle palliation.

Down Syndrome

Congenital heart disease is common in Down syndrome (DS), with an increased prevalence of atrioventricular septal defects (AVSDs), some of whom have unbalanced AVSDs (uAVSDs) and require a Fontan-type operation. There are concerns about Fontan palliation in DS due to a challenging perioperative course, a vulnerable pulmonary vasculature and airway obstruction. Whilst good outcomes have been reported [14, 15], a recent US wide study has demonstrated a five-fold increase in mortality following Fontan surgery in DS [16].

Low Birthweight

The challenges of low birthweight in the neonatal management of complex congenital heart disease are well-recognised and is a particular challenge for those with a single ventricle circulation [17, 18]. Stage 1 palliation in children <2.5 kg birthweight is associated with poor outcomes [19, 20], both in terms of survival after stage 1 and survival to Fontan completion [21].

The evolution of a hybrid catheter-based approach with stenting of the arterial duct and surgical banding of the branch pulmonary arteries has improved neonatal survival. This leads to a more complex stage 2 procedure, but long-term outcomes appear favourable [22] Increasingly, this is the pathway of choice for neonates with high-risk variants of HLHS [23–26].

Heterotaxy Syndrome

Heterotaxy syndrome, with atrial isomerism and a single ventricle is a highly complex condition with considerable variation in anatomical features. Whilst there are some forms of left atrial isomerism in which a biventricular repair is possible, this is rarely the case with right atrial isomerism. Venous connections are varied and complex, especially in right atrial isomerism which is typically associated with anomalous pulmonary venous drainage and bilateral SVC and dextrocardia. The anatomical complexities can lead to challenging surgery in early life, and an adverse outcome following neonatal palliation compared to other forms of single ventricle anatomy [7, 27, 28]. Mortality following Fontan completion remains low in heterotaxy (4.8%), but that is still 4 times the rate of the Fontan population as a whole [29]. Survival beyond Fontan surgery is broadly similar to patients with other single ventricle anatomies [30, 31].

The complex nature of the atrioventricular valve in heterotaxy syndrome results in significant AVV regurgitation in many, and this is associated with an adverse outcome if not repaired [32]. Repair before a cavopulmonary shunt procedure is associated with a poor outcome, but good outcomes are reported for those with repair during the cavopulmonary shunt procedure, or at the time of the Fontan surgery [33, 34].

Late outcomes in adults with heterotaxy who have undergone Fontan palliation are not well described. Arrhythmias appear to be common, both tachy and bradycardias [35]. The abnormal venous connections complicate arrhythmia management, e.g. when considering approaches for pacing or electrophysiology studies.

Type of Fontan Procedure Performed

Fontan and Kreutzer described similar but fundamentally different procedures [36, 37]. Fontan's use of valve homograft material was based on the belief that retrograde flow was a disadvantage; however, the resulting venous hypertension downstream was detrimental. This method was replaced by a modification of Kreutzer's second case, whereby the right atrial appendage was directly sutured to the disconnected pulmonary trunk, with a valveless systemic venous circulation. The modified atriopulmonary (AP) Fontan became the standard operation until the late 1980s, when Marc de Leval and colleagues published their initial experience of the lateral tunnel (LT) total cavopulmonary connection (TCPC). Their approach was based on bench work and mathematical modelling of the atriopulmonary Fontan, that demonstrated marked energy loss in the circuit at the level of the atrial chamber. They devised an approach whereby a tunnel could be formed by means of a patch in the lateral portion

of the systemic venous atrium, redirecting inferior vena cava (IVC) flow. The superior end of the tunnel was anastomosed with the underside of the pulmonary artery, while a bidirectional cavopulmonary anastomosis directed SVC flow directly to the pulmonary artery. In doing so, the turbulent flow observed in the AP Fontan was streamlined into a more laminar flow within the lateral tunnel. This led to marked improvements in the fluid dynamics within the circulation, with reduced energy loss and postulated improved survival [38]. Marcelletti and colleagues developed the concept further, with the interposition of a synthetic conduit between the IVC and the pulmonary artery, completely outside the heart, the so-called extra-cardiac (EC) TCPC. The concept was that, by using a conduit, you could optimise the flow characteristics and further reduce power loss in the Fontan circulation [39].

Both LT and EC TCPC Fontan operations became rapidly adopted and were crucial to the development and success of the staged palliation of hypoplastic left heart syndrome, described by Norwood and colleagues [40].

Survival following the different types of Fontan surgery likely follows the era in which these procedures were performed, with improvements in perioperative care that also contributed to the long-term survival (Fig. 30.1). AP Fontan procedures were typically performed until the late 1980s, while EC TCPC and LT TCPC Fontan were performed thereafter. Survival following Fontan completion with either of the TCPC procedures is better than the AP Fontan [41], but there is no difference between EC TCPC and LT TCPC [42]. Whether further innovations will lead to further survival advantages remains to be determined. However, operative mortality in the current era of Fontan completion remains very low.

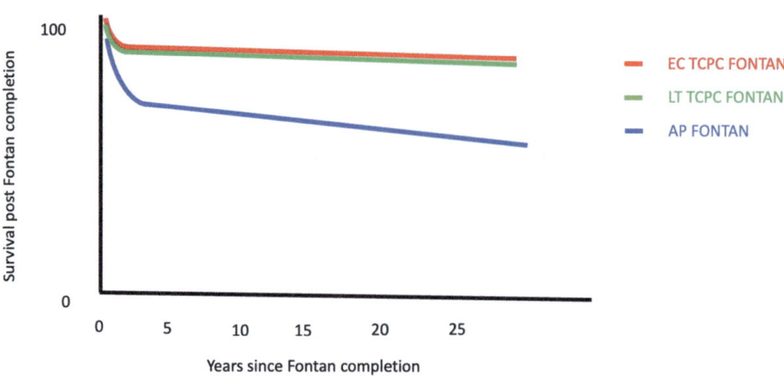

Fig. 30.1 Typical survival curves following Fontan completion based on Fontan procedure performed

Ten Commandments

Early experience of Fontan and colleagues demonstrated the importance of certain characteristics associated with a good outcome, which became known as the 'Ten Commandments': sinus rhythm, normal venous return, a mean pulmonary artery pressure less than 15 mmHg, a pulmonary vascular resistance less than 4 units. m², good sized pulmonary arteries, normal ventricular function and no atrioventricular valve incompetence [43]. We subsequently highlighted the importance of good ventricular function and a low pulmonary vascular resistance on Fontan outcomes in our series [44].

Ventricular Morphology

It was assumed that ventricular morphology (right vs left) would impact on the long-term survival and morbidity, but this has not been demonstrated consistently [45, 46]. For all HLHS, in whom the systemic ventricle is typically morphologically right, the survival from neonatal diagnosis remains poor and much worse than other forms of univentricular anatomy. This is, however, largely due to the requirement for neonatal intervention with a stage 1 Norwood, a highly complex procedure with a high mortality even in established large-volume units. The risk of Fontan completion surgery (Stage 3 Norwood) is remarkably low regardless of underlying anatomy, and survival is not determined by anatomical characteristics alone.

Pulmonary Artery Size

Early series reported by Fontan showed that smaller pulmonary arteries were associated with worse outcomes [47]. The smallest pulmonary artery size at which a Fontan procedure can be performed is not established. The Mayo Clinic demonstrated an increased risk of prolonged effusions and reintervention after AP Fontan in patients with a lower indexed size [48]. Nakata described a method of sizing pulmonary arteries based on angiographic data, suggesting a cut off of 250 mm²/m² for selection for the Fontan procedure. Subsequent studies did not clearly demonstrate that size alone could be used as a determinant of survival [49–53]. It is recognised that pulmonary artery growth is limited following Fontan completion [54, 55] or following cavopulmonary shunt [56, 57]. Concerns remain that failure of growth of the pulmonary arteries following Fontan completion will lead to increased resistance in the pulmonary circulation in later life, but this requires further investigation.

Catheter-Based Interventions

Catheter based interventions following Fontan surgery are typically either for arrhythmia management (with implantation of pacing systems or electrophysiology studies with ablation) or for structural interventions [58]. Arrhythmias are frequent events in adult life and interventional procedures are often used in expert centres, in combination with antiarrhythmic medication

[59]. Structural interventions are either performed as part of a planned catheter-based Fontan completion, or more commonly to optimise the haemodynamics of the Fontan circulation. Such interventions include manipulation of the Fontan fenestration, dilatation/stenting of a portion of the Fontan pathway to reduce restriction to flow [60], or stenting of a compressed left pulmonary artery as it passes behind the Damus-Kaye-Stansel connection [61]. Indeed, even a mild stenosis can impact significantly on flow in the Fontan circulation, and stent implantation is an effective management strategy. Balloon dilatation and stenting may also be required following Norwood stage 1 arch reconstruction for recoarctation [62].

A fenestration between the Fontan conduit/lateral tunnel and the pulmonary venous atrium is performed routinely at the time of Fontan surgery. Manipulation of the fenestration to either enlarge it or preserve it, is often considered in a patient with Fontan failure, at the expense of cyanosis [63]. Embolisation of venovenous [64] or venoarterial collaterals [65] may be performed during or following staged Fontan palliation in an attempt to reduce cyanosis.

Whilst the impact of specific interventions on long term survival is not known, survival and freedom from failure are worse in patients requiring an intervention following Fontan completion [66].

Quality of Life Outcomes

Several studies have assessed quality of life late after Fontan surgery. Fontan survivors generally report lower health-related quality of life measures relating to physical health and education [67]. Whilst impaired exercise capacity predicted quality of life in adolescents, this was less apparent in adult life, suggesting an adaptation to life with a Fontan circulation in the adult population [68]. Patients post Fontan surgery have a more negative perception of their heart defect than those with simple repaired congenital heart lesions [69]. Sexual wellbeing is impacted, with male Fontan patients reporting physical limitations and female Fontan patients being significantly impacted by psychosocial factors [70]; many adult Fontan patients report not being in a long-term relationship [71, 72] and the lack of long-term data causes a feeling of uncertainty about their own life expectancy [73].

The perception of what is a good outcome after Fontan surgery depends on the point of view. Paediatric cardiologists are rightly optimistic, given the improvements in survival for all patients born with a univentricular heart, thanks to innovations in neonatal and perioperative management, and improved surgical techniques. Adult congenital heart services focus on monitoring for the inevitable late effects of childhood surgery, managing cardiac and noncardiac complications and helping women with a Fontan circulation through pregnancy. From a patient perspective, while survival to adult life is likely, the path beyond this remains less clear, posing significant physical and psychological challenges. The role of medical therapies is limited, with a lack of randomised data even for fundamental issues, such as thromboprophylaxis. Enhanced collaboration between specialist centres, the medical devices and pharmaceutical industry, and the patients will no doubt lead to further advances and improved patient outcomes.

References

1. Trusler GA, Williams WG. Long-term results of shunt procedures for tricuspid atresia. Ann Thorac Surg. 1980;29(4):312–6.
2. de Brux JL, et al. Tricuspid atresia. Results of treatment in 115 children. J Thorac Cardiovasc Surg. 1983;85(3):440–6.
3. La Corte MA, et al. Left ventricular function in tricuspid atresia. Angiographic analysis in 28 patients. Circulation. 1975;52(6):996–1000.
4. Fontan F, et al. Repair of tricuspid atresia in 100 patients. J Thorac Cardiovasc Surg. 1983;85(5):647–60.
5. Bezuska L, et al. 30-year experience of Fontan surgery: single-centre's data. J Cardiothorac Surg. 2017;12(1):67.
6. Rogers LS, et al. 18 years of the Fontan operation at a single institution: results from 771 consecutive patients. J Am Coll Cardiol. 2012;60(11):1018–25.

7. Gentles TL, et al. Fontan operation in five hundred consecutive patients: factors influencing early and late outcome. J Thorac Cardiovasc Surg. 1997;114(3):376–91.

8. Giannico S, et al. Clinical outcome of 193 extracardiac Fontan patients: the first 15 years. J Am Coll Cardiol. 2006;47(10):2065–73.

9. Mair DD, Puga FJ, Danielson GK. The Fontan procedure for tricuspid atresia: early and late results of a 25-year experience with 216 patients. J Am Coll Cardiol. 2001;37(3):933–9.

10. Dabal RJ, et al. The modern Fontan operation shows no increase in mortality out to 20 years: a new paradigm. J Thorac Cardiovasc Surg. 2014;148(6):2517–2523.e1.

11. Knott-Craig CJ, et al. The modified Fontan operation. An analysis of risk factors for early postoperative death or takedown in 702 consecutive patients from one institution. J Thorac Cardiovasc Surg. 1995;109(6):1237–43.

12. Downing TE, et al. Long-term survival after the Fontan operation: twenty years of experience at a single center. J Thorac Cardiovasc Surg. 2017;154(1):243–253.e2.

13. McGuirk SP, et al. Staged surgical management of hypoplastic left heart syndrome: a single institution 12 year experience. Heart. 2006;92(3):364–70.

14. Colquitt JL, et al. Survival in children with Down syndrome undergoing single-ventricle palliation. Ann Thorac Surg. 2016;101(5):1834–41.

15. Furukawa T, et al. Outcome of univentricular repair in patients with Down syndrome. J Thorac Cardiovasc Surg. 2013;146(6):1349–52.

16. Allen P, et al. Trisomy 21 patients undergoing cavopulmonary connections need improved preoperative and postoperative care. Ann Thorac Surg. 2021;112(6):2012–9.

17. Liu MY, et al. Longitudinal assessment of outcome from prenatal diagnosis through Fontan operation for over 500 fetuses with single ventricle-type congenital heart disease: the Philadelphia fetus-to-Fontan cohort study. J Am Heart Assoc. 2018;7(19):e009145.

18. Alsoufi B, et al. Single ventricle palliation in low weight patients is associated with worse early and midterm outcomes. Ann Thorac Surg. 2015;99(2):668–76.

19. Surendran S, et al. Influence of weight at the time of first palliation on survival in patients with a single ventricle. Cardiol Young. 2017;27(9):1778–85.

20. Oh TH, et al. The New Zealand Norwood procedure experience: 22-year cumulative review. Heart Lung Circ. 2017;26(7):730–5.

21. Gelehrter S, et al. Outcomes of hypoplastic left heart syndrome in low-birth-weight patients. Pediatr Cardiol. 2011;32(8):1175–81.

22. Yerebakan C, et al. Hybrid therapy for hypoplastic left heart syndrome: myth, alternative, or standard? J Thorac Cardiovasc Surg. 2016;151(4):1112–21, 1123.e1–5.

23. DiBardino DJ, et al. Intermediate results of hybrid versus primary Norwood operation. Ann Thorac Surg. 2015;99(6):2141–7; discussion 2147–9.

24. Murphy MO, et al. Hybrid procedure for neonates with hypoplastic left heart syndrome at high-risk for Norwood: midterm outcomes. Ann Thorac Surg. 2015;100(6):2286–90; discussion 2291–2.

25. Galantowicz M, et al. Hybrid approach for hypoplastic left heart syndrome: intermediate results after the learning curve. Ann Thorac Surg. 2008;85(6):2063–70; discussion 2070–1.

26. Schranz D, et al. Fifteen-year single center experience with the "Giessen hybrid" approach for hypoplastic left heart and variants: current strategies and outcomes. Pediatr Cardiol. 2015;36(2):365–73.

27. Alsoufi B, et al. Outcomes of multistage palliation of infants with functional single ventricle and heterotaxy syndrome. J Thorac Cardiovasc Surg. 2016;151(5):1369–77.e2.

28. Bartz PJ, et al. Early and late results of the modified Fontan operation for heterotaxy syndrome 30 years of experience in 142 patients. J Am Coll Cardiol. 2006;48(11):2301–5.

29. Jacobs JP, et al. Heterotaxy: lessons learned about patterns of practice and outcomes from the congenital heart surgery database of the society of thoracic surgeons. World J Pediatr Congenit Heart Surg. 2011;2(2):278–86.

30. Marathe SP, et al. Outcomes of the Fontan operation for patients with heterotaxy: a meta-analysis of 848 patients. Ann Thorac Surg. 2020;110(1):307–15.

31. Atz AM, et al. Functional state of patients with heterotaxy syndrome following the Fontan operation. Cardiol Young. 2007;17(Suppl 2):44–53.

32. Culbertson CB, et al. Factors influencing survival of patients with heterotaxy syndrome undergoing the Fontan procedure. J Am Coll Cardiol. 1992;20(3):678–84.

33. Imai K, et al. Long-term outcome of patients with right atrial isomerism after common atrioventricular valve plasty. Eur J Cardiothorac Surg. 2017;51(5):987–94.

34. Misumi Y, et al. Long-term outcomes of common atrioventricular valve plasty in patients with functional single ventricle. Interact Cardiovasc Thorac Surg. 2014;18(3):259–65.

35. Broda CR, et al. Outcomes in adults with congenital heart disease and heterotaxy syndrome: a single-center experience. Congenit Heart Dis. 2019;14(6):885–94.

36. Fontan F, Baudet E. Surgical repair of tricuspid atresia. Thorax. 1971;26(3):240–8.

37. Kreutzer G, et al. An operation for the correction of tricuspid atresia. J Thorac Cardiovasc Surg. 1973;66(4):613–21.

38. de Leval MR, et al. Total cavopulmonary connection: a logical alternative to atriopulmonary connection for complex Fontan operations. Experimental studies and early clinical experience. J Thorac Cardiovasc Surg. 1988;96(5):682–95.
39. Marcelletti C, et al. Inferior vena cava-pulmonary artery extracardiac conduit. A new form of right heart bypass. J Thorac Cardiovasc Surg. 1990;100(2):228–32.
40. Norwood WI Jr, Jacobs ML, Murphy JD. Fontan procedure for hypoplastic left heart syndrome. Ann Thorac Surg. 1992;54(6):1025–9; discussion 1029–30.
41. Rijnberg FM, et al. A 45-year experience with the Fontan procedure: tachyarrhythmia, an important sign for adverse outcome. Interact Cardiovasc Thorac Surg. 2019;29(3):461–8.
42. Lin Z, et al. Comparison of extracardiac conduit and lateral tunnel for functional single-ventricle patients: a meta-analysis. Congenit Heart Dis. 2017;12(6):711–20.
43. Choussat A, Fontan F, Besse P. Selection criteria for Fontan's procedure. In: Shinebourne EA, Anderson RH, editors. Pediatric cardiology. Edinburgh: Churchill Livingstone; 1978. p. 559–66.
44. Hosein RB, et al. Factors influencing early and late outcome following the Fontan procedure in the current era. The 'Two Commandments'? Eur J Cardiothorac Surg. 2007;31(3):344–52; discussion 353.
45. Schwartz I, et al. Late outcomes after the Fontan procedure in patients with single ventricle: a meta-analysis. Heart. 2018;104(18):1508–14.
46. McGuirk SP, et al. The impact of ventricular morphology on midterm outcome following completion total cavopulmonary connection. Eur J Cardiothorac Surg. 2003;24(1):37–46.
47. Fontan F, et al. The size of the pulmonary arteries and the results of the Fontan operation. J Thorac Cardiovasc Surg. 1989;98(5 Pt 1):711–9; discussion 719–24.
48. Knott-Craig CJ, et al. Pulmonary artery size and clinical outcome after the modified Fontan operation. Ann Thorac Surg. 1993;55(3):646–51.
49. Chun DS, et al. Incidence, outcome, and risk factors for stroke after the Fontan procedure. Am J Cardiol. 2004;93(1):117–9.
50. Bridges ND, et al. Pulmonary artery index. A nonpredictor of operative survival in patients undergoing modified Fontan repair. Circulation. 1989;80(3 Pt 1):I216–21.
51. Adachi I, et al. Preoperative small pulmonary artery did not affect the midterm results of Fontan operation. Eur J Cardiothorac Surg. 2007;32(1):156–62.
52. Lehner A, et al. Influence of pulmonary artery size on early outcome after the Fontan operation. Ann Thorac Surg. 2014;97(4):1387–93.
53. Baek JS, et al. Pulmonary artery size and late functional outcome after Fontan operation. Ann Thorac Surg. 2011;91(4):1240–6.
54. Ovroutski S, et al. Absence of pulmonary artery growth after Fontan operation and its possible impact on late outcome. Ann Thorac Surg. 2009;87(3):826–31.
55. Tatum GH, et al. Pulmonary artery growth fails to match the increase in body surface area after the Fontan operation. Heart. 2006;92(4):511–4.
56. Reddy VM, et al. Pulmonary artery growth after bidirectional cavopulmonary shunt: is there a cause for concern? J Thorac Cardiovasc Surg. 1996;112(5):1180–90; discussion 1190–2.
57. Kansy A, et al. Pulmonary artery growth in univentricular physiology patients. Kardiol Pol. 2013;71(6):581–7.
58. Downing TE, et al. Surgical and catheter-based reinterventions are common in long-term survivors of the Fontan operation. Circ Cardiovasc Interv. 2017;10(9):e004924.
59. Moore BM, et al. Ablation of atrial arrhythmias after the atriopulmonary Fontan procedure: mechanisms of arrhythmia and outcomes. JACC Clin Electrophysiol. 2018;4(10):1338–46.
60. Hagler DJ, et al. Fate of the Fontan connection: mechanisms of stenosis and management. Congenit Heart Dis. 2019;14(4):571–81.
61. Griselli M, et al. Fate of pulmonary arteries following Norwood procedure. Eur J Cardiothorac Surg. 2006;30(6):930–5.
62. Reinhardt Z, et al. Catheter interventions in the staged management of hypoplastic left heart syndrome. Cardiol Young. 2014;24:212–9.
63. Bhole V, et al. Transcatheter interventions in the early postoperative period after the Fontan procedure. Catheter Cardiovasc Interv. 2011;77(1):92–8.
64. Lluri G, Levi DS, Aboulhosn J. Systemic to pulmonary venous collaterals in adults with single ventricle physiology after cavopulmonary palliation. Int J Cardiol. 2015;189:159–63.
65. Banka P, et al. Practice variability and outcomes of coil embolization of aortopulmonary collaterals before Fontan completion: a report from the Pediatric Heart Network Fontan Cross-Sectional Study. Am Heart J. 2011;162(1):125–30.
66. Daley M, et al. Reintervention and survival in 1428 patients in the Australian and New Zealand Fontan registry. Heart. 2020;106(10):751–7.
67. Marshall KH, et al. Health-related quality of life in children, adolescents, and adults with a Fontan circulation: a meta-analysis. J Am Heart Assoc. 2020;9(6):e014172.
68. Suter B, et al. Does reduced cardiopulmonary exercise testing performance predict poorer quality of life in adult patients with Fontan physiology? Cardiol Young. 2021;31(1):84–90.

69. Holbein CE, et al. A multinational observational investigation of illness perceptions and quality of life among patients with a Fontan circulation. Congenit Heart Dis. 2018;13(3):392–400.
70. Wolff D, et al. Quality of life and sexual well-being in patients with a Fontan circulation: an explorative pilot study with a mixed method design. Congenit Heart Dis. 2018;13(2):319–26.
71. Pike NA, et al. Clinical profile of the adolescent/adult Fontan survivor. Congenit Heart Dis. 2011;6(1):9–17.
72. Bordin G, et al. Clinical profile and quality of life of adult patients after the Fontan procedure. Pediatr Cardiol. 2015;36(6):1261–9.
73. du Plessis K, et al. "How long will I continue to be normal?" Adults with a Fontan circulation's greatest concerns. Int J Cardiol. 2018;260:54–9.

Part VIII

A Multi-system Disorder

Electrophysiology Considerations and Management of Arrhythmias After the Fontan Operation

Sabine Ernst and Jeremy P. Moore

Introduction

Arrhythmias are common in patients with a univentricular heart and their frequency and nature depend on the type of surgical palliation performed. Acute and long-term management should focus on restoration of coordinated atrioventricular activation. Catheter ablation should be considered as a potentially curative procedure. Detailed anatomical understanding of the arrhythmic substrate is essential and can be obtained using 3D imaging to guide the operator (3D "roadmap"). Access to cardiac chambers can be difficult in Fontan patients and can be facilitated using remote magnetic navigation.

Types of Arrhythmia

Univentricular heart patients after the Fontan operation are affected by multiple electrical abnormalities (See Fig. 19.1). The issues most frequently observed include:

- Atrial tachycardias, most commonly intra-atrial reentrant tachycardia
- Sinus node dysfunction
- Sudden cardiac death
- Ventricular dyssynchrony

The Effects of Atrial Arrhythmias in Fontan Patients

Over the last five decades, advances in surgery have produced a number of palliative (Fontan) operations, that initially involved the right atrium (RA) being connected to the pulmonary artery (PA): RA appendage directly anastomosed to the PA, or by use of a conduit (atriopulmonary (AP) Fontan). De Leval and colleagues developed the technique of a total cavopulmonary connection (TCPC), which meanwhile has also undergone modifications, resulting in intra- or extracardiac tunnels (see previous chapters) [1–4].

All surgical interventions for univentricular hearts have in common extensive surgical incisions, which often result in scar-related re-entrant arrhythmias. In addition, dilatation of atrial chambers (especially the RA in AP Fontan) increases the risk of arrhythmias, both re-entrant and focal. Typically, arrhythmias occur 2–3 decades after surgery and account for 40% of admissions for Fontan patients [5–9].

A fast heart rate combined with the lack of coordinated sequential atrial and ventricular

S. Ernst (✉)
Department of Cardiology, Royal Brompton Hospital, London, UK
e-mail: S.Ernst@rbht.nhs.uk

J. P. Moore
Department of Pediatric Cardiology, UCLA Medical Center, Los Angeles, CA, USA
e-mail: JPMoore@mednet.ucla.edu

© The Author(s), under exclusive license to Springer Nature Switzerland AG 2023
P. Clift et al. (eds.), *Univentricular Congenital Heart Defects and the Fontan Circulation*,
https://doi.org/10.1007/978-3-031-36208-8_31

activation during atrial tachyarrhythmias can be highly detrimental to Fontan patients and may result in hemodynamic compromise and heart failure, that typically brings patients to the emergency department.

Restoration of sinus rhythm can be achieved by DC cardioversion or class III anti-arrhythmic medication (providing the patient is not acutely unwell and cannot, thus, wait for antiarrhythmics to act) [10]. Rate control is less desirable, as it does not restore coordinated sequential activation. Moreover, medication used for rate control may be detrimental to the systemic ventricle.

Another important consequence of sustained arrhythmia is the increased risk of spontaneous thrombus formation [11]. This risk is especially high in patients with classical AP Fontan, where the RA can be extremely large and blood flow is particularly sluggish. Spontaneous echo contrast can be observed even in patients exhibiting SR, but sustained atrial arrhythmia is believed to enhance the risk of thrombus formation significantly [12].

Catheter ablation should be considered as a long-term option, and has the potential chance to eliminate or suppress the arrhythmia substrate for long periods [13–15].

Arrhythmia Substrates in Univentricular Hearts After Surgery

Most Fontan patients present with atrial arrhythmias due to the multiple atrial incisions performed during the Fontan and conversion operations [16, 17]. Moreover, the raised central venous and RA pressures in AP Fontan result in severe dilatation of the RA, with RA wall stretch and fibrosis that creates anatomic conduction barriers and areas of functional block.

Patients can also present with a "simpler" arrhythmia substrate, e.g. an accessory pathway-mediated tachycardia or AV nodal reentrant circuits [18]. A growing number of patients (especially in the presence of a massively enlarged RA) are now presenting with paroxysmal or even persistent atrial fibrillation [19, 20].

Detailed 3D anatomical data, integrated with information from surgical notes (surgical incisions) and electrophysiological mapping, are important in understanding the nature of the intra-atrial reentrant circuits and planning ablation [21].

Arrhythmia After "Classical" Atriopulmonary Fontan Operations

Patients after any type of AP Fontan operation typically, present with a very enlarged RA. In addition, there is usually a large atriotomy scar on the free wall. However, the most frequently encountered arrhythmia is a re-entrant circuit around the tricuspid annulus. In case of a double inlet right or left ventricle, part of the surgical "creation" of the Fontan may be a patch that occludes the tricuspid annulus. However, this divides the so-called RA isthmus in two parts, with the "hidden" part only accessible via a retrograde approach using remote magnetic navigation (see below) [22]. Despite the obvious scar-related re-entrant mechanisms, there is also clear evidence of focal tachycardia and micro-reentry substrates.

Arrhythmia After TCPC Conversion

After TCPC conversion (Table 31.1), access to the native atrial chambers is difficult, as all venous accesses will lead to the lateral or intra-

Table 31.1 Fontan conversion: indications and contraindications

Indications

Atrial arrhythmia

Fontan pathway obstruction

Ventricular dysfunction related to arrhythmia

AV valve insufficiency[a]

Cyanosis-causing pulmonary AV fistulas

Residual intracardiac shunts

Disconnected pulmonary arteries

Circular venous flow

Aortic aneurysms/aortic regurgitation

Anomalous systemic venous drainage

Contraindications

Severe ventricular dysfunction not related to arrhythmia or pathway obstruction

Non-compensated protein-losing enteropathy

Multiple organ dysfunction

[a] When successful AV valve repair considered likely

cardiac tunnel. Some atrial tachycardia can indeed originate within this compartment, as there is persisting atrial tissue of the IVC and SVC connection or even the entire RA posterior wall (in case of an intracardiac hemi-tunnel); but most of the arrhythmias originate in the native atrial chambers. Trans-baffle access through the artificial tunnel material is technically challenging, as there is usually significant calcification [23, 24]. As an alternative, remote magnetic navigation can reach all native atrial chambers retrogradely via a transaortic approach (see below) [18, 25, 26].

Besides the obvious scar-related re-entrant substrate for arrhythmia, an even bigger challenge are 1:1 narrow QRS complex tachycardias (AV nodal re-entrant or AV re-entrant tachycardias). This is mostly due to the fact, that in case of AV nodal damage, the only access to the ventricles is via the aortic valve. In case of permanent AV nodal block, this would result in a further surgical procedure to secure epicardial pacing leads.

Arrhythmia in Heterotaxy Syndrome (Isomerism)

In addition to the already discussed "common" arrhythmia substrates, the special feature of patients with heterotaxy syndrome is that the conduction system can be duplicated [24, 27, 28]. This leads to two different narrow QRS complexes. If there is additionally a connecting "Moenckeberg" sling, then twin AV nodal re-entrant tachycardia (AVNRT) is a further possible tachycardia substrate. Once the mechanism of the twin AVNRT is proven, ablation of the "weaker" AV node is the treatment of choice. Key to the identification of this kind of AVNRT is the demonstration of two separate His recording areas (typically on opposing aspects along an atrioventricular septal defect with a common AV valve).

Pharmacological Options

Arrhythmias typical of Fontan patients, and pharmacologic options for rate or rhythm control are shown on Table 31.2. Depending on the type of arrhythmia, there is a limited choice of pharmacologic agents that can be employed to manage recurrent arrhythmias.

In the presence of reduced ventricular function, Class IC drugs are rarely recommended, leaving Class III drugs as the only viable option for rhythm control in recurrent arrhythmia [10].

Table 31.2 Intra-atrial reentrant tachycardia (IART)

Epidemiology

• Classic Fontan and subsequent modifications:
  – Associated with a very high risk of atrial arrhythmia
  – Development of significant atrial arrhythmia in ~50% at 10–15 years [19–22]
• Lateral Tunnel (LT) Fontan
  – Postoperative IART observed in ~25% at 10 years [20]
  – Significantly lower atrial arrhythmia burden as compared to classic/modified Fontan
  – Ongoing concern for atrial arrhythmia based on a preclinical studies in dogs [23]
• Extracardiac conduit (EC) Fontan
  – Introduced to further reduce atrial arrhythmia
  – Initial work did not support a difference in arrhythmia between the 2 techniques (LT vs EC), but
  – Recently, a two- to three-fold reduction in atrial arrhythmia has been shown by longer follow-up and meta-analysis [10, 24]

Management of atrial arrhythmia

• Development of atrial arrhythmia is associated with increased mortality and adverse events; hence, aggressive management is recommended [25]
• Therapeutic approaches:
  1. **Fontan conversion** (Table 31.3) **with arrhythmia surgery**
     – Generally indicated for drug-refractory atrial arrhythmia and good hemodynamics; patient selection is critical
     – A modified right atrial Maze should be employed for all patients and a modified Cox III Maze for documented AF
     – In-hospital mortality rates range from 3 to 10% [26–29] with an additional 10% at 1-year in one study [27]
     – Recurrent arrhythmia occurs in 10–20% at 5 years [26, 27]
  2. **Catheter ablation**
     – Modified AP Fontan (see Fig. 19.4)
         Highly variable, although atriotomy and IVC circuits are common [30, 31]
         Modest success, although improving with contemporary mapping technologies [31]
         Tachycardia recurrence in up 30%; often novel substrates; [21, 32] multiple procedures may be required
     – LT Fontan
         Direct access to the lateral tunnel is possible, with trans-baffle puncture usually required for access to the pulmonary venous atrium. Magnetic navigation with a retrograde approach is an alternative
         Catheter ablation outcomes are favorable with the cavo-tricuspid isthmus being the most frequent target, followed by the LT chamber [33]
     – EC Fontan
         As opposed to other Fontan variants, the EC conduit poses significant challenge for access to the pulmonary venous atrium
         Approaches include trans-conduit, [34] trans-caval, [35] and retrograde access (remote magnetic navigation) (see Fig. 19.5)
         The cavotricuspid isthmus (CTI) is the most frequent ablation target, with the exception of patients that have undergone Fontan conversion, in whom substrates tend to be highly variable [36]
         Outcome data are lacking
  3. **Anti-tachycardia pacing**
     – Some studies support its efficacy and safety for congenital heart disease patients, [37] however, few Fontan cases reported in the literature
     – Often useful as part of the Fontan conversion strategy [26]
  4. **Drug therapy**
     – Class III drugs (sotalol, dofetilide, or amiodarone)
     – Generally considered poorly effective in the Fontan population [29]

Non-pharmacologic Arrhythmia Management Options

Prerequisites for Invasive EP Procedures

Understanding the underlying cardiac anatomy is key for successful catheter arrhythmia ablation in all ACHD patients. In addition, surgical operation notes should be reviewed to understand any surgical modification of the anatomy and the likely set of surgical lesion/scars. 3D reconstruction of advanced imaging, either contrast computed tomography (CT) or cardiac magnetic resonance (CMR), can delineate the patient's individual anatomy quite accurately and can be merged with 3D electroanatomical maps (Table 31.3, and Figs. 31.1 and 31.2) [27, 29].

Vascular access planning is also important for reaching the target chamber [13]. Femoral vein access is standard for non-ACHD patients; however, previous surgery or intervention may mean that many ACHD patients have occluded femoral or iliac veins. A superior access (e.g. internal jugular) may be equally difficult and, in many Fontan patients, does not provide access to target cardiac chambers; e.g. in TCPC patients, all central venous access leads to the TCPC pathway and, in the absence of a fenestration, trans-baffle puncture is required to reach the atria.

Table 31.3 Overview on the available 3D imaging options for 3D reconstruction of individual anatomy

	Advantage	Disadvantage
Contrast computed tomography (CT) scan	• Easy reconstruction of contrast-enhanced cardiac chambers excellent depiction of coronary arteries • Late iodine enhancement • Thinning of myocardium	• Imaging of contrast-filled chambers only • Requires large contrast volumes and long acquisitions (= large radiation exposure) due to long transit times • Limited imaging window (= heart only) • Burden of contrast in kidney disease
3D cardiac magnetic resonance imaging (CMR) roadmap	• Detailed 3D reconstruction of all cardiac chambers • Window can be enlarged beyond the heart to image access routes • Combination with late gadolinium enhancement (LGE) allows scar depiction	• Exclusion of patients with non-CMR compatible implants • Longer acquisition times • Artefacts from stents, implantable loop recorders (ILRs), valves • Artefacts from turbulent flow
3D intracardiac echocardiography (ICE)	• Excellent intraprocedural imaging tool • Requires expertise	• Large access necessary • Invasive imaging (no procedural planning) • Costs

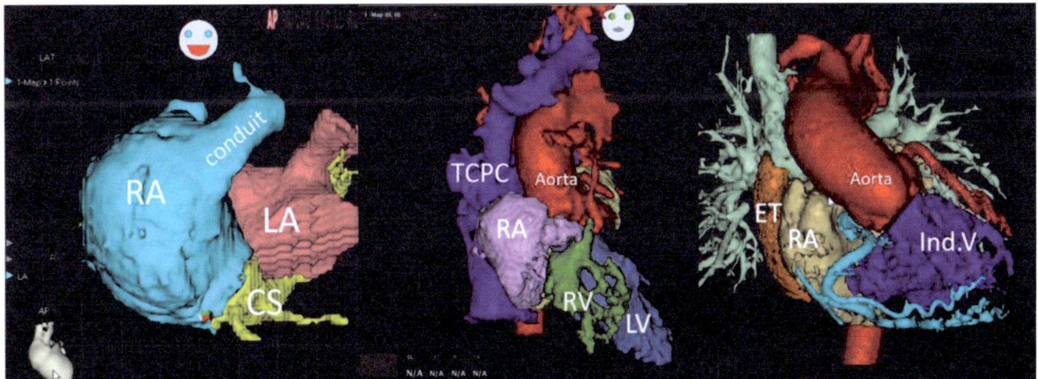

Fig. 31.1 Examples of AP Fontan, TCPC and heterotaxy syndrome 3D reconstructions

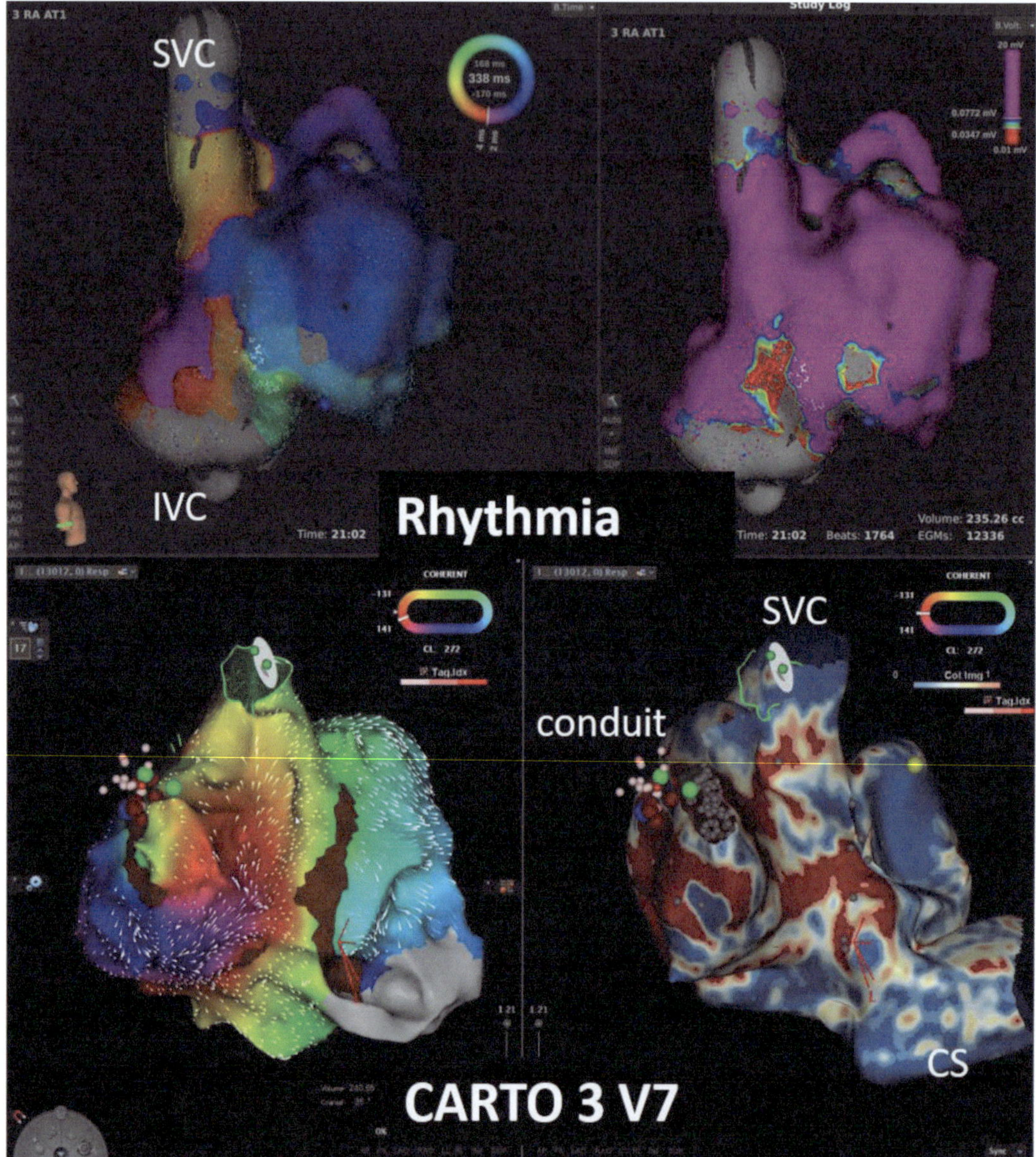

Fig. 31.2 3D electroanatomical maps using the Rhythmia and CARTO 3 (V7) systems

Remote Magnetic Navigation in Difficult Access Cases

As an alternative to potentially technically challenging trans-baffle punctures, remote magnetic navigation has been shown to facilitate retrograde access to the native atrial chambers [30, 31]. The system consists of two permanent magnets, which allow navigation of a very soft, magnetically equipped ablation catheter. A further strength of the system is the potential of the navigation platform for 3D image integration, which facilitates the ablation procedure.

High-Resolution Mapping to Better Delineate the arrhythmia Substrate

The main limitations of sequential "point-by-point" mapping using the ablation catheter is the size of the distal electrode (typically 3.5- or 4-mm tip), which only collects a relatively imprecise electric signal, and the shear time is takes to collect meaningful mapping information in Fontan patients.

A recent evolution has been the use of dedicated mapping catheters that have multiple small electrodes mounted (basket or "flower"-shaped catheters) [32, 33]. These allow fast collection of several thousand data-points (rather than a few hundred) and automated annotation algorithms facilitate the identification of the tachycardia substrate. However, direct catheter access is necessary to collect all the information (may be difficult in Fontan patients) and the arrhythmia needs to be sustained long enough in the catheter lab to allow a complete 3D map. Figure 31.2 compares multielectrode mapping using the Rhythmia system to electroanatomical mapping using the CARTO system.

Sinus Node Dysfunction (SND)

Fontan Physiology and the Importance of Sinus Rhythm

- Cardiac output in Fontan physiology is dependent on downstream pressure in the pulmonary venous atrium, as determined by
  - atrial relaxation properties,
  - diastolic and systolic function of the single ventricle,
  - function of the atrioventricular (AV) valve, and
  - presence of AV synchrony
- The majority of pulmonary blood flow in patients who are in sinus rhythm after Fontan surgery occurs during ventricular systole, driven by:
  - Atrial relaxation
  - Downward descent of the closed AV valve, with a suction-like effect
- Junctional rhythm results in loss of forward systolic flow by:
  - Simultaneous atrial and ventricular contraction
  - Systolic flow reversal in the pulmonary veins

  - Pulmonary venous pressure transiently exceeding the Fontan pressure, compromising cardiac output [34, 35].
- Junctional rhythm after Fontan operation is poorly tolerated:
  - May result in the development of Fontan failure and protein-losing enteropathy
  - It is reversible, with atrial pacing [36–38].

Scope of the Problem

Potential etiologies of SND after Fontan surgery are described on Table 31.4.

- To a degree, mild and asymptomatic sinus bradycardia is expected after the Fontan operation and does not require treatment [39, 40].
- Maintenance of sinus rhythm (or even sinus bradycardia) is, however, critical.
- Junctional rhythm is present in 5–6% of Fontan patients at baseline [41].
- Clinically significant bradycardia or need for pacemaker placement is observed in ~15% of TCPC patients at 10 years after surgery [42, 43].
- In Fontan patients with total cavopulmonary connection (TCPC), no difference between lateral tunnel (LT) and extracardiac conduit (EC) has been demonstrated in terms of SND.

Pacemaker Implantation

- Pacemaker implantation can be achieved by either the surgical or transvenous route, depending on anatomy.

Table 31.4 Causes of sinus node dysfunction after Fontan surgery

Timing	Etiology
Operative	Manipulation at cavo-atrial junction
	Surgical autonomic denervation
	Trauma to sinus node artery
Post-operative	Progressive dilation and fibrosis of the right atrium

- Surgical approach
  - The right-sided atrium is often densely scarred, with poor pacing characteristics; left-sided atrial myocardium preferred [44].
  - Left thoracotomy approach is often utilized to reach viable tissue at the dome of the left atrium.
  - Recent data suggest higher rates of lead failure and more frequent need for generator replacement as compared to transvenous route after Fontan operation [45, 46].
  - Potential complications include pain, prolonged pleural drainage, pocket infection, prolonged hospital stay [47].
- Transvenous approach (See Figs. 19.2 and 19.3):
  - Transvenous implantation, with placement of pacing leads within the Fontan circulation, is considered safe and effective after the Fontan operation, with similar risk for thromboembolism as compared to the surgical approach; [47–49] however chronic anticoagulation required.
  - Direct venous route for atrial pacing is possible for atriopulmonary (AP) and LT tunnel to the epicardial atrial surface, are necessary for patients who have undergone extracardiac Fontan operation [50, 51].
  - Ventricular pacing is possible, but is usually approached surgically

Sudden Cardiac Death

Epidemiology and Risk Factors

- Sudden death is uncommon in Fontan patients, with an incidence of 3–5% at 10 years follow up. [5]
- Modes of death include IART with rapid AV conduction, ventricular tachycardia, AV block, and thromboembolism.
- Predictive risk factors have included surgical AV valve repair, postoperative Fontan pressure >20 mmHg, and absence of sinus rhythm [52, 53].
- Non sustained ventricular tachycardia (NSVT)—but not sudden death—can be predicted by MRI late gadolinium enhancement [53].

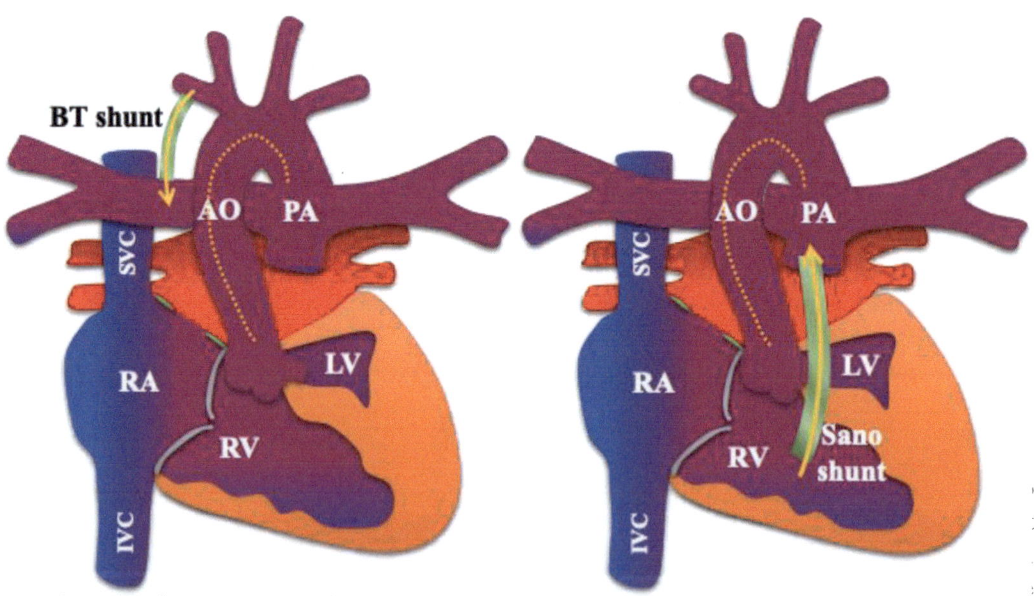

Fig. 31.3 The Norwood procedure with a Blalock-Taussig (BT) shunt (left) or Sano shunt (right) for hypoplastic left hearts. (Courtesy of Prof K. Dimopoulos)

may be proarrhythmic, although this has not yet been demonstrated [54].

Prevention of Sudden Cardiac Death

- ICD implantation is indicated for Fontan patients with aborted cardiac arrest or sustained ventricular tachycardia [55]
- Primary prevention indications are lacking
- ICD implantation is either surgical, or most recently, subcutaneous
- Initial subcutaneous ICD (SICD) experience is favorable [55, 56]:
  - Fontan patients are often good candidates for SICD
  - Technology is safe and effective
  - Caveats:
      Bradycardia pacing is not available
      Anti-tachycardia pacing is not available

Ventricular Dyssynchrony

Scope of the Problem

- Negative impact of ventricular pacing appreciated very early in the Fontan experience [57].
- Recently, increased attention has been paid to this phenomenon.
- Greater than 50% pacing appears to be a strong predictor of negative outcomes: [58–60]
  - Systemic ventricular dysfunction
  - Moderate-to-severe AV valve regurgitation
  - Death or transplantation

Resynchronization Strategies

- Multisite pacing: [57]
  - Improvement in NYHA class and/or systemic EF in two-thirds of patients after Fontan [61].
  - Greater freedom from death/transplantation as compared to single-site pacing,

however borderline statistical difference at 5-years of follow up. [62]
- Apical pacing:
  - Likely superior to single site pacing, however not well studied.

References

1. Ho SY, Zuberbuhler JR, Anderson RH. Pathology of hearts with a univentricular atrioventricular connection. Perspect Pediatr Pathol. 1988;12:69–99.
2. Fontan F, Baudet E. Surgical repair of tricuspid atresia. Thorax. 1971;26:240–8.
3. Marcelletti C, Corno A, Giannico S, Marino B. Inferior vena cava-pulmonary artery extracardiac conduit. A new form of right heart bypass. J Thorac Cardiovasc Surg. 1990;100:228–32.
4. de Leval MR, Kilner P, Gewillig M, Bull C. Total cavopulmonary connection: a logical alternative to atriopulmonary connection for complex Fontan operations. Experimental studies and early clinical experience. J Thorac Cardiovasc Surg. 1988;96:682–95.
5. Khairy P, Fernandes SM, Mayer JE, et al. Long-term survival, modes of death, and predictors of mortality in patients with Fontan surgery. Circulation. 2008;117:85–92.
6. d'Udekem Y, Iyengar AJ, Galati JC, et al. Redefining expectations of long-term survival after the Fontan procedure: twenty-five years of follow-up from the entire population of Australia and New Zealand. Circulation. 2014;130:S32–8.
7. Pundi KN, Johnson JN, Dearani JA, et al. 40-year follow-up after the Fontan operation: long-term outcomes of 1,052 patients. J Am Coll Cardiol. 2015;66:1700–10.
8. Diller G-P, Giardini A, Dimopoulos K, et al. Predictors of morbidity and mortality in contemporary Fontan patients: results from a multicenter study including cardiopulmonary exercise testing in 321 patients. Eur Heart J. 2010;31:3073–83.
9. Lasa JJ, Glatz AC, Daga A, Shah M. Prevalence of arrhythmias late after the Fontan operation. Am J Cardiol. 2014;113:1184–8.
10. Khairy P, Van Hare GF, Balaji S, et al. PACES/HRS expert consensus statement on the recognition and management of arrhythmias in adult congenital heart disease: developed in partnership between the Pediatric and Congenital Electrophysiology Society (PACES) and the Heart Rhythm Society (HRS). Endorsed by the governing bodies of PACES, HRS, the American College of Cardiology (ACC), the American Heart Association (AHA), the European Heart Rhythm Association (EHRA), the Canadian Heart Rhythm Society (CHRS), and the International Society for Adult Congenital Heart Disease (ISACHD). Can J Cardiol. 2014;30:e1–e63.

11. Masuda K, Ishizu T, Niwa K, et al. Increased risk of thromboembolic events in adult congenital heart disease patients with atrial tachyarrhythmias. Int J Cardiol. 2017;234:69–75.

12. Mantziari L, Babu-Narayan SV, Suman-Horduna I, Rigby ML, Ernst S. Atrial arrhythmia after Fontan surgery leads to giant thrombus: opening Pandora's box. Int J Cardiol. 2013;166:e23–4.

13. Triedman JK, Alexander ME, Love BA, et al. Influence of patient factors and ablative technologies on outcomes of radiofrequency ablation of intra-atrial re-entrant tachycardia in patients with congenital heart disease. J Am Coll Cardiol. 2002;39:1827–35.

14. Yap S-C, Harris L, Silversides CK, Downar E, Chauhan VS. Outcome of intra-atrial re-entrant tachycardia catheter ablation in adults with congenital heart disease: negative impact of age and complex atrial surgery. J Am Coll Cardiol. 2010;56:1589–96.

15. de Groot NMS, Atary JZ, Blom NA, Schalij MJ. Long-term outcome after ablative therapy of postoperative atrial tachyarrhythmia in patients with congenital heart disease and characteristics of atrial tachyarrhythmia recurrences. Circ Arrhythm Electrophysiol. 2010;3:148–54.

16. de Groot NMS, Lukac P, Blom NA, et al. Long-term outcome of ablative therapy of postoperative supraventricular Tachycardias in patients with Univentricular heart. Circ Arrhythm Electrophysiol. 2009;2:242–8.

17. de Groot NMS, Zeppenfeld K, Wijffels MC, et al. Ablation of focal atrial arrhythmia in patients with congenital heart defects after surgery: role of circumscribed areas with heterogeneous conduction. Heart Rhythm. 2006;3:526–35.

18. Upadhyay S, Marie Valente A, Triedman JK, Walsh EP. Catheter ablation for atrioventricular nodal reentrant tachycardia in patients with congenital heart disease. Heart Rhythm. 2016;13:1228–37.

19. Guarguagli S, Kempny A, Cazzoli I, et al. Efficacy of catheter ablation for atrial fibrillation in patients with congenital heart disease. Europace. 2019;21:1334–44.

20. Sohns C, Nürnberg J-H, Hebe J, et al. Catheter ablation for atrial fibrillation in adults with congenital heart disease: lessons learned from more than 10 years following a sequential ablation approach. JACC Clin Electrophysiol. 2018;4:733–43.

21. Stephenson EA, Lu M, Berul CI, et al. Arrhythmias in a contemporary Fontan cohort: prevalence and clinical associations in a multicenter cross-sectional study. J Am Coll Cardiol. 2010;56:890–6.

22. Ueda A, Horduna I, Rubens M, Ernst S. Reaching the ventricular aspect of the inferior isthmus in a Fontan patient using magnetic navigation. Heart Rhythm. 2013;10:1094–5.

23. Krause U, Backhoff D, Klehs S, Schneider HE, Paul T. Transbaffle catheter ablation of atrial re-entrant tachycardia within the pulmonary venous atrium in adult patients with congenital heart disease. Europace. 2016;18:1055–60.

24. Loomba RS, Aggarwal S, Gupta N, et al. Arrhythmias in adult congenital patients with bodily isomerism. Pediatr Cardiol. 2016;37:330–7.

25. Ueda A, Suman-Horduna I, Mantziari L, et al. Contemporary outcomes of supraventricular tachycardia ablation in congenital heart disease: a single-center experience in 116 patients. Circ Arrhythm Electrophysiol. 2013;6:606–13.

26. Ernst S, Babu-Narayan SV, Keegan J, et al. Remote-controlled magnetic navigation and ablation with 3D image integration as an alternative approach in patients with intra-atrial baffle anatomy. Circ Arrhythm Electrophysiol. 2012;5:131–9.

27. Suman-Horduna I, Babu-Narayan SV, Ueda A, et al. Magnetic navigation in adults with atrial isomerism (heterotaxy syndrome) and supraventricular arrhythmias. Europace. 2013;15:877–85.

28. Levine JC, Walsh EP, Saul JP. Radiofrequency ablation of accessory pathways associated with congenital heart disease including heterotaxy syndrome. Am J Cardiol. 1993;72:689–93.

29. Keegan J, Jhooti P, Babu-Narayan SV, Drivas P, Ernst S, Firmin DN. Improved respiratory efficiency of 3D late gadolinium enhancement imaging using the continuously adaptive windowing strategy (CLAWS). Magn Reson Med. 2014;71:1064–74.

30. Wu J, Pflaumer A, Deisenhofer I, Hoppmann P, Hess J, Hessling G. Mapping of atrial tachycardia by remote magnetic navigation in postoperative patients with congenital heart disease. J Cardiovasc Electrophysiol. 2010;21:751–9.

31. Akca F, Bauernfeind T, Witsenburg M, et al. Acute and long-term outcomes of catheter ablation using remote magnetic navigation in patients with congenital heart disease. Am J Cardiol. 2012;110:409–14.

32. Ernst S, Cazzoli I, Guarguagli S. An initial experience of high-density mapping-guided ablation in a cohort of patients with adult congenital heart disease. Europace. 2019;21:i43–53.

33. Martin CA, Yue A, Martin R, et al. Ultra-high-density activation mapping to aid isthmus identification of atrial tachycardias in congenital heart disease. JACC Clin Electrophysiol. 2019;5:1459–72.

34. Hasselman T, Schneider D, Madan N, Jacobs M. Reversal of fenestration flow during ventricular systole in Fontan patients in junctional or ventricular paced rhythm. Pediatr Cardiol. 2005;26:638–41.

35. Rychik J, Fogel MA, Donofrio MT, et al. Comparison of patterns of pulmonary venous blood flow in the functional single ventricle heart after operative aortopulmonary shunt versus superior cavopulmonary shunt. Am J Cardiol. 1997;80:922–6.

36. Cohen MI, Bridges ND, Gaynor JW, et al. Modifications to the cavopulmonary anastomosis do

not eliminate early sinus node dysfunction. J Thorac Cardiovasc Surg. 2000;120:891–900.

37. Barber BJ, Burch GH, Tripple D, Balaji S. Resolution of plastic bronchitis with atrial pacing in a patient with Fontan physiology. Pediatr Cardiol. 2004;25:73–6.

38. Dodge-Khatami A, Rahn M, Prêtre R, Bauersfeld U. Dual chamber epicardial pacing for the failing atriopulmonary Fontan patient. Ann Thorac Surg. 2005;80:1440–4.

39. Evans WN, Acherman RJ, Restrepo H. Normal sinus rhythm-sinus bradycardia is common in young children post-extracardiac Fontan. Pediatr Cardiol. 2016;37:1377–9.

40. Blaufox AD, Sleeper LA, Bradley DJ, et al. Functional status, heart rate, and rhythm abnormalities in 521 Fontan patients 6 to 18 years of age. J Thorac Cardiovasc Surg. 2008;136:100–7, 107.e1.

41. Anderson PAW, Sleeper LA, Mahony L, et al. Contemporary outcomes after the Fontan procedure: a pediatric heart network multicenter study. J Am Coll Cardiol. 2008;52:85–98.

42. Balaji S, Daga A, Bradley DJ, et al. An international multicenter study comparing arrhythmia prevalence between the intracardiac lateral tunnel and the extracardiac conduit type of Fontan operations. J Thorac Cardiovasc Surg. 2014;148:576–81.

43. Ben Ali W, Bouhout I, Khairy P, Bouchard D, Poirier N. Extracardiac versus lateral tunnel Fontan: a meta-analysis of long-term results. Ann Thorac Surg. 2019;107:837–43.

44. Ramesh V, Gaynor JW, Shah MJ, et al. Comparison of left and right atrial epicardial pacing in patients with congenital heart disease. Ann Thorac Surg. 1999;68:2314–9.

45. Huntley GD, Deshmukh AJ, Warnes CA, Kapa S, Egbe AC. Longitudinal outcomes of epicardial and endocardial pacemaker leads in the adult Fontan patient. Pediatr Cardiol. 2018;39:1476–83.

46. Egbe AC, Huntley GD, Connolly HM, et al. Outcomes of cardiac pacing in adult patients after a Fontan operation. Am Heart J. 2017;194:92–8.

47. Hansky B, Blanz U, Peuster M, et al. Endocardial pacing after Fontan-type procedures. Pacing Clin Electrophysiol. 2005;28:140–8.

48. Takahashi K, Cecchin F, Fortescue E, et al. Permanent atrial pacing lead implant route after Fontan operation. Pacing Clin Electrophysiol. 2009;32:779–85.

49. Segar DE, Maldonado JR, Brown CG, Law IH. Transvenous versus epicardial pacing in Fontan patients. Pediatr Cardiol. 2018;39:1484–8.

50. Moore JP, Shannon KM. Transpulmonary atrial pacing: an approach to transvenous pacemaker implan-tation after extracardiac conduit Fontan surgery. J Cardiovasc Electrophysiol. 2014;25:1028–31.

51. Arif S, Clift PF, De Giovanni JV. Permanent trans-venous pacing in an extra-cardiac Fontan circulation. Europace. 2016;18:304–7.

52. Pundi KN, Pundi KN, Johnson JN, et al. Sudden cardiac death and late arrhythmias after the Fontan operation. Congenit Heart Dis. 2017;12:17–23.

53. Rathod RH, Prakash A, Powell AJ, Geva T. Myocardial fibrosis identified by cardiac magnetic resonance late gadolinium enhancement is associated with adverse ventricular mechanics and ventricular tachycardia late after Fontan operation. J Am Coll Cardiol. 2010;55:1721–8.

54. Wilson WM, Valente AM, Hickey EJ, et al. Outcomes of patients with hypoplastic left heart syndrome reaching adulthood after Fontan palliation: multi-center study. Circulation. 2018;137:978–81.

55. Moore JP, Mondésert B, Lloyd MS, et al. Clinical experience with the subcutaneous implantable cardioverter-defibrillator in adults with congenital heart disease. Circ Arrhythm Electrophysiol. 2016;9:9.

56. Garside H, Leyva F, Hudsmith L, Marshall H, de Bono J. Eligibility for subcutaneous implantable cardioverter defibrillators in the adult congenital heart disease population. Pacing Clin Electrophysiol. 2019;42:65–70.

57. Paridon SM, Karpawich PP, Pinsky WW. The effects of rate responsive pacing on exercise performance in the postoperative univentricular heart. Pacing Clin Electrophysiol. 1993;16:1256–62.

58. Bulic A, Zimmerman FJ, Ceresnak SR, et al. Ventricular pacing in single ventricles—a bad combination. Heart Rhythm. 2017;14:853–7.

59. Poh CL, Celermajer DS, Grigg LE, et al. Pacemakers are associated with a higher risk of late death and transplantation in the Fontan population. Int J Cardiol. 2019;282:33–7.

60. Kodama Y, Kuraoka A, Ishikawa Y, et al. Outcome of patients with functional single ventricular heart after pacemaker implantation: what makes it poor, and what can we do? Heart Rhythm. 2019;16:1870–4.

61. Cecchin F, Frangini PA, Brown DW, et al. Cardiac resynchronization therapy (and multisite pacing) in pediatrics and congenital heart disease: five years experience in a single institution. J Cardiovasc Electrophysiol. 2009;20:58–65.

62. O'Leary ET, Gauvreau K, Alexander ME, et al. Dual-site ventricular pacing in patients with Fontan physiology and heart block: does it mitigate the detrimental effects of single-site ventricular pacing? JACC Clin Electrophysiol. 2018;4:1289–97.

A Multi-system Disorder: Extracardiac Complications

Rachael L. Cordina and David S. Celermajer

Introduction

The Fontan operation leads to a complex physiology with wide ranging effects on multiple organ systems as summarized in Fig. 32.1. Some have important implications and are readily measurable and appreciated; other effects are more subtle.

R. L. Cordina (✉) · D. S. Celermajer
Department of Cardiology, Royal Prince Alfred Hospital, Sydney, Australia

Sydney Medical School, University of Sydney, Sydney, Australia
e-mail: rachael.cordina@sydney.edu.au; David.Celermajer@health.nsw.gov.au

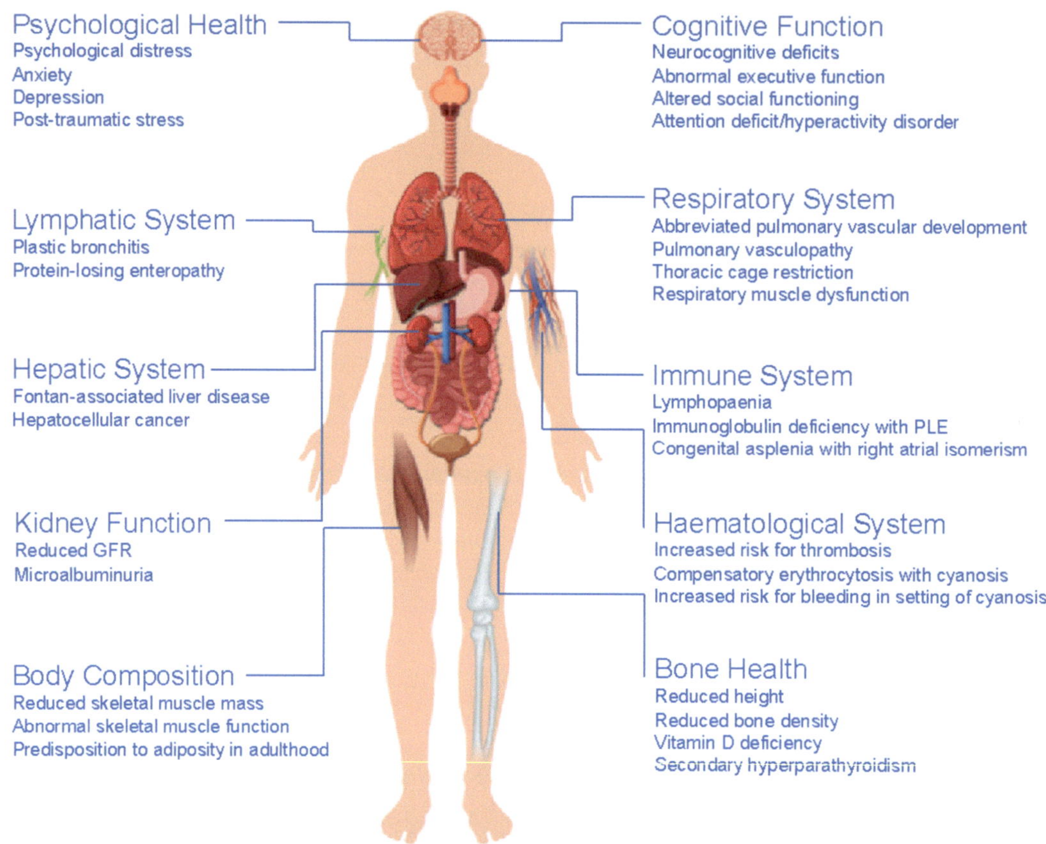

Fig. 32.1 *GFR* Glomerular filtration rate, *PLE* Protein-losing enteropathy

Fontan Associated Liver Disease

Liver injury is recognised as a universal feature of Fontan physiology [1]. Chronically elevated systemic venous pressure that leads to hepatic congestion and lymphatic dysfunction is probably the primary mediator of Fontan-associated liver disease but other factors such as perioperative hepatic injury, reduced cardiac output and chronic hypoxaemia may also contribute [2].

The majority of people living with a Fontan circulation will demonstrate at least one biochemical derangement of liver function; raised gamma glutamyl transferase (GGT) is the most common [3]. By adulthood, hepatic fibrosis is evident in the majority of patients [4, 5]. Although ultrasound is not sensitive for detecting early fibrotic change, it is useful for assessing progressive fibrosis and changes suggestive of portal hypertension that occur in more advanced disease. In adults, serial ultrasound and measurement of alpha-fetoprotein (AFP) levels are important to screen for hepatocellular carcinoma, a rare but devastating complication of Fontan-related hepatic injury [6–8].

Hepatic CT and MRI may also provide important information on hepatic structure in more advanced liver disease. Elastography, a measure of hepatic stiffness, is an evolving tool to aid in the assessment of liver disease. Since stiffness reflects both fibrosis and congestion, readings are generally increased in the setting of a Fontan circulation, even with relatively minor fibrosis and, thus, results should be interpreted cautiously until more data are available [9, 10].

In people who have evidence for synthetic liver dysfunction or advanced fibrosis on imaging, biopsy may be indicated. This is particularly relevant in the setting of perioperative risk or cardiac transplant assessment.

Most of the Fontan population do not develop decompensated cirrhosis [11, 12], although with increasing numbers of late Fontan survivors, this may become a more common problem. Currently, aside from interventions to optimise hemodynamics and, possibly, reduce venous pressure, evidence-based therapies for Fontan-associated liver disease do not exist. Minimising exposure to liver toxins, such as alcohol, maintaining a healthy weight and diet, avoiding smoking, and vaccination for hepatitis B are likely to be beneficial.

Kidney Function

The impact of the Fontan circulation on the renal system has only been recognised recently and, thus, comprehensive data are lacking. A mild reduction in the glomerular filtration rate and/or microalbuminuria are common [9] and may be unmasked during illness or surgery.

The pathophysiology is likely to relate to chronic venous hypertension as well as perioperative damage [13].

Renal function should be monitored regularly in adults. In children, cystatin C may be a more reliable measure of glomerular function than creatinine-based assessments due to the high prevalence of reduced skeletal muscle mass in the Fontan population [14, 15].

The significance of microalbuminuria in this setting, the need for serial monitoring, and effective medical therapies remain unknown. General measures such as maintaining optimal hydration, treating systemic hypertension, avoiding smoking and maintaining a healthy weight and diet, are likely to be beneficial. Nephrotoxins should be avoided when possible, especially when there is evidence of kidney disease.

The Lymphatic System

Abnormal lymphatic function is an important contributor to plastic bronchitis and protein-losing enteropathy, two very serious complications of Fontan physiology affecting 5–10% of this population [16, 17]. Abnormal lymphatic drainage may also contribute to end-organ damage in other systems.

Although the pathophysiology is not well-established, increased lymphatic pressure related to systemic venous hypertension, with secondary increase in lymphatic production and reduced reabsorption, appear to drive the lymphatic derangement observed in Fontan patients. Congenital abnormalities of lymphatic structure may also contribute.

Plastic bronchitis typically, occurs early in life, soon after Fontan completion, whereas protein-losing enteropathy can occur at any time. Both diagnoses are associated with an increased risk for premature death [18, 19].The diagnosis and management of plastic bronchitis and protein-losing enteropathy are described in Table 32.1.

Plastic bronchitis usually presents as dyspnoea, hypoxaemia and a productive cough. Thick casts of inflammatory cells and mucous are characteristic.

Protein-losing enteropathy may be detected by the presence of hypoalbuminaemia on blood testing, or may present with diarrhoea, ascites, immunodeficiency and/or growth failure in young patients. Protein-losing enteropathy is formally diagnosed by the presence of an elevated stool alpha-1-antitrypsin on a single sample, or a 24-h stool collection if a single sample is non-

Table 32.1 Principles of management for the extra-cardiac complications of the Fontan circulation

Condition	Strategy	Objective
Diagnostic evaluation		
Protein-losing enteropathy and plastic bronchitis	Cardiac imaging and catheterisation	Identify anatomic and haemodynamic issues
	Lymphatic imaging with T2-weighted MRI and lymphangiography	Characterise lymphatic anatomy and possible decompression channels
	ECG and Holter monitor	Identify important arrhythmia
Medical management		
Protein-losing enteropathy and plastic bronchitis	Correct significant anaemia	Treat severe anaemia [24]
	Diuretics	Reduce venous and lymphatic congestion
	Aldosterone inhibition	Possible direct effect on lymphatic congestion [25, 26]
	Pulmonary vasodilators (phosphodiesterase inhibitors, endothelin-1 receptor antagonists)	Reduce pulmonary vascular resistance with secondary reduction in lymphatic congestion [27]
Protein-losing enteropathy	Subcutaneous heparin	Reduce intestinal membrane permeability and inflammation [28, 29]
	Oral budesonide	Reduced intestinal inflammation and restore intestinal integrity [30, 31]
	Octreotide	?Altered mesenteric blood flow [32]
	Vasopressin	?Altered mesenteric blood flow [33]
Plastic bronchitis	Aerosolised tissue plasminogen activator	Break down bronchial casts and reduce production [34, 35]
	Chest physiotherapy	Assist with clearing casts
Intervention		
Protein-losing enteropathy and plastic bronchitis	Cardiac pacing	Establish appropriate heart rate and cardiac output if important brady arrhythmia or heart block [36]
	Fontan fenestration	Reduce systemic venous pressure and increase cardiac output [37]
	Catheter-based intervention	Address Fontan pathway/pulmonary artery obstruction
	Catheter-based lymphatic intervention	Identify pathways of lymphatic decompression and occlude if possible [17, 22]
	Surgical intervention	Address important obstructive and/or valvar lesions Fontan takedown Heart transplantation
Protein-losing enteropathy	Surgical rerouting of innominate vein or thoracic duct to left atrium	Decompress lymphatic system [38]
Plastic bronchitis	Thoracic duct ligation	Redirect lymphatic drainage away from airway decompression channels [39]

Adapted from Rychik et al. [40]

diagnostic [20, 21]. Lymphatic imaging and interventions are emerging as promising diagnostic and therapeutic tools [22].

Detailed evaluation for correctable problems that may be adversely impacting the circulation should be undertaken in patients with protein-losing enteropathy, as outlined in Table 32.1. Any potentially reversible issues should be aggressively treated and may lead to resolution. Protein loss may result in a thrombophilic state and, thus, anticoagulation may be warranted in the setting of severe disease. A high-protein diet, substituting long with medium chain fatty acids, may help to optimise nutritional status [23].

The Respiratory System

The pulmonary circulation is abnormal in the setting of Fontan physiology, which has important implications for circulatory function; indeed, even a slight increase in the transpulmonary gradient can have catastrophic implications in this setting. Numerous factors contribute to abnormal pulmonary vascular structure and function including:

- Pulmonary vascular flow profile changes that occur at Fontan completion when flow changes from pulsatile to non-pulsatile. These alterations cause pulmonary vascular development to slow or cease, which may cause an increase in pulmonary vascular resistance [41].
- Disproportionate flow favouring one lung due to anatomical issues within the Fontan pathways, further impacting vascular growth.
- Congenital hypoplasia and scarring of the pulmonary arteries from previous surgical shunts which may impact on pulmonary artery size.
- Small aortopulmonary collateral vessels which may have an impact in a subset of patients, but data are lacking.
- The lack of pulsatile pulmonary blood flow which causes an endotheliopathy, characterised by intimal proliferation and a further increase in pulmonary vascular resistance [42, 43].

Some trials studying the impact of pulmonary vasodilator drugs on Fontan physiology have demonstrated an improvement in pulmonary vascular resistance and a modest increase in peak oxygen uptake [44]. Despite this, most experts currently use these drug only in a small subset of Fontan patients with additional indications (e.g. refractory heart failure, protein-losing enteropathy).

Restrictive lung function (a reduction in lung volumes) is common, likely predominantly related to recurrent sternotomies and/or thoracotomies, even though intrinsic respiratory muscle dysfunction may also play a role [45]. Restrictive lung defects has been shown to contribute to exercise limitation; this is particularly relevant to patients with a Fontan circulation, which is highly dependent on effective inspiration and expiration for cardiac filling and augmenting cardiac output [46]. Inspiratory muscle training improves ventilatory efficiency and cardiac filling in Fontan patients, with a modest benefit on exercise capacity [47, 48].

Cognitive Function

People living with a Fontan circulation are at risk of important neurocognitive deficits [49–51] although most have an intelligence quotient within normal range, and many individuals are highly functioning [52, 53]. It is likely that a complex interplay of factors contribute to the recognised neurocognitive issues in the Fontan population, including genetics, low birth weight, prematurity, altered fetal and neonatal haemodynamics, surgical factors and environmental influences [54–57]. The impact of recurrent cardiac surgery (associated with cerebral hypoxia as well as macro and microembolic events) on the developing and already 'at risk' brain is increasingly recognised [58]. Chronic cyanosis may also affect brain development [59].

Cerebral imaging with magnetic resonance imaging is frequently abnormal in Fontan patients: reduced brain volume and white matter abnormalities are common, with more obvious ischaemic abnormalities also frequently evident. The extent of white matter injury has been found to be (inversely) associated with intelligence scores and cognitive processing speed [60].

Abnormal executive function, attention-deficit/hyperactivity disorder and social cognition problems, which are especially common in this population [61, 62], can have an enormous impact on relationships, careers and integration into the community, as well as medical attendance and compliance.

Neurodevelopmental screening and assessment throughout childhood is essential to aid early detection and intervention that can optimise individual potential [49, 63, 64]. Support and education for families is also very important.

Psychological Health

Surviving with a Fontan circulation involves living with memories of recurrent hospitalisations, periods of major illness, chronic physical limitation and deep uncertainty about the future. Not surprisingly, mental health issues are frequent in people who have a Fontan circulation compared with their peers; some reports suggest that up to two thirds of the population are affected. Anxiety, post-traumatic stress and depressive symptoms are especially common [65, 66].

Risk factors for psychological distress include male sex, lower birth weight, lower intelligence and longer duration of deep hypothermic arrest [65, 67, 68]. Family members also experience high rates of psychological distress [67, 69, 70]. Fontan-specific data are lacking in this area, but based on evidence in other populations, early recognition of psychological distress in patients and their families, with appropriate psychological support, is likely to be highly beneficial. Optimised transition services to alleviate the trauma and uncertainty of moving to adult care is critical [71].

Musculoskeletal Health and Body Composition

A healthy skeletal muscle bulk is important for optimal functioning of the Fontan circulation: muscle contraction "squeezes" blood out of the peripheral vasculature and assists venous return, accounting for the majority of increased venous return during exercise [14, 72–74]; Leg muscle contractions may even generate pulsatile pulmonary blood flow in some patients [75].

However, people living with a Fontan circulation often have reduced skeletal muscle mass (Fontan-associated myopenia) [14, 76, 77], with dysfunctional skeletal muscle aerobic metabolism [14, 78] and impaired sympathetic reflex responses [79]. The aetiology of Fontan-associated myopenia is not well characterised, but likely relates to attenuated skeletal muscle blood flow, as well as chronic venous hypertension and neurohormonal activation. The role of factors present prior to Fontan completion is unclear.

Obesity, on the other hand, is likely to have important detrimental effects on Fontan physiology, due to its impact on thoracic "suction" force, as well as on pulmonary and systemic vascular resistance, although data are lacking in this area. The prevalence of obesity (based on body mass index) in the setting of a Fontan circulation is similar to the broader community [80]. However, due to the high prevalence of skeletal muscle deficiency, body mass index frequently underestimates adiposity in people who have a Fontan circulation, because muscle is denser than fat [77]. Increased adiposity assessed by dual X-ray absorptiometry, is common in adolescents and adults with a Fontan circulation [77], and is associated with a lower in exercise capacity and poor clinical outcomes [81]. Low adiposity in the setting of Fontan-associated malnourishment is also a poor prognostic sign.

Exercise training has been shown to improve skeletal muscle function and body composition in the setting of the Fontan circulation [79, 82]. A healthy diet is also likely to be important, but nutritional interventions have not been investigated, other than in the setting of protein-losing enteropathy.

In addition to abnormal body composition, bone health and growth are also affected in Fontan patient. Somatic growth may be impacted and short stature has been associated with poorer physical and psychosocial function [83]. Bone density is frequently reduced in adults and children [84–86]. There are many possible contributors to abnormal bone health including:

- Vitamin D deficiency and secondary hyperparathyroidism which are common and have been shown to correlate with bone density abnormalities in Fontan adults [86].
- Chronic cyanosis, neurohormonal activation, reduced blood flow and physical activity which may also contribute to skeletal abnormalities [86].

- Important hepatic dysfunction and protein-losing enteropathy.
- Drugs, such warfarin [87].

Time outdoors, adequate levels of physical activity, maintenance of adequate vitamin D levels and high dietary calcium intake are established measures for optimizing bone health in the general population and are also likely to be of benefit for the Fontan population.

The Immune System

The impact of the Fontan circulation on the immune system is poorly understood. Lymphopaenia is common and may contribute to delayed viral clearance [88]. In the setting of protein-losing enteropathy, lymphopaenia may be more marked and immunogloblin levels are frequently reduced due to gastrointestinal protein loss, resulting in inadequate immune responses to vaccinations, and predisposing to important infections [89].

People who have right atrial isomerism (congenital asplenia) have an increased risk for infections, particularly related to encapsulated bacteria, and should be vaccinated accordingly. Although controlling infection early is important for anyone living with a Fontan circulation, it is of particular importance in this subset of patients. In early life, daily penicillin prophylaxis may be warranted.

The Haematological System

Major haematological considerations in Fontan physiology relate to thrombosis, bleeding and anaemia. The Fontan circulation is particularly predisposed to thrombosis due to slow venous blood flow, stasis and endothelial dysfunction (especially in patients with atriopulmonary Fontan, large pulmonary artery stumps and akinetic cardiac chambers) [90] In addition, atrial arrhythmias and cardiac chamber enlargement contribute to the risk for clot formation [91]. Patients with an atriopulmonary-type Fontan cir-culation may have massive right atrial dilatation and can develop clots within the atrium, even when in sinus rhythm.

Thrombosis can have especially catastrophic implications for a Fontan patients [12, 92, 93] because:

- Pulmonary embolism may cause an abrupt increase in pulmonary vascular resistance, resulting in a sudden drop in cardiac output that may be incompatible with life.
- Venous thromboembolism may manifest as a stroke in Fontan patients with a fenestration or other right-to-left shunt

Cyanotic patients typically present with an appropriate compensatory erythrocytosis, which is associated with an increased blood viscosity, but also increased consumption of clotting factors and platelets that may also increase the risk for major bleeding [94]. Advanced Fontan-associated liver disease may result in reduced production of clotting factors and hypersplenism due to portal hypertension with a low platelet count that further increases bleeding risk.

Current data and expert opinion suggest that thromboprophylaxis is important for people with Fontan physiology [95]. In the absence of high risk features, such as previous thromboembolic event, atrial arrhythmias, large right to left shunt or massive atrial dilatation, many experts use single or dual antiplatelet therapy. Anticoagulation with warfarin is generally used in higher-risk patients, including all patients with atriopulmonary Fontan [90, 96]. The safety and efficacy of direct acting oral anticoagulants in this setting is not yet established, even though new promising data are emerging (see chapter by Rafiq et al.).

Cyanosis is common in Fontan physiology, typically due to a fenestration in the Fontan pathway or systemic-to-pulmonary venous collaterals that may develop to decompress the systemic veins. Compensatory erythrocytosis is an appropriate haematological response to support the delivery of oxygen to the tissues and relies on adequate iron stores to produce increased levels of haemoglobin concentration. Anaemia (or "relative anaemia") may not be obvious on blood testing in this setting: results may still fall within the laboratory "normal" levels, yet haemoglobin concentration may be far lower than what is expected for the severity of the cyanosis. For example, in a patient with resting oxygen saturation in the mid 80s, haemoglobin concentration is expected to be 20 g/dL or above. Such patients should be kept well hydrated at all times to minimise the risk of hyperviscosity symptoms or other complications.

Iron stores should be regularly monitored in cyanotic patients: ferritin and transferrin saturation levels should be maintained within the normal range by iron supplementation (oral or intravenous) in patients with lower-than-expected haemoglobin concentration for their resting saturations (seek expert opinion). This is likely to help optimise exercise capacity and reduce unnecessary haemodynamic loading [97]. Air emboli should be avoided when giving intravenous iron or other intravenous medication or fluids to cyanotic patients with a right-left shunt. In people with important chronic iron deficiency, it is important to consider whether there is gastrointestinal loss and/or address menorrhagia that may be exacerbated by anticoagulation.

References

1. Goldberg DJ, Surrey LF, Glatz AC, et al. Hepatic fibrosis is universal following Fontan operation, and severity is associated with time from surgery: a liver biopsy and hemodynamic study. J Am Heart Assoc. 2017;6:6.
2. Pundi K, Pundi KN, Kamath PS, et al. Liver disease in patients after the Fontan operation. Am J Cardiol. 2016;117:456–60.
3. van Nieuwenhuizen RC, Peters M, Lubbers LJ, Trip MD, Tijssen JG, Mulder BJ. Abnormalities in liver function and coagulation profile following the Fontan procedure. Heart. 1999;82:40–6.
4. Wilson TG, d'Udekem Y, Winlaw DS, et al. Hepatic and renal end-organ damage in the Fontan circulation: a report from the Australian and New Zealand Fontan registry. Int J Cardiol. 2018;273:100–7.
5. Nandwana SB, Olaiya B, Cox K, Sahu A, Mittal P. Abdominal imaging surveillance in adult patients after Fontan procedure: risk of chronic liver disease and hepatocellular carcinoma. Curr Probl Diagn Radiol. 2018;47:19–22.
6. Elder RW, McCabe NM, Hebson C, et al. Features of portal hypertension are associated with major adverse events in Fontan patients: the VAST study. Int J Cardiol. 2013;168:3764–9.
7. Asrani SK, Warnes CA, Kamath PS. Hepatocellular carcinoma after the Fontan procedure. N Engl J Med. 2013;368:1756–7.
8. Ghaferi AA, Hutchins GM. Progression of liver pathology in patients undergoing the Fontan procedure: chronic passive congestion, cardiac cirrhosis, hepatic adenoma, and hepatocellular carcinoma. J Thorac Cardiovasc Surg. 2005;129:1348–52.
9. Wilson TG, Udekem Y, Winlaw DS, et al. Hepatic and renal end-organ damage in the Fontan circulation: a report from the Australian and New Zealand Fontan registry. Int J Cardiol. 2018;273:100–7.
10. Hilscher MB, Johnson JN, Cetta F, et al. Surveillance for liver complications after the Fontan procedure. Congenit Heart Dis. 2017;12:124–32.
11. Dennis M, Zannino D, du Plessis K, et al. Clinical outcomes in adolescents and adults after the Fontan procedure. J Am Coll Cardiol. 2018;71:1009–17.
12. Khairy P, Fernandes SM, Mayer JE Jr, et al. Long-term survival, modes of death, and predictors of mortality in patients with Fontan surgery. Circulation. 2008;117:85–92.
13. Velpula M, Sheron N, Guha N, Salmon T, Hacking N, Veldtman GR. Direct measurement of Porto-systemic gradient in a failing Fontan circulation. Congenit Heart Dis. 2011;6:175–8.
14. Cordina R, O'Meagher S, Gould H, et al. Skeletal muscle abnormalities and exercise capacity in adults with a Fontan circulation. Heart. 2013;99:1530–4.
15. Opotowsky AR, Baraona FR, Mc Causland FR, et al. Estimated glomerular filtration rate and urine biomarkers in patients with single-ventricle Fontan circulation. Heart. 2017;103:434–42.
16. Menon S, Chennapragada M, Ugaki S, Sholler GF, Ayer J, Winlaw DS. The lymphatic circulation in adaptations to the Fontan circulation. Pediatr Cardiol. 2017;38:886–92.
17. Itkin MG, McCormack FX, Dori Y. Diagnosis and treatment of lymphatic plastic bronchitis in adults using advanced lymphatic imaging and percutaneous embolization. Ann Am Thorac Soc. 2016;13:1689–96.
18. Meadows J, Jenkins K. Protein-losing enteropathy: integrating a new disease paradigm into recommendations for prevention and treatment. Cardiol Young. 2011;21:363–77.
19. Allen KY, Downing TE, Glatz AC, et al. Effect of Fontan-associated morbidities on survival with intact Fontan circulation. Am J Cardiol. 2017;119:1866–71.
20. Miranda C, Taqatqa A, Chapa-Rodriguez A, Holton JP, Awad SM. The use of fecal calprotectin levels in the Fontan population. Pediatr Cardiol. 2018;39:591–4.
21. Breatnach CR, Cleary A, Prendiville T, Crumlish K, Murchan H, McMahon CJ. Prevalence of subclinical enteric alpha-1-antitrypsin loss in children with univentricular circulation following total cavopulmonary connection. Pediatr Cardiol. 2018;39:33–7.

22. Itkin M, Piccoli DA, Nadolski G, et al. Protein-losing enteropathy in patients with congenital heart disease. J Am Coll Cardiol. 2017;69:2929–37.
23. John AS, Johnson JA, Khan M, Driscoll DJ, Warnes CA, Cetta F. Clinical outcomes and improved survival in patients with protein-losing enteropathy after the Fontan operation. J Am Coll Cardiol. 2014;64:54–62.
24. Yetman AT, Everitt MD. The role of iron deficiency in protein-losing enteropathy following the Fontan procedure. Congenit Heart Dis. 2011;6:370–3.
25. Ringel RE, Peddy SB. Effect of high-dose spironolactone on protein-losing enteropathy in patients with Fontan palliation of complex congenital heart disease. Am J Cardiol. 2003;91:1031–2, A9.
26. Okano S, Sugimoto M, Takase M, Iseki K, Kajihama A, Azuma H. Effectiveness of high-dose spironolactone therapy in a patient with recurrent protein-losing enteropathy after the Fontan procedure. Intern Med. 2016;55:1611–4.
27. Reinhardt Z, Uzun O, Bhole V, et al. Sildenafil in the management of the failing Fontan circulation. Cardiol Young. 2010;20:522–5.
28. Ryerson L, Goldberg C, Rosenthal A, Armstrong A. Usefulness of heparin therapy in protein-losing enteropathy associated with single ventricle palliation. Am J Cardiol. 2008;101:248–51.
29. Donnelly JP, Rosenthal A, Castle VP, Holmes RD. Reversal of protein-losing enteropathy with heparin therapy in three patients with univentricular hearts and Fontan palliation. J Pediatr. 1997;130:474–8.
30. Thacker D, Patel A, Dodds K, Goldberg DJ, Semeao E, Rychik J. Use of oral budesonide in the management of protein-losing enteropathy after the Fontan operation. Ann Thorac Surg. 2010;89:837–42.
31. Schumacher KR, Cools M, Goldstein BH, et al. Oral budesonide treatment for protein-losing enteropathy in Fontan-palliated patients. Pediatr Cardiol. 2011;32:966–71.
32. John AS, Phillips SD, Driscoll DJ, Warnes CA, Cetta F. The use of octreotide to successfully treat protein-losing enteropathy following the Fontan operation. Congenit Heart Dis. 2011;6:653–6.
33. Friedland-Little JM, Gajarski RJ, Schumacher KR. Dopamine as a potential rescue therapy for refractory protein-losing enteropathy in Fontan-palliated patients. Pediatr Transplant. 2017;21:e12925.
34. Costello JM, Steinhorn D, McColley S, Gerber ME, Kumar SP. Treatment of plastic bronchitis in a Fontan patient with tissue plasminogen activator: a case report and review of the literature. Pediatrics. 2002;109:e67.
35. Do TB, Chu JM, Berdjis F, Anas NG. Fontan patient with plastic bronchitis treated successfully using aerosolized tissue plasminogen activator: a case report and review of the literature. Pediatr Cardiol. 2009;30:352–5.
36. Cohen MI, Rhodes LA, Wernovsky G, Gaynor JW, Spray TL, Rychik J. Atrial pacing: an alternative treatment for protein-losing enteropathy after the Fontan operation. J Thorac Cardiovasc Surg. 2001;121:582–3.
37. Jacobs ML, Rychik J, Byrum CJ, Norwood WI Jr. Protein-losing enteropathy after Fontan operation: resolution after baffle fenestration. Ann Thorac Surg. 1996;61:206–8.
38. Antonio M, Gordo A, Pereira C, Pinto F, Fragata I, Fragata J. Thoracic duct decompression for protein-losing enteropathy in failing Fontan circulation. Ann Thorac Surg. 2016;101:2370–3.
39. Shah SS, Drinkwater DC, Christian KG. Plastic bronchitis: is thoracic duct ligation a real surgical option? Ann Thorac Surg. 2006;81:2281–3.
40. Rychik J, Atz AM, Celermajer DS, et al. Evaluation and management of the child and adult with Fontan circulation: a scientific statement from the American Heart Association. Circulation. 2019;140:e234–84.
41. Ovroutski S, Ewert P, Alexi-Meskishvili V, et al. Absence of pulmonary artery growth after Fontan operation and its possible impact on late outcome. Ann Thorac Surg. 2009;87:826–31.
42. Kurotobi S, Sano T, Kogaki S, et al. Bidirectional cavopulmonary shunt with right ventricular outflow patency: the impact of pulsatility on pulmonary endothelial function. J Thorac Cardiovasc Surg. 2001;121:1161–8.
43. Khambadkone S, Li J, de Leval MR, Cullen S, Deanfield JE, Redington AN. Basal pulmonary vascular resistance and nitric oxide responsiveness late after Fontan-type operation. Circulation. 2003;107:3204–8.
44. Wang W, Hu X, Liao W, et al. The efficacy and safety of pulmonary vasodilators in patients with Fontan circulation: a meta-analysis of randomized controlled trials. Pulm Circ. 2019;9:2045894018790450.
45. Greutmann M, Le TL, Tobler D, et al. Generalised muscle weakness in young adults with congenital heart disease. Heart. 2011;97:1164–8.
46. Ginde S, Bartz PJ, Hill GD, et al. Restrictive lung disease is an independent predictor of exercise intolerance in the adult with congenital heart disease. Congenit Heart Dis. 2013;8:246–54.
47. Laohachai K, Winlaw D, Selvadurai H, et al. Inspiratory muscle training is associated with improved inspiratory muscle strength, resting cardiac output, and the ventilatory efficiency of exercise in patients with a Fontan circulation. J Am Heart Assoc. 2017;6:6.
48. Wu FM, Opotowsky AR, Denhoff ER, et al. A pilot study of inspiratory muscle training to improve exercise capacity in patients with Fontan physiology. Semin Thorac Cardiovasc Surg. 2018;30:462–9.
49. Marino BS, Lipkin PH, Newburger JW, et al. Neurodevelopmental outcomes in children with congenital heart disease: evaluation and management: a scientific statement from the American Heart Association. Circulation. 2012;126:1143–72.
50. Latal B. Neurodevelopmental outcomes of the child with congenital heart disease. Clin Perinatol. 2016;43:173–85.

51. Verrall C, Blue G, Loughran-Fowlds A, et al. Big issues in neurodevelopment in congenital heart disease. Open Heart. 2019;6(2):e000998.
52. Gaynor JW, Ittenbach RF, Gerdes M, et al. Neurodevelopmental outcomes in preschool survivors of the Fontan procedure. J Thorac Cardiovasc Surg. 2014;147:1276–82; discussion 1282–1283.e5.
53. Cordina R, du Plessis K, Tran D, d'Udekem Y. Super-Fontan: is it possible? J Thorac Cardiovasc Surg. 2018;155:1192–4.
54. Martinez-Biarge M, Jowett VC, Cowan FM, Wusthoff CJ. Neurodevelopmental outcome in children with congenital heart disease. Semin Fetal Neonatal Med. 2013;18:279–85.
55. Gaynor JW, Stopp C, Wypij D, et al. Neurodevelopmental outcomes after cardiac surgery in infancy. Pediatrics. 2015;135:816–25.
56. Wernovsky G. Current insights regarding neurological and developmental abnormalities in children and young adults with complex congenital cardiac disease. Cardiol Young. 2006;16(Suppl 1):92–104.
57. Goldberg CS, Mussatto K, Licht D, Wernovsky G. Neurodevelopment and quality of life for children with hypoplastic left heart syndrome: current knowns and unknowns. Cardiol Young. 2011;21(Suppl 2):88–92.
58. Ohye RG, Sleeper LA, Mahony L, et al. Comparison of shunt types in the Norwood procedure for single-ventricle lesions. N Engl J Med. 2010;362:1980–92.
59. Cordina R, Grieve S, Barnett M, Lagopoulos J, Malitz N, Celermajer DS. Brain volumetric, regional cortical thickness and radiographic findings in adults with cyanotic congenital heart disease. Neuroimage Clin. 2014;4:319–25.
60. Watson CG, Stopp C, Wypij D, Bellinger DC, Newburger JW, Rivkin MJ. Altered white matter microstructure correlates with IQ and processing speed in children and adolescents post-Fontan. J Pediatr. 2018;200:140–149.e4.
61. Calderon J, Bellinger DC. Executive function deficits in congenital heart disease: why is intervention important? Cardiol Young. 2015;25:1238–46.
62. Bellinger DC, Watson CG, Rivkin MJ, et al. Neuropsychological status and structural brain imaging in adolescents with single ventricle who underwent the Fontan procedure. J Am Heart Assoc. 2015;4:e002302.
63. Walker K, Holland AJ, Halliday R, Badawi N. Which high-risk infants should we follow-up and how should we do it? J Paediatr Child Health. 2012;48:789–93.
64. Supporting the long-term developmental needs of children with congenital heart disease and their families. Queensland Health. 2018. https://www.childrens.health.qld.gov.au/wp-content/uploads/PDF/pink-book.pdf. Accessed Apr 2019.
65. DeMaso DR, Calderon J, Taylor GA, et al. Psychiatric disorders in adolescents with single ventricle congenital heart disease. Pediatrics. 2017;139:e20162241.
66. Pike NA, Evangelista LS, Doering LV, Eastwood JA, Lewis AB, Child JS. Quality of life, health status, and depression: comparison between adolescents and adults after the Fontan procedure with healthy counterparts. J Cardiovasc Nurs. 2012;27:539–46.
67. Kasparian NA, Winlaw DS, Sholler GF. "Congenital heart health": how psychological care can make a difference. Med J Aust. 2016;205:104–7.
68. Spijkerboer AW, De Koning WB, Duivenvoorden HJ, et al. Medical predictors for long-term behavioral and emotional outcomes in children and adolescents after invasive treatment of congenital heart disease. J Pediatr Surg. 2010;45:2146–53.
69. Woolf-King SE, Anger A, Arnold AE, Weiss SJ, Teitel D. Mental health among parents of children with critical congenital heart defects: a systematic review. J Am Heart Assoc. 2017;6:e004862.
70. Sharpe D, Rossiter L. Siblings of children with a chronic illness: a meta-analysis. J Pediatr Psychol. 2002;27:699–710.
71. Uzark K, Wray J. Young people with congenital heart disease—transitioning to adult care. Prog Pediatr Cardiol. 2018;48:68–74.
72. Shafer KM, Garcia JA, Babb TG, Fixler DE, Ayers CR, Levine BD. The importance of the muscle and ventilatory blood pumps during exercise in patients without a subpulmonary ventricle (Fontan operation). J Am Coll Cardiol. 2012;60:2115–21.
73. Hjortdal VE, Emmertsen K, Stenbog E, et al. Effects of exercise and respiration on blood flow in total cavo-pulmonary connection: a real-time magnetic resonance flow study. Circulation. 2003;108:1227–31.
74. Avitabile CM, Goldberg DJ, Leonard MB, et al. Leg lean mass correlates with exercise systemic output in young Fontan patients. Heart. 2018;104:680–4.
75. Cordina R, Celermajer DS, d'Udekem Y. Lower limb exercise generates pulsatile flow into the pulmonary vascular bed in the setting of the Fontan circulation. Cardiol Young. 2018;28:732–3.
76. Avitabile CM, Leonard MB, Zemel BS, et al. Lean mass deficits, vitamin D status and exercise capacity in children and young adults after Fontan palliation. Heart. 2014;100:1702–7.
77. Tran D, D'Ambrosio P, Verrall C, et al. Body composition abnormalities in adults with a Fontan circulation. Heart Lung Circulation. 2019;28:S148–9.
78. Inai K, Saita Y, Takeda S, Nakazawa M, Kimura H. Skeletal muscle hemodynamics and endothelial function in patients after Fontan operation. Am J Cardiol. 2004;93:792–7.
79. Brassard P, Poirier P, Martin J, et al. Impact of exercise training on muscle function and ergoreflex in Fontan patients: a pilot study. Int J Cardiol. 2006;107:85–94.
80. Chung ST, Hong B, Patterson L, Petit CJ, Ham JN. High overweight and obesity in Fontan patients: a 20-year history. Pediatr Cardiol. 2016;37:192–200.
81. Ohuchi H, Negishi J, Miike H, et al. Positive pediatric exercise capacity trajectory predicts better adult Fontan physiology rationale for early establishment of exercise habits. Int J Cardiol. 2018;274:80–7.

82. Cordina RL, O'Meagher S, Karmali A, et al. Resistance training improves cardiac output, exercise capacity and tolerance to positive airway pressure in Fontan physiology. Int J Cardiol. 2013;168:780–8.

83. Cohen MS, Zak V, Atz AM, et al. Anthropometric measures after Fontan procedure: implications for suboptimal functional outcome. Am Heart J. 2010;160:1092–8, 1098.e1.

84. Avitabile CM, Goldberg DJ, Zemel BS, et al. Deficits in bone density and structure in children and young adults following Fontan palliation. Bone. 2015;77:12–6.

85. Bendaly EA, DiMeglio LA, Fadel WF, Hurwitz RA. Bone density in children with single ventricle physiology. Pediatr Cardiol. 2015;36:779–85.

86. D'Ambrosio P, Tran D, Verrall CE, et al. Prevalence and risk factors for low bone density in adults with a Fontan circulation. Congenit Heart Dis. 2019;14:987–95.

87. Rezaieyazdi Z, Falsoleiman H, Khajehdaluee M, Saghafi M, Mokhtari-Amirmajdi E. Reduced bone density in patients on long-term warfarin. Int J Rheum Dis. 2009;12:130–5.

88. Morsheimer MM, Rychik J, Forbes L, et al. Risk factors and clinical significance of lymphopenia in survivors of the Fontan procedure for single-ventricle congenital cardiac disease. J Allergy Clin Immunol Pract. 2016;4:491–6.

89. Magdo HS, Stillwell TL, Greenhawt MJ, et al. Immune abnormalities in Fontan protein-losing enteropathy: a case-control study. J Pediatr. 2015;167:331–7.

90. Monagle P, Cochrane A, Roberts R, et al. A multicenter, randomized trial comparing heparin/warfarin and acetylsalicylic acid as primary thromboprophylaxis for 2 years after the Fontan procedure in children. J Am Coll Cardiol. 2011;58:645–51.

91. Pessotti CF, Jatene MB, Jatene IB, et al. Comparative trial of the use of antiplatelet and oral anticoagulant in thrombosis prophylaxis in patients undergoing total cavopulmonary operation with extracardiac conduit: echocardiographic, tomographic, scintigraphic, clinical and laboratory analysis. Rev Bras Cir Cardiovasc. 2014;29:595–605.

92. Monagle P, Cochrane A, McCrindle B, Benson L, Williams W, Andrew M. Thromboembolic complications after Fontan procedures—the role of prophylactic anticoagulation. J Thorac Cardiovasc Surg. 1998;115:493–8.

93. van den Bosch AE, Roos-Hesselink JW, Van Domburg R, Bogers AJ, Simoons ML, Meijboom FJ. Long-term outcome and quality of life in adult patients after the Fontan operation. Am J Cardiol. 2004;93:1141–5.

94. Cordina RL, Celermajer DS. Chronic cyanosis and vascular function: implications for patients with cyanotic congenital heart disease. Cardiol Young. 2010;20:242–53.

95. Alsaied T, Alsidawi S, Allen CC, Faircloth J, Palumbo JS, Veldtman GR. Strategies for thromboprophylaxis in Fontan circulation: a meta-analysis. Heart. 2015;101:1731–7.

96. McCrindle BW, Manlhiot C, Cochrane A, et al. Factors associated with thrombotic complications after the Fontan procedure: a secondary analysis of a multicenter, randomized trial of primary thromboprophylaxis for 2 years after the Fontan procedure. J Am Coll Cardiol. 2013;61:346–53.

97. Tay EL, Peset A, Papaphylactou M, et al. Replacement therapy for iron deficiency improves exercise capacity and quality of life in patients with cyanotic congenital heart disease and/or the Eisenmenger syndrome. Int J Cardiol. 2011;151:307–12.

The Failing Adult Fontan Patient

Andrew Constantine, Isma Rafiq, Paul Clift, and Konstantinos Dimopoulos

Abbreviations

ACE	Angiotensin-converting enzyme
(A)CHD	(Adult) Congenital heart disease
ERA	Endothelin receptor antagonist
FALD	Fontan-associated liver disease
MRA	Mineralocorticoid receptor antagonist
PDE-5	Phosphodiesterase-5
PVR	Pulmonary vascular resistance
RCT	Randomized controlled trial
TPR	Total pulmonary resistance
VE/VCO$_2$	Minute ventilation/carbon dioxide production
VO$_2$	Oxygen uptake

A. Constantine (✉) · I. Rafiq · K. Dimopoulos
Adult Congenital Heart Centre and Centre for Pulmonary Hypertension, Royal Brompton Hospital, London, UK

National Heart and Lung Institute, Imperial College, London, UK

P. Clift
Department of Cardiology, Queen Elizabeth Hospital, University Hospitals Birmingham NHS Foundation Trust, Birmingham, UK

Pathophysiology

Concept of Fontan Failure

Optimal functioning of the Fontan circulation requires adequate non-pulsatile blood to flow through the pulmonary vascular bed, in the absence of a subpulmonary pump (ventricle). This relies on a moderately raised systemic venous pressure, low pulmonary vascular resistance (PVR) and an unobstructed route from the systemic veins to the pulmonary circulation. Problems anywhere within and beyond the Fontan circuit causing inefficiencies and obstruction of blood flow can lead to worsening systemic venous hypertension, and a drop in cardiac output, fluid overload, cyanosis and exercise intolerance (see 'Managing the pulmonary circulation' chapter). The resulting state of chronic cardiac and multiorgan decompensation is termed "Fontan failure", a term that is used widely by experts, though lacking a formal definition [1].

Complications and clinical deterioration occurring soon after Fontan completion (e.g., within 1 year) are differentiated from complications occurring several years after the establishment of a Fontan circulation i.e., "early" versus "late" Fontan failure. Instances of early Fontan failure usually stem from pre-existing anatomical features or surgical complications, which usually herald a poor outcome, including ventricular dysfunction, atrioventricular valve regurgitation, pre-existing pulmonary vascular disease, pulmonary vein obstruction, or thromboembolism. [2] In contrast, late Fontan failure occurs several years or decades after Fontan palliation, with progressive exercise intolerance, new or progressive pulmonary vascular disease, arrhythmias, and/or multi-organ dysfunction.

To understand the causes of Fontan failure, we must first assess the determinants of optimal cardiac functioning in this unique physiology.

Determinants of Cardiac Output and Exercise Intolerance

Preload has a dominant role in determining cardiac output in the Fontan circulation, due to the direct connection of the systemic venous return via the caval veins to the pulmonary arteries, without a subpulmonary ventricle to actively generate a right-sided cardiac output. The pulmonary circulation is effectively interposed between the systemic venous return and the single ventricle, forming a neoportal system: the systemic venous capillary bed drains into a second (pulmonary) capillary bed before returning to the heart. This has multiple downstream effects:

- Flow of blood from the systemic veins, across the pulmonary capillary bed and into the systemic ventricle requires a passive gradient i.e., systemic venous pressure high enough to overcome resistance in the Fontan circuit, and total pulmonary resistance (TPR):

$$TPR\left(\text{Wood units}\right) = \frac{\text{Mean pulmonary artery pressure}}{\text{Cardiac output}}$$

- It follows that, to function optimally, the Fontan circulation requires a moderately elevated systemic venous resistance and a low PVR, with no obstruction in the Fontan circulation, normal systemic ventricular function, and no hemodynamic lesions (see section below).
- Increased impedance over time in the Fontan pathway and pulmonary vasculature creates a circulation bottleneck that reduces the preload of the systemic ventricle and an inability

to effectively augment cardiac output on exercise (reduced preload reserve). Inadequate preload and preload reserve is, in most situations, the main determinant of cardiac output rather than inadequate contractility, heart rate or afterload (Fig. 33.1) [3–5]. Variables that alter ventricular preload and contractility, heart rate and ventricular afterload can have an impact on cardiac output, chronically or acutely. Indeed, acute clinical situations and medication cause rapid changes in physiology, with the risk of hypotension and circulatory collapse, e.g.:

- Prolonged fasting (e.g., in preparation for cardiac catheterisation, intervention or surgery), dehydration (e.g. hot weather, diarrhoea or vomiting), sepsis, excessive diuresis and anaesthetic agents all reduce preload, which can negatively impact on cardiac output, with disastrous consequences.
- Brady- or tachyarrhythmias, loss of atrioventricular synchrony, and beta-blockade can negatively influence cardiac output by altering the heart rate or impacting on systemic ventricular function.
- Afterload-reducing drugs, such as angiotensin-converting enzyme (ACE)-inhibitors, reduce afterload and can also reduce systemic venous resistance, which can lower cardiac output and cause hypotension.

Additionally, cardiac output can be affected by chronic changes that may occur late after Fontan repair, including a rise in PVR, systemic ventricular impairment, chronotropic incompetence, and the presence of residual haemodynamic lesions.

Several factors can affect the ability of Fontan patients to augment cardiac output during exercise, with a high prevalence of exercise intolerance in the Fontan population (see Chap. 49 on 'Physiological testing and basics of cardiac catheterisation in Fontan patients'). Again, limited preload is an important variable, which is linked to and compounded by systolic and/or diastolic ventricular dysfunction, persistent haemody-

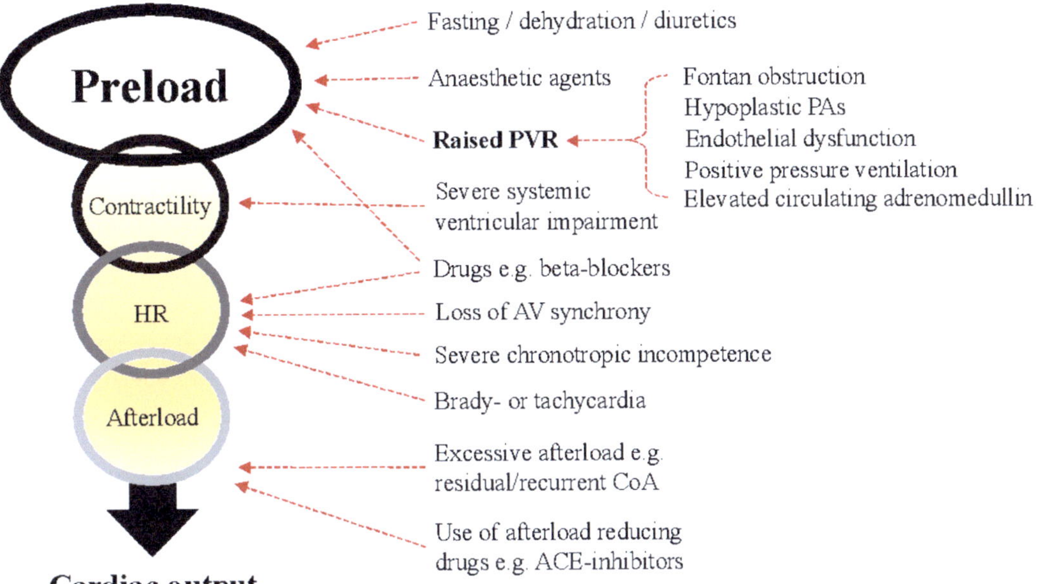

Fig. 33.1 Determinants of cardiac output in patients following Fontan-type repair. The "underloaded" ventricle of the Fontan patient, characterised by a decreased or absent preload reserve, is the main determinant of circulatory output in this setting, unlike in biventricular circulations. Changes in contractility and heart rate (HR) usually play a negligible role unless there is severe systemic ventricular dysfunction or significant brady- or tachyarrhythmia. Part of the compensatory mechanism for the reduced resting circulatory output is an elevation in systemic vascular resistance, but afterload reduction in the setting of an absent preload reserve will not increase cardiac output [3]. The variables listed on the right increase the importance of a given component to the cardiac output; even modest rises in pulmonary vascular resistance (PVR), for example, have a detrimental effect on the ventricular preload and therefore on the cardiac output. *ACE* angiotensin-converting enzyme, *AV* atrioventricular, *CoA* coarctation of the aorta, *PA* pulmonary artery

namic lesions, chronotropic incompetence, ventilation-perfusion mismatch and an impaired ventilatory response to exercise.

The Estimation and Importance of a Low Pulmonary Vascular Resistance

PVR is a critical determinant of pulmonary blood flow in the Fontan circulation due to the reliance on a passive pressure gradient to maintain an effective cardiac output. Even a marginal rise in PVR is poorly tolerated in this setting, compromising ventricular filling and leading to a chronically low cardiac output as well as an excessively high central venous pressure, the hallmarks of Fontan failure. [6]

Pulmonary hypertension (PH) in the setting of complex CHD, including patients with a Fontan-type circulation, is classified in the international PH guidelines as group 5 pulmonary hypertension i.e., PH with multifactorial or unclear mechanisms [7]. Indeed, even in the presence of pulmonary vascular disease, the formal definition of PH (mean pulmonary artery pressure >20 mmHg) is infrequently fulfilled in Fontan patients due to the lack of a subpulmonary ventricle and low pulmonary blood flow, despite a rise in PVR. [8–12]

Assessment of "Failing Fontan" Patients

Careful stepwise assessment of specific hemodynamic parameters is important:

- Raised pressures within the Fontan circuit should initiate a search for possible reversible causes e.g., pathway or pulmonary artery stenosis.

- It is important to remember that even small gradients of a few mmHg across a Fontan pathway or pulmonary artery stenosis may be clinically relevant, given the low blood flow.
- Ventricular end-diastolic pressure and/or pulmonary artery wedge pressure should be measured carefully, especially in the setting of ventricular dysfunction, systemic atrioventricular valvular regurgitation or outflow tract obstruction/aortic regurgitation. Indeed, a post-capillary rise in pressure requires a different management strategy.
- Estimation of the transpulmonary gradient, pulmonary blood flow and PVR is desirable, even though accurate calculation of PVR may be difficult in Fontan patients.

Estimation of pulmonary blood flow and PVR in Fontan patients at cardiac catheterization is challenging due to variable access to either or both pulmonary arteries, reduced non-pulsatile blood flow and multiple sources of pulmonary blood flow (e.g., in patients with a bidirectional or classical Glenn shunt). Vascular access needs to be planned carefully, also considering other anatomical features such as interruption of the inferior vena cava in cases of left atrial isomerism or left / bilateral superior vena cavae. Furthermore, the presence of extra-cardiac shunts, either as venovenous collaterals or pulmonary arteriovenous malformations, alter the 'effective' pulmonary blood flow and complicate PVR estimation and shunt fraction calculation. Hybrid cardiac MRI catheterization can provide accurate estimates of pulmonary as well as systemic blood flow in Fontan patients but is not widely available.

The mechanisms causing pulmonary vasculopathy in Fontan patients remain unclear, but multiple mechanisms are thought to contribute in individual patients:

- Various degrees of abnormal pulmonary artery growth, or abnormal arborization, often with abnormal proximal pulmonary arteries, which may be discontinuous, small or stenosed.
- The absence of pulsatile pulmonary blood flow, at least in animal models, associated with reduced release of endothelium-derived nitric oxide and decreased recruitment of the small arterioles and capillaries [13, 14]. This may contribute to endothelial dysfunction and cause a rise in PVR late after Fontan operation [10].
- Silent or subclinical thromboemboli have also been implicated, based on coagulation abnormalities and relative venous stasis observed in patients following Fontan repair, especially in patients with an atriopulmonary Fontan repair and a severely dilated right atrium [15].

Diastolic and Systolic Dysfunction of the Systemic Ventricle

As described above, the ventricular loading conditions are abnormal in the Fontan circulation. Flow through the neoportal system, modulated by PVR, limits the ventricular preload and, therefore, cardiac output. The (systemic) ventricle is volume underloaded after an initial period of volume overload in early life i.e., prior to the Fontan operation. Reduced myocardial contractility and systolic dysfunction are less likely to play a prominent role in determining cardiac output, unless severely depressed [8]. There is evidence of neurohormonal activation in many patients late after Fontan repair with autonomic and endothelial dysfunction, however, and when significant systolic dysfunction occurs it worsens Fontan haemodynamics [16, 17].

Diastolic dysfunction is an underrecognized component of Fontan failure, which may occur in the presence or absence of systolic ventricular dysfunction [18]. Diastolic dysfunction is usually occult in the setting of a Fontan circulation, masked by the underfilled state of the single ventricle, with a systemic ventricular end-diastolic pressure usually <15 mmHg. A fluid challenge (e.g., of 7 mL/kg) can often unmask diastolic dysfunction [19]. Increased end-diastolic pressures are poorly tolerated in the palliated single ventricle due to the reliance on passive blood flow across the pulmonary vascular bed. When ventricular filling pressures rise, atrial pressure increases, reducing the transpulmonary gradient, pulmonary blood flow and cardiac output.

The factors contributing to progressive diastolic dysfunction after the Fontan operation are not fully understood, but several variables have been postulated to contribute to myocardial stiffness in this setting:

- Myocardial dyssynchrony [20]
- Altered ventricular geometry (through increased sphericity, wall stress and impaired diastolic filling) [21]
- Myocardial fibrosis/scarring, including from previous surgical procedures
- Ventricular morphology i.e., right versus left
- Decreased ventricular preload and increased afterload
- Long-standing ventricular volume overload prior to Fontan repair
- Ventricular volume overload after Fontan repair e.g., due to progressive atrioventricular valve regurgitation, aortic or pulmonary valve regurgitation, Fontan pathway leaks causing right-left shunting, and pulmonary arteriovenous malformations.
- Hypoxia.

The standard for the diagnosis of diastolic dysfunction remains cardiac catheterization, with the addition of acute volume loading in cases of borderline ventricular end-diastolic pressure, where occult diastolic dysfunction is suspected. Serial cardiac catheterization is not without risk, hence, initial assessment by non-invasive means is desirable. On echocardiography, diastolic dysfunction has been identified through prolonged isovolumetric relaxation time and decreased E and A wave deceleration times, which remained highly abnormal late after Fontan palliation [22]. However, standard markers of diastolic dysfunction on pulse wave and tissue Doppler assessment used in patients with biventricular circulation (E/A ratio, deceleration time, E'), have been show to correlate poorly to end-diastolic pressure in Fontan patients [23]. Other markers of diastolic function, such as speckle tracking, have been shown to correlate with invasive pressure-volume loop analysis, and may be more useful [24].

Chronotropic Response

Unlike in normal individuals, augmentation of cardiac output during exercise in Fontan patients is dependent on increases in heart rate rather than stroke volume. A reduced heart rate response to exercise is commonly observed and better predicts survival in Fontan patients than other exercise-derived parameters [25]. In a subset of Fontan patients there can be primary chronotropic incompetence due to sinus node dysfunction, either from birth or as a result of multiple surgeries. However, recent work using exercise cardiac magnetic resonance has found that the reduced heart rate response seen in well-functioning Fontan patients is not chronotropic incompetence in the sense of a primary electrical phenomenon (i.e. failure of the sinoatrial node to respond appropriately to varying workloads), but rather chronotropic limitation consequent to inadequate systemic ventricular filling, inappropriate ventricular contraction and impaired ability to augment cardiac output [26]. Indeed, the increase in heart rate relative to workload is normal or even supranormal in most Fontan patients, but exercise exhaustion, manifest by an early and marked reduction in stroke volume, causes the diminished and prematurely attained maximum heart rate. In this setting of an inherently limited cardiac contractile reserve, [27] augmenting the heart rate further may result in a fall in stroke volume and would therefore be poorly tolerated.

Based on these results, it has been hypothesised that therapies limiting the chronotropic response in these patients may improve exercise capacity by enhancing diastolic filling and could serve as a novel therapeutic target in certain Fontan patients, but this needs to tested in further studies.

Causes of Fontan Failure

Multiple clinical variables feed into the main physiological drivers of the failing Fontan circulation, namely a low cardiac output and chronic, excessively raised systemic venous pressure, leading to multi-system downstream effects, exercise intolerance and poor survival (Fig. 33.2). A meta-analysis of 7536 patients following Fontan repair identified late Fontan failure as the predominant cause of mortality, responsible for one third of deaths; the 20-year survival was 82% [28].

Identifying the precise cause of new or progressive clinical deterioration in a Fontan patient is challenging, as there is a multitude of ways in which the Fontan circulation may fail: Chronic "attrition" of the Fontan circulation, e.g., through inefficient flow dynamics, progressive pulmonary artery distortion, collaterals or endothelial dysfunction, can manifest over several years, whereas sudden changes in physiology, e.g. arrhythmia or thromboembolism, can lead to acute clinical deterioration. Furthermore, extra-cardiac organ failure can be subtle and requires a high index of suspicion, as well as regular, routine surveillance.

Anatomical and clinical risk factors of Fontan failure and late mortality have been studied in both adult and paediatric patients (Table 33.1). In the largest longitudinal study to date, d'Udekem et al. examined over 1000 survivors of the Fontan operation, representing the entire Fontan population of Australia and New Zealand. In this study, failure was defined as death, transplantation, Fontan takedown or conversion, NYHA functional class III/IV, or PLE/plastic bronchitis. Freedom from failure was 83% (95% CI:79–86%) at 15 years and 56% (95% CI: 44–66%) at 25 years. Patients with hypoplastic left heart syndrome were at increased risk of Fontan failure and had a higher mortality than patients with other morphologies [29, 30].

Other risk factors for Fontan failure have been inconsistently identified, including heterotaxy, a systemic right ventricle, high central venous pressure, and portal hypertension [30–35]. The presence of pulmonary vascular disease, with even modest elevations of PVR, also identifies Fontan patients at risk of failure; patients who

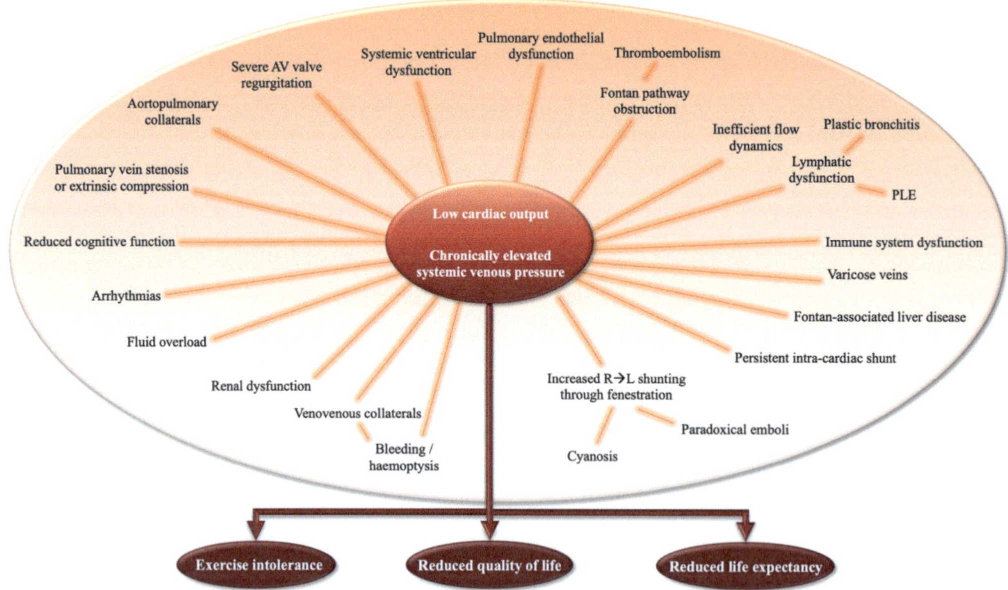

Fig. 33.2 Contributing factors, physiological drivers, and complications of Fontan failure. *PLE* protein losing enteropathy, *R–L* right-to-left

Table 33.1 Anatomical and clinical risk factors for Fontan failure and late mortality

Fontan failure	Late mortality
Demographic/anatomical	
Hypoplastic left heart syndrome	Male sex
Systemic right ventricle	Hypoplastic left heart syndrome
Heterotaxy	Atriopulmonary Fontan
Clinical	
Raised PVR (>2 WU)[a]	Older age at Fontan surgery
Raised central venous pressure[a]	Prolonged pleural effusions post-Fontan surgery
Portal hypertension[a]	Requirement for permanent pacing
Protein losing enteropathy[a]	Higher right atrial pressure
	Increased ventricular EDV
	Protein losing enteropathy

EDV end-diastolic volume, *PVR* pulmonary vascular resistance, *WU* Wood Units

[a] Identified as risk factors for Fontan failure in exclusively adult patient cohorts

develop pulmonary vascular disease are more likely to be older, have an atriopulmonary Fontan and take higher diuretic doses [6].

The presentation of patients with Fontan failure varies widely, from sudden haemodynamic deterioration (e.g., Fontan pathway obstruction or arrhythmia), to an insidious process of progressive extra-cardiac disease that may be completely asymptomatic for years before manifesting clinically. Fontan patients, therefore, require regular, specialist assessment that focuses on identifying symptoms, signs, and biochemical/imaging markers consistent with suboptimal haemodynamics, multiorgan failure, or overt Fontan failure.

Presentation and Assessment of the Patient with Fontan Failure

The Medical History and Symptoms of Fontan Failure

The symptoms of Fontan failure are often non-specific and may not be volunteered by patients. Significant expertise is, therefore, required to collect all the relevant information from the clinical assessment and investigations, with specialist surveillance at regular intervals commensurate with the physiological stage of the patient [36].

The clinical history forms the basis of the clinical assessment and directs the strategy of investigation and management (Table 33.2). Eliciting a history from several sources is especially important for paediatric patients, including the patient and their parents, carers, close relations, and other specialists. In Fontan patients, the severity of disease in early life and initial presentation help to determine the surgical management strategy. Long-standing or slowly progressive symptoms may be ignored or downplayed by the adult patient; it is often the partner who volunteers information about a change in exercise tolerance or new fatigue.

When assessing adolescent or adult patients for the presence of exercise intolerance, it is important to ask them to compare themselves to their peers and family. The use of landmarks is also advisable, noting their ability to walk to their local bus or train station, up 1 or more flight of stairs at home, school or work, exercise at home or at the gym. For patients with more advanced disease, milder "ordinary" activities should be discussed, ranging from washing and dressing to shopping or playing with children.

A detailed surgical history is essential when assessing Fontan patients, including all surgeries or interventions, the age and year they took place, and any intraoperative findings or perioperative complications they may have occurred. Operative notes are a particularly rich source of information, with valuable insights into morphology and variations to the surgical technique used, including the presence and position of surgical fenestration, type of prosthetic material used, details of the arrhythmia surgery performed.

Questions should aim to explore and quantify the following symptoms:

1. Functional impairment/reduced exercise tolerance

    Objective measures of exercise capacity, from cardiopulmonary exercise testing, demonstrate severe limitation in most Fontan patients [40]. Despite this, many patients do

Table 33.2 Important information to collect from the medical and surgical history during assessment of an adult Fontan patient

Medical history *(history of presenting complaint)*

Exercise tolerance (relate to daily activities/exercise compared to peers, log ability to perform more demanding household tasks such as vacuuming, and distance/speed one can walk on flat or uphill, flights of stairs)

Palpitations

Cyanosis and usual resting oxygen saturation (if known/measured at home)

Leg swelling

Increasing abdominal girth

Hyperviscosity symptoms (*rare*), including headaches, dizziness, paraesthesia, tinnitus, myalgia, visual disturbance

Unexpected weight loss: red flag caused by cardiac cachexia, associated malignancy, advanced extra-cardiac disease

Diarrhoea or pale, malodorous stools

Fatigue

Haemoptysis

Varicose veins, common in lower limbs, but new varicosities, especially over abdomen may indicate Fontan pathway obstruction or portal hypertension

Surgical history *(from operative notes where possible)*

Timing of/age at each surgical procedure

Pre-Fontan interventions

    Stage 1—Altered pulmonary blood flow

      Augmentation (e.g., central shunt, L/R modified Blalock-Taussig shunt)

      Reduction (e.g., pulmonary artery banding)

    Stage 2—Superior cavo-pulmonary shunt (e.g., classical vs. bidirectional Glenn)

Fontan-type procedure

    Type of Fontan connection (atriopulmonary, lateral tunnel, extracardiac conduit)

    Presence of modifications, including valved conduits, RA-RV outflow tract connection (Björk Fontan), patency of native RV-pulmonary artery connection

      Presence of fenestration/inter-atrial communication

Indications, timing and type of Fontan takedown, revision, or conversion

Additional procedures e.g., CoA repair, valve repair, ligation of MAPCAs

Peri-operative complications, including ventricular failure, requirement of post-operative ECMO, prolonged pleural effusions, arrhythmias

Fontan clinic checklist

Exercise—encourage a regular exercise program appropriate to their abilities and in line with exercise prescription guidelines [37]

Alcohol consumption—quantify in units per week, promote abstinence if any FALD

Smoking/recreational drug use—smoking cessation advice, referral for additional support

Occupation/current education—any modifications/help required to promote health?

Driving—does the licencing authority need to be made aware? Are there symptoms that will affect safe driving?

Medical insurance—travel insurance with disclosure of medical condition encouraged, support life insurance applications with medical information if required

Family planning/contraception—discuss safe contraception options, referral to Pregnancy and Heart Disease service in active planning phase i.e. pre-pregnancy [38]

Vaccination—e.g., annual influenza vaccination

Dental hygiene—education on merits of good dental and skin hygiene, including regular dental visits. Antibiotic prophylaxis is required for high-risk dental procedures only in patients at increased risk: prosthetic valves or prosthetic material used for valve repair, uncorrected cyanotic CHD, or prosthetic material or device implanted within the last 6 months, residual shunts in proximity of prosthetic material/device, previous endocarditis [39]

not perceive themselves as being functionally limited [41]. Directed questioning aimed at discerning one's ability to perform tasks which pose a haemodynamic burden is useful to tease out exercise intolerance e.g. recreational sport, walking uphill, gardening, housework, such as vacuum cleaning. New or changing exercise intolerance is a common, but non-specific, feature of Fontan failure. Clarification of the degree and progression of exertional intolerance should be followed by clinical examination to establish whether there are features of Fontan failure (see 'signs of Fontan failure' section below).

2. Leg swelling and increasing abdominal girth

   The typical history is of leg swelling, starting at the end of the day or after long periods of sitting. Also usual is a history of an increase in "stomach size" and an inability to wear shoes, without the patient recognising the link with fluid overload. Escalating doses of loop diuretics or the need for adjunctive thiazide diuretics e.g., metolazone may be the first sign of a problem. Other causes of fluid overload include cardiac decompensation due to progressive ventricular dysfunction, AV valve regurgitation, pulmonary vascular disease, arrhythmias, or Fontan pathway obstruction. Extra-cardiac sequelae, such as protein losing enteropathy (PLE), progressive renal dysfunction or advanced liver disease with portal hypertension can also cause leg swelling and ascites and should be ruled out. Chronic venous insufficiency with or without varicose veins affects most adults with Fontan physiology and does not necessarily indicate Fontan failure. Patients may complain of itching and discolouration of the lower extremities, and/or varicose veins. Advanced skin changes, however, including diffuse lower leg pigmentation, lipodermatosclerosis, or healed/active ulceration, occur more frequently in older Fontan patients, those with a diagnosis of heart failure or on diuretics, as well as following repeated cardiac catheterisations from the femoral approach [42].

3. Palpitations

   A history of palpitations should form part of every clinical contact with a Fontan patient; supraventricular tachycardia (SVT) and bradyarrhythmia, from sinus node dysfunction and chronotropic incompetence, are common in this population. Atrial arrhythmias, typically macro-re-entrant atrial tachycardias, are common in Fontan patients. Review of the clinical record may identify predictors of SVT, such as the presence of an AP Fontan, the presence of a heterotaxy syndrome, atrial dilatation and AV valve regurgitation. [29, 31] Sustained SVT is poorly tolerated in Fontan patients and should be treated as a medical emergency, requiring urgent inpatient rhythm control with trans-oesophageal echocardiographic guidance to exclude intra-cardiac thrombus under guidance of a CHD specialist (see Chap. 64).

4. Cyanosis

   Hypoxaemia and resulting central cyanosis can be found in the presence of an iatrogenic or residual intra-cardiac shunt without indicating Fontan failure. A fenestration, residual intra-atrial connection, baffle leak or previous surgical unroofing of the coronary sinus into the left atrium, can cause resting desaturation. New or worsening hypoxaemia and cyanosis, however, should prompt a search for raised right-sided pressures (obstruction of the Fontan circuit downstream of an existing shunt, pulmonary vascular disease, co-existing restrictive lung disease) or the formation of new right-to-left shunts. The latter can be a result of systemic venous collaterals draining into the pulmonary veins, left atrium or coronary sinus, increased shunting through dilated Thebesian veins, or pulmonary arteriovenous malformations (AVMs). Patients in whom hepatic venous return bypasses the lungs, e.g. following a classical Glenn or Kawashima repair, are prone to the development of pulmonary AVMs [43, 44].

   Erythrocytosis is a common sequela of long-standing cyanosis, although this is rarely associated with hyperviscosity. The symptoms of hyperviscosity: headaches, dizziness, paraesthesia, tinnitus, myalgia and visual disturbance, are closely related to those of iron deficiency, which is common in cyanotic CHD patients [45].

Signs of Fontan Failure

Examination findings in patients after the Fontan operation are variable and depend on anatomic and surgical factors, including the type of Fontan surgery (Table 33.3).

Fontan failure may be indicated by the following signs:

Table 33.3 Examination findings in adults following a Fontan operation

Clinical finding	Underlying morphology/mechanism
Peripheral oxygen saturation > 94%	Well-functioning; absence of a fenestration or residual shunt
Peripheral oxygen saturation ≤ 94%	Presence of a fenestration, baffle leak, residual inter-atrial connection, pulmonary vein compression by dilated RA, veno-venous collaterals, pulmonary AVM
Non-pulsatile, mildly raised JVP	Systemic venous hypertension, total cavo-pulmonary connection
Thoracotomy scar(s)	Previous Blalock-Taussig shunt(s) or PA banding, co-existence of surgically managed CoA
Single second heart sound	Typical, may be loud if aorta positioned anteriorly
No murmur	Typical
Loud systolic murmur	Significant AV valve regurgitation, central shunt, left ventricular outflow obstruction, aortic pathology, residual forward flow across the pulmonary valve
Ascites	Worsening Fontan haemodynamics, PLE, chronic liver disease with portal hypertension (rarely), obstruction of Fontan circuit
Pedal oedema	Worsening Fontan haemodynamics, PLE, obstruction of Fontan circuit
Varicose veins	Typical over lower limbs; present on trunk with circuit obstruction or portal hypertension

AV arteriovenous, *AVM* arterio-venous malformations, *CoA* coarctation of the aorta, *JVP* jugular venous pressure, *PA* pulmonary artery, *PLE* protein losing enteropathy, *RA* right atrium

- New or progressive cyanosis due to an inter-atrial communication/fenestration, pulmonary arteriovenous malformations (patients at increased risk when the pulmonary blood flow bypasses the liver i.e., in the presence of a classical Glenn shunt), venovenous collaterals (e.g. to the pulmonary veins), or coronary sinus drainage to the left atrium.
- Progressive elevation of the jugular venous pulse.
- The presence of a cardiac murmur is often not expected, and may indicate atrioventricular valve, aortic or pulmonary regurgitation, ventricular outflow tract obstruction.
- Lack of hepatomegaly may indicate advanced liver disease/cirrhosis.
- Ascites and leg oedema, which are usually signs of advanced heart failure, Fontan circuit obstruction or protein losing enteropathy.
- Varicose veins, which are expected in the lower limbs, but if present on the trunk may be associated with Fontan pathway obstruction or portal hypertension.
- Cardiac cachexia.

Extra-cardiac Involvement in Fontan Failure

The pathophysiology of extra-cardiac involvement in patients with a Fontan circulation is covered fully elsewhere (see Sect. 13: A multisystem disorder: Extracardiac complication). The extra-cardiac sequelae of a low cardiac output state and/or excessively elevated systemic venous pressures include protein-losing enteropathy, plastic bronchitis, Fontan-associated liver disease (FALD), and renal dysfunction. These comorbidities contribute to the multi-organ dysfunction of a failing Fontan circulation. The symptoms and signs of these conditions can be non-specific and usually manifest late in the course of disease, often with a prolonged period of subclinical derangement that can be identified through directed surveillance:

- Protein-losing enteropathy, a devastating complication affecting patients following

Fontan surgery, is characterised by the loss of serum proteins, primarily albumin, into the intestinal tract. The diagnosis is suspected by a history of progressive peripheral oedema, with leg swelling and increasing abdominal girth, although there may be an absence of symptoms altogether. A minority of patients experience gastrointestinal symptoms, including diarrhoea and pale, malodorous stool. This latter symptom is caused by malabsorption due to gut wall oedema. Recent viral respiratory infections are common triggers to a disease flare. Physical examination reveals fluid overload, with peripheral oedema, ascites, pleural or pericardial effusions.

- FALD usually has a very long pre-clinical course, often with an absence of symptoms for several years. Therefore, timely identification and management of FALD requires regular, proactive screening. When symptoms do arise, they are frequently non-specific: Ascites, for example, is commonly encountered as part of anasarca. Hepatomegaly may also arise due to congestive hepatopathy, and an absence of hepatomegaly may signify cirrhosis and advanced liver disease. Clinical features or sequelae of decompensated liver disease, including variceal bleeding, jaundice, or hepatic encephalopathy, rarely manifest. In the absence of routine screening, new or progressive symptoms of chronic liver disease, along with unintentional weight loss, fatigue, nausea, vomiting and abdominal pain, should prompt a search for hepatocellular carcinoma.

- Renal dysfunction is common in Fontan patients, contributing to a third of deaths in one long-term follow-up study [46]. Renal dysfunction typically becomes apparent and drives clinical decision making in patients with advanced "Fontan failure". Clinical signs and symptoms are initially absent or vague and, even when present, are often underappreciated by patients. Fatigue may be the only symptom and can be a consequence of progression in the underlying cardiac disease, combined with anaemia of renal disease. Features of uraemia occur later and indicate significant renal impairment but may occur with lower serum levels of urea and creatinine due to the lower muscle mass (in the case of creatinine) and cardiorespiratory reserve in this population.

Clinical Work-Up of the Patient with Fontan Failure

The diagnostic work-up of patients with a Fontan-type circulation starts with a basic set of non-invasive diagnostic/screening tests that make up the routine panel of tests performed in every Fontan patient at regular intervals in line with European and American guidelines. Patients with evidence of Fontan failure are in physiological stage C or D and therefore require 3–6 monthly outpatient adult CHD (ACHD) clinical contact along with the following tests: [36, 47].

- Observations, including pulse oximetry (at each visit)
- 12-lead ECG (every 6–12 months)
- Blood tests, including haematology, serum albumin, liver, and renal function (every 12 months)
- Transthoracic echocardiography (every 12 months)
- Holter monitor (every 12 months)
- Cardiopulmonary exercise test (every 12 months)
- Cardiac MRI (every 24 months)
- Liver imaging (ultrasonography, MRI, CT) on a regular basis.

If Fontan failure is identified on routine screening, this should instigate a search for new haemodynamic abnormalities and a more detailed assessment of extra-cardiac disease (Figs. 33.3 and 33.4), initially by non-invasive means. Transthoracic echocardiography is the initial screening test of choice, but cardiac MRI can provide valuable information on Fontan pathway patency, collaterals, pulmonary veins, thrombus, atrioventricular valve regurgitation, subaortic stenosis and the location and burden of myocardial fibrosis. Patients in whom the cause of a new haemodynamic derangement has not been identified

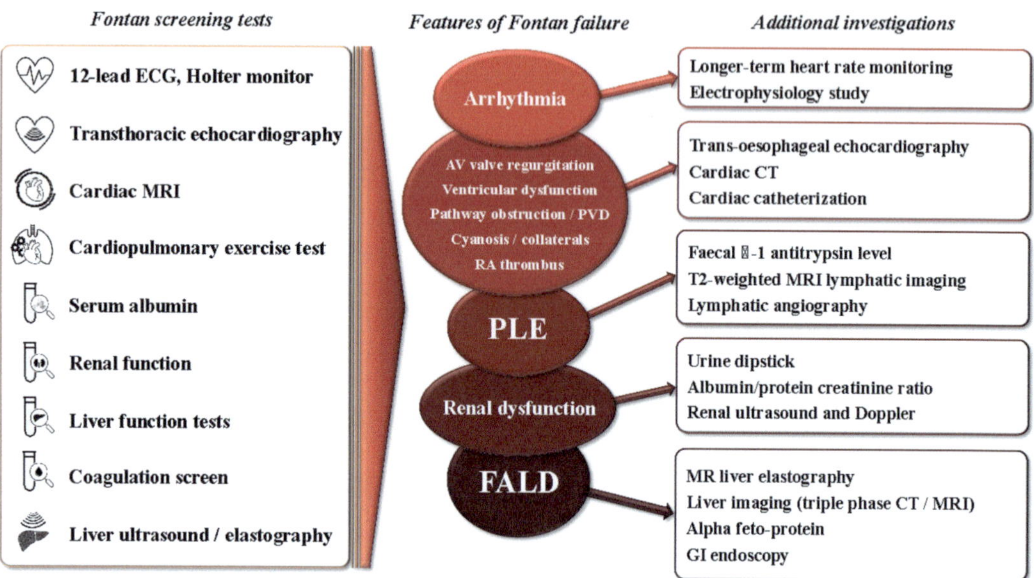

Fig. 33.3 Routine screening tests for Fontan patients (left) and additional, targeted investigations (right) based on abnormal findings. *AV* atrioventricular, *CT* computed tomography, *FALD* Fontan-associated liver disease, *GI* gastrointestinal, *MR(I)* magnetic resonance (imaging), *PLE* protein losing enteropathy, *PVD* pulmonary vascular disease, *RA* right atrial

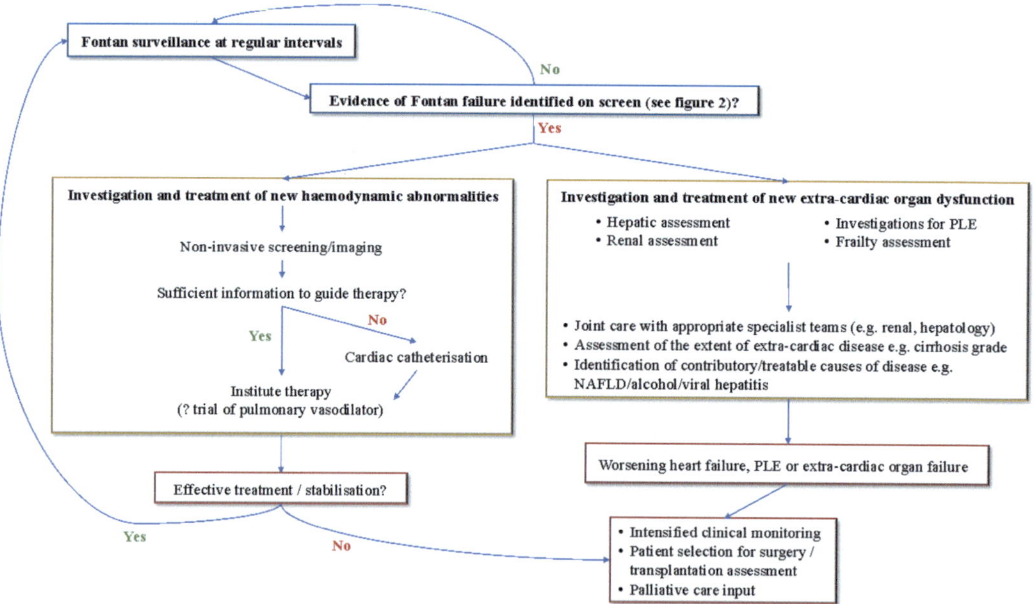

Fig. 33.4 Algorithm for the investigation and management of Fontan failure. *NAFLD* non-alcoholic fatty liver disease, *PLE* protein-losing enteropathy

should undergo invasive assessment by cardiac catheterization to establish Fontan haemodynamics, including PVR. Catheterisation can aid the assessment of Fontan obstruction, anomalous vascular connections, ventricular and valvular function; the ACHD ESC guidelines support a low threshold for cardiac catheterisation in cases of unexplained oedema, worsening exercise intolerance, new-onset arrhythmia, cyanosis, and haemoptysis [47].

A detailed evaluation of extra-cardiac disease should also be performed, including assessment for PLE, FALD and renal disease. Assessment of frailty and quality of life are often overlooked but are important components of grading overall disease burden. Findings consistent with Fontan failure, especially features associated with a guarded prognosis, such as PLE, should prompt evaluation for heart or heart-lung transplantation. Management of Fontan failure can be medical, interventional, or surgical and is directed towards managing cardiac and extra-cardiac complications.

Medical Management

Patients with a Fontan circulation require lifelong specialist ACHD follow-up, ideally in a dedicated Fontan clinic, allowing the development and testing of protocols for Fontan screening, investigation, and management. Cross-disciplinary working is essential given the complex needs of these patients and the high rate of extra-cardiac disease. This includes ACHD physicians, congenital cardiac surgeons, interventionalists, electrophysiologists, transplant physicians and surgeons, pulmonary hypertension specialists, hepatologists, renal physicians, clinical psychologists, physiotherapists, and palliative care. This may involve multidisciplinary clinic appointments, such as joint heart-liver clinics, and Fontan multi-disciplinary meetings to discuss individualised management strategies.

A proposed algorithm for the investigation and management of the patient with Fontan failure is shown in Fig. 33.4. Once a new haemodynamic abnormality responsible for a feature of Fontan failure is identified, effective therapy can stabilise the patient and allow a return to surveillance at regular intervals. Worsening heart failure or advancing extra-cardiac organ dysfunction may, however, require intensified clinical monitoring, discussion of surgical options, including advanced heart failure therapies, and should prompt consideration of palliative care input.

Medical therapy for a failing Fontan circulation is limited, but includes the management of congestive symptoms with diuretics, anticoagulation to prevent/ treat thromboembolic disease, and therapies directed at extra-cardiac disease. A trial of pulmonary vasodilators is advocated by some experts, especially when there is evidence pulmonary vascular disease.

Heart Failure Therapy

Due to the mechanisms outlined in the previous section, conventional heart failure therapy targeting contractility, chronotropy and afterload reduction do not appear to significantly influence cardiac output in a Fontan circulation. Indeed, afterload reduction in a Fontan patient may be poorly tolerated through excessive reduction in systemic venous pressure and reduced preload, possibly leading to hypotension and clinical decompensation. Most studies examining the role of ACE inhibition in patients undergoing Fontan repair have targeted infants prior to Fontan completion or are limited to short-term outcomes after Fontan repair; in these groups, most studies have shown no improvement in exercise capacity, somatic growth, ventricular function, or reduction in post-operative pleural effusions. Despite the lack of evidence for the use of ACE inhibitors in patients with Fontan physiology, a substantial number of paediatric Fontan patients receive these therapies, as an extrapolation of benefit from conventional heart failure therapy in a biventricular circulation [48]; some of these patients transitioning to adult CHD care are maintained on an ACE-inhibitor. In adolescent or adult patients presenting with systolic heart failure late after the Fontan operation, there is no evidence currently to support the use of ACE-inhibitors as heart failure therapy [49].

Beta-blockade is used in Fontan patients with atrial or ventricular arrhythmias as antiarrhythmic therapy, but there is no data to support beta-blocker therapy for patients with reduced systemic ventricular function. When required, beta-blockers should be used with caution due to the frequent association of single ventricle physiology and conduction disease.

Mineralocorticoid receptor antagonists (MRAs), such as spironolactone, are useful in Fontan patients with right-sided congestive symptoms, e.g., peripheral oedema, ascites, or pleural effusion. Evidence for a benefit in systemic ventricular remodelling or prognosis of spironolactone in Fontan patients is lacking. However, some experts report stabilisation of patients with a failing Fontan physiology treated with high-dose MRA therapy. One possible mechanism for this is through an effect on systemic venous capacitance and splanchnic venous tone, which are abnormal in other patient groups with increased circulating levels of aldosterone e.g. heart failure with preserved ejection fraction, leading to a redistribution of total blood volume from the periphery to the central compartment [50]. This can be partially reversed by aldosterone antagonism [51]. The potassium-sparing effects and relatively weak diuresis of MRAs mean that they are usually combined with a loop diuretic to manage congestion, with careful monitoring of renal function.

Pulmonary Vasodilator Therapy

According to the 2020 ESC ACHD guidelines, pulmonary vasodilators, mainly endothelin receptor antagonists (ERAs) and phosphodiesterase-5 (PDE-5) inhibitors, may be considered in selected adult patients following Fontan repair with elevated pulmonary pressure or resistance in the absence of elevated ventricular end-diastolic pressure (class IIb indication, level of evidence C) [47]. Prior to initiating pulmonary vasodilator therapy, therefore, it is essential to exclude causes of "post-capillary pulmonary hypertension" (even though mean pulmonary pressure is unlikely to exceed 20 mmHg in Fontan patients, the current threshold for defining pulmonary hypertension). Indeed, such therapies are contraindicated in patients with significant systemic ventricular systolic (or diastolic) dysfunction, systemic atrioventricular valve regurgitation, or outflow tract obstruction. Thus, a careful, step-wise assessment of the Fontan circulation is essential (see below).

Pulmonary vasodilators have been proposed in two different settings in Fontan patients:

- as routine therapy in stable patients, to reduce complications and improve prognosis,
- in the face of clinical deterioration and Fontan failure, mainly for symptomatic benefit.

Data supporting either of these uses are very limited, especially in patients with Fontan failure who are usually excluded from clinical studies. In this group, only paediatric case series have provided evidence of potential benefit, [52–54] while a single, small, open label study of bosentan in adult Fontan patients failed to show any improvement in the primary outcome of oxygen saturations at rest and on exercise [55].

In contrast, most studies of pulmonary vasodilators in stable adolescent and adult Fontan patients have examined the effect on exercise capacity with mixed results: 14-weeks of therapy with the ERA bosentan was associated with a small improvement in peak oxygen uptake (VO_2) in a small randomized controlled trial (RCT) of stable patients who were able to perform a bicycle exercise test [56]. This was not replicated, however, in a randomized, open label study of bosentan in unselected patients from 5 tertiary centres, 88% of whom were in NYHA functional class I or II [57].

PDE-5 inhibitors have also been used in an effort to improve exercise capacity in these patients, both in the acute setting with sildenafil [58] and following chronic administration of udenafil [59]. This study, the largest RCT of pulmonary vasodilator therapy in Fontan patients to date, included 400 patients across 30 centres in

North America and the Republic of Korea. Udenafil therapy was not associated with a significant difference in the change in peak VO_2 but was associated with improvements in markers of submaximal exercise capacity, i.e., VO_2 at ventilatory anaerobic threshold or the minute ventilation/carbon dioxide production (VE/VCO_2) slope, and myocardial performance index.

Finally, prostanoid therapy used in a small group of Fontan patients aged 12–47 years led to small improvements in peak VO_2 [60].

A meta-analysis of pulmonary vasodilator therapy after the Fontan procedure, including both paediatric and adult patients, found no evidence of an improvement in exercise capacity with these drugs [61].

The safety of pulmonary vasodilator therapies in Fontan patients has been confirmed in several studies; a 2021 meta-analysis showed no significant difference between the drug and control arms in the pooled analysis [61]. In particular, there is no evidence for the theoretical concern of an increased risk of liver dysfunction following prescription of ERAs to Fontan patients, although this has not been studied specifically in patients with Fontan-associated liver disease [56].

In a retrospective multicentre study examining clinical practice in the United Kingdom, pulmonary vasodilator therapies were reserved to a small proportion (<5%) of Fontan patients who were more likely to exhibit features of a failing Fontan circulation compared to age- and sex-matched patients, including a greater degree of exercise intolerance, fluid overload and protein losing enteropathy. [62] Notably, pulmonary vasodilators were started on a non-elective basis in a third of cases and were mainly used to improve quality of life. This contrasts to the use of pulmonary vasodilators in randomized controlled trials to date, that have recruited stable, "well" patients.

Medical Therapy for Extra-cardiac Features of Fontan Failure

The medical management of extracardiac complications related to Fontan failure is mainly targeted at lymphatic dysfunction i.e., protein losing enteropathy or plastic bronchitis, Fontan-associated liver disease and renal dysfunction. Principles of successful management of any extra-cardiac disease in Fontan failure include the following:

- A multidisciplinary approach with the appropriate speciality, which ideally involves collaboration and joint assessment and management e.g., in joint specialist clinics
- Optimisation of Fontan haemodynamics by stepwise identification and management, either medical, interventional, or surgical, of complications responsible for a reduced cardiac output and excessive systemic venous hypertension
- Serial evaluation of extra-cardiac disease with intensified monitoring appropriate to the physiological stage of disease
- Consideration of early transplant assessment before extra-cardiac organ dysfunction becomes advanced and precludes heart-only transplantation.

The medical management of protein losing enteropathy and plastic bronchitis is discussed elsewhere.

Fontan-associated liver disease is increasingly recognised in patients with a Fontan circulation, although there is uncertainty about how to address problems once identified. The following management principles represent current thinking, and assessment should be performed at regular intervals guided by local guidelines and multi-disciplinary input: [1, 36, 47].

- Assess for the presence and severity of fibrosis and cirrhosis
- Assess for the complications of chronic liver disease, including a baseline gastroscopy for oesophageal varices/hypertensive gastropathy
- Test portal synthetic function at least annually (International Normalized Ratio and albumin measurement)
- Test for thrombocytopenia and/or splenomegaly, which can indicate increased portal venous pressure and splenic consumption

- Conduct surveillance for hepatocellular carcinoma with serial imaging and serum alpha-feto protein levels
- Identify and treat other, contributory causes of liver dysfunction, including avoiding alcohol, obesity (i.e., non-alcoholic fatty liver disease) and viral hepatitis
- Review and, if possible, stop hepatotoxic drugs e.g., amiodarone
- Consider liver biopsy in patients with non-invasive evidence of cirrhosis, especially if under consideration for heart transplantation.

Evidence-based therapies for the management of renal dysfunction specific to Fontan patients are lacking, but the following principles of care can be drawn from acquired heart failure and other forms of renal dysfunction:

- Ensure accurate estimation of renal function/glomerular filtration rate. Estimation from serum creatinine concentration remains the most widely used method, but there is evidence (in paediatric Fontan patients) that cystatin C may provide a more reliable measure of glomerular function than creatinine [63]. In patients with severe cardiac cachexia undergoing transplantation assessment, 24-h urine collection for calculation of creatine clearance may be considered,
- Stop nephrotoxins e.g., ibuprofen
- Identify and treat other, contributory causes of renal dysfunction, including diabetes mellitus, hypertension, and obesity
- Identify and quantify proteinuria, as nephrotic-range proteinuria may point to alternative causes of renal dysfunction. The significance of microalbuminuria is not yet established in the Fontan population
- Assess and treat complications of chronic kidney disease, including anaemia (which may be relative in the setting of cyanosis) and may require therapy with erythropoietin and metabolic bone disease
- Optimise fluid status, with careful titration of diuretics, to improve cardiac output and reduce renal venous hypertension while maintaining adequate preload.

References

1. Rychik J, Atz AM, Celermajer DS, et al. Evaluation and management of the child and adult with Fontan circulation: a scientific statement from the American Heart Association. Circulation. 2019;140:E234–84.
2. Kotani Y, Chetan D, Zhu J, et al. Fontan failure and death in contemporary Fontan circulation: analysis from the last two decades. Ann Thorac Surg. 2018;105:1240–7.
3. Gewillig M, Brown SC, Eyskens B, Heying R, Ganame J, Budts W, La Gerche A, Gorenflo M. The Fontan circulation: who controls cardiac output? Interact Cardiovasc Thorac Surg. 2010;10:428–33.
4. Gewillig M, Brown SC. The Fontan circulation after 45 years: update in physiology. Heart. 2016;102:1081–6.
5. Veldtman GR, Opotowsky AR, Wittekind SG, Rychik J, Penny DJ, Fogel M, Marino BS, Gewillig M. Cardiovascular adaptation to the Fontan circulation. Congenit Heart Dis. 2017;12:699–710.
6. Egbe AC, Connolly HM, Miranda WR, Ammash NM, Hagler DJ, Veldtman GR, Borlaug BA. Hemodynamics of Fontan failure: the role of pulmonary vascular disease. Circ Heart Fail. 2017;10:e004515.
7. Rosenzweig EB, Abman SH, Adatia I, Beghetti M, Bonnet D, Haworth S, Ivy DD, Berger RMF. Paediatric pulmonary arterial hypertension: updates on definition, classification, diagnostics and management. Eur Respir J. 2019;53:1801916. https://doi.org/10.1183/13993003.01916-2018.
8. Gewillig M, Goldberg DJ. Failure of the Fontan circulation. Heart Fail Clin. 2014;10:105–16.
9. Rychik J. Forty years of the Fontan operation: a failed strategy. Semin Thorac Cardiovasc Surg. 2010;13:96–100.
10. Khambadkone S, Li J, de Leval MR, Cullen S, Deanfield JE, Redington AN. Basal pulmonary vascular resistance and nitric oxide responsiveness late after Fontan-type operation. Circulation. 2003;107:3204–8.
11. Mori H, Park I-S, Yamagishi H, Nakamura M, Ishikawa S, Takigiku K, Yasukochi S, Nakayama T, Saji T, Nakanishi T. Sildenafil reduces pulmonary vascular resistance in single ventricular physiology. Int J Cardiol. 2016;221:122–7.
12. Agnoletti G, Gala S, Ferroni F, Bordese R, Appendini L, Pace Napoleone C, Bergamasco L. Endothelin inhibitors lower pulmonary vascular resistance and improve functional capacity in patients with Fontan circulation. J Thorac Cardiovasc Surg. 2017;153:1468–75.
13. Presson RG, Baumgartner WA, Peterson AJ, Glenny RW, Wagner WW. pulmonary capillaries are recruited during pulsatile flow. J Appl Physiol (1985). 2002;92:1183–90.
14. Henaine R, Vergnat M, Bacha EA, Baudet B, Lambert V, Belli E, Serraf A. Effects of lack of pulsatility on pulmonary endothelial function in the Fontan circulation. J Thorac Cardiovasc Surg. 2013;146:522–9.

15. Alsaied T, Alsidawi S, Allen CC, Faircloth J, Palumbo JS, Veldtman GR. Strategies for thromboprophylaxis in Fontan circulation: a meta-analysis. Heart. 2015;101:1731–7.
16. Lambert E, d'Udekem Y, Cheung M, et al. Sympathetic and vascular dysfunction in adult patients with Fontan circulation. Int J Cardiol. 2013;167:1333–8.
17. Hjortdal VE, Stenbøg EV, Ravn HB, Emmertsen K, Jensen KT, Pedersen EB, Olsen KH, Hansen OK, Sørensen KE. Neurohormonal activation late after cavopulmonary connection. Heart. 2000;83:439–43.
18. Budts W, Ravekes WJ, Danford DA, Kutty S. Diastolic heart failure in patients with the Fontan circulation: a review. JAMA Cardiol. 2020;5:590–7.
19. Averin K, Hirsch R, Seckeler MD, Whiteside W, Beekman RH, Goldstein BH. Diagnosis of occult diastolic dysfunction late after the Fontan procedure using a rapid volume expansion technique. Heart. 2016;102:1109–14.
20. Rösner A, Khalapyan T, Dalen H, McElhinney DB, Friedberg MK, Lui GK. Classic-pattern dyssynchrony in adolescents and adults with a Fontan circulation. J Am Soc Echocardiogr. 2018;31:211–9.
21. Rösner A, Khalapyan T, Pedrosa J, Dalen H, McElhinney DB, Friedberg MK, Lui GK. Ventricular mechanics in adolescent and adult patients with a Fontan circulation: relation to geometry and wall stress. Echocardiography. 2018;35:2035–46.
22. Cheung YF, Penny DJ, Redington AN. Serial assessment of left ventricular diastolic function after Fontan procedure. Heart. 2000;83:420–4.
23. Margossian R, Sleeper LA, Pearson GD, Barker PC, Mertens L, Quartermain MD, Su JT, Shirali G, Chen S, Colan SD. Assessment of diastolic function in single-ventricle patients after the Fontan procedure. J Am Soc Echocardiogr. 2016;29:1066–73.
24. Steflik D, Butts RJ, Baker GH, Bandisode V, Savage A, Atz AM, Chowdhury SM. A preliminary comparison of two-dimensional speckle tracking echocardiography and pressure-volume loop analysis in patients with Fontan physiology: the role of ventricular morphology. Echocardiography. 2017;34:1353–9.
25. Diller G-P, Giardini A, Dimopoulos K, et al. Predictors of morbidity and mortality in contemporary Fontan patients: results from a multicenter study including cardiopulmonary exercise testing in 321 patients. Eur Heart J. 2010;31:3073–83.
26. Claessen G, La Gerche A, Van De Bruaene A, et al. Heart rate reserve in Fontan patients: chronotropic incompetence or hemodynamic limitation? J Am Heart Assoc. 2019;8:e012008.
27. Senzaki H, Masutani S, Ishido H, Taketazu M, Kobayashi T, Sasaki N, Asano H, Katogi T, Kyo S, Yokote Y. Cardiac rest and reserve function in patients with Fontan circulation. J Am Coll Cardiol. 2006;47:2528–35.
28. Poh CL, d'Udekem Y. Life after surviving Fontan surgery: a meta-analysis of the incidence and predictors of late death. Heart Lung Circ. 2018;27:552–9.
29. d'Udekem Y, Iyengar AJ, Galati JC, et al. Redefining expectations of long-term survival after the Fontan procedure. Circulation. 2014;130:S32–8.
30. Iyengar AJ, Winlaw DS, Galati JC, et al. The extracardiac conduit Fontan procedure in Australia and New Zealand: hypoplastic left heart syndrome predicts worse early and late outcomes. Eur J Cardiothorac Surg. 2014;46:465–73; discussion 473.
31. Khairy P, Fernandes SM, Mayer JE, Triedman JK, Walsh EP, Lock JE, Landzberg MJ. Long-term survival, modes of death, and predictors of mortality in patients with Fontan surgery. Circulation. 2008;117:85–92.
32. Hebson CL, McCabe NM, Elder RW, et al. Hemodynamic phenotype of the failing Fontan in an adult population. Am J Cardiol. 2013;112:1943–7.
33. Elder RW, McCabe NM, Veledar E, Kogon BE, Jokhadar M, Rodriguez FH, McConnell ME, Book WM. Risk factors for major adverse events late after Fontan palliation. Congenit Heart Dis. 2015;10:159–68.
34. Nakano T, Kado H, Tatewaki H, Hinokiyama K, Oda S, Ushinohama H, Sagawa K, Nakamura M, Fusazaki N, Ishikawa S. Results of extracardiac conduit total cavopulmonary connection in 500 patients †. Eur J Cardiothorac Surg. 2015;48:825–32.
35. Ono M, Kasnar-Samprec J, Hager A, et al. Clinical outcome following total cavopulmonary connection: a 20-year single-centre experience†. Eur J Cardiothorac Surg. 2016;50:632–41.
36. Stout KK, Daniels CJ, Aboulhosn JA, et al. 2018 AHA/ACC guideline for the management of adults with congenital heart disease: a report of the American College of Cardiology/American Heart Association task force on clinical practice guidelines. Circulation. 2018;139:e698–800.
37. Pelliccia A, Sharma S, Gati S, et al. 2020 ESC guidelines on sports cardiology and exercise in patients with cardiovascular disease. Eur Heart J. 2021;42:17–96.
38. Regitz-Zagrosek V, Roos-Hesselink JW, Bauersachs J, et al. 2018 ESC guidelines for the management of cardiovascular diseases during pregnancy. Eur Heart J. 2018;39:3165–241.
39. Habib G, Lancellotti P, Antunes MJ, et al. 2015 ESC guidelines for the management of infective endocarditis. The task force for the management of infective endocarditis of the European Society of Cardiology (ESC) endorsed by: European Association for Cardio-Thoracic Surgery (EACTS), the European Association of Nuclear Medicine (EANM). Eur Heart J. 2015;36:3075–128.
40. Kempny A, Dimopoulos K, Uebing A, Moceri P, Swan L, Gatzoulis MA, Diller G-P. Reference values for exercise limitations among adults with congenital heart disease. Relation to activities of daily life—single centre experience and review of published data. Eur Heart J. 2012;33:1386–96.
41. Dennis M, Zannino D, du Plessis K, et al. Clinical outcomes in adolescents and adults after the Fontan procedure. J Am Coll Cardiol. 2018;71:1009–17.

42. Valente AM, Bhatt AB, Cook S, et al. The CALF (congenital heart disease in adults lower extremity systemic venous health in Fontan patients) study. J Am Coll Cardiol. 2010;56:144–50.

43. Mathur M, Glenn WW. Long-term evaluation of cava-pulmonary artery anastomosis. Surgery. 1973;74:899–916.

44. McFaul RC, Tajik AJ, Mair DD, Danielson GK, Seward JB. Development of pulmonary arteriovenous shunt after superior vena cava-right pulmonary artery (Glenn) anastomosis. Report of four cases. Circulation. 1977;55:212–6.

45. Spence MS, Balaratnam MS, Gatzoulis MA. Clinical update: cyanotic adult congenital heart disease. Lancet. 2007;370:1530–2.

46. Pundi KN, Johnson JN, Dearani JA, et al. 40-year follow-up after the Fontan operation: long-term outcomes of 1,052 patients. J Am Coll Cardiol. 2015;66:1700–10.

47. Baumgartner H, De Backer J, Babu-Narayan SV, et al. 2020 ESC guidelines for the management of adult congenital heart disease. Eur Heart J. 2021;42:563–645.

48. Wilson TG, Iyengar AJ, d'Udekem Y. The use and misuse of ACE inhibitors in patients with single ventricle physiology. Heart Lung Circ. 2016;25:229–36.

49. Kouatli AA, Garcia JA, Zellers TM, Weinstein EM, Mahony L. Enalapril does not enhance exercise capacity in patients after Fontan procedure. Circulation. 1997;96:1507–12.

50. Maurer MS, Packer M. Impaired systemic venous capacitance: the neglected mechanism in patients with heart failure and a preserved ejection fraction? Eur J Heart Fail. 2020;22:173–6.

51. Drüppel V, Kusche-Vihrog K, Grossmann C, Gekle M, Kasprzak B, Brand E, Pavenstädt H, Oberleithner H, Kliche K. Long-term application of the aldosterone antagonist spironolactone prevents stiff endothelial cell syndrome. FASEB J. 2013;27:3652–9.

52. Haseyama K, Satomi G, Yasukochi S, Matsui H, Harada Y, Uchita S. Pulmonary vasodilation therapy with sildenafil citrate in a patient with plastic bronchitis after the Fontan procedure for hypoplastic left heart syndrome. J Thorac Cardiovasc Surg. 2006;132:1232–3.

53. Uzun O, Wong JK, Bhole V, Stumper O. Resolution of protein-losing enteropathy and normalization of mesenteric Doppler flow with sildenafil after Fontan. Ann Thorac Surg. 2006;82:e39–40.

54. Morchi GS, Ivy DD, Duster MC, Claussen L, Chan K-C, Kay J. Sildenafil increases systemic saturation and reduces pulmonary artery pressure in patients with failing Fontan physiology. Congenit Heart Dis. 2009;4:107–11.

55. Ovaert C, Thijs D, Dewolf D, Ottenkamp J, Dessy H, Moons P, Gewillig M, Mertens L. The effect of bosentan in patients with a failing Fontan circulation. Cardiol Young. 2009;19:331–9.

56. Hebert A, Mikkelsen UR, Thilen U, Idorn L, Jensen AS, Nagy E, Hanseus K, Sørensen KE, Søndergaard L. Bosentan improves exercise capacity in adolescents and adults after Fontan operation: the TEMPO (treatment with endothelin receptor antagonist in Fontan patients, a randomized, placebo-controlled, double-blind study measuring peak oxygen consumption) study. Circulation. 2014;130:2021–30.

57. Schuuring MJ, Vis JC, van Dijk APJ, van Melle JP, Vliegen HW, Pieper PG, Sieswerda GT, de Bruin-Bon RHACM, Mulder BJM, Bouma BJ. Impact of bosentan on exercise capacity in adults after the Fontan procedure: a randomized controlled trial. Eur J Heart Fail. 2013;15:690–8.

58. Giardini A, Balducci A, Specchia S, Gargiulo G, Bonvicini M, Picchio FM. Effect of sildenafil on haemodynamic response to exercise and exercise capacity in Fontan patients. Eur Heart J. 2008;29:1681–7.

59. Goldberg DJ, Zak V, Goldstein BH, et al. Results of the Fontan udenafil exercise longitudinal (FUEL) trial. Circulation. 2020;141:641–51.

60. Rhodes J, Ubeda-Tikkanen A, Clair M, Fernandes SM, Graham DA, Milliren CE, Daly KP, Mullen MP, Landzberg MJ. Effect of inhaled iloprost on the exercise function of Fontan patients: a demonstration of concept. Int J Cardiol. 2013;168:2435–40.

61. Li D, Zhou X, An Q, Feng Y. Pulmonary vasodilator therapy after the Fontan procedure: a meta-analysis. Heart Fail Rev. 2021;26:91–100.

62. Constantine A, Jenkins P, Oliver JJ, et al. Multicentre study on pulmonary arterial hypertension therapies in Fontan patients, under-utilised or of limited use? 2020.

63. Opotowsky AR, Baraona FR, Mc Causland FR, Loukas B, Landzberg E, Landzberg MJ, Sabbisetti V, Waikar SS. Estimated glomerular filtration rate and urine biomarkers in patients with single-ventricle Fontan circulation. Heart. 2017;103:434–42.

Jamil Aboulhosn and Weiyi Tan

Introduction

Over the past three decades, advances in surgical technique and refinements in the Fontan operation have led to improved short and medium-term survival for patients with single ventricle physiology [1]. Overall survival rates at 20 years post-Fontan procedure are as high as 87% in some cohorts [1]. Nevertheless, freedom from late complications of the Fontan procedure is low, and one study observed that 50% of patients with a Fontan circulation suffered a complication related to the Fontan circuit over a period of 20 years [1]. When compared to age and gender-matched patients with congenital heart disease and biventricular function, Fontan patients are admitted to the hospital more frequently (22 versus 55 per 100 patient-years) [2]. Fontan patients are mainly hospitalized for arrhythmia-related or heart failure-related issues (44% of all hospitalizations) [2], and complications related to their Fontan include ventricular dysfunction, thromboembolism, arrhythmia, protein-losing enteropathy, plastic bronchitis, collaterals and arteriovenous malformations [1]. To improve survival and quality of life, many adult Fontan patients undergo catheter-based interventions to treat these complications (Fig. 34.1). We will highlight a few of these interventions and the reasons for these interventions (Table 34.1).

J. Aboulhosn (✉) · W. Tan
Ahmanson/UCLA Adult Congenital Heart Disease Center, David Geffen School of Medicine at UCLA, Los Angeles, CA, USA
e-mail: JAboulhosn@mednet.ucla.edu; WeiyiTan@mednet.ucla.edu

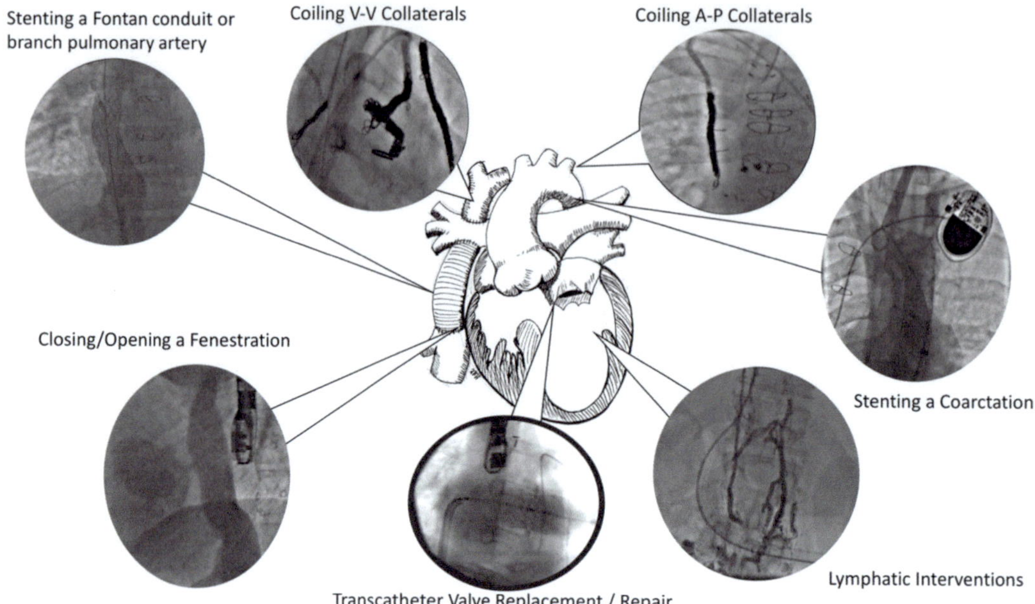

Fig. 34.1 Overview of the various catheter-based interventions available for an adult patient with a failing Fontan

Table 34.1 Catheter-based interventions for a failing adult Fontan patient

Intervention	Indication	Pre-interventional imaging	Interventional imaging with TEE	Complexity	Comments
Stent of Fontan conduit, branch pulmonary artery	Relieve obstruction	CTA or MRI	–	a	Improves Fontan hemodynamics, can treat PLE or FALD
Stent of residual coarctation/ left-sided obstructions	Relieve obstruction	CTA or MRI	–	b	Improves Fontan hemodynamics, can treat PLE or FALD
Occlusion of V-V collaterals	Improve cyanosis	CTA	–	b	Increases systemic venous pressure
Occlusion of A-P collaterals	Reduce volume overload	CTA	–	b	Reduces pulmonary blood flow
Fenestration closure	Prevent stroke, improve cyanosis	Not necessary	+	a	Increases systemic venous pressure and reduces ventricular preload/cardiac output
Fenestration creation	Improve cardiac output and ventricular preload, reduce systemic venous pressure	Not necessary	+	b	Increases stroke risk and worsens cyanosis
Lymphatic embolization	Treat PLE, PB	MRI	–	c	While effective in the short-term, lymphatic interventions do not alter underlying hemodynamics of the Fontan and complications may recur
Transcatheter valve replacement or percutaneous valve repair	Treat valvular dysfunction, relieve obstruction	CTA or MRI	+	d	Limited experience, but may have significant future potential indications

CTA computed tomography angiography, *MRI* magnetic resonance imaging, *PLE* protein losing enteropathy, *FALD* Fontan associated liver disease, *PB* plastic bronchitis

Reasons to Intervene in the Failing Adult Fontan Patient

Relieve Obstruction

A Fontan patient has no subpulmonary ventricle, and thus all pulmonary blood flow relies on a high systemic venous pressure driving flow through a low resistance circuit. Any obstruction in this circuit, even a 1 mmHg gradient, may be hemodynamically significant.

Prevent Overcirculation

Arteriopulmonary (A-P) collaterals are common in Fontan patients. The cause of all these arteriopulmonary connections is not quite known, but some hypothesize that mild hypoxia may stimulate collateral formation to increase pulmonary blood flow.

Narrowed or small pulmonary arteries may also play a role in arteriopulmonary collateral formation [3]. These abnormal connections will increase pulmonary blood flow. Over time, however, due to an increased volume load on the single ventricle and pulmonary venous atrium, these vessels will eventually cause heart failure [4, 5].

Improve Cardiac Output and Reduce Systemic Venous Pressure

As a consequence of the Fontan circuit, which places blood flow in a series instead of in a parallel circuit, the single ventricle becomes preload limited, and the ability to augment cardiac output is blunted [6]. As patients with Fontan physiology start to get older, diastolic dysfunction may increase the ventricular end-diastolic filling pressure, which reduces the passive flow to the ventricle from the pulmonary bed even further, thus resulting in even further decreases in cardiac output and increases in systemic venous pressure [6].

Create or Redirect Pulmonary Blood Flow (PBF)

The Fontan circulation creates a bottleneck at the neo-portal system within the lungs [6]. Systemic venous pressure increases as a necessary driver of pulmonary blood flow. One of the consequences of this physiology is the creation of veno-venous (V-V) collaterals as a "pop-off" or relief valve for high systemic venous pressures, bypassing the pulmonary circulation, providing preload for the single ventricle and increasing cardiac output at the expense of cyanosis.

Furthermore, if hepatic vein flow is unevenly distributed to one part of the branch pulmonary arteries, the other lung may develop significant pulmonary arteriovenous malformations from lack of hepatic factor. Interventions to coil veno-venous collaterals, occlude pulmonary arteriovenous malformations, or redirect hepatic vein flow [7] are all different ways to force blood through the pulmonary bed and improve oxygen saturation.

Relieve Cyanosis

Cyanosis is common in Fontan patients and is associated with dyspnea and decreased exercise tolerance. There are multiple causes for cyanosis in Fontan patient, from pulmonary arteriovenous malformations, veno-venous collaterals, and surgically placed fenestrations in the Fontan circuit [8].

Catheter based procedures to occlude veno-venous collaterals [9], treat arteriovenous malformations [10], and close fenestrations [11] have all reported, but these interventions have the cost of increasing systemic venous pressure. Each case has to be considered on an individual basis, as some studies have suggested that treatment of cyanosis may increase mortality [12].

Address Valvular Dysfunction

Over time, some Fontan patients will develop significant atrioventricular valve regurgitation, which is a significant risk factor for long-term morbidity and mortality in this patient population [13].

Surgical repair or replacement of the atrioventricular valve regurgitation remains the standard of care, as medical therapies are usually minimally effective [14]. Transcatheter valve replacement in certain Fontan patients has been reported. New transcatheter technologies, such as the MitraClip (Abbott, Chicago, IL), have been very effective at treating mitral valve regurgitation in patients with heart failure [15], and may be applied to Fontan patients in the near future.

Prevent Stroke

Thromboembolism and stroke are known late complications in the Fontan population [1, 8, 14]. These ischemic neurologic events are usually secondary to thrombi that travel to the brain from existing right-to-left shunts, such as a Fontan fenestration.

Closure of these shunts is performed to prevent future events [10].

Treat Complications Specific to the Fontan Circulation

- All patients with Fontan circulation can eventually develop Fontan-associated liver disease (FALD), which has features similar to end-stage cirrhosis: varices, ascites, thrombocytopenia, and encephalopathy [14].
- Protein-Losing enteropathy (PLE) is also a known manifestation of Fontan failure and, while the exact pathophysiology of PLE is still incompletely characterized, lymphatic abnormalities and congestion are associated with the condition.
- Plastic bronchitis (PB), while rare in patients with Fontan circulation, is also thought to be caused by abnormal lymphatic-bronchial connections.

These three classic complications of the Fontan circulation are byproducts of chronically elevated systemic venous pressure [6, 14]. Interventions to improve Fontan hemodynamics, such as treating atrioventricular valve regurgitation, relieving obstructions in the Fontan pathway, or creating a fenestration may improve these conditions [8, 14].

Another new and potentially effective treatment is percutaneous lymphatic embolization: identify pathways of lymphatic decompression and occlude these abnormal channels to treat PLE and plastic bronchitis [16].

Prepare for Transplant

Patients who are at the end-stage of their Fontan palliation will sometimes be referred for heart transplantation or even combined heart-liver transplantation. A lot of these patients will need pre-operative catheterization and liver biopsy for risk stratification, as well as pre-operative coil embolization/occlusion of significant arteriopulmonary or veno-venous collaterals that may cause life-threatening perioperative bleeding during the transplant operation.

Interventions in the Failing Adult Fontan Patient

Balloon Angioplasty/Stent in the Fontan Circuit, Branch Pulmonary Arteries, or Residual Coarctation of the Aorta

These interventions are meant to relieve Fontan pathway obstructions, minimise afterload to the ventricle (e.g. from residual coarctation) and treat complications of a failing Fontan, such as PLE or FALD. See Figs. 34.2 and 34.3.

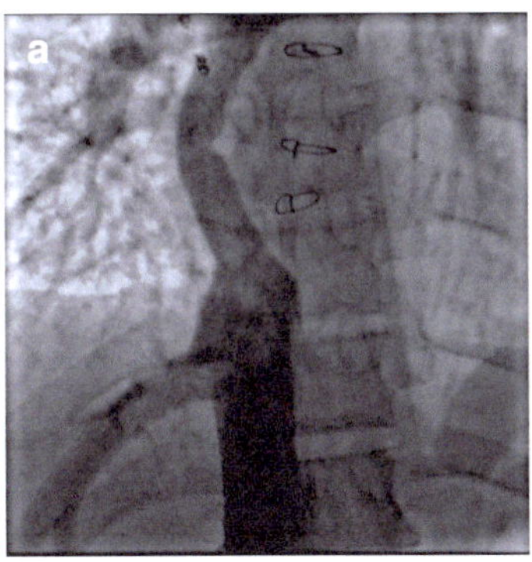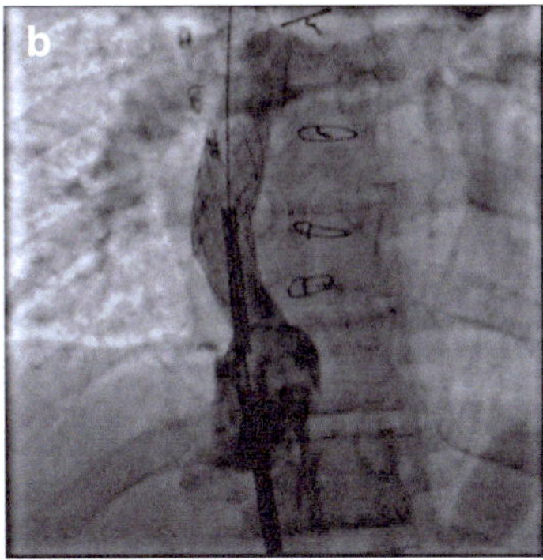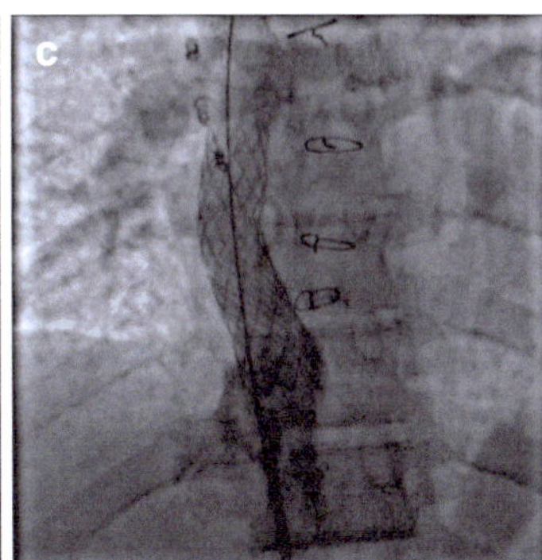

Fig. 34.2 (**a**) Angiogram of an 18 mm extracardiac Fontan conduit demonstrating a discrete 8 mm narrowing in the antero-posterior view. The initial gradient between the proximal and distal portion of the conduit was 2 mmHg. (**b**) Angiogram of the Fontan conduit after placement of a Palmaz P4010 (Cordis, Santa Clara, CA) stent inflated with a 20 mm Balloon-in-Balloon (pfm medical, Cologne, Germany) delivery system. (**c**) Angiogram of the Fontan conduit after placement of a second Palmaz P4010 stent inflated with a 20 mm Balloon-in-Balloon delivery system with no residual narrowing within the conduit. The final gradient was 0 mmHg

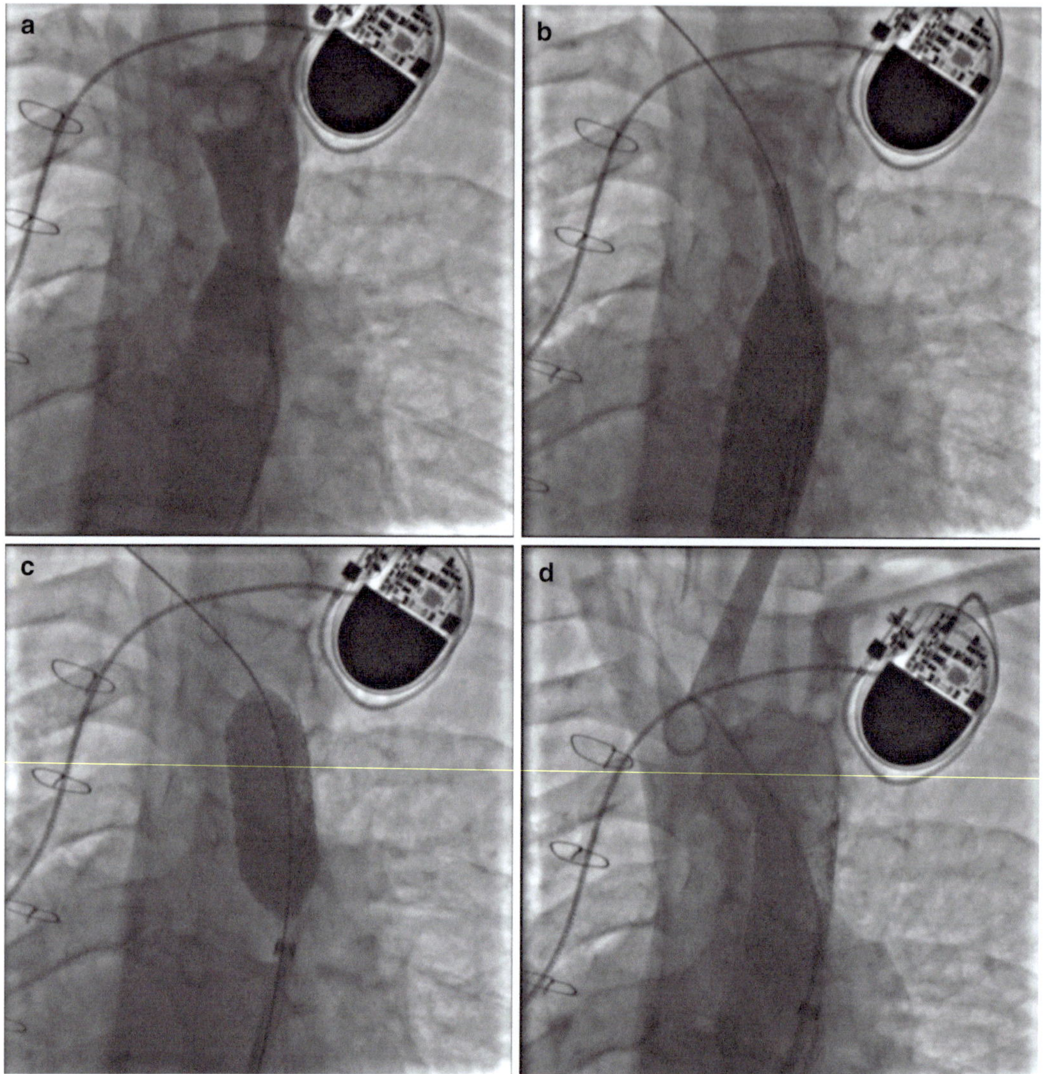

Fig. 34.3 (**a**) Angiogram of a residual coarctation of the aorta in a Fontan patient, with a peak-to-peak gradient of 20 mmHg across the narrowing, which measured 9–10 mm in diameter on angiography. The aorta measured 18 mm at the diaphragm. (**b**) Positioning an 18 × 36 mm Maxi LD EV-3 stent over an 18 mm Balloon-in-Balloon catheter. (**c**) Inflation of the 18 mm Balloon-in-Balloon delivery system to 5 atmospheres. There was no residual waist and the stent was noted to be fully expanded. (**d**) Angiogram of the aorta after stenting. The stent was fully apposed to the aorta and the aortic arch was widely patent. There was no residual coarctation and the gradient across the stent was 0 mmHg

Occlusion of Veno-Venous Collaterals

Treatment of veno-venous collaterals can improve cyanosis [9] and prevent perioperative bleeding at the time of transplant, but at the expense of increased systemic venous pressure and reduction in systemic ventricular preload. Some studies show an increase in long-term mortality after these procedures [12] (Fig. 34.4). Moreover, this intervention may fail to improve oxygen saturations as new veno-venous collaterals often appear after intervention.

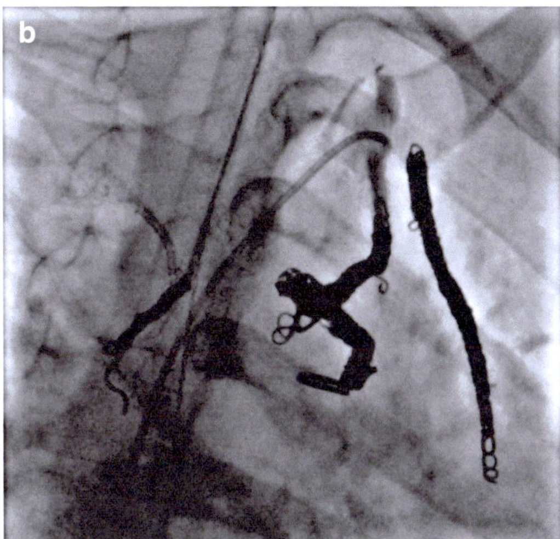

Fig. 34.4 (**a**) Angiogram of a veno-venous collateral originating from the innominate vein, draining into a left pulmonary vein. (**b**) Angiogram of the same veno-venous collateral after occlusion of the vessel with multiple POD System (Penumbra Inc., Alameda, CA) packing coils. There was no residual veno-venous flow. Note the previously coiled left internal mammary artery, which was providing collateral flow to the left pulmonary artery

Occlusion of Arteriopulmonary Collaterals

While these abnormal collateral vessels increase pulmonary blood flow, they will chronically volume load the single ventricle, which may trigger ventricular remodeling and increased end-diastolic pressure; this eventually leads to ventricular dysfunction and failure. While practice varies across institutions, [17] coiling of arterio-pulmonary collaterals is a very common procedure [11] to relieve overcirculation, treat hemoptysis, and prepare patients for transplant by reducing their perioperative bleeding risk. See Fig. 34.4.

Coiling Pulmonary Macro-Arteriovenous Malformations

These catheter-based procedures are meant to improve pulmonary blood flow and treat cyanosis.

Creation of a Fenestration

Fenestrations can be made in Fontan patients to reduce high systemic venous pressure and to provide more cardiac output by increasing systemic ventricular preload [18]. This can provide a short-term solution to a failing Fontan patient, such as someone with PLE, but at the expense of cyanosis and increased risk of systemic thromboembolism.

Closure of a Fenestration

Many Fontan patients with existing fenestrations have their fenestrations closed via transcatheter devices to prevent recurrent stroke and improve cyanosis (Fig. 34.5).

Percutaneous Lymphatic Embolization

These interventions require special techniques, including magnetic resonance lymphangiograms [19], but can be very effective at treating patients with plastic bronchitis or PLE due to abnormal lymphatic perfusion and aberrant lymphatic flow [16] (Fig. 34.6).

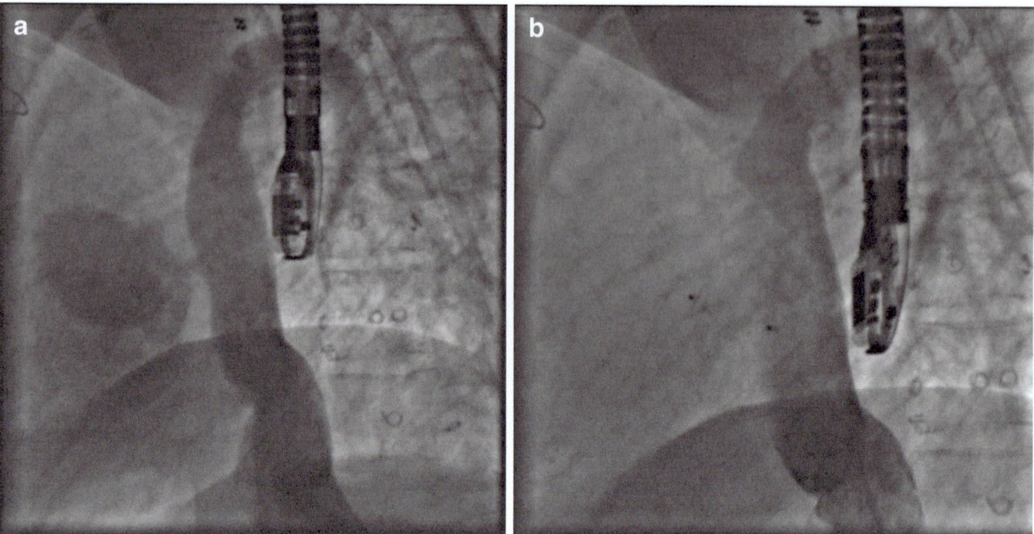

Fig. 34.5 (**a**) Angiogram of a 20 mm extracardiac Fontan conduit from the lateral projection demonstrating contrast extravasation into the left atrium from a fenestration that measured 4 mm in diameter. (**b**) Angiogram after occlu-sion of the fenestration with an 8 mm AVP II vascular plug (Abbott Inc., Chicago, IL). There was no residual shunt-ing through the fenestration and the Fontan conduit remained unobstructed

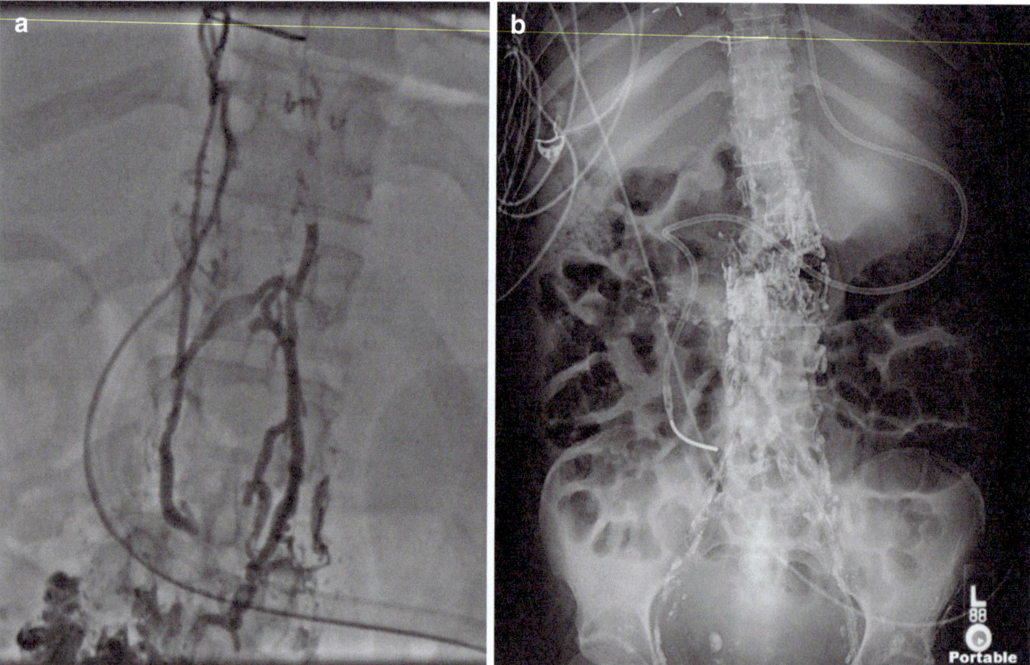

Fig. 34.6 (**a**) Occlusion of abnormal right and left lum-bar lymphatics using a mixture of 1:5 glue to ethiodized oil via retrograde access from the thoracic duct in a patient with significant chylous pleural effusions and chylous ascites. (**b**) An x-ray of the abdomen after the procedure demonstrated fully occluded lumbar lymphatics

Transcatheter Valve Replacement/Repair

There are certain cases where transcatheter valve replacement in a Fontan patient may be applicable. For example, there are reports of successful transcatheter tricuspid valve replacements in patients with tricuspid atresia who have undergone a right atrial to RV connection (Bjork Fontan modification) [20]. These procedures are effective at relieving obstructions and treating valvular dysfunction. Further adaptation of newer technologies, such as the MitraClip, may be effective tools in future interventions for high-risk Fontan patients with failing physiology. See Fig. 34.7.

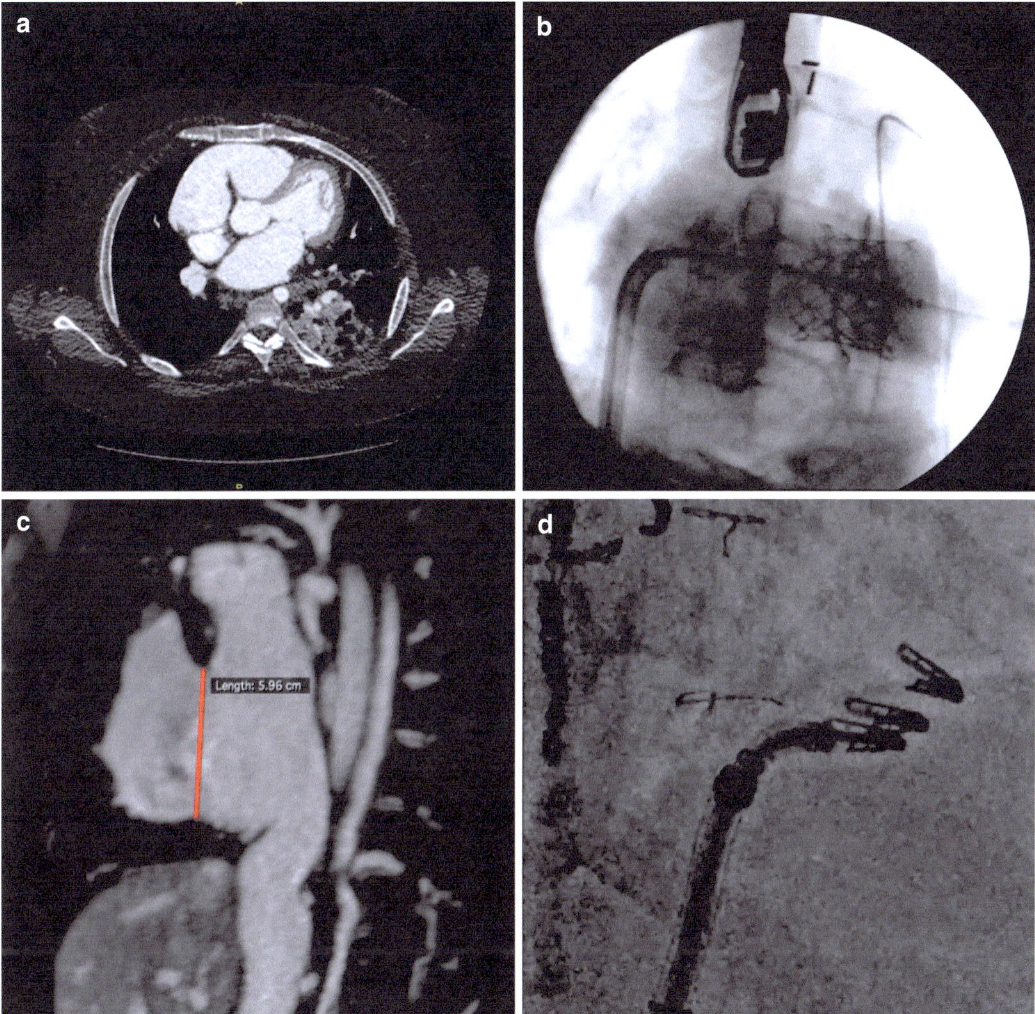

Fig. 34.7 (**a**) Computed tomography angiography image in the axial plane of a Bjork modification of the Fontan operation, with an enlarged right atrial-right ventricle (RA-RV) connection. The connection had no valve. (**b**) Fluoroscopy during a hybrid procedure where a 34 mm Carpentier-Edwards (Edwards Lifesciences, Irvine, CA) tricuspid valve ring was surgically sutured on the outside of the RA-RV connection to create an adequate landing zone for the transcatheter valve. The 29 mm Sapien S3 (Edwards Lifesciences, Irvine, CA) was then deployed with 31 mL of volume. (**c**) Magnetic resonance image in the sagittal plane of another Fontan patient who underwent a percutaneous edge-to-edge repair of a common atrioventricular valve with a MitraClip (Abbott, Chicago, IL) device. (**d**) Fluoroscopy of the third MitraClip being deployed between the anterior and inferior bridging leaflets of the common atrioventricular valve, to create a "zipper"

References

1. Kotani Y, Chetan D, Zhu J, et al. Fontan failure and death in contemporary Fontan circulation: analysis from the last two decades. Ann Thorac Surg [Internet]. 2018;105(4):1240–1247. https://doi.org/10.1016/j.athoracsur.2017.10.047.
2. Egbe A, Khan AR, Al-Otaibi M, et al. Outcomes of hospitalization in adults with Fontan palliation: the Mayo Clinic experience. Am Heart J [Internet]. 2018;198:115–122. https://doi.org/10.1016/j.ahj.2017.12.012.
3. Latus H, Gummel K, Diederichs T, et al. Aortopulmonary collateral flow is related to pulmonary artery size and affects ventricular dimensions in patients after the Fontan procedure. PLoS One. 2013;8(11):1–9.
4. Kanter KR, Vincent RN. Management of aortopulmonary collateral arteries in Fontan patients: occlusion improves clinical outcome. Pediatr Card Surg Annu. 2002;5(1):48–54.
5. Kanter KR, Vincent RN, Raviele AA. Importance of acquired systemic-to-pulmonary collaterals in the Fontan operation. Ann Thorac Surg. 1999;68(3):969–74.
6. Gewillig M, Brown SC. The Fontan circulation after 45 years: update in physiology. Heart. 2016;102(14):1081–6.
7. Adamson GT, Peng LF, Lui GK, et al. Transcatheter redirection of hepatic venous blood to treat unilateral pulmonary arteriovenous malformations in a Fontan circulation by short-term total exclusion of the unaffected lung. Catheter Cardiovasc Interv. 2019;93(4):660–3.
8. Kay WA, Moe T, Suter B, et al. Long term consequences of the Fontan procedure and how to manage them. Prog Cardiovasc Dis [Internet]. 2018;61(3–4):365–376. https://doi.org/10.1016/j.pcad.2018.09.005.
9. Lluri G, Levi DS, Aboulhosn J. Systemic to pulmonary venous collaterals in adults with single ventricle physiology after cavopulmonary palliation. Int J Cardiol [Internet]. 2015;189(1):159–163. https://doi.org/10.1016/j.ijcard.2015.04.065.
10. Lafuente MV, Alonso J, Pibernus JL, et al. Percutaneous interventions in patients with Fontan circulation. Rev Argent Cardiol. 2016;84(3):228–34.
11. Downing TE, Allen KY, Goldberg DJ, et al. Surgical and catheter-based reinterventions are common in long-term survivors of the Fontan operation. Circ Cardiovasc Interv. 2017;10(8):1–9.
12. Poterucha JT, Johnson JN, Taggart NW, et al. Embolization of veno-venous collaterals after the Fontan operation is associated with decreased survival. Congenit Heart Dis. 2015;10(5):E230–6.
13. King G, Gentles TL, Winlaw DS, et al. Common atrioventricular valve failure during single ventricle palliation. Eur J Cardiothorac Surg. 2017;51(6):1037–43.
14. Rychik J, Atz AM, Celermajer DS, et al. Evaluation and management of the child and adult with Fontan circulation: a scientific statement from the American Heart Association. Circulation. 2019;140:e234–84.
15. Stone GW, Lindenfeld JA, Abraham WT, et al. Transcatheter mitral-valve repair in patients with heart failure. N Engl J Med. 2018;379(24):2307–18.
16. Dori Y, Keller MS, Rome JJ, et al. Percutaneous lymphatic embolization of abnormal pulmonary lymphatic flow as treatment of plastic bronchitis in patients with congenital heart disease. Circulation. 2016;133(12):1160–70.
17. Banka P, Sleeper LA, Atz AM, et al. Practice variability and outcomes of coil embolization of aortopulmonary collaterals before Fontan completion: a report from the Pediatric Heart Network Fontan Cross-Sectional Study. Am Heart J [Internet]. 2011;162(1):125–130. https://doi.org/10.1016/j.ahj.2011.03.021.
18. Rupp S, Schieke C, Kerst G, et al. Creation of a transcatheter fenestration in children with failure of Fontan circulation: focus on extracardiac conduit connection. Catheter Cardiovasc Interv. 2015;86(7):1189–94.
19. Biko DM, Smith CL, Otero HJ, et al. Intrahepatic dynamic contrast MR lymphangiography: initial experience with a new technique for the assessment of liver lymphatics. Eur Radiol. 2019;29:5190–6.
20. Ghobrial J, Aboulhosn J. Transcatheter valve replacement in congenital heart disease: the present and the future. Heart. 2018;104:1629–36.

Phil Botha and Milind Chaudhari

Introduction

Fontan physiology is disadvantaged by non-pulsatile pulmonary blood flow, systemic venous hypertension, chronic preload depletion, and a low cardiac output state. The marked heterogeneity of the anatomical substrate with its inherent or acquired myocardial, conduction and vascular abnormalities leads to a cascade of pathophysiological changes that adversely affect multiple organ systems in the long term. Although overall survival has improved to 90% at 30 years, and 80% at 40 years of age, major concerns remain about functional capacity, and serious complications in adult survivors of the Fontan operation [1]. Only 53% of patients from the Australia-New Zealand Fontan registry were reported to be in New York Heart Association Functional Class I (asymptomatic) at age 40 years, and freedom from serious adverse events was only 41% [2]. Time-dependent attrition in the efficiency of the Fontan circulation can result in a multisystem disorder with cardiac arrhythmia, heart failure, thromboembolic events, protein-losing enteropathy, plastic bronchitis, renal dysfunction and Fontan associated liver disease (FALD).

Together with the presence of multiple previous sternotomies and often vascular mediastinal adhesions due to collateral formation in the setting of chronic cyanosis, re-operation in these patients can be a formidable undertaking. Re-interventions are frequently performed in adult Fontan survivors to maintain the efficiency of circulation and achieve the dual objectives of higher cardiac output at the lowest possible central venous pressure. In a large cohort of contemporary Fontan patients, 40% required catheter-based interventions and an additional 25% required surgical interventions within 20 years after the operation [3, 4].

Surgical reinterventions play an important role in the prevention of Fontan failure as well as in Fontan conversion and transplantation when the circulation does fail (Fig. 35.1).

P. Botha · M. Chaudhari (✉)
Birmingham Children's Hospital, Birmingham, UK
e-mail: p.botha@nhs.net; milind.chaudhari@nhs.net

© The Author(s), under exclusive license to Springer Nature Switzerland AG 2023
P. Clift et al. (eds.), *Univentricular Congenital Heart Defects and the Fontan Circulation*,
https://doi.org/10.1007/978-3-031-36208-8_35

<table>
<tr><td>

Fontan Optimization

Anatomy:
- Relieve obstruction in Fontan pathways or systemic outflow tract
- Treat valvar (AV/VA) regurgitation

Physiology:
- ↓ Systemic venous pressure :
  - Create fenestration
  - Block collaterals
- Restore A-V synchrony:
  - Pacemaker / Ablation / Device Therapy
- Lymphatic System Interventions

</td><td>

Mechanical Cardiac Support

- ECMO for emergencies
- LVAD for pump failure
- ?BIVAD for Fontan Failure
- Total Artificial Heart

Indications
- Bridge to recovery
- Bridge to decision
- Bridge to transplantation

</td></tr>
<tr><td>

Fontan Conversion

Arrhythmia surgery plus conversion to TCPC and Pacemaker

Indications
- Failing AP or LT Fontan with intractable atrial arrhythmias / thrombo-embolic complications and preserved ventricular function

</td><td>

Transplantation

Type
- Heart
- Heart/Lung
- Heart/Liver/Kidney

Indications
End-Stage Fontan failure with no correctable anatomical or electrical cause

</td></tr>
</table>

Fig. 35.1 Surgical interventions in the Fontan circulation. *AV* Atrioventricular, *VA* Ventriculo-arterial, *ECMO* Extra-corporeal membrane oxygenation, *LVAD* Left ventricular assist device, *BiVAD* Bi-ventricular assist device, *AP* Atriopulmonary, *LT* Lateral tunnel, *TCPC* Total cavopulmonary connection

Surgical Interventions to Optimize the Fontan Circulation

General Principles

A complex interplay of multiple electrical, mechanical and physiological factors leads to circulatory failure in the ageing Fontan circulation and contributes to a significant proportion of late deaths in this cohort [2, 5]. Comprehensive surveillance coupled with judicious use of electrophysiological, catheter, and surgical interventions play a crucial role in optimizing the efficiency of the Fontan circulation and reducing mortality in the long term.

Surgical interventions in the setting of Fontan failure are high risk undertakings and present several unique challenges, mandating a detailed pre-operative assessment (Fig. 35.2). The limited experience and lack of an evidence-based approach to planning and performing such procedures needs to be acknowledged. The balance of risks and benefits is often not as clear-cut as would be for surgical procedures in patients with a biventricular circulation.

Cardiac Arrhythmias and Pacemaker Therapy

Cardiac arrhythmias are frequently encountered in Fontan patients and closely related to the anatomical substrate, type of Fontan operation and the duration of follow up. The AP Fontan operation is associated with a significantly higher incidence of sinus node dysfunction (46%) and atrial tachy-arrhythmias (40%) [2, 5]. The overall arrhythmia burden in lateral tunnel (LT) and ECC Fontan groups is similar (20–25%) [2, 5, 6].

The onset of arrhythmia and loss of atrioventricular synchrony often precipitates rapid clinical decline. Arrhythmia impacts on ventricular

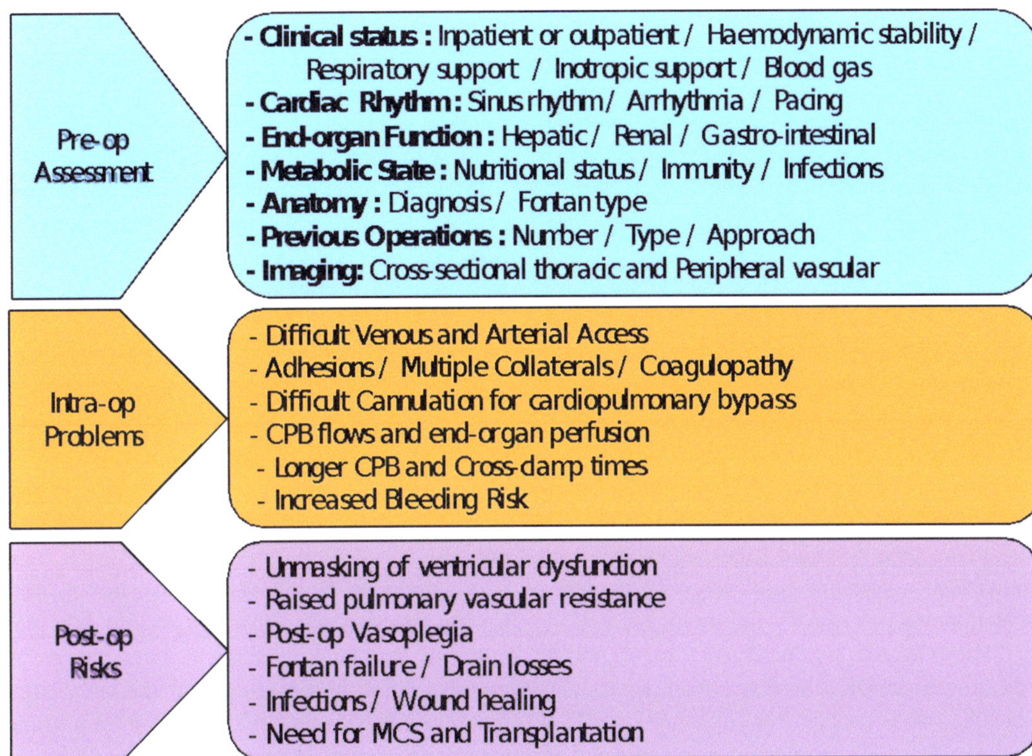

Fig. 35.2 Re-operations in the adult Fontan—general considerations. *CPB* Cardiopulmonary bypass, *MCS* Mechanical circulatory support

function and atrioventricular valve regurgitation, and is associated with an increased risk of thromboembolism, which can lead to Fontan failure or sudden death. Unsurprisingly, pacemaker implantation/revision is the commonest surgical procedure performed in this subgroup of patients and accounts for up to 42% of the total surgical interventions [2–5]. Device therapy is also used in the management of atrial tachycardia, ventricular tachycardia and rarely for cardiac resynchronisation. Although the morbidity of pacemaker procedures is relatively low, the requirement for a pacemaker is a predictor of poor long-term survival in patients with Fontan circulation [7].

In the presence of a fenestration, placement of endocardial pacing leads can be challenging, and the risk of clot formation with systemic embolisation is a concern. Implantation of epicardial leads is the conventional approach to pacing in Fontan patients, but repeated previous surgical procedures, with epicardial scar formation, can lead to higher rates of lead failure [8, 9]. When a concomitant surgical procedure is being planned, epicardial pacing remains the preferred option. When pacemaker therapy is needed in isolation, endocardial lead placement provides superior durability and avoids the need for sternotomy [8, 9]. Careful anatomical assessment is required to determine if baffle puncture is feasible and can provide adequate positioning of pacing wires.

An alternative to these options is video-assisted thoracoscopic or a mini-thoracotomy approach, although little published evidence exists to guide decision making and select between these approaches.

Surgery for Atrioventricular Valve Failure

A normally functioning atrioventricular valve (AVV) is one of the original "ten commandments" for patient selection and successful outcome after Fontan operation [10]. Significant AVV regurgitation adversely affects the outcome of patients with a functionally single ventricle. Indeed, early or concomitant AVV repair procedures are routinely undertaken during various stages of surgical palliation to improve long term Fontan outcomes.

Late development of AVV regurgitation is a unique problem in adult survivors of the Fontan operation and is seen in nearly 33% of patients by 30 years of age [11]. The etiology is often multifactorial, with inherent or acquired abnormalities affecting both ventricular and valvar morphology and function. A common AVV (complete atrioventricular septal defect) in association with isomerism, or a systemic tricuspid valve in the presence of a systemic right ventricle are independent predictors of AVV failure [5, 11, 12].

If left untreated, significant AVV regurgitation leads to ventricular volume overload, ventricular dilatation and progressive dysfunction. This results in elevated central venous pressure and an increased incidence of cardiac arrhythmias, which further exacerbate circulatory failure. Patients with AVV failure are twice as likely to develop failure of the Fontan circulation than those with competent valves [11, 12].

Medical management alone is of limited value. The timing and nature of surgical interventions are debatable and, historically, outcomes following valve surgery in the presence of established Fontan failure and ventricular dysfunction have been poor. There is, however, emerging consensus in favour of earlier surgical intervention to treat moderate-severe or severe AVV regurgitation in patients with a Fontan circulation [11]. A more aggressive approach is likely to preserve ventricular function and prevent late Fontan failure [12].

Accurate multimodality assessment of ventricular function and valve morphology is a prerequisite to planning surgical intervention. A protocol based on assessment of the ventricular function and valve morphology can help guide the nature of surgical intervention (Fig. 35.3).

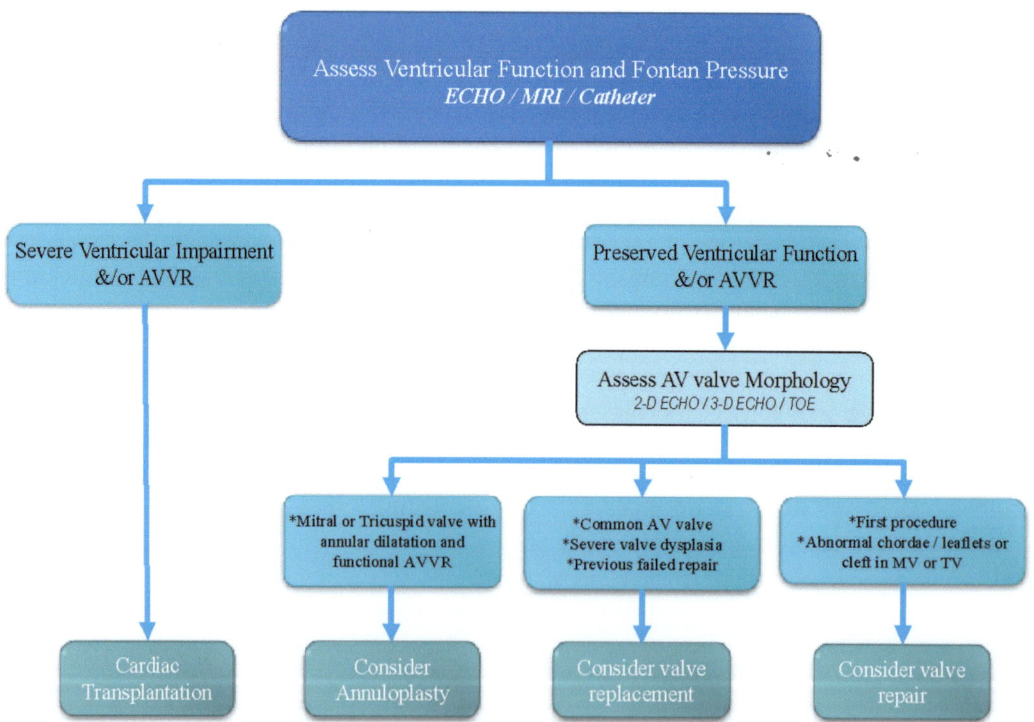

Fig. 35.3 Management of atrioventricular valve regurgitation in the Adult Fontan patient. *MRI* Magnetic resonance imaging, *AVVR* Atrioventricular valve regurgitation, *2D* Two dimensional, *3D* Three dimensional, *TOE* Transoesophageal echocardiogram, *MV* Mitral valve, *TV* Tricuspid Valve

Optimization of the Fontan Pathway

In the current era, surgical revision of the Fontan circulation to optimize its anatomy or physiology (e.g. by relieving obstruction or creating a fenestration) is rarely performed. Patient-specific modelling of fluid dynamics holds promise in improving the energetics of the Fontan circulation on an anatomically individualised basis but, at present, evidence of improved outomes from this approach is lacking.

Minimally invasive catheter interventions, including balloon dilation or stenting to relieve Fontan pathway obstruction, creation or closure of a fenestration and embolization of arterial or venous collaterals, are well established methods for improving hemodynamics and avoiding surgery, with its associated morbidity and mortality [3, 4]. Up to 50% of Fontan patients undergo catheter-based intervention by 20 years of age to optimise Fontan physiology [3, 4].

Systemic Outflow Tract Intervention

Subaortic stenosis can complicate double inlet left ventricle or tricuspid atresia with ventriculo-arterial discordance and usually takes the form of a subaortic fibromuscular tissue or restrictive VSD [13]. Early aorto-pulmonary amalgamation through the Damus-Kay-Stansel (DKS) procedure at initial stages of palliation is the preferred management strategy (Fig. 35.4) [14]. Rarely, obstruction develops late after Fontan completion. In this scenario, direct relief of subaortic obstruction by enlarging the VSD and /or subaortic chamber may be the preferred option but risks complete heart block, aortic valve regurgitation and recurrent obstruction in later life [15].

Progressive aortic root dilatation observed in genetic connective tissue disorders like Marfan syndrome is also well documented in congenital heart disease with bicuspid aortic valve, contotruncal abnormalities and procedures involving surgical reconstruction of the aortic root [16]. In

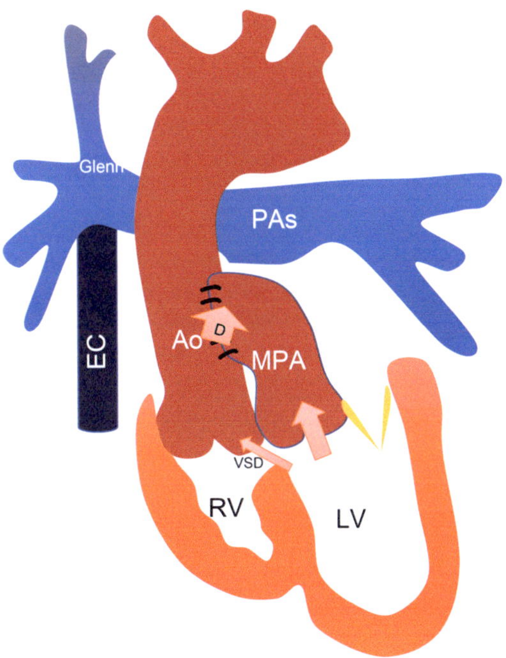

Fig. 35.4 Damus-Kaye-Stansel (DKS) operation (courtesy of K. Dimopoulos). In the presence of transposed great arteries, a small VSD may obstruct flow from the systemic (dominant) ventricle to the aorta (thin arrow), acting as subaortic stenosis. The DKS operation is an end -to-side anastomosis of the main pulmonary artery (MPA, which is disconnected from the branch pulmonary arteries) to the ascending aorta. Hence blood flow from the systemic ventricle crosses the pulmonary valve and reaches the ascending aorta through the DKS anastomosis. *Ao* aorta, *ECC* extracardiac conduit (total cavopulmonary connection), *Glenn* Glenn anastomosis of the superior vena cava to the right pulmonary artery, *LV* left ventricle, *MPA* main pulmonary artery, *RV* right ventricle, *VSD* ventricular septal defect

most CHD cases, aortopathy is mild and reflect abnormalities of the aortic wall in combination with haemodynamic and other genetic factors. Aneurysmal dilatation of the ascending aorta in the setting of Fontan circulation is rarely reported to cause aortic dissection, aortic regurgitation or compression of Fontan pathways necessitating surgical intervention to preserve Fontan physiology [17–19]. Aortic root replacement with an aortic tube graft and a mechanical or tissue valve or valve sparing aortic root replacement [19] are the surgical options in this scenario.

Lymphatic System Interventions

Persistent chylothorax, protein losing enteropathy and plastic bronchitis are serious life-threatening complications of the failing Fontan circulation. Emerging evidence from studies using magnetic resonance lymphangiography have identified an important role for lymphatic hypertension and abnormal lymphatic drainage in the pathogenesis of these disorders [20]. Catheter-based lymphatic interventions or surgical thoracic duct decompression using innominate vein takedown procedures [21] are promising innovative treatment options in selected cases.

Fontan Conversion

De Leval's experiments demonstrated in vitro that the compliance chamber of the AP Fontan leads to energy loss due to turbulent blood flow, and that the pulsatility of the RA exaggerates this effect [22]. Conversion of AP Fontan circulations to an extracardiac conduit TCPC has been shown to improve symptoms and outcomes in numerous series [23–25]. Exemplary results have been demonstrated in experienced centres by combining this with atrial reduction plasty, liberal application of cryo-ablation to treat arrhythmia, and insertion of an epicardial pacing system to manage the high incidence of sino-atrial node dysfunction after the procedure.

Important risk factors for mortality have been identified as right or indeterminate ventricular morphology, protein-losing enteropathy, ascites, cardiopulmonary bypass (CPB) time >240 minutes, and bi-atrial arrhythmia operation [23]. Long-term follow-up has demonstrated durable improvements in symptoms and improved survival. A review of all publications on the topic, however, demonstrates the complicated nature of conversion surgery, with mortality rates varying from 0 to 21% between centres in the collective published experience of 1182 patients [26]. It should also be born in mind that, as the population of AP Fontan patients is dwindling, older patients with a greater degree of end-organ dysfunction and co-morbidity are becoming the norm and are at greater perioperative risk compared to patients undergoing earlier conversion.

Those most experienced with the procedure advise against Fontan conversion in the setting of protein-losing enteropathy (without significant pathway stenoses) or with ventricular impairment not related directly to recent-onset arrhythmia. Additionally, it is also recommended that patients with ascites, right or indeterminate ventricular morphology should be considered for heart transplantation.

Transplantation

Transplantation in adults with failing Fontan circulation is challenging for numerous reasons, including:

- Multiple previous sternotomies with difficult re-entry and dissection are the norm, as well as difficult post-operative haemostasis,
- Anatomical variations necessitating more extensive vascular reconstruction,
- Co-existent hepatic dysfunction,
- Pre-operative assessment of pulmonary vascular resistance is challenging in the absence of a sub-pulmonary ventricle and the adverse vascular changes induced by the Fontan paradox can result in post-transplant right ventricular failure.
- Many potential candidates may have become highly sensitised to human leucocyte antigens by exposure to blood transfusions and homograft material, excluding many potential donors and resulting in longer waiting times and further end-organ attrition on the waiting list.
- Careful pre-operative assessment of all important venous and arterial connections on cross-sectional imaging is mandatory, as is careful surgical planning to limit the duration of CPB and graft ischaemic time. Importantly, the careful coordination of donor and recipient procedures is required to allow the necessary time for dissection without increasing ischaemic time to the detriment of surgical risk [27].

Although results of transplantation in children with the Fontan circulation have been good, and similar overall to outcomes of transplantation for children with biventricular congenital heart disease, some early results in adults have been less satisfactory. Single-centre reports have demonstrated early mortality of up to 50% [28]. Fortunately, recent registry analyses have suggested that results are improving. Although mortality remained considerably higher than that in patients without Fontan circulation (5.3%), a US nationwide sample showed 93 transplants in adults with a Fontan circulation over the past decade [29]. Mortality in this group was 26% (OR 18.1, CI 5.1–65.0) and post-operative extracorporeal membrane oxygenation (ECMO, OR 5.3) and bleeding (OR 5.3) were common. In the same sample, 10 patients were identified that underwent liver transplant during the same admission, with no mortality identified in this group. Single-centre studies have identified Fontan failure with preserved ventricular function and heterotaxy to be significant risk factors for mortality [30, 31].

The improvement in outcomes demonstrated in more recent reports has been attributed to earlier recognition of the post-operative systemic vasoplegia syndrome and increasing use of rescue ECMO in this setting. Advanced hepatic or renal dysfunction may necessitate combined heart and liver or kidney transplantation. Combined heart-kidney transplantation has increased in US practice and improves survival in patients in the lowest glomerular filtration rate quintile [32]. Little evidence on this practice exists beyond the demonstration of feasibility in the adult Fontan population.

Mechanical Circulatory Support (MCS)

Although all standard modalities of MCS have been utilised in the setting of Fontan failure, risks of complications and mortality are considerably higher than in cardiomyopathy. Analysis of the United network for organ sharing (UNOS) registry has demonstrated that adults transplanted for congenital heart disease are, therefore, less likely to be supported mechanically prior to transplantation [33].

As in cardiac failure from biventricular congenital heart disease, end-organ dysfunction increases the risk of bleeding complications from ECMO. Overall survival to hospital discharge has been very poor in the small number of adults included in single-centre reports [34]. The difficulties with haemostasis after resternotomy in the patient on ECMO increases the risk of a bridge-to-bridge or bridge-to-transplant strategy considerably. The development of specialised cannulas to facilitate extracorporeal cavopulmonary assist in the Fontan circulation remain at present at the pre-clinical stage [35, 36].

Several series exist of MCS in children and adolescents with Fontan failure; both pulsatile and continuous flow devices have been utilised in this setting (see also Chap. 76) [37] [38]. A smaller number of reports have emerged detailing centrifugal support device implantation in adults with Fontan failure [39, 40].

Total artificial heart support has been demonstrated in adolescents with Fontan, but with a high morbidity [41]. Notably, the duration of support has been relatively short in some reports, but it has been demonstrated that support in excess of 200 days is feasible.

The feasibility of true long-term mechanical support in the setting of a Fontan circulation remains uncertain. Implantable MCS of the cavopulmonary circulation remains the topic of considerable research, especially appropriate patient selection, as patients with preserved ventricular function and Fontan failure are unlikely to benefit to the same extent from mechanical assistance of the systemic ventricle.

The only clinical report of successful cavopulmonary support in an adult (a 27 year old patient converted from AP Fontan to a extracardiac conduit connected via a Berlin Heart extracorporeal pulsatile VAD to the pulmonary arteries) remains singular more than a decade later [42]. Several existing continuous flow devices have been tested in the in vitro setting [43], and purpose-made pumps are eagerly awaited, despite well over a decade of research [44].

References

1. d'Udekem Y, Iyengar AJ, Galati JC, et al. Redefining expectations of long-term survival after the Fontan procedure: twenty-five years of follow-up from the entire population of Australia and New Zealand. Circulation. 2014;130:S32–8.
2. Dennis M, Zannino D, du Plessis K, Bullock A, Disney PJS, Radford DJ, et al. Clinical outcomes in adolescents and adults after the Fontan procedure. J Am Coll Cardiol. 2018;71(9):1009–17.
3. Downing TE, Allen KY, Goldberg DJ, Rogers LS, Ravishankar C, Rychik J, et al. Surgical and catheter-based Reinterventions are common in long-term survivors of the Fontan operation. Circ Cardiovasc Interv. 2017;10:10.
4. Daley M, du Plessis K, Zannino D, et al. Reintervention and survival in 1428 patients in the Australian and New Zealand Fontan registry. Heart. 2020;106(10):751–7.
5. Pundi KN, Johnson JN, Dearani JA, Pundi KN, Li Z, Hinck CA, Dahl SH, et al. 40-year follow-up after the Fontan operation: long-term outcomes of 1,052 patients. J Am Coll Cardiol. 2015;66:1700–10.
6. Balaji S, Daga A, Bradley DJ, Etheridge SP, Law IH, Batra AS, et al. An international multicenter study comparing arrhythmia prevalence between the Intracardiac lateral tunnel and the extracardiac conduit type of Fontan operations. J Thorac Cardiovasc Surg. 2014;148(2):576–81.
7. Poh CL, Celermajer DS, Grigg LE, et al. Pacemakers are associated with a higher risk of late death and transplantation in the Fontan population. Int J Cardiol. 2019;282:33–7.
8. Egbe AC, Huntley GD, Connolly HM, Ammash NM, Deshmukh AJ, Khan AR, Said SM, Akintoye E, Warnes CA, Kapa S. Outcomes of cardiac pacing in adult patients after a Fontan operation. Am Heart J. 2017;194:92–8.
9. Segar DE, Maldonado JR, Brown CG, Law IH. Transvenous versus epicardial pacing in Fontan patients. Pediatr Cardiol. 2018;39(7):1484–8.
10. Choussat A, Fontan F, Besse P, Vallot F, Chauve A. Selection criteria for Fontan's procedure. In: Anderson R, Shinebourne E, editors. Pediatric cardiology. Edinburgh: Churchill Livingstone; 1978. p. 559–66.
11. King G, Ayer J, Celermajer D, Zentner D, Justo R, Disney P, Zannino D, d'Udekem Y. Atrioventricular valve failure in Fontan palliation. J Am Coll Cardiol. 2019;73(7):810–22.
12. Stephens EH, Dearani JA. Management of the bad atrioventricular valve in Fontan…time for a change. J Thorac Cardiovasc Surg. 2019;158(6):1643–8.
13. Freedom RM. Subaortic obstruction and the Fontan operation. Ann Thorac Surg. 1998;66(2):649–52.
14. Tchervenkov CI, Shum-Tim D, Beland MJ, Jutras L, Platt R. Single ventricle with systemic obstruction in early life: comparison of initial pulmonary artery banding versus the Norwood operation. Eur J Cardiothorac Surg. 2001;19(5):671–7.
15. Razzouk AJ, Freedom RM, Cohen AJ, Williams WG, Trusler GA, Coles JG, Burrows PE, Rebeyka IM. The recognition, identification of morphologic substrate, and treatment of subaortic stenosis after a Fontan operation. An analysis of twelve patients. J Thorac Cardiovasc Surg. 1992;104(4):938–44.
16. Niwa K. Aortic dilatation in complex congenital heart disease. Cardiovasc Diagn Ther. 2018;8(6):725–38.
17. Egan M, Phillips A, Cook SC. Aortic dissection in the adult Fontan procedure with aortic root enlargement. Pediatr Cardiol. 2009;30:562–3.
18. Stolla M, Sweeney A, Alfieris GM, et al. Aortic aneurysm with a ruptured dissection in a 15-year-old boy with hypoplastic left heart syndrome. J Thorac Cardiovasc Surg. 2014;147:e35–6.
19. Erez E, Tam VK, Galliani C, Lashus A, Doublin NA, Peretti J. Valve-sparing aortic root replacement for patients with a Fontan circulation. J Heart Valve Dis. 2012;21(2):175–80.
20. Biko DM, DeWitt AG, Pinto EM, Morrison RE, Johnstone JA, Griffis H, et al. MRI evaluation of lymphatic abnormalities in the neck and thorax after Fontan surgery: relationship with outcome. Radiology. 2019;291(3):774–80.
21. Hraska V, Mitchell ME, Woods RK, Hoffman GM, Kindel SJ, Ginde S. Innominate vein Turn-down procedure for failing Fontan circulation. Semin Thorac Cardiovasc Surg Pediatr Card Surg Annu. 2020;23:34–40.
22. de Leval MR, Kilner P, Gewillig M, Bull C. Total cavopulmonary connection: a logical alternative to atriopulmonary connection for complex Fontan operations. Experimental studies and early clinical experience. J Thorac Cardiovasc Surg. 1988;96:682–95.
23. Backer CL. Rescuing the late failing Fontan: focus on surgical treatment of dysrhythmias. Semin Thorac Cardiovasc Surg Pediatr Card Surg Annu. 2017;20:33–7.
24. Hoashi T, Shimada M, Imai K, Komori M, Kurosaki K, Ohuchi H, Ichikawa H. Long-term therapeutic effect of Fontan conversion with an extracardiac conduit. Eur J Cardiothorac Surg. 2019;101:717.
25. Blitzer D, Habib AS, Brown JW, Kean AC, Lin J-HI, Turrentine MW, Rodefeld MD, Herrmann JL, Kay WA. Early conversion of classic Fontan conversion may decrease term morbidity: single centre outcomes. Cardiol Young. 2019;29:1045–50.
26. Brida M, Baumgartner H, Gatzoulis MA, Diller G-P. Early mortality and concomitant procedures related to Fontan conversion: quantitative analysis. Int J Cardiol. 2017;236:132–7.
27. Russo MJ, Chen JM, Sorabella RA, et al. The effect of ischemic time on survival after heart transplantation varies by donor age: an analysis of the United Network for Organ Sharing database. J Thorac Cardiovasc Surg. 2007;133:554–9.
28. Davies RR, Sorabella RA, Yang J, Mosca RS, Chen JM, Quaegebeur JM. Outcomes after transplantation

for "failed" Fontan: a single-institution experience. J Thorac Cardiovasc Surg. 2012;143:1183–1192.e4.

29. Hernandez GA, Lemor A, Clark D, et al. Heart transplantation and in-hospital outcomes in adult congenital heart disease patients with Fontan: a decade nationwide analysis from 2004 to 2014. J Card Surg. 2020;35(3):603–8.

30. Murtuza B, Hermuzi A, Crossland DS, Parry G, Lord S, Hudson M, Chaudhari MP, Haynes S, O'Sullivan JJ, Hasan A. Impact of mode of failure and end-organ dysfunction on the survival of adult Fontan patients undergoing cardiac transplantation. Eur J Cardiothorac Surg. 2017;51:135–41.

31. Griffiths ER, Kaza AK, Wyler von Ballmoos MC, Loyola H, Valente AM, Blume ED, del Nido P. Evaluating failing Fontans for heart transplantation: predictors of death. Ann Thorac Surg. 2009;88:558–64.

32. Karamlou T, Welke KF, McMullan DM, Cohen GA, Gelow J, Tibayan FA, Mudd JM, Slater MS, Song HK. Combined heart-kidney transplant improves post-transplant survival compared with isolated heart transplant in recipients with reduced glomerular filtration rate: analysis of 593 combined heart-kidney transplants from the United Network Organ Sharing Database. J Thorac Cardiovasc Surg. 2014;147:456–61.

33. Davies RR, Russo MJ, Yang J, Quaegebeur JM, Mosca RS, Chen JM. Listing and transplanting adults with congenital heart disease. Circulation. 2011;123:759–67.

34. Booth KL, Roth SJ, Thiagarajan RR, Almodovar MC, del Nido PJ, Laussen PC. Extracorporeal membrane oxygenation support of the Fontan and bidirectional Glenn circulations. Ann Thorac Surg. 2004;77:1341–8.

35. Wang D, Gao G, Plunkett M, Zhao G, Topaz S, Ballard-Croft C, Zwischenberger JB. A paired membrane umbrella double-lumen cannula ensures consistent cavopulmonary assistance in a Fontan sheep model. J Thorac Cardiovasc Surg. 2014;148:1041–7; discussion 1047.

36. Lin WCP, Doyle MG, Roche SL, Honjo O, Forbes TL, Amon CH. Computational fluid dynamic simulations of a cavopulmonary assist device for failing Fontan circulation. J Thorac Cardiovasc Surg. 2019;158:1424–33.

37. Woods RK, Ghanayem NS, Mitchell ME, Kindel S, Niebler RA. Mechanical circulatory support of the Fontan patient. Semin Thorac Cardiovasc Surg Pediatr Card Surg Annu. 2017;20:20–7.

38. Morales DLS, Adachi I, Heinle JS, Fraser CD. A new era: use of an intracorporeal systemic ventricular assist device to support a patient with a failing Fontan circulation. J Thorac Cardiovasc Surg. 2011;142:e138–40.

39. Shah NR, Lam WW, Rodriguez FH, Ermis PR, Simpson L, Frazier OH, Franklin WJ, Parekh DR. Clinical outcomes after ventricular assist device implantation in adults with complex congenital heart disease. J Heart Lung Transplant. 2013;32:615–20.

40. Lorts A, Villa C, Riggs KW, Broderick J, Morales DLS. First use of HeartMate 3 in a failing Fontan circulation. Ann Thorac Surg. 2018;106:e233–4.

41. Rossano JW, Goldberg DJ, Fuller S, Ravishankar C, Montenegro LM, Gaynor JW. Successful use of the total artificial heart in the failing Fontan circulation. Ann Thorac Surg. 2014;97:1438–40.

42. Prêtre R, Häussler A, Bettex D, Genoni M. Right-sided univentricular cardiac assistance in a failing Fontan circulation. Ann Thorac Surg. 2008;86:1018–20.

43. Zhu J, Kato H, Fu YY, Zhao L, Foreman C, Davey L, Weisel RD, Van Arsdell GS, Honjo O. Cavopulmonary support with a microaxial pump for the failing Fontan physiology. ASAIO J. 2015;61:49–54.

44. Rodefeld MD, Marsden A, Figliola R, Jonas T, Neary M, Giridharan GA. Cavopulmonary assist: long-term reversal of the Fontan paradox. J Thorac Cardiovasc Surg. 2019;158:1627–36.

Palliative Care Strategies in Adult Patients

Daniel Tobler

Introduction

Fontan palliation is a life-limiting condition with markedly reduced average life expectancy in many of the affected individuals [1, 2]. There is an urgent need for a more proactive approach to discussing advance care planning (ACP) and end-of-life issues in Fontan patients and a more appropriate use of palliative care in clinical practice. This chapter we will focus on practical recommendations of ACP discussions and end-of-life strategies in adult Fontan patients.

Terminology and the Concept of Advance Care Planning

- Advance care planning is a process that "enables individuals to define goals and preferences for future medical treatment and care, to discuss these goals and preferences with family and health-care providers, and to record and review these preferences if appropriate" [3].
- Palliative care is a specialized form of medical care that focuses on treatment of symptom relief and comfort rather that curing the illness [4]. It can be used alongside curative treatments and has been shown to improve patient satisfaction and quality of life [5].
- End-of-life care is the care given to people who are near the end of life and may have stopped treatment to cure or control their disease. The goal of end-of-life care is to control pain and other symptoms, so the patient can be as comfortable as possible. End-of-life care may include palliative care, supportive care, and hospice care.

The goal of ACP in Fontan patients is to guide medical teams and family members about future care, should a patient become incapable to speak for him- or herself. It enhances patient autonomy and self-determination in important aspects, such as end-of-life care. It may prevent overly aggressive or futile treatment at the end of life, for which Fontan patients are at particularly high risk [6].

ACP and palliative care integrate continuously into each other and complement the specific cardiac therapy. Greutmann and Tobler et al. offer a conceptualization of "comprehensive care" in CHD [7], which is also applicable to Fontan patients (Fig. 36.1).

D. Tobler (✉)
University Hospital Basel, University of Basel, Basel, Switzerland

Department of Cardiology, Basel, Switzerland
e-mail: daniel.tobler@usb.ch

© The Author(s), under exclusive license to Springer Nature Switzerland AG 2023
P. Clift et al. (eds.), *Univentricular Congenital Heart Defects and the Fontan Circulation*,
https://doi.org/10.1007/978-3-031-36208-8_36

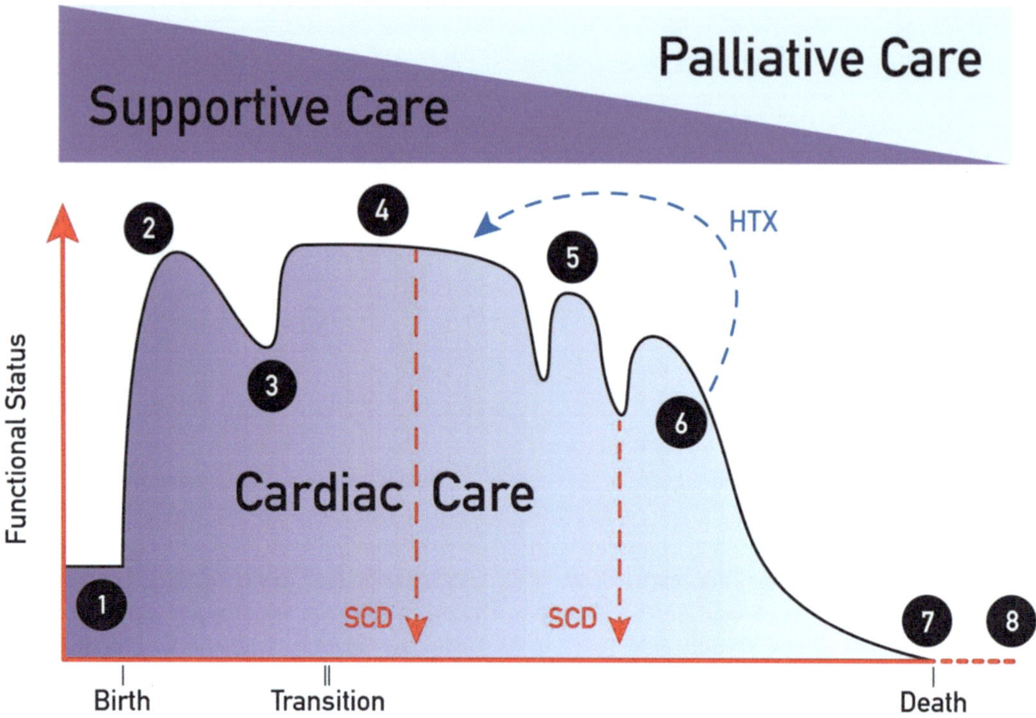

Fig. 36.1 Illustration of the comprehensive care model with stages of disease in patients with congenital heart disease. (Modified from Greutmann and Tobler et al. with permission) [7]. Disease stages in congenital heart disease covering the entire life-span (x-axis). The y-axis depicts the functional status along the different disease stages. Numbers 1–8 represent the several stages of comprehensive care in patients with congenital heart disease: (1) Parental prenatal support, (2) Initial surgical repair/palliation, (3) Re-interventions during childhood or adolescence, (4) Plateau of variable lengths in adulthood, (5) Variable adverse cardiac events and functional decline with variable slope, intermittent exacerbations that respond to rescue efforts and/or adult re-interventions or procedures, (6) Refractory symptoms and limited function, (7) End-of-life care, (8) Bereavement care. The concept of comprehensive care combines cardiac care, supportive care including advanced care planning and measures of palliative care adjusted and matched to the individual patient's stage of disease and circumstances of living. The different categories of care are by no means exclusive or sequential but rather complement each other in every stage of cardiac disease. Dotted line with arrowhead represents possible occurrence of sudden cardiac death events. *SCD* Sudden cardiac death, *CHD* congenital heart disease, *HTX* heart transplantation

Initiation of Advance Care Planning Discussions in Fontan Patients

Only limited data exist about the patient preference on when to start ACP discussions [8]. In principle, ACP can be performed at any time, yet the focus usually shifts according to the rate of deterioration of their health [3].

- Ideally, ACP discussions should start early in the disease course, before life-threatening events occur [8]. Initiating ACP discussions during unplanned hospital admissions and around acute cardiac complications is not ideal. Despite this, only a minority of Fontan patients have documented end-of-life discussions prior to an emergency admission [6].

- Initiating ACP discussions should be approached as a teamwork. While, generally, patients prefer having discussions about ACP with their ACHD physician [8], other healthcare professionals have other kinds of contacts with patients. Different members of the healthcare team can be prompted to broach the subject of ACP by different triggers and may then help patients and physicians to engage in the discussion.

- Every Fontan patient who asks for additional information on future health and care plans should be invited to talk about ACP with their ACHD specialist.
- Disease progression and worsening prognosis may be important triggers to initiate ACP discussions.
- All interventions that carry a risk of major complications (cardiac surgery, ICD-implantation, catheter-based or other therapeutic interventions) should provide an opportunity to talk about ACP [9].

- Changes in the patient's social support system, such as death of a spouse or close family members, may trigger ACP discussions [10, 11].

Practical Recommendations on ACP and Effective Communication Regarding ACP

Practical recommendations on how ACP should be designed are based on literary sources and the author's experience. Box 36.1 summarizes the most important recommendations, which should be implemented individually for each patient.

Practical recommendations for effective communication about ACP or end-of-life issues are outlined in Table 36.1, modified with permission from Kovacs et al. [12]

Table 36.1 The Ask-Tell-Ask Cycle (modified, with permission from Kovacs et al. [12])

Ask	*Ask what patients currently understand about their disease and what they would like to know*	• Tell me what you understand about Fontan palliation, and what you expect? • What have other doctors or nurses told you about what to expect down the road? • What would you like to know about your health? • How would you like decisions to be made about your health care? • What have you told your family or other doctors you would want if your heart or breathing stops? • What worries do you have?
Tell	*Provide information that is requested by the patients or is important to communicate to them*	• You asked about how long I think you will live. Based upon how your health is now, we would expect that you have several months/a few years/a few decades. Of course, this is not easy to predict and some patients live longer (or less) than expected • When your heart or breathing stops, we can either attempt to revive you, or allow you to die naturally • I am afraid we have reached a phase in your illness, when you may be nearing the end of your life • We are at a turning point in your condition, and there are choices to be made regarding which road to take • I try to talk with all patients about what they would like to happen when they become very ill and/or near-death. These might not be easy topics to discuss, but it is very important that we know of your preferences for end-of-life care and whether there is a person you would want to be involved in making decisions about your health if you become unable to do so. Talking about this now, will help your family if they ever need to make decisions on your behalf
Ask	*Confirm an understanding of what was said and provide an opportunity for patients to ask follow-up questions*	• It is important that I explain things clearly to you • Please tell me what you understood • What questions do you have?

Box 36.1 Practical Recommendations for Advanced Care Planning in Clinical Practice

- Offer ACP discussions to patients irrespective of disease complexity, early in the disease course, but acknowledge that a minor proportion of patients is not (yet) ready for these conversations.
- Consider scheduling a visit to discuss ACP issues. Give patients enough time to prepare for these discussions and to discuss with their relatives and friends.
- Normalize ACP discussions. Information about ACP can be provided using standardized written format.
- Provide information in the simplest and clearest language possible.
- Document ACP discussions and advance directives documents. These documents, once completed, should be made readily available at any time and it may be wise to flag such documents in the patient's chart.
- Ensure sensitivity to a patient's cultural background and be aware of the cognitive and developmental abilities of an individual patient; tailor ACP discussions accordingly.
- Repeat ACP discussions as necessary. These discussions should not be regarded as a single event but rather an on-going process.
- Patients should be encouraged to identify a trusted person that may be approached by the medical team to assist with decision-making when the patient is unable to communicate.

Special Considerations of Palliative Care Management in Fontan Patients

Fontan patients are confronted with unusual situations that complicate the palliative care management:

- Prognostication models, similar to those developed for heart failure due to acquired heart disease [13, 14], do not exist for Fontan patients and thus, prognostication in individual Fontan patients remains difficult.
- The lack of reliable prognostication models has been shown to be one of the major barriers for the initiation of conversations with patients about prognosis, ACP and end-of-life care [7].
- Intensive care and palliative care specialists are often not familiar with the complex anatomy of Fontan patients. Hemodynamics should be explained—drawing a picture/diagram and explaining potential pitfalls in care.
- Fontan patients tend to die younger than patients with acquired heart disease [15]. The death of these young patients can be particularly difficult/distressing for families and healthcare providers [16]
- Fontan patients often expect to have a near-normal life expectancy [17] and many of them lack awareness and understanding of their Fontan-specific risks.
- Younger patients might be at particular risk of receiving overly aggressive or futile treatment before death ensues [6].
- Adult cardiologists are not used to caring for dying young patients, nor with families comprising of the patients' parents, grandparents, and young children [18].
- It may be difficult to recognize when a Fontan patient is nearing end-of-life, which may impact on the quality of care. Prognostication in "failing Fontan" patients with extracardiac features, such as liver disease or protein-loosing-enteropathy, may be even more difficult.
- The social and professional/employment circumstances of Fontan patients are often very different to those of elderly patients seen in heart failure clinics. Functional decline in Fontan patients often interrupts careers long before retirement age and may occur within complex family systems. Financial difficulties and lack of appropriate insurance in many countries may add to the distress of dying.

Palliative and End-of-Life Care Strategies (Modified and Reprinted with Permission [19])

- Consider identifying a primary attending physician for an inpatient facing death who can provide continuity of care (and communication) in settings in which attending (senior) staff typically rotates.
- Ensure that end-of-life discussions are well-documented, and all members of the outpatient and inpatient care team are informed.
- Include health providers on the care team who can attend to the physical, emotional, and spiritual needs of patients facing death
- Consider referral to palliative care—making sure that the complex anatomy and hemodynamics are understood.
- Consider bioethics consultations in challenging situations.
- Use interpreters, as necessary, to ensure that information is provided in the patient's language.
- When an adult Fontan patient dies, consider informing the patient's pediatric providers.

References

1. Diller GP, Kempny A, Alonso-Gonzalez R, Swan L, Uebing A, Li W, Babu-Narayan S, Wort SJ, Dimopoulos K, Gatzoulis MA. Survival prospects and circumstances of death in contemporary adult congenital heart disease patients under follow-up at a large tertiary centre. Circulation. 2015;132:2118–25.
2. Greutmann M, Tobler D, Kovacs AH, Greutmann-Yantiri M, Haile SR, Held L, Ivanov J, Williams WG, Oechslin EN, Silversides CK, Colman JM. Increasing mortality burden among adults with complex congenital heart disease. Congenit Heart Dis. 2015;10:117–27.
3. Rietjens JAC, Sudore RL, Connolly M, van Delden JJ, Drickamer MA, Droger M, van der Heide A, Heyland DK, Houttekier D, Janssen DJA, Orsi L, Payne S, Seymour J, Jox RJ, Korfage IJ, European Association for Palliative Care. Definition and recommendations for advance care planning: an international consensus supported by the European Association for Palliative Care. Lancet Oncol. 2017;18:e543–51.
4. Munoz-Mendoza J. Competencies in palliative care for cardiology fellows. J Am Coll Cardiol. 2015;65:750–3.
5. Lowey SE. Palliative care in the management of patients with advanced heart failure. Adv Exp Med Biol. 2018;1067:295–311.
6. Tobler D, Greutmann M, Colman JM, Greutmann-Yantiri M, Librach LS, Kovacs AH. End-of-life care in hospitalized adults with complex congenital heart disease: care delayed, care denied. Palliat Med. 2012;26:72–9.
7. Greutmann M, Tobler D, Colman JM, Greutmann-Yantiri M, Librach SL, Kovacs AH. Facilitators of and barriers to advance care planning in adult congenital heart disease. Congenit Heart Dis. 2013;8:281–8.
8. Tobler D, Greutmann M, Colman JM, Greutmann-Yantiri M, Librach LS, Kovacs AH. End-of-life in adults with congenital heart disease: a call for early communication. Int J Cardiol. 2012;155:383–7.
9. Denvir MA, Murray SA, Boyd KJ. Future care planning: a first step to palliative care for all patients with advanced heart disease. Heart. 2015;101:1002–7.
10. Dunlay SM, Strand JJ, Wordingham SE, Stulak JM, Luckhardt AJ, Swetz KM. Dying with a left ventricular assist device as destination therapy. Circ Heart Fail. 2016;9:e003096.
11. Clayer MT. Clinical practice guidelines for communicating prognosis and end-of-life issues with adults in the advanced stages of a life-limiting illness, and their caregivers. Med J Aust. 2007;187:478.
12. Kovacs AH, Landzberg MJ, Goodlin SJ. Advance care planning and end-of-life management of adult patients with congenital heart disease. World J Pediatr Congenit Heart Surg. 2013;4:62–9.
13. Lee DS, Austin PC, Rouleau JL, Liu PP, Naimark D, Tu JV. Predicting mortality among patients hospitalized for heart failure: derivation and validation of a clinical model. JAMA. 2003;290:2581–7.
14. Levy WC, Mozaffarian D, Linker DT, Sutradhar SC, Anker SD, Cropp AB, Anand I, Maggioni A, Burton P, Sullivan MD, Pitt B, Poole-Wilson PA, Mann DL, Packer M. The Seattle heart failure model: prediction of survival in heart failure. Circulation. 2006;113:1424–33.
15. Verheugt CL, Uiterwaal CS, van der Velde ET, Meijboom FJ, Pieper PG, van Dijk AP, Vliegen HW, Grobbee DE, Mulder BJ. Mortality in adult congenital heart disease. Eur Heart J. 2010;31:1220–9.
16. Badger JM. Factors that enable or complicate end-of-life transitions in critical care. Am J Crit Care. 2005;14:513–21.
17. Reid GJ, Webb GD, Barzel M, McCrindle BW, Irvine MJ, Siu SC. Estimates of life expectancy by adolescents and young adults with congenital heart disease. J Am Coll Cardiol. 2006;48:349–55.
18. de Stoutz ND, Leventhal M. Adult age with congenital heart disease—quo vadis. Kardiovaskulaere Medizin. 2009;9(2):38–44.
19. Kovacs AH, Dipchand AI, Greutmann M, Tobler D. End-of-life care in pediatric and congenital heart disease. In: Goodlin S, Rich M, editors. End-of-life care in cardiovascular disease. London: Springer; 2015.

Role of Mechanical Support for Failing Single Ventricle

37

Massimo Griselli and Rebecca Ameduri

Mechanical circulatory support (MCS) is a complex and challenging issue for all patients, but particularly for failing single ventricle (SV) patients. SV physiology can result from a variety of congenital heart anomalies, all of which lead to one of the ventricles being absent or too small to support one of the circulations. Classically, these patients undergo a series of palliative surgical procedures from infancy aimed to make the SV the systemic pumping chamber, with deoxygenated blood flowing passively to the pulmonary circulation to achieve ultimately what is called "Fontan circulation" [1]. It is well established that many SV patients develop heart failure at some point in their lives and at any stage of their palliation.

When SV patients develop heart failure refractory to treatment, the only management option for them is heart transplantation (HTx) [2, 3]. These patients often need MCS as a bridge to HTx therapy, but SV anatomy and physiology create some unique challenges for MCS support [4]. The three main types of MCS used to aid the failing SV are veno-arterial extracorporeal membrane oxygenator (VA-ECMO) for short-term support, ventricular assist devices (VADs) or Total Artificial Heart (TAH) for both mid- and long-term support [4] (Fig. 37.1).

The most used MCS in children with SV, particularly in acute setting, is VA-ECMO. VA-ECMO is similar to a cardiopulmonary bypass system where the blood is drained from the systemic venous atrium or a large peripheral vein like the jugular or the femoral vein, pumped through an oxygenator and a heat exchanger, and eventually returned to the patient via the ascending aorta or a large peripheral artery like the femoral or carotid artery [4]. In most cases, VA-ECMO can be deployed quickly and provides support for both the cardiac and respiratory systems and can adequately support the patients for a short-term, usually no more than 2 or 3 weeks in our experience before complications may occur [4]. From VA-ECMO, patients can be weaned off if recovery of heart failure has been accomplished or to go directly to heart transplantation, if an organ becomes available. However, most commonly patients on VA-ECMO are moved to a long-term support represented by the VADs [4]. In addition to adult mechanical devices, VADs suitable for children have become available in the last 20 years [4]. The disadvantage of VA-ECMO support compared to VADs is that the device is not as stable, and patients often need to be sedated and are not able to rehabilitate while awaiting transplant. VA-ECMO also has high infection and bleeding/stroke complication

M. Griselli (✉)
King Abdullah bin Abdulaziz University Hospital, Riyadh, Saudi Arabia
e-mail: mgriselli@kauauh.edu.sa

R. Ameduri
Mayo Clinic, Rochester, MN, USA
e-mail: Ameduri.Rebecca@mayo.edu

P. Clift et al. (eds.), *Univentricular Congenital Heart Defects and the Fontan Circulation*,
https://doi.org/10.1007/978-3-031-36208-8_37

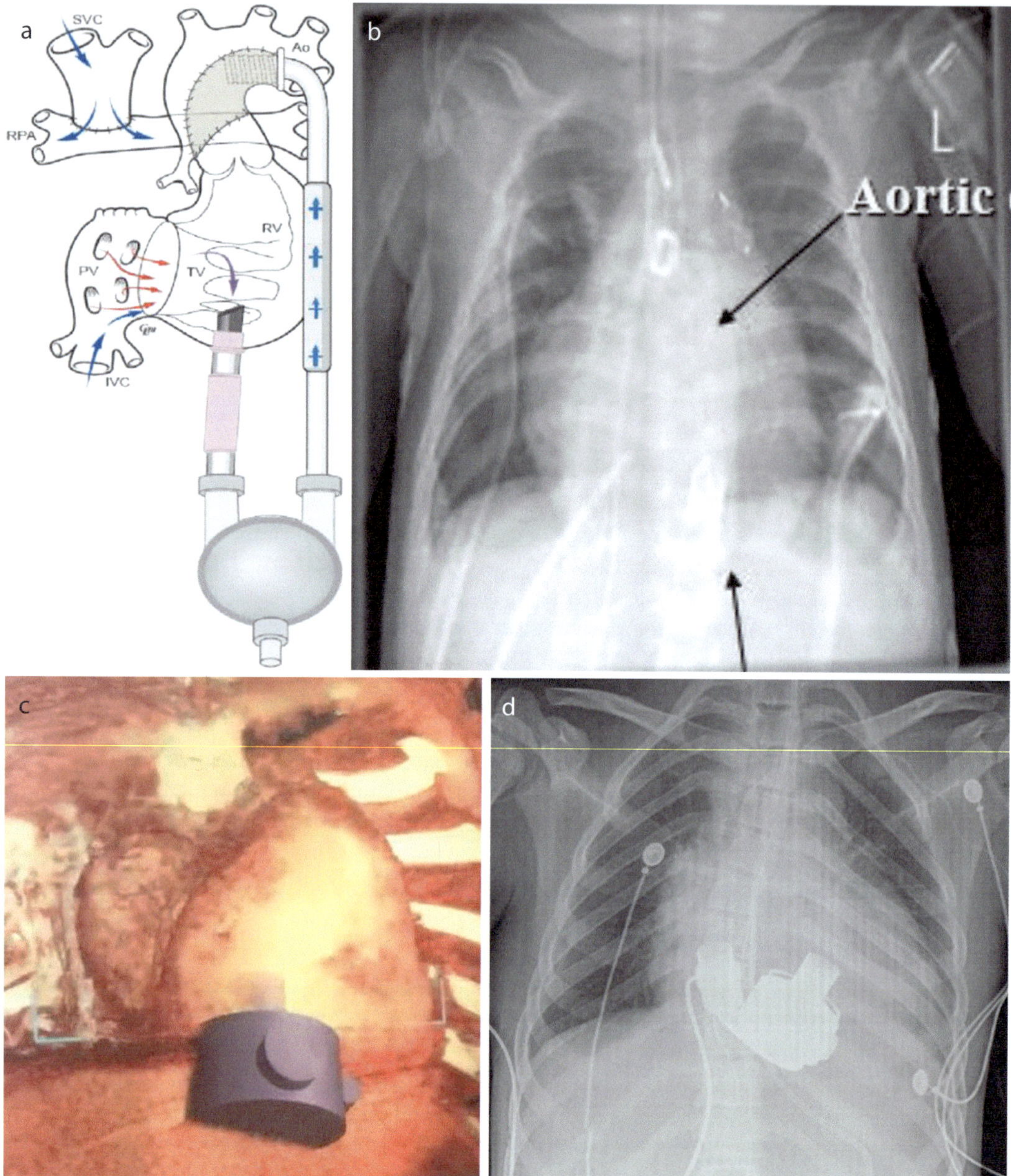

Fig. 37.1 Images and schematics of some of the types of MCS that can be utilized in single ventricle patients. (**a**) Diagram of cannulation strategy for HLHS after superior cavo-pulmonary connection (Glenn shunt) with the Berlin Heart Excor® (BHE) Device. (**b**) Chest x ray after BHE cannulation (**c**) 4D Computerized Tomography recon- struction to determine the ideal placement of a Heartmate III in a Fontan patient with underlying diagnosis of hypo- plastic left heart syndrome (HLHS). (**d**) Chest x ray fol- lowing placement of Heartmate III showing the device placed in an ideal position based on virtual fit from the 4D reconstruction

rates, hence the device is limited to short-term support [4]. Furthermore, children with superior cavo-pulmonary connection needing VA-ECMO represent a real challenge to the surgeons because of lack of large peripheral vein suitable for cannulation and chest re-opening is often required, and patients with failing Fontan circulation who are supported with VA-ECMO have a low (35%) survival rate to discharge [5].

As we said, in the current era, pediatric VADs are available, and we have gained more experience in their management in the pediatric heart failure community. VADs are now commonly used to support SV patients as a bridge to HTx [6] and have important advantages over VA-ECMO: they can be used as longer-term therapy, are associated with a lower complication rate and improved survival to transplantation and post-transplantation, and allow patients to be ambulatory or even be discharged to home while awaiting HTx [7, 8]. There are various types of VADs that can be implanted depending on patient size and clinical scenario: extra-corporeal VADs (Berlin Heart Excor®, the only one available nowadays) or intra-corporeal VADs with the Heartmate III® being the most used across the surgical community. The Berlin Heart Excor® is the most used VAD in pediatric patients and consists of an external polyurethane pneumatic-driven pump with different sizes options able to support patients from neonatal age to adult size: 10 cc, 15 cc, 25 cc, 30 cc, 50 cc, 60 cc, and 80 cc [9]. Intra-corporeal VADs cannot be used in small pediatric patients, but can be used in bigger children, adolescents, and adults with a SV. The choice of VAD depends on the anatomy, clinical situation and risk factors for bleeding/stroke and infection.

Total Artificial Heart (TAH) is another type of intra-corporeal MCS and the TAH replaces all the ventricular mass and valves [10]. The 70 cc version has been used for adult-sized patients, and the 50 cc version was developed to support smaller patients [10]. The advantage of the TAH is that it is the only option that provides biventricular support for patients with SV anatomy [11]. However, it is a complex surgery that requires extensive reconstruction at the time of the implant, particularly in patients with SV anatomy, and requires an experienced congenital heart surgeon.

The process of managing SV failure is challenging for surgeons because it involves complex pathophysiology. The size of the patient, timing and mechanism of SV failure are the important factors in determining the management strategy. Implementing MCS for patients with SV failure is possible and is being utilized ever more, as the lack of appropriate donors for transplantation remains an ongoing problem. The development of new devices with a better risk profile will undoubtedly translate to an increasing number of SV patients supported with MCS for both the short and long-term in the future.

One of the major challenges of MCS in SV patients is that each case is unique; therefore, there is no optimal support device for the entire SV population, but MCS needs to be tailored to each patient. MCS devices are summarized in Table 37.1, to help with decision making regarding which device is optimal to use in each situation.

Table 37.1 Summary of the different types of mechanical circulatory support devices that can be used in both biventricular circulation and single ventricle circulation

Mechanical device	Indications	Duration of use	Advantages	Disadvantages
ECMO	Acute cardiac and respiratory failure	2–4 weeks	Supports cardiac and respiratory systems	Short term use, patients are typically sedated
Berlin Heart Excor	Cardiac failure in children	0–6 months	Only device for small children, cannulas stable	Extracorporeal device and risks of infection/bleeding, high rates of stroke especially in small children, patients must remain hospitalized
Heartmate II	Cardiac failure in adults	0–10 years	Many years of experience with this device, continuous flow so may be better to support Fontan circulation, patients can go home with this device	Large device for adult size patients only[a]
Heartware HVAD	Cardiac failure in adults or children	0–5 years	Smaller than HM II, can be used in children and adolescents, continuous flow so can support Fontan circulation, patients can go home with this device	Slightly higher stroke rates than HM II[b]
Heartmate III	Cardiac failure in adults or children	0–5 years	Newest device, has some features for "pulsing" even though is a continuous flow device, patients can go home with this device	Less outcomes data available as it is newest device, limited experience in single ventricle patients
Total artificial heart	Cardiac failure and failure of Fontan circulation	0–3 years	Only device that provides pump for pulmonary and systemic circulation, patients can go home with this device	Complexity of the surgery in single ventricle patient, limited to larger patients >50 kg, limited experience in single ventricle patients

[a]No longer used as this been replaced by HM III
[b]No longer available for use due to recall for mechanical failure rates

References

1. Fontan F, Baudet E. Surgical repair of tricuspid atresia. Thorax. 1971;26:240.
2. Chakrabarti S, Keeton BR, Salmon AP, Vettukattil JJ. Acquired combined immunodeficiency associated with protein losing enteropathy complicating fontan operation. Heart. 2003;89:1130–1.
3. Carey JA, Hamilton JRL, Hilton CJ, Dark JH, Forty J, Parry G, Hasan A. Orthotopic cardiac transplantation for the failing fontan circulation. Eur J Cardiothorac Surg. 1998;14:7–14.
4. Griselli M, Sinha R, Jang S, Perri G, Adachi I. Mechanical circulatory support for single ventricle failure. Front Cardiovasc Med. 2018;5:115.
5. Rood KL, Teele SA, Barrett CS, Salvin JW, Rycus PT, Fynn-Thompson F, Laussen PC, Thiagarajan RR. Extracorporeal membrane oxygenation support after the fontan operation. J Thorac Cardiovasc Surg. 2011;142:504–10.
6. Rossano JW, Woods RK, Berger S, et al. Mechanical support as failure intervention in patients with cavopulmonary shunts (MFICS): rationale and aims of a new registry of mechanical circulatory support in single ventricle patients. Congenit Heart Dis. 2013;8:182–6.
7. Humpl T, Furness S, Gruenwald C, Hyslop C, Van Arsdell G. The Berlin heart EXCOR pediatrics-the SickKids experience 2004-2008. Artif Organs. 2010;34:1082–6.
8. Irving CA, Cassidy JV, Kirk RC, Griselli M, Hasan A, Crossland DS. Successful bridge to transplant with the Berlin heart after cavopulmonary shunt. J Heart Lung Transplant. 2009;28:399–401.
9. Miera O, Schmitt KRL, Delmo-Walter E, Ovroutski S, Hetzer R, Berger F. Pump size of Berlin heart EXCOR pediatric device influences clinical outcome in children. J Heart Lung Transplant. 2014;33:816–21.
10. Cook JA, Shah KB, Quader MA, Cooke RH, Kasirajan V, Rao KK, Smallfield MC, Tchoukina I, Tang DG. The total artificial heart. J Thorac Dis. 2015;7:2172.
11. Rossano JW, Goldberg DJ, Fuller S, Ravishankar C, Montenegro LM, Gaynor JW. Successful use of the Total artificial heart in the failing fontan circulation. Ann Thorac Surg. 2014;97:1438–40.

Marny Fedrigo, Ilaria Barison,
Massimo A. Padalino, Liliana Chemello,
Giovanni di Salvo, and Annalisa Angelini

Key Points

- Solid organ remodelling is happening even before Fontan surgery.
- Era and time from Fontan to complications and death are key elements.
- Technical and post surgical management improvements have changed dramatically the outcome.
- Late complications are unchanged between early era and nowadays.
- All Fontan patients will experience in the follow-up some degree of Fontan failure.

- Mode of death is characterized by heart failure, sudden death, thromboembolism, multi-organ failure and sepsis.
- Patients with a long-standing Fontan circuit develop liver fibrosis without obvious inflammation.
- Sinusoidal fibrosis and sinusoidal dilatation in the liver are costant features.

In this chapter we discuss the autopsy findings of Fontan patients with reference to how, when and why Fontan patients die and how they are evaluated at autopsy and what the pathologists should know before approaching post-Fontan patients. There are few published reports of the results of autopsy in post-Fontan patients [1–4].

The pathologist performing the autopsy in a patient after a Fontan Surgical procedure should understand the many variants of the Fontan operation. Francis Fontan first described a direct connection between the right atrial appendage to the pulmonary trunk. Many modifications of the Fontan procedure have occurred but the principle remains that the systemic and pulmonary circulations are placed in series and there is a single ventricle that supports the systemic circulation, but provides the power to the whole circulation.

The key physiological changes are upstream venous congestion and downstream decreased cardiac output. Pulmonary vascular resistance will influence the pulmonary venous return and

M. Fedrigo · I. Barison · A. Angelini (✉)
Cardiovascular Pathology, Department of Cardiac,
Thoracic and Vascular Sciences and Public Health,
University of Padua, Padua, Italy
e-mail: marny.fedrigo@aopd.veneto.it; annalisa.angelini@unipd.it

M. A. Padalino
Cardiac Surgery, Department of Cardiac, Thoracic
and Vascular Sciences and Public Health, University
of Padua, Padua, Italy
e-mail: massimo.padalino@unipd.it

L. Chemello
Hepatology Unit, Department of Medicine,
University of Padua, Padua, Italy
e-mail: liliana.chemello@unipd.it

G. di Salvo
Department of Women's and Children's Health,
University of Padua, Padua, Italy
e-mail: giovanni.disalvo@unipd.it

consequently cardiac output [5–8]. A degree of hypoxia is very common following the Fontan procedure.

Moreover, it is well known that end organ remodelling is happening even before the definitive palliative procedure and can relate to previous surgical interventions or even the native congenital defect including the development of myocardial fibrosis.

The different types of surgical procedures so far introduced could be easily grouped in three main approaches: **the atrio-pulmonary connection**, where the atria is connected directly to the main pulmonary trunk, **the lateral tunnel connection or intracardiac tunnel**, where there is an intra-atrial tunnelling of the inferior vena cava to the pulmonary arteries through a complete vascular synthetic graft or a biological patch, while the superior vena cava is anastomosed directly to the pulmonary artery and **the extracardiac conduit connection**, with a complete synthetic vascular graft outside the heart, redirecting the inferior vena cava to the pulmonary arteries and the direct connection of the superior vena cava to the pulmonary arteries [9].

The outcomes in patients with Fontan surgery has dramatically improved through the years and nowadays death and subsequent autopsies occur mainly many years after the Fontan or modified Fontan procedures. Fontan operative mortality is less than 5% and midterm mortality at 10 years around 10% depending on the type of underline primary congenital defect [6]. However, the long-term outcomes are limited by numerous complications which to some extent affect nearly all patients after Fontan-type procedures [2, 10]. Only seldom are pathologists requested to perform an autopsy in the early operative period following Fontan completion, excluding early death after conversion or redo Fontan procedures (Fig. 38.1).

A major reason for intra-operative or early death relates to challenging anatomy with hypoplasia of the pulmonary arteries or stenosis of their peripheral intraparenchymal branches (Fig. 38.2). Distortion of the conduit either intracardiac or extracardiac or a stenotic vascular anastomosis, which characterized the early surgical experience, are a rare event in modern practice. Thus, the classic autopsy would be on an adolescent or an adult patient, who has been operated early in life, with a single ventricle, who has developed multiorgan failure, and in whom a heart transplantation was not an option or who has undergone an unsuccessful redo or conversion procedure.

Thus, it would be important to know the time interval between Fontan surgical procedure and death, in order to consider likely causes of death at a given time point. There are three helpful time frames: early deaths which include in hospital death (Fig. 38.3); midterm death, occurring within 1 year; and late deaths, which include

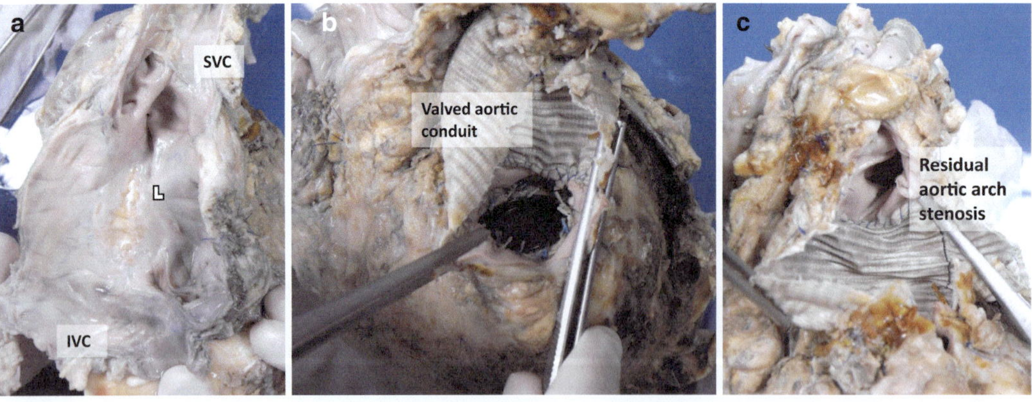

Fig. 38.1 Lateral Tunnel Connection with calcification of the patch (arrow) (**a**); valved conduit for ascending aorta and aortic valve (**b**) with residual aortic arch stenosis in a redo Fontan procedure

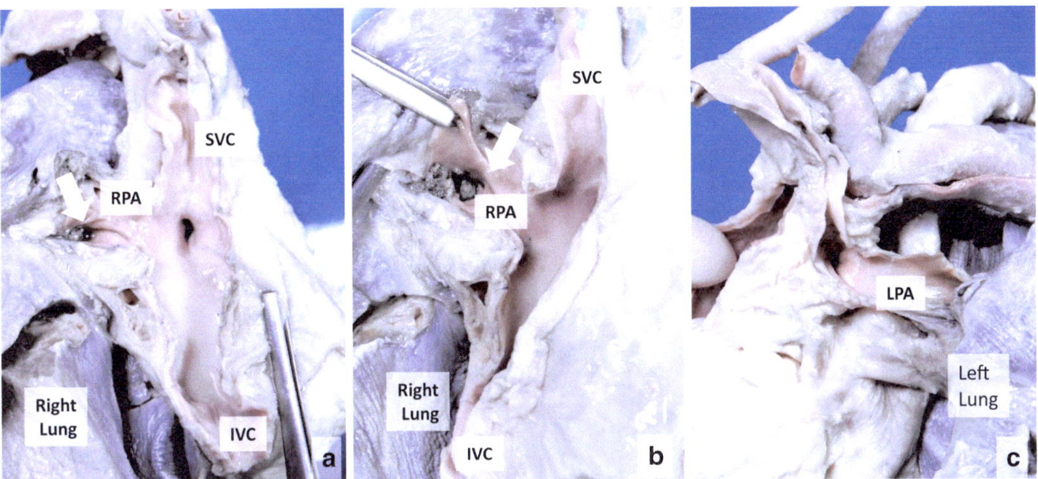

Fig. 38.2 Thrombosis in the pulmonary arteries due to hypoplasia (arrow) of peripheral pulmonary arteries in a 3-year-old boy with a cavo-pulmonary connection

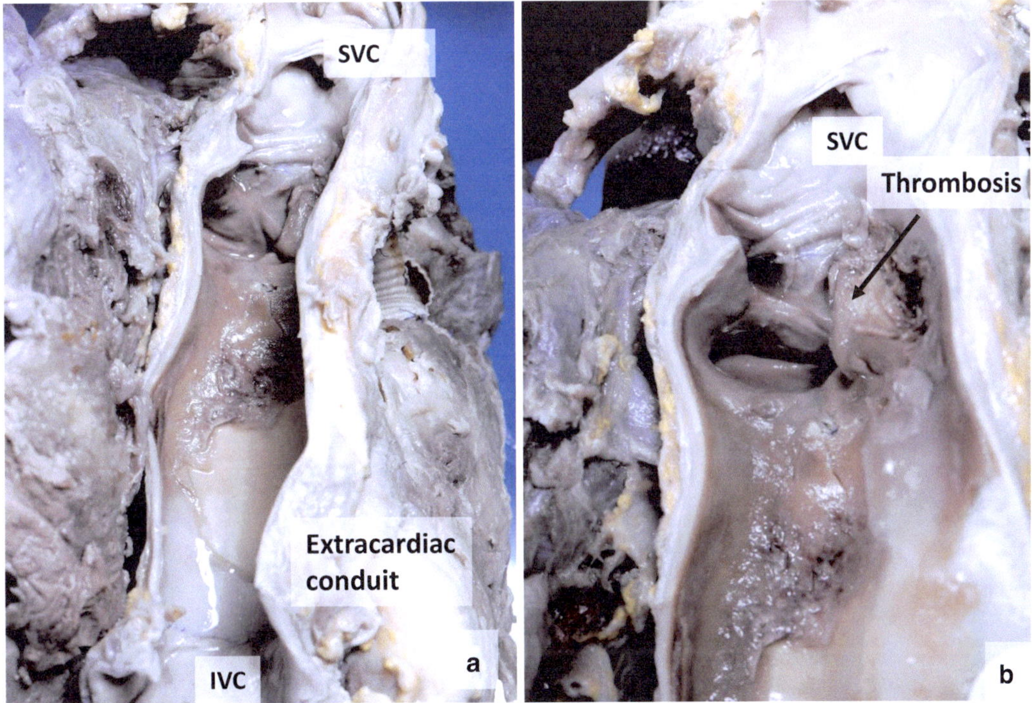

Fig. 38.3 Thrombosis at cavo-pulmonary anastomosis in extra-cardiac TCPC in a 3-year-old boy. Macroscopic view with the lateral tunnel opened longitudinally from inferior to superior vena cava (**a**). Stratified thrombosis at the superior caval junction (**b**)

those occurring after the first year and are often seen in patients with a so called failing Fontan [6] (Figs. 38.4, 38.5, and 38.6). Lastly, specific consideration should focus on deaths occurring after a redo- or conversion Fontan procedures [11] (Fig. 38.1).

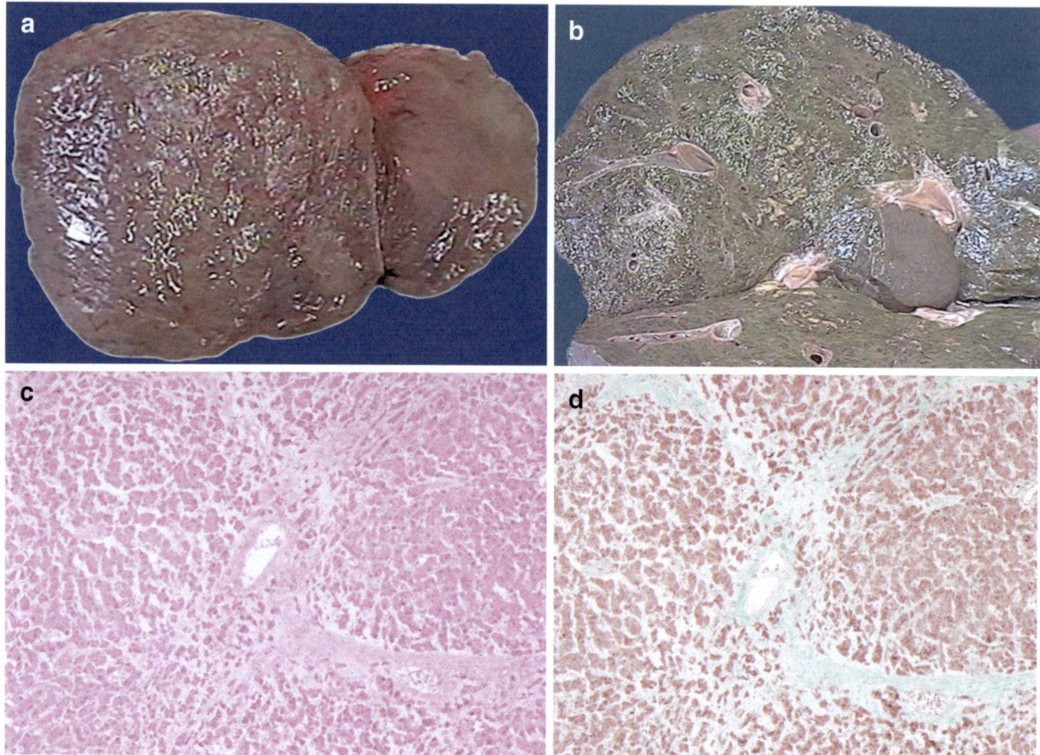

Fig. 38.4 Failing Fontan circulation with hepatic cirrhosis in a 50 year old woman, who died after a follow-up of 12 years for hemorrhagic shock and end-stage chronic liver disease: macroscopic view of the liver at autopsy, with evidence of cirrhosis (**a**, anterior view and **b**, cross section); histology showing fibrosis of the centrolobular vein and central vein—portal tract bridging fibrosis hematoxylin-eosin staining (**c**) H&E staining, magnification 80×; Masson trichrome staining highlighting the fibrosis in green (**d**), magnification 80×

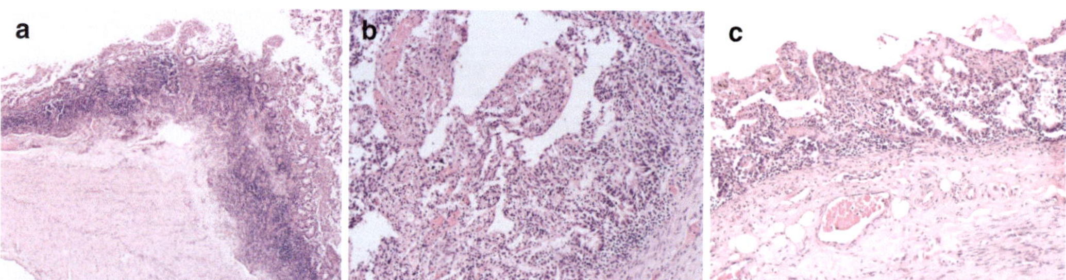

Fig. 38.5 Ileus of an 18-year-old man with protein losing enteropathy: (**a**) the mucosal inflammation damage, with moderate chronic inflammation and destruction of glandular crypt, and villi (H&E 250×; **b**) highest magnification (100×) of the ileus villi (black arrow) with oedema, lymphatic vessel dilatation (asterisk); (**c**) diffuse damage of mucosa

The modes of death vary according to the time periods: perioperative mortality relates to sudden cardiac death, thromboembolism, heart failure and sepsis [2, 6, 12]. Sudden death and cerebrovascular events due to thromboembolism were important causes of mid-term death [12] whereas heart failure related death was mostly confined to later deaths after 10 years. As reported also by Kotani, a pathological substrate in the heart such as fibrosis could determine sudden death within

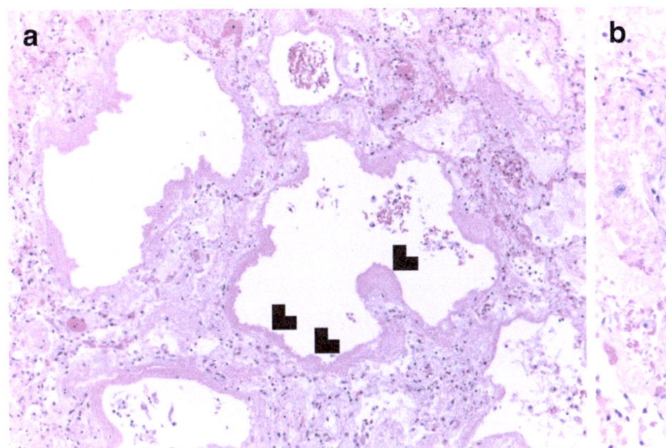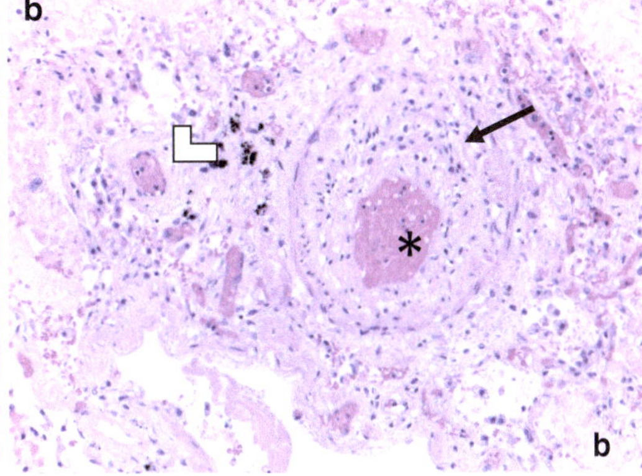

Fig. 38.6 Lung: (**a**) alveolar damage is shown with fibrinoid necrosis of alveolar cells (hyaline membranes, black head arrows) (H&E 200×) (**b**) pulmonary vascular disease with thrombosis (asterisk) and ialinosis of small artery (white head arrow) and concentric proliferation of smooth muscle cells and necrosis (arrow) in a 21-year-old man with history of multiple interventions following Norwood procedures, and extracardiac TCPC Fontan (H&E 400×)

Table 38.1 Mode of death

- Heart failure
- Multi-organ failure
- Sudden death
- Thromboembolism
- Sepsis

1 year [2]. Arrhythmias, PLE and arteriovenous malformations appear relatively late and cause late death (Table 38.1).

Early deaths are mainly related to the cardiac condition and the surgical procedures performed.

In this regard, the main complications relating to the heart can be subdivided into three main groups relating to the surgical procedure (technical aspects) or to the native congenital heart malformations:

- **Systemic venous pathway obstruction**
  - Stenotic atriopulmonary or intracardiac tunnel cavopulmonary connections
  - Lateral tunnel stenosis
  - Superior caval vein stenosis
  - Peripheral pulmonary artery and pulmonary veins stenosis and or thrombosis
  - Right atrial stenosis
- Narrowing or distortion of the TCPC/Fontan pathways (intra or extracardiac)
- Pulmonary artery thrombosis
- Pulmonary vein stenosis

- Right atriomegaly (atriopulmonary Fontan)
- Right atrial thrombus.
- Recanalization of the ligated pulmonary trunk (competing flow with the Fontan circulation)
- Systemic ventricular dysfunction (systolic or diastolic)

Related to Native congenital heart defect:
- Pulmonary artery hypoplasia, stenosis or thrombosis
- Systemic atrioventricular or aortic valve regurgitation
- Ventricular outflow tract obstruction
- **Left ventricular outflow tract obstruction with arterial ischemia**
  - Associated conditions that can cause left ventricular outflow tract obstruction
  - **Related to the surgical procedures**
- Recurrent coarctation in Norwood
- Supraaortic stenotic anastomosis in DKS operation

Native congenital heart defect
- DILV + TGA with a restricted bulboventricular foramen
- **Valvular abnormalities**
  - Associated abnormal valve on left side in tricuspid atresia
  - Common atrioventricular valve in heterotaxy
  - ccTGA with Ebstein anomaly

What is fundamental to recognize for a pathologist is that a failing Fontan is a systemic condition, which affects not only the heart, but all the organs, such as lungs (Fig. 38.6), kidneys, brain, gut (Fig. 38.5) and liver (Fig. 38.4), which should not be overlooked [13, 14] (Table 38.2).

A failing Fontan can result from elevated pulmonary resistance, pulmonary thrombi, distortion of the Fontan conduit, pulmonary arteries hypoplasia, arrhythmias, and failure of the systemic ventricle. As a consequence, the involved organs other than the heart will remodel overtime reaching end stage failure.

It could be argued that a failing Fontan is inevitable and can manifest even 20 years after the initial surgery (Table 38.2). However, the palliation provided by the Fontan procedures has to be considered effective, allowing the patients with complex congenital heart disease to grow into adulthood with a good quality of life and in some cases to be candidates for heart or heart and liver transplantion [15]. A major concern is the continuous progressive decline of systolic and diastolic function with heart failure as a major mode of death due to myocardial diffuse fibrosis.

Fontan Associated liver disease (FALD) Liver complications are common late after Fontan palliative operation, starting from hepatomegaly, cirrhosis, portal hypertension leading to hepatocellular carcinoma [16–19]. It is becoming a frequent cause of morbidity and mortality after Fontan surgery [20]. The prevalence of FALD is not well defined yet. There is evidence that liver deterioration probably starts immediately after Fontan surgery [21], with the contribution of iatrogenic damage. However, it remains hidden for years, with the only evidence of liver venous congestion and stasis, until it reveals itself with the complications due to liver cirrhosis [4].

FALD is present in all Fontan patients with differing severity [22]. Liver disease can start even before the surgical palliation is performed and its progression can be different in each patient. Patients who died early after the Fontan procedures showed some form of hepatic centrilobular, or periportal fibrosis as result of native congenital disease [1, 23–25]. Hepatic fibrosis is the result of elevated caval pressure and the lack of pulsatile flow. Thus, the heart pump failure, at preload and afterload sites, induces both stasis and ischemia in the major organs in a failing Fontan [26, 27], and is the mechanism of FALD.

Thus, all Fontan patients under follow up will have some degree of fibrosis and at 10 years half of them will have developed severe fibrosis [28] (Table 38.3). Complications of fibrosis such as gastrointestinal bleeding and laboratory liver abnormalities are uncommon and will appear very late. Many questions are still unanswered related to FALD and its outcome. It impacts on

Table 38.2 Failing Fontan

Organs	Pathological substrates
Lungs	Thromboembolism, pulmonary artery vasculopathy, plastic bronchitis
Kidneys	Glomerular sclerosis, interstitial and tubular fibrosis
Bowel	Enteric villous atrophy (protein loosing enteropathy) inflammatory cell infiltrate
Liver	Chronic cardiac cirrhosis
Brain	Cerebrovascular disease
Heart	Ventricular fibrosis remodeling

Table 38.3 Histopathological substrates of FALD with scoring system

Histological features	Semiquantitative analysis (score)	Description
Fibrosis (modified to METAVIR system)	F0–F4	Define the distribution of fibrosis from centro-lobular vein, bridges to cirrhosis
Sinusoidal fibrosis	0–3 (<1/3; 1/3–2/3; >2/3)	Sinusoidal fibrosis, neomatrix within Disse and sinusoidal space
Sinusoidal dilatation	0–3	Dilatation of sinusoidal space from perivenula region to portal space (lobular direction)
Centrolobular hemorrhagic necrosis	(0–3)	Wave front necrosis from centrolobular vein to parenchyma
Ductal reaction	(0–3)	Degree of bile duct reaction
Iron deposition	(0–3)	Degree of iron deposition

decisions regarding transplantation, i.e. whether a patient undergoes heart transplantation first, with possible later liver transplantation or to go for a combined heart and liver transplantation remains uncertain, and there is no simple way of determining the optimal strategy. Liver biopsy remains the gold standard diagnostic procedure for definition of extent and severity of fibrosis and to guide the therapeutic approach [10, 29, 30].

The histopathology findings in FALD are sinusoidal dilatation, centrolobular hemorrhagic necrosis, perisinusoidal fibrosis, ductular reaction, perivenular fibrous septa, central fibrous bridges, nodular regenerative hyperplasia and late hepatocellular carcinoma. (Fig. 38.4).

Of interest the distribution of the fibrosis in the space of Disse, is a characteristic of FALD as compared with other forms of hepatic congestion [29, 31]. Bridging fibrosis starts from the centrolobular veins and reach out to the portal tract. No periportal inflammation is present [4]. There are multiple regenerative hypervascular nodules usually located at the periphery of the liver. In advanced liver disease the evolution of these nodules into hepatocellular carcinoma has been reported in a subset of patients [10]. There are many different semiquantitative scoring system which has been proposed to score the severity of liver disease [4, 21, 28, 32–34].

Protein losing enteropathy is also a complication of the Fontan circulation, usually manifesting in the medium term, thought to be triggered by chronic venous congestion, impaired intestinal lymphatic drainage and intestinal inflammation [35]. It is characterized histologically by intestinal lymphangiectasia, vascular congestion, chronic inflammation and abnormal enterocyte basal membrane structure [35] (Fig. 38.5) **Chylothorax** can be present as result of the derangement in the lymphatic drainage for venous congestions. **Plastic bronchitis** is also the result of lympathic congestions in the peritracheal space with exudation in the bronchial tree, the equivalent of PLE at the thoracic compartment.

Renal impairment is also common after Fontan procedures but is underestimated both in the early and late follow-up. It has a number of possible aetiologies, such as low cardiac output, nephrotoxic medications, cardiopulmonary bypass runs (inflammation), intravenous iodinated contrast agents, and long-standing cyanosis. Acute kidney injury can be secondary to prolonged cardiopulmonary bypass times, resulting in hemoglobinuria, perioperative low cardiac output, and systemic hypotension [14].

Lung disease: Growth and development of the pulmonary vasculature are often abnormal in patients with single-ventricle congenital cardiac malformations. Reduced pulmonary flow may originate following palliation with partial (Glenn) and total cavo-pulmonary connection [36, 37].

Overtime there is development of pulmonary fibrosis, venovenous collaterals, arteriovenous malformations and pulmonary vascular disease. Pulmonary thrombosis and hemorrhages as a consequence of hepatic insufficiency, arteriovenous malformations and venovenous collaterals are a common feature [38–40] (Fig. 38.6).

Heart Transplantation and Heart and Liver Transplantation

Heart transplantation provides us with a unique opportunity to improve our understanding of the failing Fontan. The explanted heart should be carefully examined to evaluate the myocardial fibrosis as substrate of heart failure. Mortality following heart transplantation alone is quite high (20%) and autopsy performed in these patients should focus not only on the transplanted heart, usually coming from a good donor, but on the pathological aspects involving all solid organs to identify multiorgan failure. In a literature review of 514 cases of HTx for failing Fontan from 1998 to 2013, early mortality ranged from 4 to 35%, with an average of 22% [15]. When a combined liver and heart transplantation is performed careful evaluation should be directed to extensive evaluation not only of the heart but also of the liver to characterize the pathology of the liver and the degree of cirrhosis, nodular hyperplasia or HCC [15, 16, 20].

References

1. Johnson JA, Cetta F, Graham RP, et al. Identifying predictors of hepatic disease in patients after the Fontan operation: a postmortem analysis. J Thorac Cardiovasc Surg. 2013;146(1):140–5.

2. Kotani Y, Chetan D, Zhu J, et al. Fontan failure and death in contemporary Fontan circulation: analysis from the last two decades. Ann Thorac Surg. 2018;105(4):1240–7.

3. Ghaferi AA, Hutchins GM, Surrey LF, et al. Progression of liver pathology in patients undergoing the Fontan procedure: chronic passive congestion, cardiac cirrhosis, hepatic adenoma, and hepatocellular carcinoma. J Thorac Cardiovasc Surg. 2005;57(6):1348–52.

4. Padalino MA, Chemello L, Cavalletto L, Angelini A, Fedrigo M. Prognostic value of liver and spleen stiffness in patients with Fontan associated liver disease (FALD): a case series with histopathologic comparison. J Cardiovasc Dev Dis. 2021;8:30.

5. Gewillig M, Brown SC. The Fontan circulation after 45 years: update in physiology. Heart. 2016;102(14):1081–6.

6. Kverneland LS, Kramer P, Ovroutski S. Five decades of the Fontan operation: a systematic review of international reports on outcomes after univentricular palliation. Congenit Heart Dis. 2018;13(2):181–93.

7. Rychik J, Atz AM, Celermajer DS, et al. Evaluation and management of the child and adult with Fontan circulation: a scientific statement from the American Heart Association. Circulation. 2019;140:e234–84.

8. Gewillig M, Brown SC, Eyskens B, et al. The Fontan circulation: who controls cardiac output? Interact Cardiovasc Thorac Surg. 2010;10(3):428–33.

9. Aboulhosn J, Child JS. The adult with a Fontan operation. Curr Cardiol Rep. 2007;9(4):331–5.

10. Téllez L, Rodríguez-Santiago E, Albillos A. Fontan-associated liver disease: a review. Ann Hepatol. 2018;17(2):192–204.

11. Park HK, Shin HJ, Park YH. Outcomes of Fontan conversion for failing Fontan circulation: mid-term results. Interact Cardiovasc Thorac Surg. 2016;23(1):14–7.

12. Khairy P, Fernandes SM, Mayer JE, et al. Long-term survival, modes of death, and predictors of mortality in patients with Fontan surgery. Circulation. 2008;117(1):85–92.

13. Rychik J, Goldberg DJ. Late consequences of the Fontan operation. Circulation. 2014;30:1525–8.

14. Byrne RD, Weingarten AJ, Clark DE, et al. More than the heart: hepatic, renal, and cardiac dysfunction in adult Fontan patients. Congenit Heart Dis. 2019;14(5):765–71.

15. Backer CL, Russell HM, Pahl E, et al. Heart transplantation for the failing Fontan. Ann Thorac Surg. 2013;96(4):1413–9.

16. Emamaullee J, Zaidi AN, Schiano T, et al. Fontan-associated liver disease: screening, management, and transplant considerations. Circulation. 2020;142(6):591–604.

17. Ghaferi AA, Hutchins GM. Progression of liver pathology in patients undergoing the Fontan procedure: chronic passive congestion, cardiac cirrhosis, hepatic adenoma, and hepatocellular carcinoma. J Thorac Cardiovasc Surg. 2005;129(6):1348–52.

18. Kogiso T, Tokushige K. Fontan-associated liver disease and hepatocellular carcinoma in adults. Sci Rep. 2020;10(1):1–14.

19. Possner M, Gordon-Walker T, Egbe AC, et al. Hepatocellular carcinoma and the Fontan circulation: clinical presentation and outcomes. Int J Cardiol. 2021;322:142–8.

20. Wu FM, Kogon B, Earing MG, et al. Liver health in adults with Fontan circulation: a multicenter cross-sectional study. J Thorac Cardiovasc Surg. 2017;153(3):656–64.

21. Bedossa P, Poynard T. An algorithm for the grading of activity in chronic hepatitis C. Hepatology. 1996;24(2):289–93.

22. Camposilvan S, Milanesi O, Stellin G, Pettenazzo A, Zancan L, D'Antiga L. Liver and cardiac function in the long term after Fontan operation. Ann Thorac Surg. 2008;86(1):177–82.

23. Schwartz MC, Glatz AC, Daniels K, et al. Hepatic Abnormalities Are Present Before and Early After the Fontan Operation. The annals of Thoracic Surgery. 2015;100(6):2298–304.

24. Schwartz MC, Sullivan L, Cohen MS, et al. Hepatic pathology may develop before the Fontan operation in children with functional single ventricle: an autopsy study. J Thorac Cardiovasc Surg. 2012;143(4):904–9.

25. Goldberg DJ, Surrey LF, Glatz AC, et al. Hepatic fibrosis is universal following Fontan operation, and severity is associated with time from surgery: a liver biopsy and hemodynamic study. J Am Heart Assoc. 2017;6(5):1–8.

26. Fredenburg TB, Johnson TR, Cohen MD. The Fontan procedure: anatomy, complications, and manifestations of failure. Radiographics. 2011;31(2):453–63.

27. Daniels CJ, Bradley EA, Landzberg MJ, et al. Fontan-associated liver disease: proceedings from the American College of Cardiology Stakeholders Meeting, October 1 to 2, 2015, Washington DC. J Am Coll Cardiol. 2017;70(25):3173–94.

28. Gordon-Walker TT, Bove K, Veldtman G. Fontan-associated liver disease: a review. J Cardiol. 2019;74(3):223–32.

29. Surrey LF, Russo P, Rychik J, et al. Prevalence and characterization of fibrosis in surveillance liver biopsies of patients with Fontan circulation. Hum Pathol. 2016;57:106–15.

30. Perucca G, de Lange C, Franchi-Abella S, et al. Surveillance of Fontan-associated liver disease: current standards and a proposal from the European

Society of Paediatric Radiology Abdominal Task Force. Pediatr Radiol. 2021;51(13):2598–606.

31. Koehne de Gonzalez AK, Lefkowitch JH. Heart disease and the liver: pathologic evaluation. Gastroenterol Clin North Am. 2017;46(2):421–35.

32. Dai DF, Swanson PE, Krieger EV, Liou IW, Carithers RL, Yeh MM. Congestive hepatic fibrosis score: a novel histologic assessment of clinical severity. Mod Pathol. 2014;27(12):1552–8.

33. Goodman ZD. Grading and staging systems for inflammation and fibrosis in chronic liver diseases. J Hepatol. 2007;47(4):598–607.

34. Kendall TJ, Stedman B, Hacking N, et al. Hepatic fibrosis and cirrhosis in the Fontan circulation: a detailed morphological study. J Clin Pathol. 2008;61(4):504–8.

35. Johnson JN, Driscoll DJ, O'Leary PW. Protein-losing enteropathy and the Fontan operation. Nutr Clin Pract. 2012;27(3):375–84.

36. Mitchell MB, Campbell DN, Ivy D, et al. Evidence of pulmonary vascular disease after heart transplantation for Fontan circulation failure. J Thorac Cardiovasc Surg. 2004;128(5):693–702.

37. Becker K, Uebing A, Hansen JH. Pulmonary vascular disease in Fontan circulation-is there a rationale for pulmonary vasodilator therapies? Cardiovasc Diagn Ther. 2021;11(4):1111–21.

38. Ridderbos FJS, Wolff D, Timmer A, et al. Adverse pulmonary vascular remodeling in the Fontan circulation. J Heart Lung Transplant. 2015;34(3):404–13.

39. Ishida H, Kogaki S, Ichimori H, et al. Overexpression of endothelin-1 and endothelin receptors in the pulmonary arteries of failed Fontan patients. Int J Cardiol. 2012;159(1):34–9.

40. Dimopoulos K, Wort SJ, Gatzoulis MA. Pulmonary hypertension related to congenital heart disease: a call for action. Eur Heart J. 2014;35(11):691–700.

Index

A

Adaptations, 255
Adult congenital heart disease (ACHD), 165, 239, 253
Advanced care planning (ACP), 348, 350
Anatomy, 31, 32, 39, 45, 53, 55, 59, 62, 64, 69, 72, 78,
83, 84, 95, 99, 101, 151, 179, 182, 191, 197,
208, 213–214, 219, 222, 231, 232, 234, 246,
247, 273, 274, 276, 287, 289, 298, 341, 350,
351, 353, 355, 358
Antenatal, 51, 52, 62, 64, 87
Antiarrhythmic drugs, 207, 276, 284, 322
Anticoagulation, 102, 108, 113, 164, 165, 171, 180, 201,
207, 220, 260, 265–267, 269, 290, 298, 301,
302, 321
Anxiety, 89, 151, 152, 156, 198, 207, 209, 210, 253–255
Aorta, 14–21, 25, 38, 41, 42, 55, 56, 62, 63, 69, 77, 83,
106–108, 117–120, 126, 132, 178, 179, 191,
214, 218, 219, 225, 233, 235, 246, 248, 311,
318, 331–332, 341, 353, 358
Arrhythmia, 3, 4, 88, 99, 101, 102, 111, 163, 165,
172–174, 199, 225–226, 275, 276, 283–289,
298, 314, 315, 321, 327, 337, 338, 342
Arterial saturations, 181
Arterial saturations while, 181
Atresia/mitral, 39
Atrial flutter, 172
Atrio-pulmonary (AP), 3, 99–101, 111, 113, 162, 163,
178, 213, 214, 219, 223, 225–227, 234,
246–247, 269, 275, 283, 284, 290, 301, 312,
315, 316, 361
Autopsy, 117, 357, 358, 360, 363

B

Balloon angioplasty, 85, 118, 331–332
Barriers, 156–157, 284, 350
Brain volume neuropsychological tests, 147

C

Cardiac, 207
Cardiac catheterization, 74, 110, 135, 144, 186, 246–249,
312, 313, 321

Cardiac CT, 59
Cardiac pacing, 219, 298
Cardiac resynchronization, 174, 291
Cardiac transplantation, 3, 4, 87, 181, 187, 188, 192,
199, 222
Cardiopulmonary bypass (CPB), 46, 83, 95, 102,
108, 109, 111, 118, 124, 126, 144, 186,
342, 353, 363
Cardiopulmonary exercise testing (CPET), 239, 240,
263, 315
Career advice, 197, 200
Catheter ablation, 172–174, 283, 284, 286, 288
Cavo-pulmonary connection, 245, 363
Closure, 330
Cognitive-behavioral therapy, 255
Collateral occlusion, 330
Collaterals, 38, 62, 110, 112, 163, 179, 192, 213,
219, 221, 227, 231, 235, 247, 248, 264,
277, 301, 312, 314, 317–319, 327, 329,
330, 341, 363
Computed tomography (CT), 4, 55, 64, 83, 110, 174,
207, 210, 214, 221, 222, 225, 227, 231–237,
264, 287, 296, 319, 354
Congenital heart disease (CHD), 4, 12, 31, 32, 37, 38,
74, 87, 95, 134, 156, 165, 191, 198–201, 221,
231, 254, 261, 262, 274, 286, 327, 341, 343,
348, 362
Connections, 213
Contraception, 199, 200, 207, 209, 259, 260, 263,
267, 316
Contraception counselling, 199
Contrast, 2, 52, 81, 131, 135, 181, 182, 222, 227,
231–237, 246, 266, 284, 287, 310, 322, 323,
334, 363
Conversion Fontan, 359
Counselling, 39, 43, 45–46, 56, 57, 199, 200, 207, 263,
265, 267
Cross sectional imaging, 55, 221, 342
Cyanosis, 3, 13, 95, 110, 113, 144, 147, 163, 173,
178, 180, 181, 189, 200, 227, 240, 243, 245,
249, 260, 261, 264, 273, 277, 285, 299–301,
309, 316–318, 321, 324, 329, 330, 332, 333,
337, 363

I

Impella, 103
Implantable cardioverter-defibrillator (ICD), 174, 207, 291
Interventions, 31, 45, 46, 55–56, 75, 77, 81, 88, 89, 120, 126, 135–137, 146, 151, 158, 187, 188, 192, 197, 198, 220, 222, 231, 240, 243, 246, 254, 276, 277, 283, 297, 298, 300, 315, 316, 327–331, 333, 335, 337, 338, 340–342, 349, 358, 361
Intra-cardiac repair, 95

L

Late complications, 3, 5, 209, 213, 327, 330
Lateral tunnel (LT), 3, 96, 100–102, 111–113, 143, 163, 164, 171–173, 178, 185, 214, 219, 220, 223, 226, 227, 233, 237, 245, 275, 277, 286, 289, 316, 338, 358, 359, 361
Lateral tunnel TCPC, 226
Left heart syndrome, 223
Lifestyle, 4, 197–199, 255
Liver, 3, 4, 88, 144, 148, 152, 161, 163, 166, 187–190, 199, 206–210, 222, 226, 231, 232, 260, 296, 297, 301, 317–319, 323, 324, 331, 343, 350, 360, 362, 363
Liver dysfunction, 323
Lymphatic, 3, 132, 189, 190, 210, 296–298, 329, 331, 333–335, 342, 360, 363
Lymphatic dysfunction, 323
Lymphatic intervention, 298, 329, 342

M

Magnetic resonance imaging (MRI), 41, 55, 59, 64, 102, 134, 146–147, 174, 182, 192, 207–210, 214, 221, 223, 226, 227, 263, 264, 290, 296, 298, 299, 312, 319, 329, 335
Measurement, 74, 124, 192, 246, 248, 249, 296, 323
Mechanical cardiac support (MCS), 187, 192
Mechanical circulatory support (MCS), 343, 353–356
Mental health, 4, 254–256, 300
Mitral atresia, 15, 16, 18, 31, 81, 118, 225
Modification, 3, 100, 118, 171, 236, 246, 275, 287, 335
Modified, 95, 107, 108, 119, 120, 172, 177, 186, 232, 234, 235, 244, 246, 275, 286, 316, 349, 351, 358, 362
Multidisciplinary, 4, 197, 205–207, 209, 210, 266, 321, 323
Multi-organ failure, 222, 315, 358, 361, 363
Musculoskeletal, 300

N

Natural, 39
Neonate, 59, 74, 77, 78, 85, 87–89, 108, 117, 120, 126, 274
Neurodevelopment, 46–47, 120, 126, 144–148, 152, 210, 299
Norwood modifications, 117–120

Norwood procedure, 32, 110, 117, 118, 120, 126, 144, 192, 290, 361
Nutrition, 74, 77–78, 187, 207

O

Optimization, 76, 323, 341
Outcome, 3, 25, 26, 41, 42, 44–47, 55, 56, 64, 77, 85, 88, 143–145, 147, 173, 180, 186, 190, 192, 199, 222, 246, 263, 267–269, 273–277, 286, 309, 322, 340, 362

P

PA/IVS, 41
Pacemaker, 113, 145, 171, 221, 222, 267, 289–290, 338–339
Palliative care, 46, 56, 87–90, 123, 321, 347, 348, 350, 351
Pathway, 12, 41, 44–47, 54, 60, 83, 102, 111, 126, 144, 148, 151, 154, 158, 161, 163, 178, 179, 181, 197, 213–215, 220, 222–224, 227, 246, 247, 254, 274, 277, 284, 298, 299, 301, 310–313, 319, 331, 341, 342, 361
Pathway obstruction, 134, 173, 178, 214, 285, 315–318, 331, 341, 361
Pathway/pulmonary artery obstruction, 298
Physiology, 4, 69, 70, 85, 96, 123, 131, 144–145, 147, 151, 153, 154, 158, 170, 181, 192, 198, 199, 201, 207, 213, 231, 240, 243, 246, 262, 289, 295, 297, 299–301, 310, 314, 317, 321, 322, 327, 330, 335, 337, 341
Plastic bronchitis (PB), 188, 190, 207, 297, 298, 323, 327, 331, 333, 337, 363
Pre-conception assessment, 263, 265, 267
Pregnancy, 26, 31, 32, 37–39, 41–45, 47, 51, 57, 87, 163, 165, 199, 200, 207, 259–269, 277
Pregnancy counselling, 199–200
Preload, 11, 102, 105, 112, 132, 134, 136, 137, 181, 186, 242, 264, 310–313, 321, 324, 329, 330, 332, 333, 337, 362
Prenatal diagnosis, 31, 37, 44–47, 53, 74, 87
Prognosis, 38–40, 43, 46, 51, 53–55, 65, 88, 95, 96, 113, 187, 222–227, 321, 322, 349, 350
Protein losing enteropathy (PLE), 3, 4, 88, 161, 163, 170, 173, 188, 190, 265, 285, 289, 296–301, 314, 315, 317, 318, 321, 323, 327, 329, 331, 333, 337, 342, 360, 361, 363
Protocol, 3–5, 206, 213–220, 222, 233, 234, 239, 244, 263, 340
Pulmonary artery (PA), 2, 12, 15, 21, 27, 28, 38, 40, 41, 43, 53, 62–65, 69, 70, 78, 83–85, 95, 99–101, 105–111, 117–120, 123, 124, 132, 162, 164, 172, 173, 177–179, 186, 187, 191, 213, 214, 219, 222, 224, 233, 246–248, 274–276, 283, 285, 290, 299, 310–312, 314, 316, 329–333, 341, 343, 358, 359, 361, 362
Pulmonary artery stenosis, 311
Pulmonary artery stenting, 207
Pulmonary atresia with intact ventricular septum (PA/IVS), 12, 22, 26, 41–42, 54

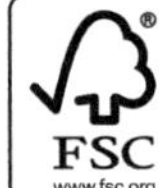